HIV Nursing and Symptom Management

Jones and Bartlett Series in Oncology

Biotherapy: A Comprehensive Overview, Rieger
Bone Marrow Transplantation: Administrative Strategies and Clinical Concerns, Buschel/Whedon
Blood and Marrow Stem Cell Transplantation: Second Edition, Whedon/Wujick
Cancer and HIV Clinical Nutrition Pocket Guide, Second Edition, Wilkes
Cancer Chemotherapy: A Nursing Process Approach, Second Edition, Barton Burke, et al.
Cancer Nursing: Principles and Practice, CD-ROM, Groenwald, et al.
Cancer Nursing: Principles and Practice, Fourth Edition, Groenwald, et al.
Cancer Pain Management, Second Edition, McGuire/Yarbro/Ferrell
A Cancer Source Book for Nurses, Seventh Edition, American Cancer Society
Cancer Symptom Management, Groenwald, et al.
Cancer Symptom Management, Patient Self-Care Guides, Groenwald, et al.
Chemotherapy Care Plans Handbook, Barton Burke, et al.
A Clinical Guide to Stem Cell and Bone Marrow Transplantation, Shapiro, et al.
Comprehensive Cancer Nursing Review, Fourth Edition Groenwald, et al.
Contemporary Issues in Breast Cancer, Hassey Dow
Handbook of Oncology Nursing, Third Edition, Johnson/Gross
A Clinical Companion for Biotherapy, Rieger
Homecare Management of the Blood Cell Transplant Patient, Third Edition, Kelley, et al.
Hospice and Palliative Care, Sheehan/Forman
Memory Bank for Chemotherapy, Third Edition, Preston/Wilfinger
Oncogenes, Cooper
1997–1998 Oncology Nursing Drug Handbook, Wilkes, et al.
Oncology Nursing Homecare Handbook, Barton Burke
Oncology Nursing in the Ambulatory Setting: Issues and Models of Care, Buschel/Yarbro
Oncology Nursing Society's Building a Legacy: Voices of Oncology Nurses, Nevidjon
Oncology Nursing Society's Instruments for Clinical Health-Care Research, Frank-Stromborg/Olsen
Oncology Nursing Society's Suffering, Ferrell
Pocket Guide for Women and Cancer, Moore, et al.
Quality of Life: From Nursing and Patient Perspectives, King
Women and Cancer, Moore

HIV Nursing and Symptom Management

Edited by

Mary Ropka, Ph.D., RN, FAAN
Associate Professor of Research,
Department of Health Evaluation Sciences, School of Medicine
Research Associate Professor, Center for Survey Research
University of Virginia
Charlottesville, VA

Ann Williams, Ed.D., RN-C, FAAN
Associate Professor
School of Nursing
Yale University
New Haven, CT

JONES AND BARTLETT PUBLISHERS
Sudbury, Massachusetts
BOSTON TORONTO LONDON SINGAPORE

World Headquarters
Jones and Bartlett Publishers
40 Tall Pine Drive
Sudbury, MA 01776
978-443-5000
800-832-0034
info@jbpub.com
www.jbpub.com

Jones and Bartlett Publishers Canada
P.O. Box 19020
Toronto, ON M5S 1X1
CANADA

Jones and Bartlett Publishers International
Barb House, Barb Mews
London W6 7PA
UK

Acquisitions Editor: Karen McClure
Production Editor: Lianne B. Ames
Manufacturing Buyer: Jane Bromback
Design/Editorial Production Service/Typesetting: Modern Graphics
Cover Design: Dick Hannus
Printing and Binding: Courier
Cover Printing: Courier
Cover Image: AIDS Virus © Michael Freeman/Corbis

Library of Congress Cataloging-in-Publication Data

HIV nursing and symptom management / edited by Mary Ropka, Ann Williams.
p. cm.
Includes bibliographical references and index.
ISBN 0-7637-0544-6
1. AIDS (Disease)--Nursing. I. Ropka, Mary. II. Williams, Ann. 1945– .
[DNLM: 1. HIV Infections--nursing. 2. Acquired Immunodeficiency Syndrom--nursing. 3. AIDS-Related Opportunistic Infections--nursing. WY 153.5 H676 1998]
RC607.A26H5764 1998
616.97'92--dc21
DNLM/DLC
for Library of Congress 98–13527
CIP

The selection and dosage of drugs presented in this book are in accord with standards accepted at the time of publication. The authors, editors, and publisher have made every effort to provide accurate information. However, research, clinical practice, and government regulations often change the accepted standard in this field. Before administering any drug, the reader is advised to check the manufacturer's product information sheet for the most up-to-date recommendations on dosage, precautions, and contraindications. This is especially important in the case of drugs that are new or seldom used.

Printed in the United States
02 01 00 99 10 9 8 7 6 5 4 3 2

Contents

List of Figures and Tables

List of Figures

List of Tables

Foreword

Living with HIV infection is an immense challenge. For some, knowledge of the disease comes early, and the challenges have more to do with the psychological impact of this disease and decisions about disclosure and long-term planning for career, housing, and relationships. For others, knowledge comes later, when the impact of opportunistic infections, weight loss, medication choices, and disability have become obvious. Whenever the diagnosis is made, it is likely that one or more nurses will be involved in providing support and care.

Early in the epidemic a number of nurses and physicians commented on their sense that the clock had been turned back to the beginning of this century, or even earlier, to the time when patients with severe illnesses could look to professionals not for definitive treatment but for care and comfort throughout their illness until their death. Today, effective therapies for opportunistic infections and combination therapies that limit the replication of the virus have led some casual observers to believe that the epidemic is over. But the epidemic is far from over, especially for each individual living with the virus and learning to manage the symptoms of the disease and associated conditions.

Clinicians interested in being up to date in their patient care recommendations have had, in the case of HIV infection, an abundance of information. Articles in major professional journals, HIV-specific publications for nurses and physicians, newsletters from HIV support and advocacy organizations abstracting the professional literature, plus conferences, and the Internet all offer an abundance of material. This flood of words, however, does not always meet the need. New information is published sequentially as it emerges from laboratories and clinical trials. Descriptions of molecular-level activity in the virus appear next to emerging information regarding drug cocktails, updates on epidemiology, and descriptions of prevention methodologies. One new finding builds on prior work in a way that may seem to conflict with another finding reported in another journal. The rapid dissemination of research results and the sharing of patient experiences can leave the professional caregiver feeling perpetually behind on the information highway.

As a larger proportion of the estimated 860,000 North Americans infected with HIV[1] live longer and remain actively involved in work, and community and social activities, effective management of the symptoms associated with the infection will become even more important to them than it has been.[2] Regardless of decisions about antiretroviral therapy, protease inhibitors, or other specific therapies, nurses and other professionals providing ongoing care and support need a good grounding in the causes, natural history, and management of symptoms. Searching for information among multiple sources is not the most efficient method of acquiring information.

HIV Nursing and Symptom Management provides a well-organized review of the management of HIV infection. The material is based on the best of available research and the expertise of outstanding clinicians. The heart of the book is the management of common clinical problems, including those that are neurological, nutrition-related, gastrointestinal, respiratory, hematologic, dermatologic, psychosocial, and those related to comfort and sleep. Related material such as pathogenesis, epidemiology, pharmacological treatment, models of treatment, and discussions of special and vulnerable populations are included as necessary background or expansion on the important management core.

No single book can be a substitute for regular perusal of the emerging research literature, but this volume, with its generous use of research references, provides excellent up-to-date information. Both experienced clinicians (nurses, but also others such as dieticians, physical therapists,

[1]United Nations Program on HIV/AIDS, November 26, 1997.

[2]The North American reference is not intended to suggest that the material would not be of use to those practicing in other locales. It should be noted, however, that an immense proportion of those infected live in areas of the globe where access to any form of treatment is limited, and supporting the basic necessities of living (e.g., shelter, food) may take precedence over any medical interests.

or physicians) and new practitioners seeking to develop expertise in this important field of practice will find the text and tables of value.

At the beginning of the HIV epidemic, a handful of nurses in the epicenter cities were developing ad hoc treatment plans daily to provide needed care for those dying of a poorly understood malady. Because of the limited number of informed professionals, and the desperation of the infected to understand and control what was happening to them, patients educated themselves and joined actively in decision making at an unusually high level. Today there is no place in practice for a nurse who does not have at least a rudimentary knowledge of this blood-borne pathogen and its impact on the lives of those infected. For the nurse who only occasionally is called upon to go beyond that basic information and assist an HIV-positive person in managing her disease or support a patient with AIDS as he makes treatment and life choices, *HIV Nursing and Symptom Management* is a handy reference. The role of patients as informed decision makers has not decreased. Patients and their advocates may also find this volume of assistance as they attempt to organize and interpret the mass of information available to them.

In 1859 Florence Nightingale said that nursing "ought to signify the proper use of fresh air, light, warmth, cleanliness, quiet and the proper selection and administration of diet—all at the least expense of vital power to the patient."[3] Although the science base for our practice has grown exponentially in nearly a century and a half since these words were written, and although the specific components of diet or method of maintaining warmth and cleanliness have changed, the basic thrust of the words should ring true to any clinician interested in symptom management. No dramatic intervention to attack a virus is sufficient. We must also attend to the unnecessary drain of energy (or "vital power") that will surely occur if symptoms such as diarrhea, pain, or cough are not attended.

Mary Ropka, Ann Williams, and an impressive team of expert clinicians have assembled a resource that can support any practitioner in improving

[3]Nightingale, Florence. *Notes on Nursing: What It Is and What It Is Not* (facsimile of 1859 edition). Philadelphia: JB Lippincott; 1946:6.

the care of those infected with HIV. Their work will be supplemented by new research and should indeed stimulate more studies to improve practice. Our partnership with all of those affected by this disease will be strengthened as we use this resource effectively to expand our knowledge and to organize our approach to care.

Kristine M. Gebbie, DrPH, RN
Elizabeth Standish Gill, Associate Professor of Nursing
Director, Center for Health Policy and Health Services Research
Columbia University School of Nursing
New York, NY

Preface

Good human immunodeficiency virus (HIV) care is synonymous with good nursing care. In the beginning of the HIV epidemic, this meant exquisite attention to the management of HIV symptoms and the side effects associated with its treatment. Even before the identification of the etiologic agent of acquired immunodeficiency syndrome (AIDS), nurses cared for patients affected by the new malady by using what they had learned from other health conditions. Fever, nausea, pain, dyspnea, malnutrition, and cough were familiar symptoms to nurses, although new and terrifying to patients. Now, a decade and a half later, although fewer patients with HIV infection suffer these symptoms acutely, the need for counseling and support has increased as patients learn to live longer and try to live better with what has become a chronic disease.

HIV Nursing and Symptom Management is designed to help nurses and other health care providers who care for patients across the spectrum of HIV infection—from early disease through long-term, end-stage care—make clinical decisions based on the best evidence available. Evidence-based practice is based on a synthesis of the current health care research that has then been combined with clinical expertise when a research base does not yet exist. The research base is derived from HIV research as well as research regarding other diseases.

HIV Nursing and Symptom Management is organized as follows. Unit One provides introductory and background information fundamental to HIV infection and its treatment. Unit Two is the major thrust of the book, with the information in the other units providing supporting information. Unit Two contains state-of-the-art, evidence-based information for the management of clinical problems. The clinical problems in Unit Two are those that are common or have a significant impact on comfort or function for those individuals experiencing HIV infection and its treatment. Part of the impetus for this came from Dr. Ropka's work at the National Institute for Nursing Research (NINR) at the National Institutes of Health from 1988 to 1993, developing the NINR intramural research program and its Clinical Therapeutics Laboratory's symptom management research initiatives. Unit Three addresses special dimensions of HIV clinical practice including compliance, models of care, ethics, and legal aspects of HIV care. Finally, Unit Four highlights unique aspects of caring for the increasingly diverse populations infected and affected by HIV infection. Unit Four summarizes the differences in HIV infection in that population, and then providing specific guidance in approaching HIV care for that group.

HIV Nursing and Symptom Management is useful to nurses and other health care providers caring for people with HIV infection. We dedicate it to the many nurses around the world who have been at the forefront of response to the pandemic of AIDS. They are heroes and role models for us all.

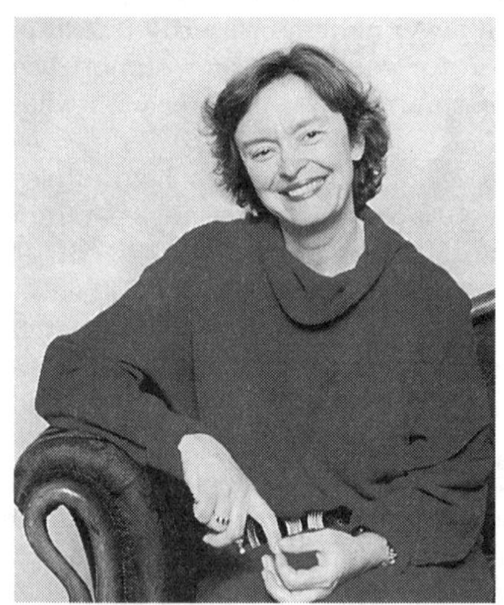

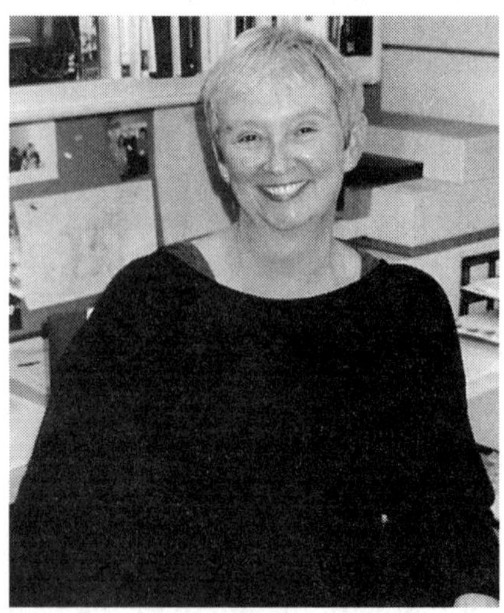

Mary Ropka

Mary E. Ropka, PhD, RN, FAAN

Ann B. Williams

Ann Williams, EdD, RN-C, FAAN

Contributors

Laurie Andrews, RN, BSN
Program Manager, AIDS Clinical Trials Unit
Yale University
New Haven, CT

Barbara Aranda-Naranjo, PhD, RN
Brigadier General Dunlap Endowed Professional Chair
University of the Incarnate Word
San Antonio, TX

Sonia Baker, PhD, RN
Assistant Professor
New York University School of Nursing
New York, NY

Alice Basch, RN, MSN, ET
Consultant in Ostomy, Wound Care, and Incontinence
San Rafael, CA

Emma J. Brown, PhD, RNC
Research Associate
University of Pennsylvania School of Nursing
Philadelphia, PA

Vivian L. Bruzzese, MD
Adjunct Assistant Professor, Internal Medicine
Medical College of Virginia/Virginia Commonwealth University
Richmond, VA

Arlene Manns Butz, RN, CPNP, ScD
Associate Professor, Division of General Pediatrics and School of Nursing
Johns Hopkins University
Baltimore, MD

Virginia Carrieri-Kohlman, RN, DNSc, FAAN
Professor
University of California at San Francisco, School of Nursing
San Francisco, CA

Cecily D. Cosby, PhD(c), FNP
University of California at San Francisco
San Francisco, CA

Patrick Coyne, RN, MSN, CS, CRNH
Clinical Nurse Specialist, Oncology-Pain Management
Massey Cancer Center, Medical College of Virginia Hospital
Richmond, VA

Evan G. DeRenzo, PhD
Senior Staff Fellow, Department of Clinical Bioethics
NIH Clinical Center
Bethesda, MD

Teri Dew, RN, MSN
Clinical Nurse Specialist, Coordinator HIV/AIDS Services
Metropolitan Health Medical Center
Cleveland, OH

Kathleen M. Doherty, RN, MS, OCN
Oncology Nurse Specialist/Nurse Practitioner
Stanford Health Services
Stanford, CA

Steven Jay Farber, PA-C, JD
Clinical Instructor, Department of Internal Medicine
Yale University
New Haven, CT

Kristine Gebbie, DrPH, RN, FAAN
Elizabeth Standish Gill, Associate Professor of Nursing
Director, Center for Health Policy and Health Services Research
Columbia University School of Nursing
New York, NY

Patty J. Hale, PhD, RN, FNP-C
Associate Professor
Lynchburg College
Lynchburg, VA

Barbara J. Holtzclaw, PhD, RN, FAAN
Director of Nursing Research
University of Texas Health Science Center at San Antonio, School of Nursing
San Antonio, TX

Mary Jo Hoyt, RN, MSN, FNP
Director, Women's Program
St. Vincent's Hospital Medical Center, Section of HIV Medicine
Manhattan, NY

Susan Janson, DNSc, RNc, ANP, FAAN
Professor, Department of Community Health Systems
University of California at San Francisco, School of Nursing
San Francisco, CA

Alain Joffe, MD
Director of Adolescent Medicine
Johns Hopkins University
Baltimore, MD

Lisa G. Kaplowitz, MD
Director, HIV/AIDS Center
Virginia Commonwealth University
Richmond, VA

Catherine S. Kay, RN, MSN
Instructor
Liberty University
Lynchburg, VA

Joyce K. Keithley, DNSc, FAAN
Professor and Practitioner-Teacher
Rush University College of Nursing
Chicago, IL

Felissa Lashley, RN, PhD, ACRN, FAAN
Dean and Professor
Southern Illinois University at Edwardsville School of Nursing
Edwardsville, IL

Wende L. Levy, RN, MS
Clinical Trials Specialist
Rockville, MD

Brenda Luna, MS, RN, CS, FNP
Nursing Administrator
Palatka Health Department
Palatka, FL

Linda Moneyham, DNS, RN
Research Associate Professor
University of South Carolina School of Nursing
Columbia, SC

Edward V. Morse, PhD
Clinical Professor of Psychiatry
Louisiana State University Medical Center
New Orleans, LA

Barbara A. Munjas, PhD, RN, FAAN
Professor
Virginia Commonwealth University School of Nursing
Richmond, VA

Catherine A. Oliver, MS, RN
Family Nurse Practitioner
Branch Medical Clinic
Mayport, FL

John Ownby, MD
Assistant Professor of Medicine, Pulmonary and Critical Care Medicine
Baylor College of Medicine
Houston, TX

Kristin Kane Ownby, PhDc, MPH, RN, OCN, ACRN
Doctoral Student
Texas Woman's University
Houston, TX

C. Fay Parpart, RN, MS, ANP, OCN
Nurse Practitioner
Salt Lake City, Utah

Joan A. Piemme, RN, MNEd, FAAN
HIV Coordinator
VA Medical Center
Martinsburg, WV

Barbara Piper, DNSc, RN, AOCN, FAAN
Associate Professor
University of Nebraska School of Nursing
Omaha, NE

JoLynn M. Pratt, MPH
Research Fellow
Department of Psychiatry, Louisiana State University Medical Center
New Orleans, LA

Tracy A. Riley, MSN, RN, CS
Instructor
University of Akron College of Nursing
Clinical Nurse Specialist
Akron General Medical Center
Akron, OH

Mary Ropka, PhD, RN, FAAN
Associate Professor
Department of Health Evaluation Sciences and Center for Survey Research
University of Virginia
Charlottesville, VA

Susan Sepples, RN, CCRN, PhD
Assistant Professor
University of Southern Maine School of Nursing
Portland, ME

Patricia M. Simon, MSW, PhD
Associate Professor of Clinical Psychiatry
Louisiana State University Medical Center
New Orleans, LA

Richard L. Sowell, PhD, RN, FAAN
Associate Professor and Chair
University of South Carolina College of Nursing
Columbia, SC

Roberta Anne Strohl, RN, MN, AOCN
Clinical Nurse Specialist, Department of Radiation Oncology
University of Maryland at Baltimore
Baltimore, MD

Mary Beth Tombes, RN, MN, OCN
Clinical Research Coordinator
Massey Cancer Center, Medical College of Virginia
Richmond, VA

Carol S. Viele, RN, MS
Clinical Nurse Specialist
University of California at San Francisco
San Francisco, CA

Gail Wilkes, RNC, MS, AOCN
Nurse Manager Hematology/Oncology and Immunodeficiency Clinics
Boston Medical Center
Boston, MA

Ann Williams EdD, RN, RN-C, FAAN
Associate Professor
School of Nursing
Yale University
New Haven, CT

UNIT ONE

HIV Infection Overview

CHAPTER 1

The Pathogenesis of HIV Infection

Laurie Andrews, RN, BSN

Chapter Preview

- HIV Structure
- Cells of the Immune System and HIV Infection
- Other Components of the Immune System
- Viral Types and Viral Dynamics
- Immune System Dynamics and Mechanisms of Immune Destruction
- HIV Natural History

Substantial progress has been made into the complex pathogenesis of HIV since the first individuals with AIDS were identified in 1981. A great deal is already known about the structure of the virus and its life cycle, and recent studies on viral dynamics and interactions with cellular targets have produced meaningful insight into the nature of HIV infection. This chapter reviews the current understanding of the virus and the mechanisms of action that lead to the devastating effects on the immune system of people with HIV infection.

The human immunodeficiency virus (HIV) is a member of the Lentivirus genus of the retroviral family. Retroviruses are so named because they carry their genetic material in the form of RNA and use an enzyme called *reverse transcriptase* (RT) to convert their RNA to DNA. The Lentivirus genus is distinguished from other retroviruses by its involvement in the nervous and immune systems, long periods of clinical latency, persistent viremia, and a more complex genomic structure than other relatives in the retroviral family. HIV is the only lentivirus that is known to infect humans.

Two types of HIV have been identified: HIV-1 is found throughout the world and is responsible for the majority of individuals with HIV infection. HIV-2 is less virulent and at this point seems to be found primarily in West Africa.

HIV Structure

The Viral Genome

HIV contains at least nine genes that are linked together to comprise its 9-kilobase RNA strand, which carries the blueprint to create new HIV particles (more than 200 million HIV particles could fit onto the head of a pin). Unlike most retroviruses, which contain only three genes (gag, pol, and env) the HIV genome also contains six additional genes: vif, vpu, vpr, tat, rev, and nef.[1] These nine structural and regulatory genes carry the specific information to create the proteins that make up a single, complete HIV particle, or *virion* (Figure 1.1).[2] For example, the env gene encodes for the envelope proteins gp120 and gp41.

The HIV-1 Virion

The HIV virion is comprised of proteins and glycoproteins, which are identified by their molecular weight (Figure 1.2).[2] Once a virion is success-

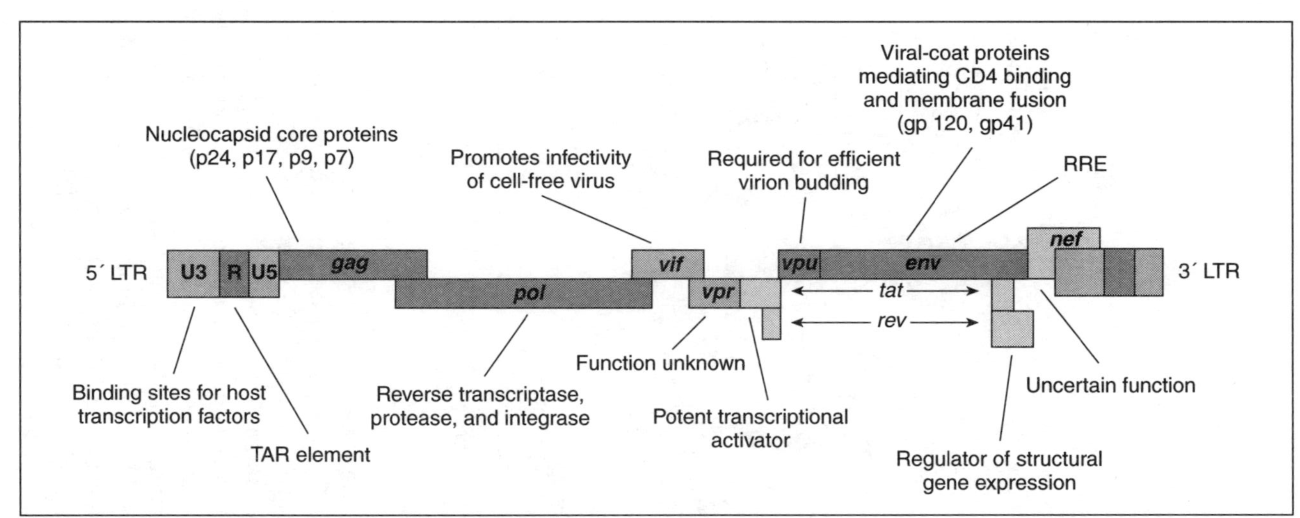

Figure 1.1 HIV Genome Map (Broder S, Merigan TC, Bolognesi D. Textbook of AIDS Medicine. Samuel Broder, M.D., 1993.)

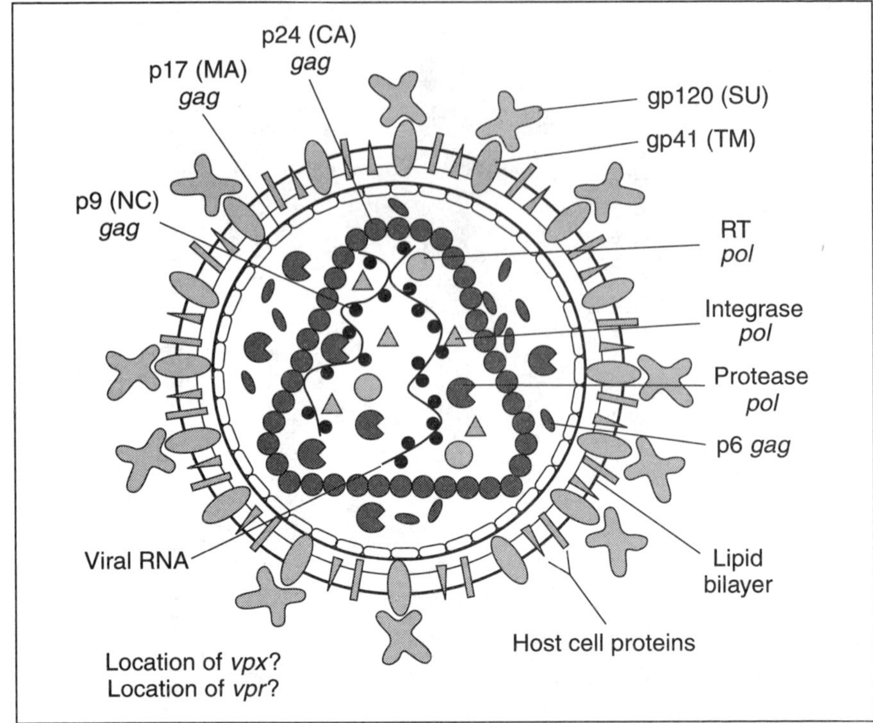

Figure 1.2 HIV Virion (Broder S, Merigan TC, Bolognesi D. Textbook of AIDS Medicine. Samuel Broder, M.D., 1993.)

fully made it carries the RNA genome, with the "orders" for additional virus particles, in its core (or *capsid*) in the form of two single strands of RNA. In addition to the two single strands of RNA, the core of a mature HIV virion also contains four nucleocapsid proteins: p9, p7, p24, and p17. The p24 protein forms a covering for the RNA strands whereas p17 bridges the interior and exterior components of the virion by forming a lipid bilayer. P7 is directly bound to the RNA strands and p9 is contained between the two RNA strands. Also contained in the core are the viral enzymes, which include RT, protease, and integrase, which play important roles in viral replication. Encasing the capsid is a glycoprotein coat or envelope with 72 external spikes. These spikes are formed by two envelope proteins gp120 and gp41 as well as major histocompatibility complex (MHC) molecules, which helps the virus to differentiate itself from other cells.

The HIV Life Cycle

HIV, like all viruses, is totally parasitic. This means that it cannot replicate on its own. The only way for a virus to reproduce, and therefore survive, is by infecting a host cell and usurping that cell's genetic machinery to replicate. The process by which the virus gains entry into its host cell, adopts the host replicative machinery, converts RNA to DNA, and then multiplies is called *the viral life cycle.* The host cell is thus transformed into a virus factory that produces viral proteins instead of the cell's normal regulatory proteins. This mechanism is depicted in Figure 1.3.[2]

The HIV life cycle begins with the binding of a virion to a susceptible host cell. The binding of gp120 spikes to the cell surface enable gp41, another envelope protein, to fuse the viral envelope to the cell membrane. Fusion appears to be mediated by a particular region of gp120 called the *V3 loop.* Attachment to the CD4 molecule on the target cell's surface no longer appears to be sufficient for viral binding and fusion as previously thought. Recent studies have identified additional molecules on the cell surface, referred to as *cofactors,* that influence the ability of a viral strain to enter a host cell.[3]

After fusion takes place, the viral core is injected into the cytoplasm of the host cell.[4] Once inside the cell the virus sheds its protein coat and the viral enzyme, RT, is activated. RT then converts the two single strands of viral RNA to a single strand of complementary DNA (cDNA). A second strand of DNA is then made, resulting in a double-stranded DNA copy of the original RNA genome.[5] The two cDNA strands then migrate into the nucleus of the cell where they are integrated into the host genome, an action that is assisted by another viral enzyme, *integrase.* The integrated cDNA is then called *proviral DNA.* This becomes a template from which new viral components are made to complete the replication cycle. However, since the proviral DNA cannot leave the nucleus it must be transcribed into messenger RNA (mRNA). This may not happen immediately since many viruses, including HIV-1, do not replicate in resting T cells.[6] Unactivated CD4+ cells or nondividing cells such as macrophages may allow the virus to lie dormant or latent in the form of proviral DNA awaiting host cell activation. Activation of lymphocytes by antigens, cytokines,

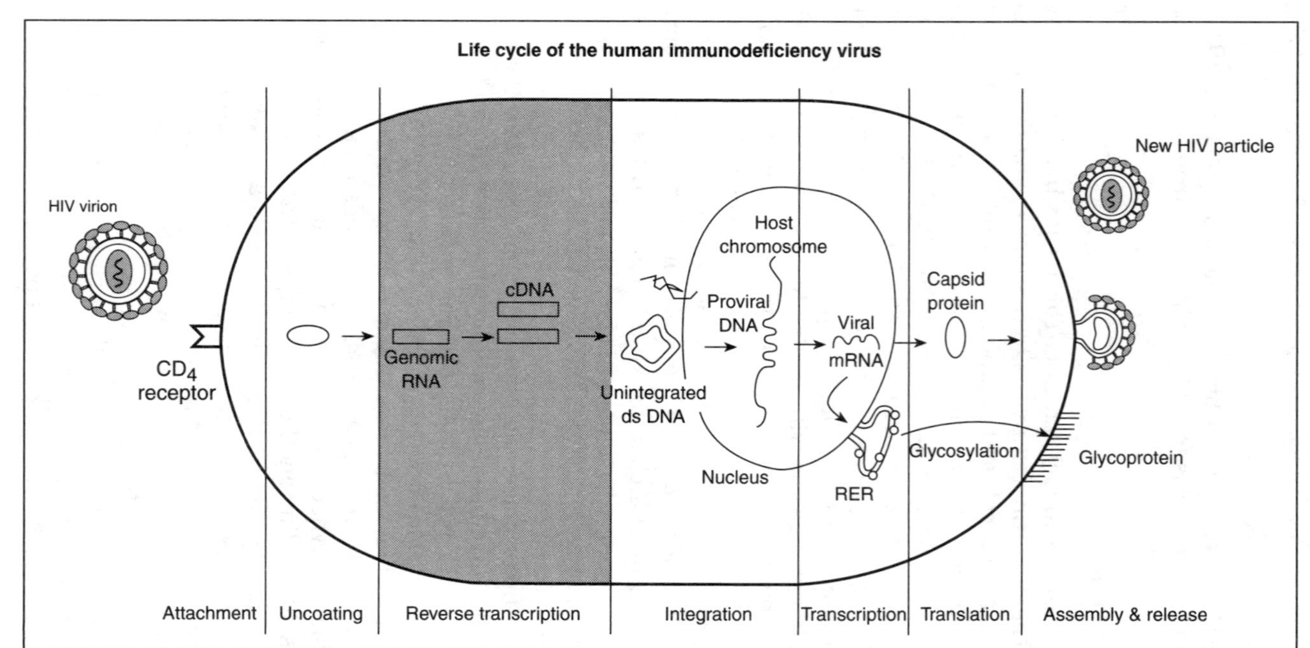

Figure 1.3 Life Cycle of HIV-1 (From Mandell G. *Atlas of Infectious Diseases.* Philadelphia: Churchill Livingston; 19.15. Reprinted with permission.)

or by various gene products creates an environment conducive to viral replication.[7]

Once the cell is activated, proviral DNA is transcribed into mRNA. Many of the factors that activate lymphocytes do so through a protein called *NF-κB*, also called the *cellular transcription nuclear factor*, that is present in all activated T cells.[8] When a cell is activated, NF-κB binds to specific sites in the viral genome to initiate transcription of the proviral DNA into the viral mRNA.

Information in the form of mRNA is transported to the ribosomes located outside the nucleus of the cell. Here the mRNA is translated into viral regulatory and structural proteins and enzymes. The viral core proteins, enzymes, and RNA gather just inside the cell's membrane, while the viral envelope proteins collect within the membrane. The core proteins, enzymes, and viral products bud off from the cell, taking the proteins to form an envelope on the way. After the immature virion buds from the cell, the protease enzyme is activated, cutting up the HIV protein chains and enabling the formation of mature virus particles.

Cells of the Immune System and HIV Infection

HIV has a high affinity for the CD4+ molecule, particularly when the cell is activated. Thus any cells that express the CD4 molecule on their surface become major cellular targets. These cells include T lymphocytes, monocytes/macrophages, and dendritic cells.[9]

T Lymphocytes

T cells are lymphocytes that are borne by the stem cell in the bone marrow but migrate to the thymus, where they mature and differentiate into subsets of T cells. T lymphocytes are identified by the receptor molecules on their surface. For example, the CD4 cell has a cluster designation 4 surface molecule. T lymphocytes play a central role in the immune response, detecting specific antigens and orchestrating a complex immune response that includes stimulating B lymphocytes to secrete antibodies, signaling killer T cells to destroy infected cells, and alerting inflammatory T cells to call in phagocytes to devour the enemy. Once the infection is controlled, the remaining helper T cells persist as memory T cells, which stand ready to respond to future attacks by the same antigen.

CD4 Cells

The CD4+ cell has been identified as the master coordinator of the body's immune response. CD4+ cells are divided by function. Th1 CD4+ cells are specialized to activate macrophages to kill antigens (inflammatory T cells) and Th2 CD4+ cells signal B cells to produce antibodies (helper T cells).[10] CD4+ cells migrate through the lymph nodes daily, where they are constantly exposed and infected with new virus—an important mechanism of HIV pathogenesis.

Cytotoxic T Cells (CTLs)

CTLs are cells that can kill other cells. Most CTLs are CD8 cells, but CD4 cells can kill in some cases.

CD8 Cells

CD8+ cells are also known as *suppressor cells* or *T8 cells*. Normally their function is to counteract the stimulatory response of the CD4+ cells. Some CD8+ cells also differentiate into CTLs. These cells zero in on cells that have become infected with viruses or cancer and kill the whole cell.[8] CTLs play a major role in the initial immune response to HIV infection, particularly at the time of primary infection because they kill cells that are involved in high-level viral replication.[11] In addition, CD8+ cells also are believed to release substances believed to suppress viral replication.

Naive and Memory Cells

The total population of CD4+ lymphocytes is characterized as naive or memory phenotypes. T cells exit the thymus as naive cells, programmed to respond to specific potential antigens. As they encounter the antigen for which they are programmed, they undergo a splicing, which enables them to generate immunologic memory by expanding into memory cells (clonal expansion).[12] Naive T lymphocytes circulate continuously from the bloodstream to the lymphoid organs, and back to the blood, making contact with many antigen-presenting cells every day. Memory T cells have a half-life of approximately 1 year and are designated *long-lived cells.* They provide protection from subsequent challenge by the same pathogen with an accelerated response. These phenotypes are not stable, however.[12] Memory cells can revert back to naive cells if they do not encounter their antigen, and naive cells can divide and not become a memory cell. In HIV infection, naive cells decline as overall CD4+ counts decline and as infection progresses, only memory cells are left. The ramifications of this are that if a patient has both naive and memory cells as treatment is initiated, both naive and memory cells can increase. However, once naive cells are lost, only memory cells can increase,[12] seriously compromising the immune response.

Monocytes and Macrophages

Monocytes and macrophages are large white blood cells with a bean-shaped nucleus and are designed to engulf bacteria, viruses, and funguses. They also have antitumor activity. They present antigens to T cells as well as produce and secrete cytokines.

Monocytes devour antigens in the blood and are precursors of macrophages. Macrophages are antigen-presenting cells that are found in most tissues of the body. Macrophages also clear away foreign particles and organisms that have been bound to antibodies. T cells secrete cytokines to communicate with macrophages and monocytes; direct their activities; and tell them to replicate, grow, or cease activity. Macrophages are important targets for HIV because they may serve as reservoirs for virus for months after infection without being destroyed. In addition, direct HIV infection of monocytes and macrophages may contribute to HIV-related dementia and other neurological syndromes by transporting the virus to neurological tissue sites.

Other Components of the Immune System

Lymph Nodes

Lymph nodes are highly organized structures that collect extracellular fluid from tissues and return it to the blood. The lymph fluid draining the extracellular spaces of the body carries antigens from the tissues to the lymph nodes. Here antigens such as HIV become trapped. Lymph nodes contain follicles, some of which have germinal centers that are areas of intense lymphocytic proliferation after activation by antigens.[8] Extensive trapping of virus in the germinal centers leads to the eventual destruction of the lymph node architecture (Figure 1.4).[10]

Dendritic Cells

Follicular dendritic cells are located in germinal centers of lymphoid tissue and filter circulating lymphocytes. Dendritic cells have threadlike tentacles that trap antigens in the periphery and migrate to lymphoid tissue where they present antigens to T cells and B cells. HIV that is detected in lymphoid tissue exists primarily on the follicular dendritic cells. (Figure 1.4)

Dendritic cells of skin and mucosa are called *Langerhans' cells.* These dendritic cells transport antigen to the lymphoid tissue, where they can activate naive T lymphocytes.[13]

Cytokines and Chemokines

Cytokines

Cytokines are proteins that include interferons, the interleukins (ILs), colony stimulating factors (CSF), and other growth factors. They are secreted by various cells, including those of the immune system, and act as chemical messengers to stimulate or inhibit the differentiation, proliferation, or function of other cells. In the immune system they are responsible for inflammation and immunity, and serve a key role in immune regulation.

When antigens are presented to T cells, T cells become activated, stimulating cytokine production and release. HIV is a continual source of immune activation in infected individuals.[14] Numerous cytokines have been linked to enhanced viral replication, including some ILs (IL-1β, IL-2, IL-3, IL-6, and IL-12), CSFs (GM-CSF and M-CSF), and the most potent inducer of HIV, tumor necrosis factors (TNF-α and -β).[15] TNF induces cellular transcription nuclear factor, NF-κB, which triggers activation of the cell and replication of the virus by mediating transcription of proviral DNA to mRNA.[16] The influence of cytokines on viral replication is evidenced during acute and chronic infections, which are associated with elevated cytokine production. Figure 1.5 shows the relationship of cytokines to HIV infection.[17] The presence of an acute opportunistic infection, for example, is associated with a substantially increased HIV viral load.[18] These transient increases

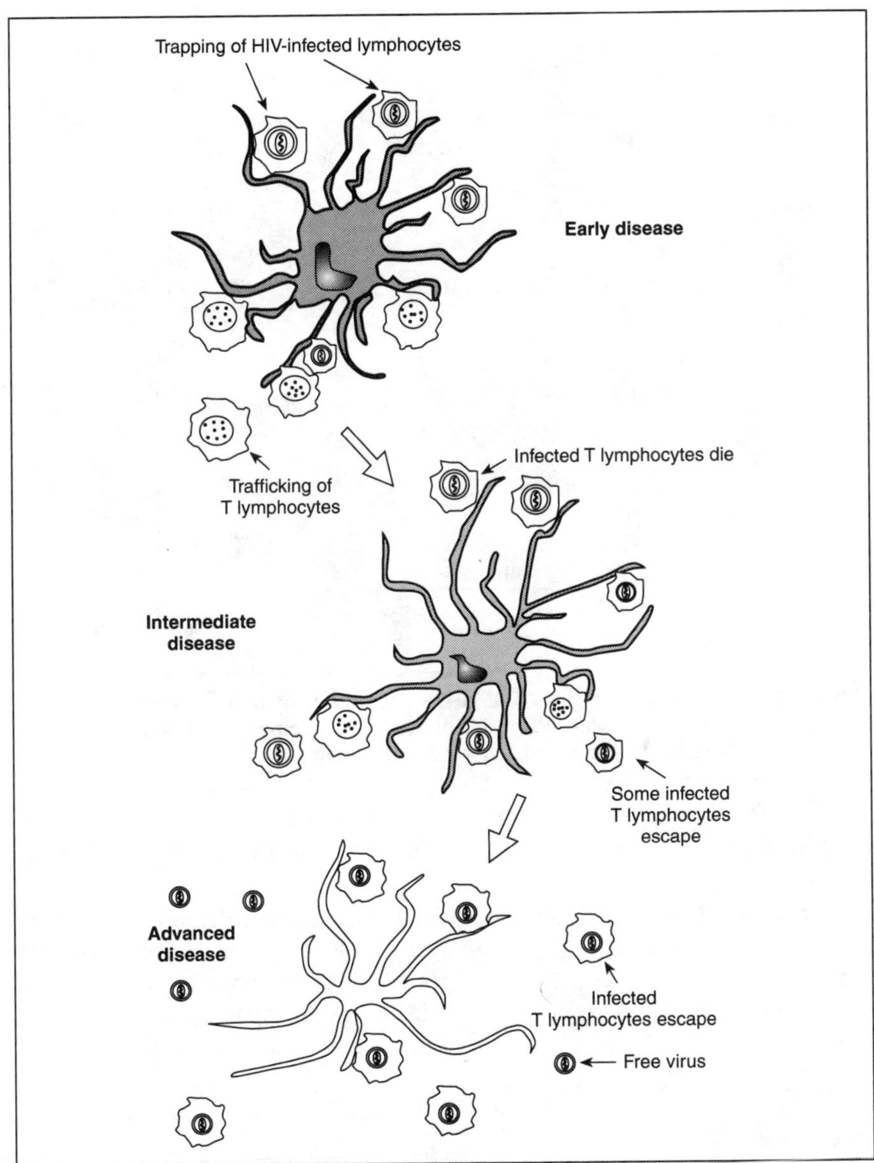

Figure 1.4 **Lymph Node Destruction** (Reprinted with permission from Fauci A. *Science* 1993:262;1011–1018. © 1993 American Association for the Advancement of Science.)

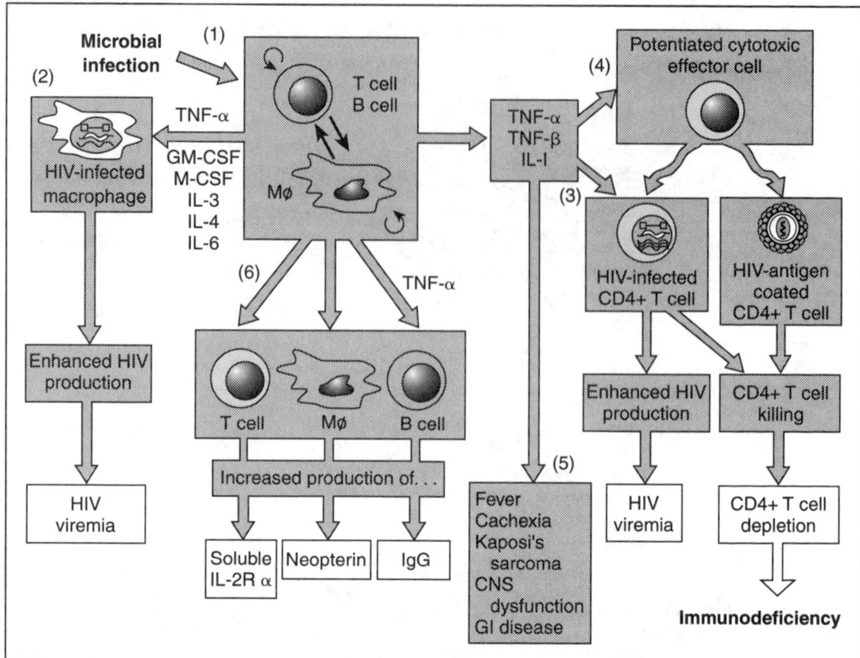

Figure 1.5 Cytokine Networks and AIDS Pathogenesis (From *AIDS* 1991, S:1405–1417, Matsuyama T, Kobayayeshi N, Yamamoto N. Rapid Science Publishers Ltd. Reprinted with permission.)

in viral load fall after the infection is treated and the cytokine response is diminished.[14]

Not all cytokines are inducers of HIV. IL-10, for example, inhibits replication in infected monocytes/macrophages by blocking the secretion of HIV-inducing cytokines.[19] Levy's early reports of HIV suppression by CD8+ T cells are now felt to be explained,[20] at least in part, by the effect of a class of cytokines called *chemokines*,[8] which have an important role in control of viral replication.

Chemokines

Chemokines are a subset of cytokines that act as chemoattractants and are secreted by a variety of cells in the immune system. They induce inflammation, direct the migration of white blood cells to sites of infection, and serve as a link between lymphocytes (T cells and B cells) and other cells in the immune system. They have a more specific function than other kinds of cytokines, focusing on inflammation and repair.[8]

Chemokines bind to specific chemokine receptors on the surface of various white blood cells, which allows signaling to occur, triggering a specific process such as, for example, the entry of a virus into a host cell. Chemokines are divided into two categories—alpha chemokines and beta chemokines—based on their structure. Alpha chemokines have two cysteine groups separated by an amino acid, and beta chemokines do not have an intervening amino acid between the cysteine groups.[20]

Each chemokine docks in a corresponding chemokine receptor. The chemokine receptors are found on the surface of various cells of the immune system and are identified by the chemokine structure with which they correspond. The alpha chemokine receptors are thus identified as *CXC* (two cysteines separated by an amino acid) and beta chemokine receptors are identified as *CC* (two cysteines next to each other).

The Role of Chemokines and HIV in HIV Infection

In 1986, Levy et al[20] proposed that there were substances secreted by CD8 cells, called *cell antiviral factor* (CAF), that inhibit HIV replication in infected cells.[19] Since then, Gallo et al[19] identified three chemokines known as Rantes and macrophage inflammatory protein (MIP) MIP-1α and MIP-1β (all beta chemokines), which are made by activated CD8+ T cells. These chemokines are able to inhibit HIV replication in vitro.[3] It is not known, however, if these three chemokines are in fact the CAF proposed by Levy.

The first chemokine, Rantes, is a moderately potent chemoattractant for monocytes and a very potent chemoattractant for memory cells. It is produced by activated CD8+ T lymphocytes and by platelets. It promotes the adherence of T cells to endothelial cells. The second chemokine, MIP-1α, is a chemoattractant for monocytes and activated T lymphocytes (particularly CD8 lymphocytes) that promote the adhesion of activated CD8 cells to endothelial cells. MIP-1β promotes the adherence of activated CD4 cells rather than CD8 cells to endothelial cells. Both MIP-1α and MIP-1β activate macrophages to be cytotoxic for tumor cells.

The Role of Chemokine Receptors in HIV Infection

Chemokine receptors are members of the seven-transmembrane G protein-coupled receptors. The three beta chemokines discovered in Gallo's laboratory bind to the corresponding receptors chemotactic chemokine receptors (CCR) CCR1, CCR2, CCR3, CCR4, and CCR5. The identification of multiple coreceptors that mediate the entry of specific viral strains clarifies for us that the CD4 molecule is necessary but not sufficient for HIV infection. In 1996 Berger et al[3] published findings on a coreceptor that allowed the entry of T-tropic (syncytium-inducing) strains of HIV. He called the receptor *Fusin* (now known as *CXCR4*).[21] CXCR4 mediates the fusion and entry of pathogenic strains of the virus that are able to induce syncytium, and are associated with a more rapid progression of disease. Its corresponding chemokine is stromal cell-derived factor (SDF) SDF-1. Since the discovery of CXCR4, additional receptors have been identified. Data from several labs have shown that the chemokine receptor CCR5 allows the fusion and entry of M-tropic (nonsyncytium-inducing) strains of HIV.[22,23] Deletion of the CCR5 coreceptor appears to influence susceptibility to infection, but is not absolutely protective. A heterozygous deletion or defect (a deletion or defect inherited from one parent but not from the other) of CCR5 or CCR2 does not seem to affect the incidence of infection but has been correlated with delayed progression to AIDS.[24] Figure 1.6 demonstrates the association of chemokine receptors to viral strains.[25]

However some people, who despite multiple high-risk exposures do not become infected with HIV, are homozygous (inherited from both parents)

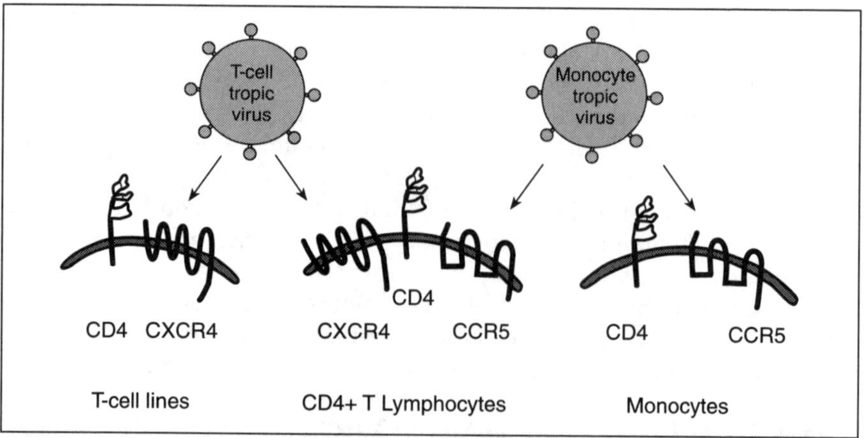

Figure 1.6 New Co-receptors for HIV-1 (From Kuritzkes D. *HIV Pathogenesis and Viral Markers.* Healthcare Communications Group, 1996. Reprinted with permission.)

for the deleted CCR5 gene.[26] Although estimates for homozygous deletions of CCR5 vary, it has been found consistently that Caucasians have a greater prevalence of these defects and deletions than other racial backgrounds. It is estimated that approximately 1% of the Caucasian population is homozygous for missing the CCR5 gene.[14] The implications for this new area of research are far reaching—from a greater understanding of viral mechanisms to added hope for new therapies and vaccines.

Viral Types and Viral Dynamics

Viral Strains

Different viral strains preferentially infect different target cells of the immune system. Some viral strains are said to be M-tropic; that is, they grow equally well in monocytes and macrophages, and T cells. Other viral strains are said to be T-cell tropic. These viruses prefer to infect T lymphocytes, but not monocytes and macrophages. Recent research[23] has linked cellular tropism to the presence of newly identified coreceptors.

The preference of a viral strain to infect particular cells is referred to as *cellular tropism.*[27] Different viral phenotypes have different characteristics, including viral tropism.

Syncytium-Inducing Viruses

Syncytium formation is a mechanism by which a few HIV-1-infected cells fuse with many uninfected CD4+ cells.[28] The result of this cell-to-cell transmission by fusion is the creation of multinucleated giant cells. Most individuals are initially infected with M-tropic viral strains that are not capable of inducing syncytia. However, syncytia-inducing strains can emerge later in infection.[29] Syncytium-inducing viruses tend to grow more rapidly and are associated with an accelerated decline in CD4+ lymphocyte counts.[30] Individuals who have syncytium-inducing strains of virus are also more likely to progress more quickly to AIDS and to death than those who do not.[31]

To summarize, HIV strains that use CXCR4 tend to infect T cells predominately and can induce syncytia, while strains that use CCR5 infect monocytes and macrophages and tend to be nonsyncytia forming. Early on in infection, M-tropic strains tend to dominate; however, as infection progresses, these strains tend to be replaced by the more pathogenic T-tropic strains.[32]

Viral Load

The battle between the virus and the immune system results in the number of virions present in the body in a given moment. The number of virions detected is referred to as the *viral load.* Assays that quantify viral particles actually measure free virus in plasma (virus that isn't in any cell). Viral load assays report these results in numbers of copies of virus detected per ml.

The value of knowing an individual's viral load has been well established.[33,34] To underscore the role of the amount of virus in the body, Coffin[34] introduced the analogy of a train approaching a cliff, in which the CD4+ cell count is the distance to the precipice and the viral load is the speed of the train (Figure 1.7). The total amount of virus detected on viral load

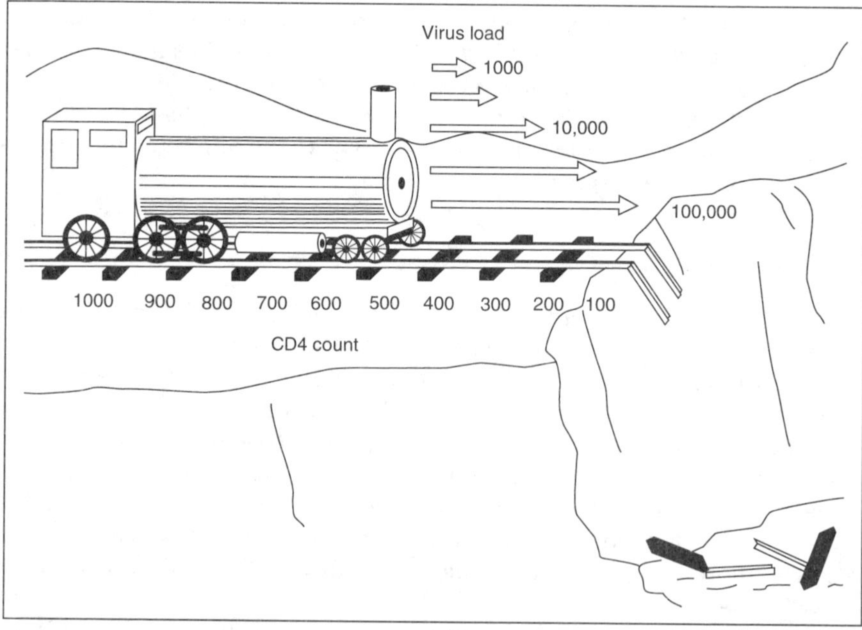

Figure 1.7 **Train Analogy Relating HIV Progression to Viral Load and CD4 Count** (From *AIDS,* 10(Suppl. 3):575–584;1996, Coffin J.M., HIV Viral dynamics, Rapid Science Publishers Ltd. Reprinted with permission.)

testing is in fact a surrogate for how quickly the virus is actually replicating. How quickly the virus replicates determines how quickly CD4+ lymphocytes are being destroyed and how hard the immune system must work to replenish the store of immune cells. Having access to viral load information has changed the practice of HIV care and the process of clinical research.

Mellors et al[32,33] analyzed viral load data from the Muticenter AIDS Cohort Study (MACS) to demonstrate further the ability of viral load, with and without CD4+ cell counts, to determine the risk of progression to AIDS and death. In their analysis, they reviewed the viral load measurements (by bDNA), CD4+ cell counts, clinical end points, and deaths from 180 of the 209 HIV-infected homosexual or bisexual men enrolled in the Pittsburgh MACS site. The relationship between baseline viral load or baseline CD4+ T cell counts was examined. The proportion of subjects who progressed either to AIDS or to death was stratified into quartiles by baseline viral load or CD4+ count. Findings are summarized as follows.[32]

- CD4+ counts are an inaccurate indicator of the level of viremia. (p. 1168)
- The risk of AIDS and death was directly related to plasma viral load at study entry. (pp 1168–69)
- Plasma viral load was a better predictor of progression to AIDS and death than the number of CD4+ cells alone. (p 1168)
- There was a significant increase in the rate of progression to AIDS in those patients with higher viral loads. (p. 1169)
- There was a significant difference in median time to death in those patients with ≤10,190 copies/ml vs. ≥10,190 copies/ml. (p. 1169)
- Individuals with a threefold higher viral load face a greater risk of death (1.5 times) within 10 years. (p. 1169)

A subsequent analysis of all participants in the four MAC centers revealed similar results. Five risk categories were identified by plasma HIV-1 RNA concentrations: 500 copies/ml or less, 501 to 3,000 copies/ml, 3,001 to 10,000 copies/ml, 10,001 to 30,000 copies/ml, and more than 30,000 copies/ml.

Highly significant differences were seen in both progression to AIDS and death in the five categories. In this more recent analysis Mellors et al[33] concluded that although viral loads provide more useful information than CD4+ cell counts alone, combined use of both of these markers yields the most useful information for patient management.[35]

Viral Dynamics

Relentless viral replication in susceptible cells is the primary mechanism of immune system destruction in HIV infection. Ho et al,[35] Wei et al,[36] and Coffin[37] have demonstrated a highly dynamic process with a rapid turnover of virus, even in asymptomatic patients.

Through the work of Ho, Perelson, and others[38] it has been estimated that 10 billion particles of HIV are produced and cleared each day in an infected individual. The rate of viral clearance is constant and does not vary depending on the stage of infection. Therefore the extent of viremia depends on the rate of viral production.[38]

After treatment, the net loss of free viral particles in plasma and the loss of virus-producing cells is known as the *viral decay rate.*[38] However, the loss of virus from these different compartments where virus lives is not uniform. For example, effective antiretroviral therapy (ART) may kill virus in less than a week in one cell but it may be able to survive for many weeks in other cells. A model for viral breakdown in each of these compartments has been developed,[38] and these compartments are shown in Figure 1.8. The compartments include (1) *productively infected CD4+ lymphocytes* (those CD4+ lymphocytes that are activated by antigen presentation and actively serve as host to replicating virus); (2) *latently infected lymphocytes* (those CD4+ cells that are infected but are not activated), which lay dormant in a proviral DNA state ready to replicate on host cell activation; (3) *uninfected but activated CD4+ cells,* which present a vulnerable target for virus; and (4) *long-lived cell populations* (places where virus can live for long periods of time; so-called *sanctuary sites*) such as monocytes and macrophages, and more recently memory cells.[39] In addition, *free virus* exists in plasma, which is what is measured in viral load. The half-life of an infectious virion in plasma is believed to be as short as 0.3 days.

Ongoing research into the decay rates in each compartment has provided valuable insight into the development of HIV therapy. The decay curve for decrease of viral load must take into consideration the different compartments in which HIV must be eliminated. The most recent model of viral decay demonstrates a two-phase slope.[38] Two different populations of cells account for these two phases. The first phase eliminates free virus and

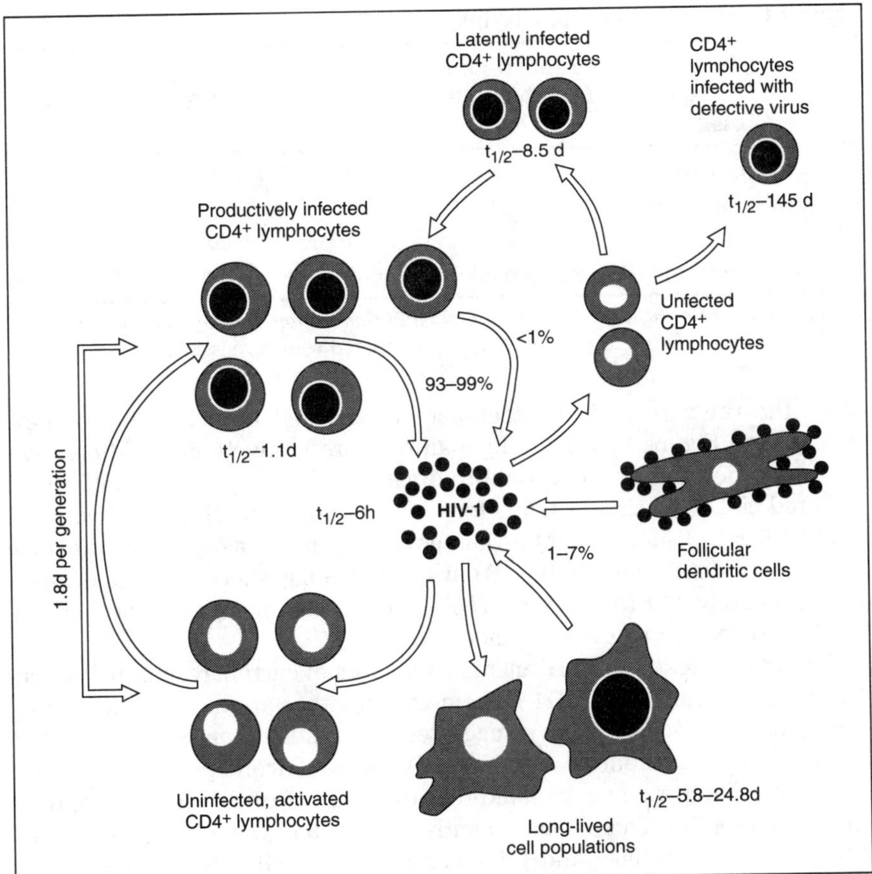

Figure 1.8 Schematic Summary of HIV-1 Infection Dynamics In Vivo (From Perelson AS, Essunger P, Ho DD. Dynamics of HIV-1 and CD4 + lymphocytes in vivo. *AIDS.* 1997;11(suppl A):522. Reprinted with permission.)

virus from productively infected cells, which accounts for about 95 to 99% of the viral load, with a mean lifetime of 1.2 days.[38] The second phase eliminates virus from latently infected cells, which accounts for 1 to 5% of the viral load, with a half-life of 2 to 3 weeks.[35,36,40] Table 1.1 presents the kinetic classes of HIV-infected cells.[41]

A mathematical model has been used to estimate the virion clearance rate, the infected cell life span, and the average viral generation time in

Table 1.1 Kinetic Classes of HIV-Infected Cells

Class	Proportion of Infected Cells (%)	No. in Body	Half-life (day)	Time to Eradicate
Productively infected	10	10^7–10^9	~1.6	38–54 days
Latently/chronically infected	1	10^6–10^9	~20	400–600 days
Defectively infected	90 (variable)	10^8–10^{11}	~100	~7–10 years

(From Coffin J. *Eradication of Infected Cells and Generation of Drug-Resistant Mutants.* Healthcare communications Group. 1997;3(2). Reprinted with permission.)

vivo (the time from viral attachment to the cell until budding of new virions; see Figure 1.8). The life span of a productively infected cell was originally determined to be approximately 2.2 days, with a half-life in infected cells (the time it takes for half the virions to clear) estimated at about 1.6 days.[38] More recent estimates on the time it takes to generate new virions was determined to be 1.8 days, which suggests that HIV undergoes approximately 140 to 200 viral replication cycles per year. One half the viral particles are lost and replaced each day.[42]

Latent viral reservoirs are an important area of current research. Particular focus has turned to CD4+ memory cells that are at rest but latently infected. Siliciano et al[39] have suggested that resting memory cells may be the longest lived source of latent HIV derived from proviral DNA yet identified. Their study calculated that the half-life of this pool is approximately 7 months. This is significantly longer than the 15- to 28-day half-life of the macrophage and follicular dendritic cell second-phase decay compartment calculated by Perelson and Ho.[38] If this is indeed a third-phase decay it implies that it could take years of treatment to eradicate virus harbored in this compartment.

Immune Systems Dynamics and Mechanisms of Immune Destruction

CD4+ Dynamics

The massive production of viral particles is paralleled by the ongoing destruction of CD4+ lymphocytes and the immune system's attempt to replenish the loss of cells. It is clear that T-cell reductions, even early on in HIV disease, are a result of their destruction and not their lack of production.[35] CD4+ cells are replaced at a rate of approximately 10^8 cells per day.[40] Mostly cells are replaced by T-cell division, and only a limited amount come directly from the thymus. Previous estimates for the dynamics of T cells have demonstrated that naive cells are believed to divide once every 3.5 years, memory cells divide once every 22 weeks, and T cells live an average of 20 years.[43] Naive cells have a greater ability to expand than memory cells, and replicate intensely to keep up with their destruction. However, it is possible that there is in fact a finite ability to continue this expansion, and clonal exhaustion may cause the ultimate failure of CD4+ cells to maintain their absolute numbers.

Additional mechanisms also contribute to the profound loss of immune response and these are discussed next.

Mechanisms of Immune Destruction

It is clear that HIV causes CD4+ cell destruction and that it does so through a complex multifactorial process. Several mechanisms have been identified thus far that lead to the mass depletion of CD4+ cells. These mechanisms include single-cell killing and apoptosis.

Single-cell killing occurs when CD4+ cells, activated by antigen presentation, permit an environment conducive to viral replication. CD4+ cells lyse or become dysfunctional from the process of viral budding and release.

Cell killing during HIV-specific immune response occurs both through antibodies as well as through cytotoxic T lymphocytes. As gp120 binds to CD4 cells, HIV-specific antibodies are alerted to destroy these complexes. Also, cytotoxic lymphocytes lyse CD4 cells that are not infected but are bound to gp120.

Apoptosis is the natural process of programmed cell death through phagocytosis. It is the normal mechanism used by the body for eliminating certain cells that might otherwise have a harmful effect. Apoptosis is one of the primary mechanisms of CD4+ cell death in HIV infection.[44] It has been shown that apoptosis occurs in substantial numbers of CD8+ cells that are not killed by HIV infection, and it occurs in CD4+ cells that are not HIV infected yet are primed to die by the presence of HIV. The reason for an increase in apoptosis is less clear than the fact that it happens. It may reflect the amplification of a normal mechanism of eliminating activated cells.[44] Other theories of apoptosis include one of abnormal signaling to kill cells after gp120/CD4+ interaction and inappropriate stimulation of CD4+ and CD8+ T cells.[44] In this explanation of apoptosis, the immune signal that would normally mediate proliferation of additional CD4+ cells actually primes the cells to die.

HIV Natural History

The course of disease in an individual who is infected with HIV is referred to as *the natural history.* It is the direct result of the interaction between HIV and the immune system. Figure 1.9 represents this relationship.[45]

Events of HIV Disease

HIV enters through the bloodstream or mucosa. High levels of viral replication occur. Individuals may experience symptoms associated with viremia and the cytokines produced in response to HIV antigen. HIV-specific cell-mediated responses are detected within weeks after infection. Levels of virus drop as virus becomes trapped in lymph nodes and CTLs kill infected cells.

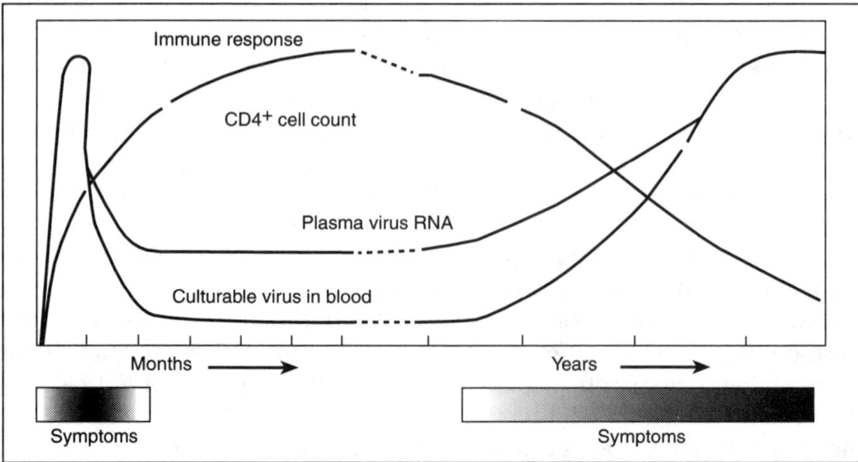

Figure 1.9 Virological and Immunologic Course of HIV Infection (From Saag MS, Holodny M, Kuritzkes DR, et al. HIV Viral load markers in clinical practice. *Nat Med.* 1996;2(6):625. Reprinted with permission.)

Seroconversion occurs as HIV antibodies are produced. Virus replicates in lymph nodes at a steady rate, with roughly 10 billion viral particles produced and cleared daily whereas 100 million CD4+ lymphocytes are produced and killed daily. Virus becomes disseminated systemically. HIV infection promotes chronic immune activation and provides the virus with an ongoing supply of new targets. Continued trapping in the lymph nodes leads to their eventual destruction and the release of virus back into the circulation. Additional mechanisms such as apoptosis and syncytia formation contribute to immune destruction. Years of assault on the CD4+ cells, the disregulation of normal T cell dynamics, and the inability of the immune system to continue replenishing them leads to their progressive decline. Dangerously low levels of CD4+ cells make individuals vulnerable to opportunistic infections and other HIV-related complications.

Stages of HIV Infection

Primary Infection

The period from infection with HIV to the development of HIV-specific antibody response is referred to as *primary infection.* Primary infection is characterized by an intense period of viral replication, high titers of virus in the blood, extensive cell killing with an associated drop in CD4+ cells, and widespread dissemination of virus throughout the body. Within a few days of infection virus is detectable in lymphocytes and monocytes, and shortly thereafter in lymph nodes. Viral load climbs during the first 2 weeks after infection.[46] Symptoms appear during the peak of viremia and occur in up to 80 to 90% of individuals.[47] Symptoms may range from mild flulike symptoms to a more severe presentation of acute viremia including fever, sore throat, skin rash, lymphadenopathy, splenomegaly, myalgia, arthritis, a mononucleosislike illness or even meningitis.[46] Table 1.2 breaks down the percentage of individuals experiencing specific signs and symptoms of primary infection.[48]

Early on, monocyte/macrophage cells present HIV antigen to CD4 cells, which alert B cells to produce HIV antibody. The production of HIV antibodies is referred to as *seroconversion* and generally occurs an average of 6 to 12 weeks after successful infection. Studies have shown that viral titers fall even before an HIV antibody response occurs, suggesting mechanisms other than an antibody response controlling viral replication.

The cell-mediated immune response is a critical determinant of viral control and presents in the form of HIV-specific cytotoxic lymphocytes

Table 1.2 Signs, Symptoms, and Laboratory Values of Primary Infection

Symptom	Percentage of Individuals Affected
Fevers	>90
Fatigue	>90
Rash	>70
Headache	32–70
Lymphadenopathy	40–70
Pharyngitis	50–70
Myalgia, arthralgia	50–70
Nausea or vomiting	30–60
Night sweats	50
Oral ulcers	10–20
Genital ulcers	5–15
Thrombocytopenia	45
Leukopenia	40
Elevated liver enzymes	21

(From Kahn J, Hecht F. Treating primary infection. *HIV Newsline.* 1996;2.)

(CD8+ cells). This response is marked by a sharp increase in the number of CD8+ cells and seems to occur at approximately day 33 after the onset of primary infection.[49] It is the contribution of this important interaction between the virus and the cytotoxic lymphocytes that probably has the greatest impact on the level of virus established when a viral equilibrium is reached. In addition, there are large numbers of virus trapped in the lymph nodes by the follicular dendritic cells.

The amount of virus that is present after the initial burst of viremia and the immune control that follows is referred to as the *viral setpoint.* This begins a period of a steady state of infection. During the steady state the amount of virus in circulation and the number of infected cells remain relatively constant, because the rate of infection of new cells equals the rate of viral clearance. This is generally maintained for years.

The events of primary infection are felt to be important indicators of an individual course of disease. The duration and intensity of symptoms are predictive of the likelihood of developing AIDS later.[50] In addition, it has been shown that the level of virus in the blood at the setpoint also predicts the likelihood of progressing to AIDS. Eight percent of patients with HIV-1 RNA levels of <4,350 copies/ml in plasma after seroconversion progressed to AIDS in 5 years compared with 62% with >36,270 copies/ml[32]. Figure 1.10 demonstrates these data.[51] Understanding the critical events of primary infection raises numerous questions about treatment during this time and the opportunity to alter the course of disease.

Clinical Latency

On reaching a viral setpoint, a chronic, clinically asymptomatic state begins. It starts with a decreased viral load and resolution of the symptoms of primary infection.[46] This typically lasts for years before outward signs of immune deficiency develop. This period of time is not, however, a period of virological latency, and is characterized by continued high rates of viral replication in the lymph nodes and chronic immune activation.

The stable viral load represents a balance in which the number of newly infected cells equals the number of cells that die; each time a virion is

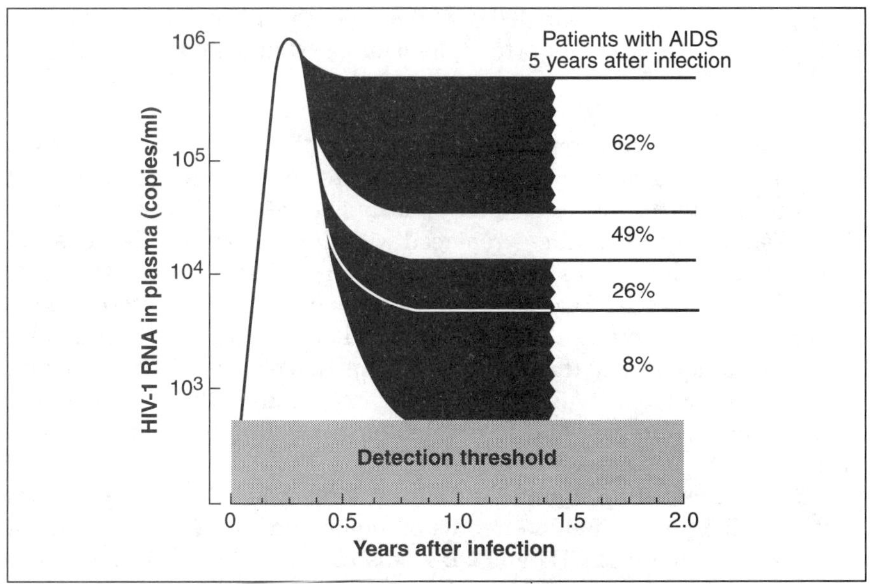

Figure 1.10 Variable Virologic Setpoints After Acute HIV-1 Infection and Their Prognostic Value (Reprinted with permission from Mellors JW. *Science* 1996:272;1124. © 1996 American Association for the Advancement of Science.)

generated one must be cleared, and each time a target cell dies one must be created.[37] However, immune activation provides a constant supply of new, susceptible targets for viral replication in the form of uninfected but activated T cells. Early seeding of monocyte/macrophage cells also serves as a long-term reservoir for latent proviral DNA.

There is substantial trapping of virus in the follicular dendritic cell (FDC) network of the germinal centers of the lymph nodes, which leads to hyperplasia of the follicles.[44] Persistent general lymphadenopathy (PGL), which can last for years, may be present as a result of the vigorous activity occurring in the lymph nodes. As CD4+ cells pass through the lymph system during the normal course of the day, they are continuously exposed to and infected with virus. Also, increased secretion of some cytokines and the depletion of others contribute to progression during this phase. In particular, an increase in TNF and a decrease in IL-2 contribute to the deterioration of the immune status.[14]

Although the individual may be asymptomatic, the level of virus in the blood may range from undetectable to hundreds of thousands. CD4 cell counts may be greater than 400 or 500/mm^3 in this phase of infection, but eventually the CD4 lymphocyte-replenishing system begins to falter.

Symptomatic HIV Disease

Eventually the viral replication process in the lymph nodes destroys the lymph node architecture and large amounts of virus are released back into the plasma. Lymphadenopathy disappears as the lymph nodes are destroyed and lymph tissue is replaced with fibrotic tissue.[52] The destruction of the lymph nodes severely cripples the body's ability to mount an immune response. Two significant consequences of the disruption of lymphoid tissue are that the FDC network is no longer able to trap virus and other antigens, and that the mechanisms that sequester virus in lymph nodes are eliminated.[44] Also, when FDCs are impaired, they can no longer present antigens to lymphocytes, which further compromises the immune response.

As viral replication continues and the viral load climbs, the immune system's ability to maintain effective immune control of the virus diminishes. The numbers of CD4 and CD8 cells also steadily decline. The viral phenotype may switch at this point to a syncytia-forming virus. All of these factors contribute to an increasing inability to protect the body from infection.

Symptoms may begin to appear as the absolute CD4+ cell counts fall to <200/mm³. As CD4+ cell counts continue to decline, sometimes into the single digits, individuals become increasingly vulnerable to the complications of AIDS.

Long-term Nonprogressors

Approximately 5 to 10% of individuals infected with HIV are clinically asymptomatic and have stable CD4 levels after 10 or more years.[53] Projections based on the MACS suggest that 20 years after infection, 10 to 17% of those infected may continue to remain free of AIDS.[53] Attempts to characterize these long-term nonprogressors (or *slow progressors*) have led to the discovery that although there are probably many differences among those who progress more slowly, a consistent pattern of viral dynamics and immune response seems to exist. The following are some of the characteristics of long-term nonprogressors:

- Decreased levels of viral replication and viral load
- Strong cellular immune response with high CD8+ levels
- Neutralizing antibodies present
- Small, intact germinal centers
- Lymph node architecture maintained
- Virus difficult to culture
- Less pathogenic viral strains

A cellular immune response occurs shortly after seroconversion in individuals with HIV infection, which is demonstrated by the presence of CD8+ cells that appear at the same time as a reduction in viral load.[54] Studies of nonprogressors have demonstrated high levels of peripheral blood CD8+ cytotoxic lymphocyte levels.[55,56] Typically their CD8+ cell levels are maintained over time,[56] are at least partially chemokine mediated, and can suppress HIV replication in virus-infected cells.[9]

Although biopsies of lymph nodes of slow progressors show varying histology, germinal centers are intact and are often smaller than in rapid progressors, and the lymph node architecture is generally preserved. Follicular dendritic cells are also maintained.

In general, those who progress more slowly have lower levels of plasma HIV RNA, as demonstrated by Mellors et al,[32] Ho and Cao et al.[57] Fauci et al[55] demonstrated that plasma HIV RNA in subjects with long-term nonprogressive disease was up to 20 times less than in those with progressive disease. Viral loads of long-term nonprogressors stayed relatively stable.[55] Viral replication levels were also 4 to 10 times lower in slow progressors.[55] In 1995 Cao et al[57] published the findings of nine slow progressors and found that repeated attempts to culture HIV in these subjects was unsuccessful.

Neutralizing antibodies against HIV-1 that arise after the initial fall of viremia have been detected. The levels of neutralizing antibodies in long-term nonprogressors are significantly higher than in typical progressors.[55]

Finally, it is possible that some long-term nonprogressors could be infected with less pathogenic strains of virus. Defects in the viral genome are under current study and nef gene deletions have been documented in some slow progressors.[58] The nef gene is believed to be required by HIV to attack and kill host cells. Defects in this gene could hamper the virus' ability to efficiently infect new cells.[59]

Viral Mutations

Viral mutations or variations are defined by the presence of changes in genomic DNA or RNA. DNA and RNA are made up of nucleotides. These nucleotides specify which amino acids should be incorportated into proteins, which are comprised of long chains of amino acids. Proteins contain specific amino acid sequences, and as discussed earlier, HIV genes encode for specific proteins, which create the HIV virion.[60]

Viral variation and the resultant genetic diversity are a natural consequence of both high levels of viral replication and an error-prone enzyme—RT. In other words, the higher the viral replication rate, the greater the number of mistakes made. Even in the absence of drug therapy, viral mutation is inevitable given the nature of HIV dynamics. A mistake in replication by RT can lead to the substitution of one amino acid for another. If a change in the amino acid results, the structure and therefore the function of the protein encoded can be altered. These amino acid changes at particular codons (a codon represents one three-nucleotide sequence on the gene) can result in changes in the strain of HIV and the viral susceptibility to a particular drug.

Newly infected individuals show little evidence of mutation. Their virus is said to be *wild-type* or in an unmutated state, like that found in nature.

Over time, the virus becomes increasingly diverse as ongoing changes become incorporated into new virus. It has been estimated that viral mutations occur about once in every 10,000 nucleotides copied by the RT enzyme. Because the genome is approximately 10,000 nucleotides in length, one such error would occur, on average, every time a viral genome is copied.[61]

Testing to determine the presence of these changes or mutations looks for the presence of altered drug susceptibility. There are two tests that are currently available to look for the presence of mutations and to determine if they affect drug susceptibility—genotypic and phenotypic testing. Genotypic testing identifies the actual changes that have occurred at the codon site. Phenotypic testing measures the amount of drug that is needed to inhibit 50 or 90 % of viral growth, referred to as (Inhibitory Concentration) *IC50* or *IC90*. As mutations occur, more drug is needed to suppress the virus. In phenotypic testing, specific levels are identified for susceptible virus. If more drug is needed than the specified level, the virus is said to be resistant.

Viral diversification is the underlying mechanism of resistance to ART. It is therefore important to have an appreciation of this phenomena so that treatment decisions can be made based on the most sound rationale. Unfortunately, the commercial resistance testing that is currently available may be limited in use because it is costly and not standardized.

References

1. Varmus H. Retroviruses. *Science.* 1988;240:1427–1435.
2. Mandell G. *Atlas of Infectious Diseases.* Philadelphia: Churchill Livingstone; 1997.
3. Feng Y, Broder CC, Kennedy PE, Berger EA. HIV-1 entry cofactor: functional cDNA cloning of a seven-transmembrane G protein-coupled receptor. *Science.* 1996;272:872–877.
4. Feinberg M, Greene W. Molecular insights into human immunodeficiency virus type 1 pathogenesis. *Curr Opin Immunol* 1992;4:446–474.
5. Devita VT, Hellman S, Rosenberg SA, eds. *AIDS, Etiology, Diagnosis, Treatment, and Prevention. Etiology of AIDS: Biology of Human Retroviruses.* Connor RI, Ho DD. 3rd ed. Philadelphia: Lippincott; 1992:13–38.
6. Cullen BR, Greene WC. Regulatory pathways governing HIV-1 replication. *Cell.* 1989;58(30):423–426.

7. Rosenberg ZF, Fauci AS. Activation of latent HIV infection. *J NIH Res* 1990;2: 41–45.
8. Janeway C, Travers P. *Immunobiology: The Immune System in Health and Disease. Failures of Host Defense Mechanisms.* 3rd ed. New York: Current Biology Ltd./Garland Publishing Inc.; 1997:10:22–10:41.
9. Levy JA. The transmission of HIV and factors influencing progression to AIDS. *Am J Med.* 1993;95:86–100.
10. Janeway C, Travers P. *Immunobiology: The Immune System in Health and Disease. Failures of Host Defense Mechanisms.* 3rd ed. New York: Current Biology Ltd./Garland Publishing Inc.; 1997:7:1–7:44.
11. Panteleo G, Cohen O, Graziosi C, et al. Immunopathogenesis of human immunodeficiency virus infection. In: Devita VT, Hellman S, Rosenberg SA, eds. *AIDS: Biology, Diagnosis, Treatment and Prevention.* 4th ed. Lippincott-Raven; 1997: 75–88.
12. Lane C. HIV pathogenesis. Highlights of advanced CME courses. Presented at the Fifth International AIDS Society. Atlanta, Georgia. 1997.
13. Frankel S, Wenig B, Allen P, et al. Replication of HIV-1 in dendritic cell-derived syncytia at the mucosal surface of the adenoid. *Science.* 1996;272:115–117
14. Fauci AS. Host factors and the pathogenesis of HIV-induced disease. *Nature.* 1996;384:529–534.
15. Poli G, Fauci AS. *Role of Cytokines in the Pathogensis of Human Immunodeficiency Virus Infection.* In: Aggarwal B, Puri RK, eds. Cambridge, MA: Blackwell Science; 1995:421–449.
16. Rosenberg Z, Fauci AS. Immunopathogenesis of HIV infection. *FASEB J* 1991; 5:2382–2387.
17. Goleti D, Weissman D, Jackson RW, et al. Effect of *Mycobacterium tuberculosis* on HIV replication. Role of immune activation. *J Immunol.* 1996;157(3): 1271–1278.
18. Denis M, Ghadirian E. *Mycobacterium avium* infection in HIV-1 infected subjects increases monokine secretion and is associated with enhanced viral load and diminished immune response to viral antigens. *Clin Exp Immunol.* 1994; 97:76–82.
19. Cocchi F, DeVico AL, Garzine-Demo A, Arya SK, Gallo RC, Lusso P. Identification of RANTES, MIP-1α and MIPβ as the major HIV-suppressive factors produced by CD8+ T cells. *Science.* 1995;270:1811–1815.
20. Walker CM, Moody DJ, Stites DP, Levy JA. CD8+ lymphocytes can control HIV infection in vitro by suppressing virus replication. *Science.* 1986;234:1563–1566.
21. Deng HK, Liu R, Ellmeier W, et al. Identification of a major co-receptor for primary isolates of HIV-1. *Nature.* 1996;381:661–666.
22. Dragic T, Litwan V, Alloway GP, et al. HIV entry into CD4+ cells is mediated by the chemokine receptor CC-CCR5. *Nature.* 1996;381:667–673.

23. Smith MW, Dean M, Carrington, et al. Contrasting genetic influence of CCR2 and CCR5 variants on HIV-1 infection and disease progression. *Science.* 1997; 277:959.
24. Kuritzkes DR. *HIV Pathogenesis and Viral Markers.* Healthcare Communications Group; 1996. Available from URL http:www.healthcg.com.
25. Liu R, Paxton WA, Choe S, et al. Homozygous defect in HIVpq coreceptor accounts for resistance of some multiply exposed individuals to HIV-1 infection. *Cell.* 1996;86:367–377.
26. Zimmerman PA, Bucklerwhite A, Alkhatib G, Spalding T, Kubofcid J, Combadiere C. Inherited resistance to HIV-1 conferred by an inactivating mutation in CC chemokine receptor 5—studies in populations with contrasting clinical phenotypes, defined racial background, and quantified risk. *Mol Med.* 1997;3: 23–36.
27. Cheng-Meyer C, Seto D, Tateno M, Levy JA. Biological features of HIV-1 that correlate with virulence in the host. *Science.* 1988;240:80–82.
28. Schuitemaker H, Koot M, Kootstra NA, et al. Biological phenotype of human immunodeficiency virus type 1 clones at different stages of infection: progression of disease is associated with a shift from monocytotropic to T-cell-tropic virus populations. *J Virol.* 1992;66:1354–1360.
29. Koot M, Keet IPM, Vos AHV, et al. Prognostic value of HIV-1 syncytium-inducing phenotype for rate of CD4+ cell depletion and progression to AIDS. *Ann Intern Med.* 1993;118:681–688.
30. Japour AJ, Welles S, D'Aquilla RT, et al. Prevalence and clinical significance of zidovudine resistance mutations in human immunodeficiency virus isolated from patients following long-term zidovudine treatment. *J Infect Dis.* 1995; 171:1172–1179.
31. McNicholl J, Smith D, Qari S, Hodge T. Host genes and HIV: the role of the chemokine receptor gene CCR5 and its allele (Δ 32 CCR5). *Emerg Infect Dis.* 1997;3:261–271.
32. Mellors JW, Rinaldo CR, Gupta P, White RM, Todd JA, Kingsley LA. Prognosis in HIV-1 infection predicted by the quantity of virus in plasma. *Science.* 1996; 272:1167–1170.
33. Mellors JW, Munoz A, Giorgi JV, et al. Plasma viral load and CD4+ lymphocytes as prognostic markers of HIV-1 infection. *Ann Intern Med.* 1997;126:946–954.
34. Coffin JM. HIV viral dynamics. *AIDS.* 1996;10(suppl 3):S75–S84.
35. Ho D, Neumann A, Perelson A, Chen W, Leonard J, Markowitz M. Rapid turnover of plasma virions and CD4 lymphocytes in HIV-1 infection. *Nature.* 1995;373:123–126.
36. Wei X, Ghosh SK, Taylor ME, et al. Viral dynamics in human immunodeficiency virus type 1 infection. *Nature.* 1995;373:117–122.

37. Coffin J. HIV population dynamics in vivo: implications for genetic variation, pathogenesis, and therapy. *Science.* 1995;267:483–489.
38. Perelson A, Neuman AU, Markowitz M, Leonard JM, Ho DD. HIV-1 dynamics in vivo: virion clearance rate, infected cell life span, and viral generation time. *Science.* 1996;271:1582–1586.
39. Sciciliano R. Unpublished abstract (91). Presented at the Sixth International Workshop on HIV Drug Resistance, Treatment Strategies and Eradication. St. Petersburg, Florida. June 25–28, 1997.
40. Perelson AS, Essunger P, Ho DD. Dynamics of HIV-1 and CD4+ lymphocytes in vivo. *AIDS.* 1997;11(suppl A):S17–S24.
41. Coffin J. *Eradication of Infected Cells and Generation of Drug-Resistant Mutants.* Healthcare Communications Group; 1997. Available from URL http: www.healthcg.com.
42. Havlir D, Eastman S, Gamsi A, Richman DD. Nevirapine-resistant human immunodeficiency virus: kinetics of replication and estimated prevalence in untreated patients. *J Virol.* 1996;70:7894–7899.
43. McLean AR, Michie CA. In vivo estimates of division and death rates of human T lymphocytes. *Proc Natl Acad Sci USA.* 1995;92:3707–3711.
44. Panteleo G, Graziosi C, Cohen OJ, Muro-Cacho C, Vaccarezza M, Fauci AS. Lymphoid organs: a window into the pathogenesis of HIV infection. *AIDS Update.* 1994;7(9):1–11.
45. Saag MS, Holodny M, Kuritzkes DR, et al. HIV viral load markers in clinical practice. *Nat Med.* 1996;2(6):625–629.
46. Daar ES, Moudgil T, Meyer RD, et al. Transient high levels of viremia in patients with primary human immunodeficiency virus type 1 infection. *N Engl J Med.* 1991;324:961–964.
47. Kinloch-de Loes S, de Saussure P, Saurat JH, et al. Symptomatic primary infection due to human immunodeficiency virus type 1: review of 31 cases. *Clin Infect Dis.* 1993;17:59–65.
48. Kahn J, Hecht F. Treating primary infection. *HIV Newsline.* 1996;2:135–141.
49. Cooper DA, et al. Characterization of T lymphocyte responses during primary infection due to human immunodeficiency virus. *J Infect Dis.* 1988;157(5): 889–896.
50. Pederson C, Lindhardt BO, Jensent BL, et al. Clinical course of primary HIV infection: consequences for subequent course of infection. *BMJ.* 1989;299: 154–157.
51. Ho DD. Viral counts count in HIV infection. *Science.* 1996;272:1124–1125.
52. Panteleo G, Graziosi C, Demarest JF, et al. Role of lymphoid organs in the pathogenesis of human immunodeficiency virus infection. *Immunol Rev.* 1994; 140:105.

53. Sheppard HW, Lang W, Ascher MS, Vittinghoff E, Winkelstein W. The characterization of nonprogressors: long-term HIV-1 infection with stable CD4+ T cell levels. *AIDS.* 1993;7:1159–1166.
54. Henrard DR, Daar E, Farzadegan H, et al. Virologic and immunologic characterization of symptomatic and asymptomatic primary HIV-1 infection. *J Acquir Immune Defic Syndr.* 1995;9:305–310.
55. Panteleo G, Menzo S, Vaccarezza M, et al. Studies in subjects with long-term nonprogressive human immunodeficiency virus infection. *N Engl J Med.* 1995; 332:209–216.
56. Haynes BF, Panteleo G, Fauci AS. Toward an understanding of the correlates of protective immunity to HIV infection. *Science.* 1996;271:324–328.
57. Cao Y, Qin L, Linqi Z, Safrit J, Ho DD. Virologic and immunologic characteristics of long-term survivors of human immunodeficiency virus type 1 infection. *N Engl J Med.* 1995;332:201–208.
58. Kirchhoff F, Greenough TC, Brettler DB, Sullivan JL, Desrosiers RC. Absence of intact nef sequences in a long-term survivor with nonprogressive HIV-1 infection. *N Engl J Med.* 1995;332:228–232.
59. Grzesiek S, Bax A, Clore GM, et al. The solution structure of HIV-1 nef reveals an unexpected fold and permits delineation of the binding surface for the SH3 domain of Hck tyrosine protein kinase. *Nat Struc Biol.* 1996;3:340–345.
60. Cooper GM. *The Cell; A Molecular Approach.* 1st ed. Washington, DC: ASM Publishers; 1997.
61. Condra JH, Emini EA. Preventing drug resistance. *Sci Med.* 1997:2–11.

CHAPTER 2

HIV Epidemiology & HIV Diagnostic Testing

Patty J. Hale, PhD, RN, FNPC • Catherine S. Kay, RN, MSN

Chapter Preview

- Epidemiology of HIV
- Diagnostic Laboratory Testing and Evaluation of HIV Infection

Well over a decade of study of the human immunodeficiency virus (HIV) has brought a new understanding of how infection with this deadly pathogen becomes the critical turning point in the lives of millions of people worldwide. As of December 1996, HIV had claimed more than 338,000 lives in the United States alone[1] and an estimated 1 million people are infected.[2,3] Early in the 1980s at the start of the epidemic, acquired immune deficiency syndrome (AIDS) was viewed as a highly acute illness with a short survival period. Discovery of the underlying viral and cellular interactions has led to a greater understanding of the disease process, enabling earlier diagnosis and intervention. This allows for better management to enhance the quality and duration of life. After infection is identified, a long-term plan for treatment can be developed even *before* clinical signs appear. Earlier intervention allows individuals to survive longer and thus has contributed to the evolution of HIV infection to a chronic condition.

Epidemiology of HIV

Acquired immunodeficiency syndrome is caused by HIV, which attacks the body's immune system and leaves it vulnerable to numerous health problems that would otherwise not develop in an individual with a healthy immune system. Among the cells attacked by HIV is a lymphocyte, the T-helper cell. This cell is also referred to as a *CD4+ lymphocyte* because the CD4+ molecule on its surface is a target for the attachment of HIV.

Two types of HIV have been identified: HIV-1 and HIV-2. HIV-1 accounts for nearly all of the infection in the United States. The greatest number of newly reported illnesses (incidence) of HIV-2 appears to be in West Africa, but it has also been found in Europe and in the United States. Prevalence, the number of existing cases during a given period in a specified population, is extremely low in the United States for HIV-2, with only 17 cases having been identified through 1991.[4] Typically those in the United States who are infected with HIV-2 have either immigrated from other countries or are US citizens who traveled to countries where HIV-2 is endemic. Although the clinical presentation for both types of the virus is similar, it appears that the HIV-2 infection is less virulent.[5,6]

Case Definition of AIDS

The standard case definition of AIDS for adolescents and adults consists of specific clinical criteria and laboratory values as determined by the

Centers for Disease Control and Prevention (CDC).[7] The case definition includes a classification system based on the number of CD4+ lymphocytes, which when used with other information also serves to guide clinical and therapeutic actions with adults and adolescents. The classification is as follows:

- **Category 1**—≥500 CD4+ T lymphocytes/mm^3
- **Category 2**—200–499 CD4+ T lymphocytes/mm^3
- **Category 3**—<200 CD4+ T lymphocytes/mm^3

The CDC case definition was further expanded in 1993 to include individuals with CD4+ lymphocyte counts of <200/mm^3 or a CD4+ lymphocyte percentage of less than 14%.[8] Prior to the 1993 revision, AIDS was determined only by the presence of specific symptoms or opportunistic infections. Because immunosuppression develops in some individuals before the manifestation of opportunistic diseases, the inclusion of a CD4+ lymphocyte count below 200 encompasses those who are immunocompromised but remain asymptomatic.[9] The 1993 modification also includes three previously unrecognized clinical conditions—pulmonary tuberculosis, recurrent pneumonia, and invasive cervical cancer.[7] Appendix A lists the additional opportunistic diseases that constitute the case definition of AIDS. (see Chapter 26 for a description of pediatric AIDS case definition).

Transmission

Transmission of HIV infection occurs through exposure to infected body fluids, which may result from sexual contact, injection drug use, blood transfusion, tissue or organ donation, perinatal transmission, or occupational exposure. Identification of risk factors in individuals is based on these potential transmission sources. Figure 2.1 shows the percent of infections attributed to each mode of transmission in adults and adolescents.[1]

HIV exhibits high comorbidity with other sexually transmitted diseases (STDs) because transmission for both occurs as a result of sexual behavior. Persons diagnosed with an STD should also be considered at risk for HIV. Presence of an STD, with or without lesions or ulcers, appears to increase transmission of HIV.[10,11] This may be due to the greater number of white blood cells in the area of the lesion that provide target cells for HIV, or

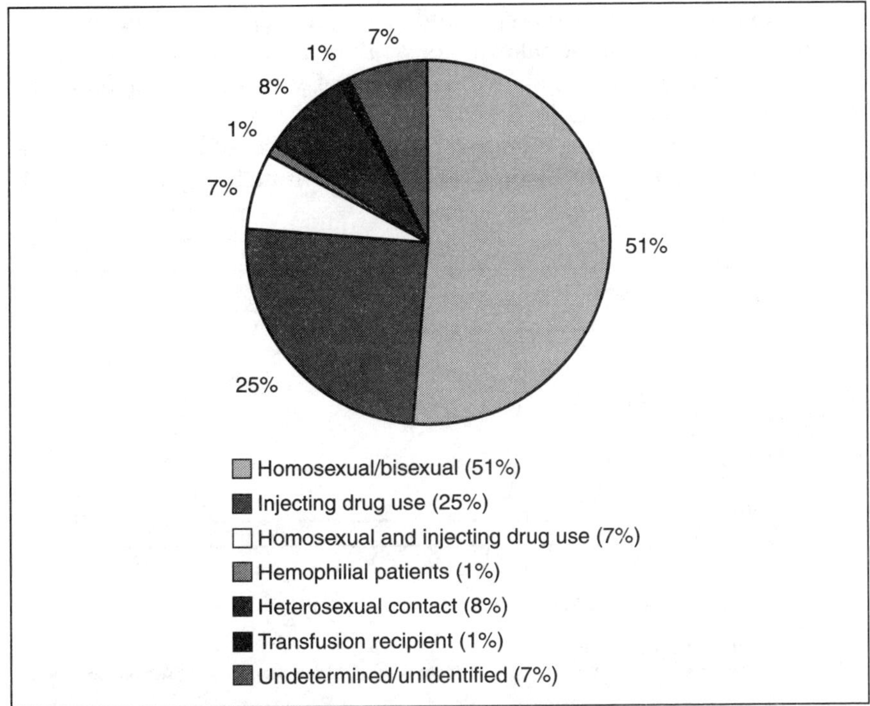

Figure 2.1 **Adult and Adolescent AIDS Patients by Exposure Category: Cumulative Totals through June 1996 for the United States**

due to breaks in the skin and mucous membrane that give ready access for HIV entry. A compromised immune system due to existing STDs can also cause the recipient to be more vulnerable to HIV.

Spectrum of Disease of Adults and Children Older Than 13 Years

In both pediatric and adult HIV infection, the spectrum of disease of HIV infection can be viewed in terms of clinical stages that correspond to the viral load and the number of CD4+ lymphocytes. These clinical stages are termed (1) early (CD4+ count of >500 cells/mm^3), (2) middle (CD4+ counts of 200–500 cells/mm^3), (3) late (CD4+ cell count of 50–199 cells/mm^3), and (4) advanced-stage disease (CD4+ cell counts <50 mm^3).[12] (A description of pediatric HIV is included in Chapter 26.) Progression to clinically apparent disease takes place as the CD4+ lymphocytes are destroyed by HIV. Figure 2.2 shows the onset of various conditions based on CD4+ count and viral load.[13]

One way of determining infection prior to the onset of actual symptoms is through HIV antibody testing. The change from being HIV antibody

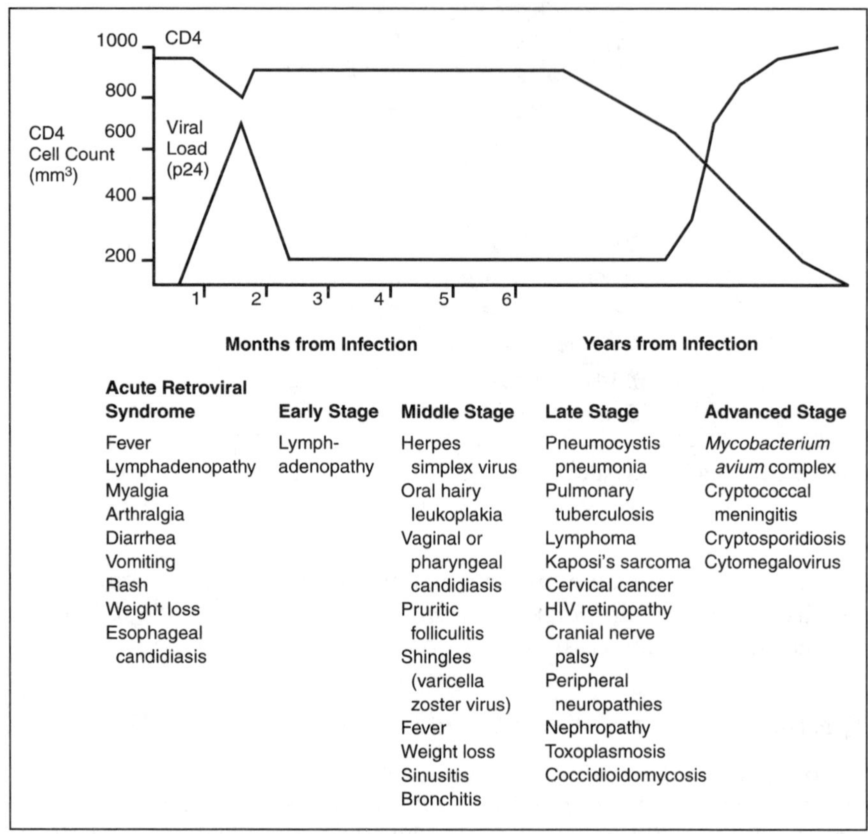

Figure 2.2 The Natural History of HIV Disease (Adapted from American College of Physicians. *Medical Knowledge Self-Assessment Program 10 (MKSAP 10).* Part A, Book 1, HIV disease. Philadelphia: American College of Physicians; 1994:6.)

negative to positive is termed *seroconversion.* Approximately 6 to 12 weeks after initial infection with HIV, antibodies are numerous enough to result in a positive enzyme-immunosorbent assay (EIA) for HIV antibody.[14,15] In some circumstances the time to seroconversion may be 6 months or longer.[15] Thus, the infection may remain asymptomatic for months or years. Delayed seroconversion appears to be linked to a weaker viral inoculum, which is partially determined by the type of exposure.[15] A positive test indicates that the person is infected with HIV and can transmit the virus, but does not mean that the person has progressed to AIDS. Thus the infection may remain asymptomatic for months or years while significant changes are taking place at the cellular level.[16]

Incubation period is defined as the "time interval beginning with invasion by an infectious agent and continuing until the organism multiplies to sufficient numbers to produce a host reaction and clinical symptoms."[17] Estimates of the length of the incubation period for HIV varies, and correlates with age of the infected individual.[18–20] Specifically, individuals older than 40 years of age when seroconverting have an estimated incubation period between 7.4 and 8.6 years.

Length of time before clinical manifestations develop is also dependent on the health of the individual's immune system at the time of initial infection. Because the immune system is already under stress, coexisting infections such as hepatitis or syphilis may result in a more rapid progression to AIDS.[10]

Some individuals experience a mononucleosis-type illness just before seroconversion termed *acute retroviral seroconversion syndrome,* which lasts about 7 to 21 days.[21] Figure 2.2 displays the signs and symptoms of this syndrome.[13] During this phase, laboratory values show reduced numbers of CD4+ and CD8 lymphocytes and a high viral load. As the acute syndrome resolves, the CD8 lymphocyte levels return to normal and the CD4+ lymphocyte count increases but remains lower than normal baseline.[12,22] If the CD4+ lymphocyte count remains suppressed, the progression to symptomatic HIV disease occurs more quickly.[12,23]

Individuals who manifest the symptoms of acute retroviral seroconversion syndrome for longer than 14 days are likely to progress more quickly to AIDS than those with an asymptomatic or briefer symptomatic primary infection.[21,24,25] As the disease progresses, the amount of virus—known as the *viral load*—increases in the body's fluids and becomes a more virulent strain. The virus mutates and produces variants that are less easily recognized by the host's immune system. Thus as HIV evolves, it becomes more pathogenic.[26] Recent attention has been directed toward whether the use of combination drug therapy, if used shortly after infection, could lead to improved suppression of HIV replication.[27]

Early-stage Disease (CD4+ count of >500 cells/mm^3)

The CD4+ lymphocyte count slowly declines at the rate of approximately 40 to 80 cells/mm^3/year. Even though dramatic changes are occurring within the immune system, individuals often remain free of symptomatic illness, whereas some may experience lymphadenopathy.[12]

Middle-stage Disease (CD4+ count of 200–500 cells/mm^3)

During this phase patients may develop any one of several conditions, as noted in Figure 2.2.[13] Opportunistic infections such as *Pneumocystis carinii* pneumonia (PCP) and oral candidiasis signal that the viral load is increasing. Due to an accompanying drop in CD4+ cells, the immune system is no longer able to fight infection. HIV has an affinity for cells of the central and peripheral nervous systems in addition to attacking the immune system, leading to neurocognitive problems such as dementia, psychosis, loss of memory, and neuropathy. Various cancers may also occur, as well as wasting (weight loss of more than 10% of usual body weight).[9] If left untreated at this stage, patients have a 20 to 30% chance of progressing to AIDS or dying within the subsequent 18- to 24-month period.[12]

Late-stage Disease (CD4+ cell count of 50–199 cells/mm^3)

At this stage, a diagnosis of AIDS can be made based on the CD4+ lymphocyte count. Common conditions are shown in Figure 2.2.[13] The most common opportunistic infection is PCP. Thus anti-PCP prophylaxis is recommended when the CD4+ count falls to 200 cells/mm^3 or less. Although lymphadenopathy may occur in the later stages of disease, the disappearance of lymphadenopathy may be a sign of impending disease progression due to the destruction of CD4+ cells. Without treatment, patients in late-stage disease have a 50 to 70% chance of dying within 18 to 24 months.[13]

In late-stage disease, the virulence of HIV increases in some individuals, resulting in a more rapid progression of immunodeficiency. This corresponds with a drop in CD4+ cells. Syncytia-inducing viruses result in cell-to-cell fusion of infected CD4+ cells, producing giant cells called *syncytia* that also fuse with uninfected CD4+ cells, resulting in additional immune destruction.[28]

Advanced-stage Disease (CD4+ cell count of <50 cells/mm^3)

Treatment for opportunistic infection is ongoing at this point to avoid probable relapse if treatments are discontinued. Neurological disease becomes more prevalent and AIDS dementia can occur with resulting cerebral atrophy and decreased cognitive functioning. Diseases occur such as disseminated *Mycobacterium avium* complex (MAC) infections, cryptococcal meningitis, and cryptosporidiosis (see Figure 2.2).[12,13]

Global and US Distribution and Trends

The World Health Organization estimates that as of July 1996, 28 million people had been infected with HIV worldwide.[29] The vast majority of these infections, fully 90%, will occur in developing countries.[30] Unlike the United States, where a majority of cases have resulted from homosexual activity (51%) and injection drug use (25%), most countries worldwide report heterosexual transmission as the primary means of spread.[2,8] Outside the United States, HIV prevalence is highest in sub-Saharan Africa.

From June 1981 through December 1996, 548,102 incident cases of AIDS were reported in the United States, with 7,296 of these in children less than 13 years of age.[1] Figure 2.3 shows the number of patients by quarter year between 1986 and 1994.[31] A total of 62% of all persons diagnosed with AIDS since 1981 have died.[1] The survival time of persons with AIDS has improved due to increasingly effective antiviral treatment, specifically protease inhibitors.[27,32] This has resulted in greater prevalence of HIV, with an estimated 223,000 persons living with AIDS in the United States in June 1996.[33] It also represents earlier recognition of HIV disease and HIV treatment progress.[32] Ultimately HIV disease is reported to approach 100% mortality.[32]

The change in AIDS definition accounted for an increase in reported cases from 1992 to 1993, because those with diagnoses that fell under the new definition were previously unreported.[33] The incidence of AIDS in men who have sex with men is declining, although it remains the most commonly reported mode of transmission. The incidence of AIDS in women and children is increasing and is expected to continue to grow as heterosexual transmission increases.[9,33]

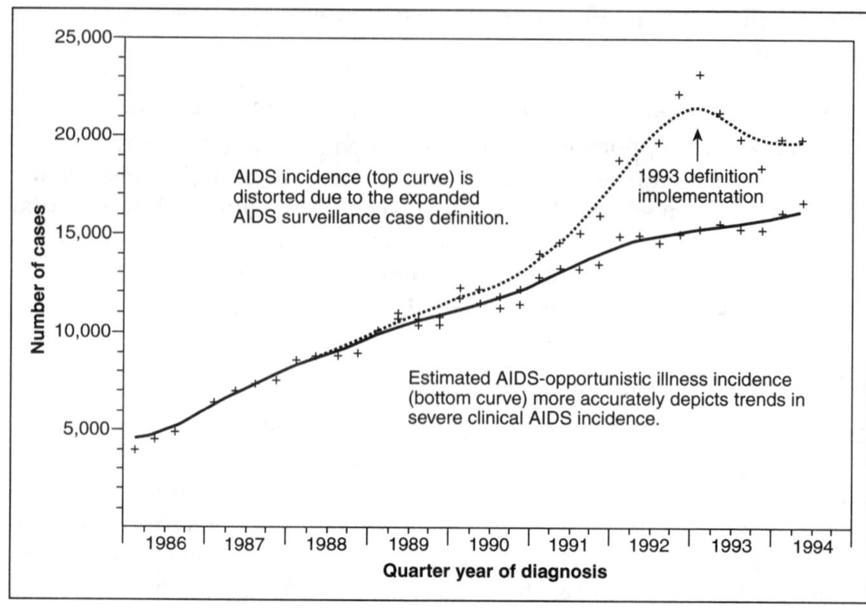

Figure 2.3 **AIDS Incidence and Estimated AIDS-Opportunistic Illness Incidence, Adjusted for Delays in Reporting, by Quarter Year of Diagnosis, January 1986 through June 1994, United States.** (Source: Centers for Disease Control. *HIV/AIDS Surveillance Report* 1994;6:1-39.)

US Geographic Distribution

At the onset of the epidemic, most US cases of AIDS were located in metropolitan areas of the United States. As the epidemic has continued, rural areas have experienced more HIV infection.[34]

Age

The age group with the largest number of cases of AIDS through June 1996 is 25- to 54-year-olds, representing 89% of all cases.[35] Given the lengthy incubation period, transmission for these individuals probably occurred 10 years before the onset of AIDS. In 1994, HIV was the leading cause of death in US men between the ages of 25 and 44 years, and the third leading cause of death in women in this age range.[36] Although pediatric AIDS represents a much smaller group, it is of concern because its incidence parallels the increase in infections in women; 90% of all pediatric AIDS cases result from vertical transmission from mother to infant/child.[8,35]

Gender

Since the start of the epidemic in the early 1980s, 85% of all reported adult AIDS cases have occurred in males.[35] This is because the major risk of transmission is men who have sex with men, which represents 51% of all AIDS cases reported since 1981. More recently, the proportion of females with AIDS is growing at a faster rate.

Ethnicity

AIDS is occurring in minority populations at a greater rate than nonminorities. In 1994, AIDS incidence in adult and adolescent African-Americans was 129.8 per 100,000 population, in adult Hispanics it was 68.2 per 100,000, and in adult Caucasians AIDS incidence was 20.8 per 100,000[31] (see Chapters 29 and 28). The epidemic among women occurs disproportionately in ethnic minorities and is primarily transmitted via sexual and injection drug use behaviors.[37,38] For African-American women between the ages of 25 and 44 years, HIV infection was the leading cause of death in 1994.[36]

Diagnostic Laboratory Testing and Evaluation of HIV Infection

Early recognition of HIV infection by laboratory testing is essential to initiate interventions that delay onset and slow progression of symptomatic HIV disease. Some of these tests are also used to follow the status of HIV infection and to guide response to treatment based on extent of disease activity. Early recognition of HIV infection also allows for notification and early treatment of partners. The three major purposes of HIV testing are (1) diagnosis of HIV infection, (2) staging and prognosis of HIV infection, and (3) guiding therapeutic decisions by following response to treatment.

Four general approaches are used in diagnostic testing for HIV infection: (1) identification of antibodies to HIV viral proteins, (2) detection of viral antigens, (3) detection of viral nucleic acids, and (4) culturing the HIV virus itself.[37]

HIV Pathogenesis and Diagnostic Tests

Understanding the laboratory tests for HIV infection is based on knowledge of HIV pathogenesis (see Chapter 1). Important events in HIV pathogenesis are (1) infection with HIV of CD4+ T cells and monocytes/macrophages and subsequent viral replication, (2) specific anti-HIV humoral and cellular immune responses, (3) lowered numbers of CD4+ T cells, (4) dysregulation through all components of the immune system, and (5) impaired immune function. [38] A "window" of approximately 3 to 4 weeks may be experienced by patients recently infected with HIV, and in some individuals this period my last up to 12 months.[19,39] During this "window," viremia is present and transmission of HIV is possible, but antibodies have not yet developed. P24 antigen is the core structural protein of the HIV. It can be detected about a week before antibodies can be measured.[40] Antibodies are detectable in 95% of HIV-infected individuals 6 months after infection.[41]

Diagnostic Test Accuracy

Diagnostic tests vary in their accuracy, which is reflected by their sensitivity, specificity, and predictive values (Figure 2.4).[42] *Sensitivity* is defined as the proportion of people with disease who have a positive test for the disease. It answers the question: Of all the people with HIV infection, what proportion have a positive test? Sensitive tests rarely miss people with the disease. *Specificity* is the proportion of people without the disease who have a negative test.[17,42] It answers the question: Of all the people who do not have HIV infection, what proportion will have a negative test? A test with high specificity rarely misclassifies people without the disease as having HIV infection. *Predictive values* are dependent on sensitivity and specificity of the test, but also on the prevalence of HIV infection in the population. The positive predictive value of an HIV diagnostic test is the probability of HIV infection in a patient with a positive test result. The negative predictive value is the probability of not having HIV infection when the test is negative.

Diagnostic tests can be used in parallel combination (all at once) or in serial (consecutively) combination to try to enhance sensitivity and specificity. With parallel tests, a positive result of any test is considered evidence of the disease. With serial test combinations, all test results must be positive for a diagnosis to occur. Tests in parallel generally increase sensitivity and the negative predictive value of either alone. Disease is less

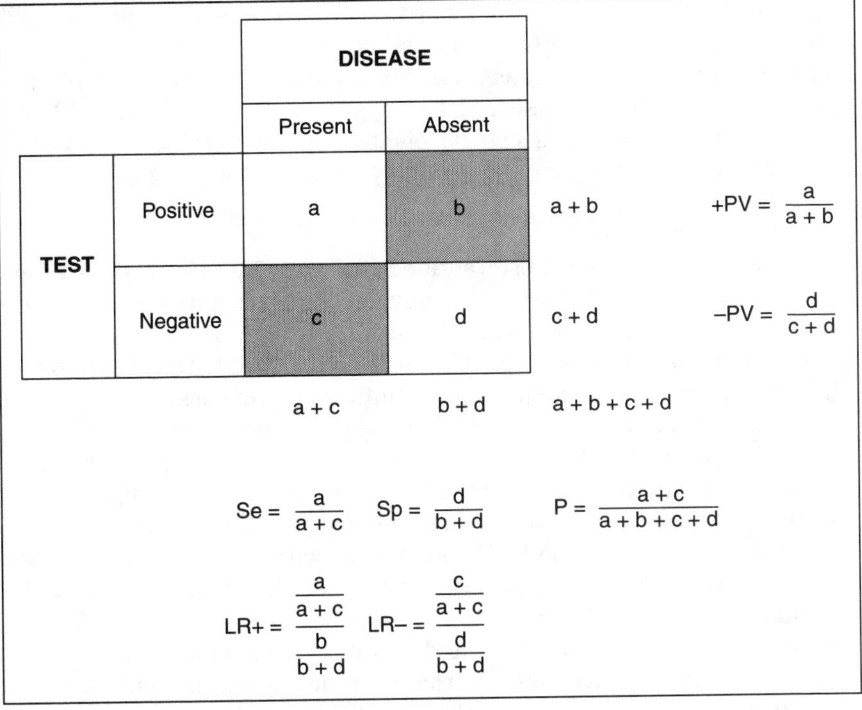

Figure 2.4 Diagnostic Test Characteristics and Definitions. Se = sensitivity; Sp = specificty; P = prevalence; PV = predictive value. (From Fletcher RH, Fletcher SN, Wagner EH. *Clinical Epidemiology: The Essentials.* 3rd ed. Baltimore: Williams & Wilkins; 1996. Reprinted with permission.)

likely to be missed with parallel testing, but false-positive results are also more likely. Serial testing is used when rapid answers are not needed or when some of the tests are expensive or risky. It maximizes specificity and positive predictive value, but lowers sensitivity and the negative predictive value.

Antibody-Based Tests

Many of the tests used for diagnosis of HIV rely on detection of the antibody response to HIV rather than detection of the virus itself because of the technical difficulty and expense of HIV culture. HIV antibodies usually appear within 2 to 3 months following first exposure to the virus, although it may take up to 6 months for antibodies to appear. The HIV genome includes three structural genes: env (envelope) for both gp120/160 and gp41; gag (core) antigens p55, p24, and p17; and pol (polymerase) p64, p51, and p32.[38] Antibodies can be elicited by each. Table 2.1 provides information about the uses and accuracy of the antigen tests.

Enzyme-Immunoassay

The two most commonly used antibody tests are the EIA and the Western blot test. An EIA is the most commonly used approach by testing centers for screening in the United States. If an EIA is reactive, it is repeated in duplicate. If either or both repeat tests are reactive, the result is positive. Then a Western blot or indirect immunofluorescence assay (IFA) is performed, on the same sample, to confirm the positive test.[43,44] The sensitivity and specificity of the EIA are >99%. False-positive results can occur in the following situations: (1) multiparous women, (2) individuals recently vaccinated against influenza or hepatitis B, (3) people who have had multiple blood transfusions, and (4) individuals with autoimmune diseases. False-negative EIAs are found very early or very late in the course of HIV infection when antibody production has fallen to very low levels. In some environments, the venipuncture and laboratory equipment necessary to run the EIA are not available. In these circumstances a whole-saliva or urine test can be used to detect the anti-HIV antibody.[45,46]

Table 2.1 Diagnostic and Screening Tests Used in Detection of HIV Disease and AIDS

Name of Test	Normal Value	Function	Purpose	Interpretation of Results	Comments
Antibody Detection					
EIA	Negative	Measures antibody to HIV-1 serum or plasma	Rules out HIV infection (not diagnosing); screens blood/ plasma or urine products	If positive, repeat to verify	Sensitivity, >99.7%; specificity, 98.5%

Table 2.1 *Continued*

Name of Test	Normal Value	Function	Purpose	Interpretation of Results	Comments
Western blot	Negative	Confirmatory test after two positive EIAs	Establishes presence of HIV antibody	Positive Western blot means a positive finding of specific protein bands p14 or p24 found in HIV	Western blot is more sensitive and specific than EIA; not used for screening, as it is time-consuming and expensive
GAC EIA (HIV IgG antibody-capture assay using whole saliva by dribble)	Negative	Detects antibody to HIV in saliva	Used for surveillance programs and screening in developing Countries	Confirmatory test required; preferable to use blood samples for confirmatory test	Sensitivity, 95–100%; specificity, 90–100%
ANTIGEN DETECTION					
p24	Negative	Detects virion particles	Determination of HIV infection during the window prior to antibody detection	Only positive prior to immune response before antibodies capture HIV antigen; positive result disappears after seroconversion	Sensitivity, 10–80% in early infection
RNA HIV (viral load); two types: PCR and bDNA	<500 viral copies/ml	Detects viral copies	Measures amount of virus in the blood; helpful for prognosis and measuring treatment effectiveness	Use same method each time on a given patient; levels of viral load <5–10,000 associated with a lower rate of HIV disease progression	PCR method, most sensitive; bDNA method, less sensitive but easier and more reliable

(continued)

Table 2.1 *Continued*

Name of Test	Normal Value	Function	Purpose	Interpretation of Results	Comments
PCR	—	Measures HIV DNA in cells by detection in serum, plasma, and CSF	Diagnosis in early disease, in neonatal infection when mother is HIV-positive and baby carries maternal antibodies, in individuals with indeterminate serology results, in patients with dual retroviral infections; determination of response to antiretroviral therapy	Detects even a few molecules of a specific HIV DNA or RNA sequence	Comparable sensitivity and specificity to viral cultures, but can be completed more quickly and less expensively
Viral culture	No viral growth	Blood cultures to determine presence of HIV	Diagnostic of HIV infection	Presence of virus indicative of infection with HIV	Very sensitive and specific, but also expensive and up to 4 weeks needed to get results
CD4+ to CD8 Ratio	Adult >0.8	Compare T-cell helper: suppressor ratio in whole blood	Defines extent of CD4 and CD8 cell loss, thus indicating the stage of HIV	Normal ratio, >2:1; early suppression, <1:0; during opportunistic disease period, <0:2	—

EIA = enzyme-immunoassay; GAC = (IgG antibody capture); IgG = immunoglobulin G; RNA = ribonucleic acid; PCR = polymerase chain reaction; bDNA = branched-chain deoxyribonucleic acid; CSF = cerebrospinal fluid.

Western Blot

When HIV antibodies are detected by EIA, then a second testing method must be used to confirm HIV infection. As previously stated, the Western blot technique is commonly used for the second test. The Western blot technique uses protein electrophoresis to separate the various HIV antigens into discrete bands to confirm the presence of antibodies to individual HIV antigens. The Western blot evaluates antibody response to protein products of three HIV gene regions: (1) the env region, gp120/160 and gp41, which are envelope proteins; (2) the pol region, p31, p51, and p66, which are reverse transcriptases (RTs) and endonucleases; and (3) the gag region, p24/55 and p17, which are core proteins. Test results may be positive, negative, or indeterminate. A positive Western blot, as defined by the guidelines established by the Association of State and Territorial Public Health Laboratory Directors and the CDC, is the presence of any two of the p24, gp41, and gp120/gp160 bands.[47] A test is considered negative when all bands are absent. A test is indeterminate when it has a single band or other bands not included in the definition of a positive test. Causes of indeterminate Western blots include (1) early in disease, only antibodies against core (p24) antigen may be seen; (2) late in disease, antibodies against core antigen may be lost; (3) cross-reaction with HIV-2 may occur; and (4) cross-reaction with autoantibodies or alloimmunization may occur.

Indirect Immunofluorescence Assay

IFA is not routinely used for diagnosis of HIV infection in clinical practice. Similar to the Western blot, IFA confirms the presence of anti-HIV antibodies in serum.

DETECTION OF VIRAL ANTIGEN Two distinct types of tests are available—those that test for the HIV antibody and those that test for the presence of the HIV antigen. Antigen detection is used to diagnose HIV infection. The three antigen-based tests are p24, polymerase chain reaction (PCR), and viral culture. Each of these tests detects actual parts of the virus and is positive earlier than any of the antibody response tests. Table 2.1 provides information about the uses and accuracy of the antigen tests.

DETECTION OF VIRAL ANTIGENS HIV antigen assays "capture" the presence of viral proteins, specifically HIV core p24 antigen, obtained from a sample (serum, plasma, or culture supernatant) on a solid-phase material.

It is then probed with an enzyme-labeled HIV antibody. The p24 antigen assay is the simplest, fastest, and least expensive virological detection method.[38] It uses a sandwich-type antigen-capture EIA technique. HIV antigen assays are primarily used as an early diagnostic aid. The Food and Drug Administration (FDA) approved it as a screening test in blood donors to reduce the window period. Immune complex-dissociated (ICD) p24 assay is probably most useful as a prognostic marker for HIV progression as opposed to diagnostic purposes. It may also have a role in diagnosing patients with passive transfer of antibodies, such as infants born to HIV-infected mothers.[48]

Viral Nucleic Acid Detection by PCR and Branched-Chain Deoxyribonucleic Acid (bDNA) Assays

Minute quantities of HIV nucleic acids can be detected by PCR and bDNA assays. Detection of HIV ribonucleic acid (RNA) is useful as a reflection of HIV plasma viremia, which is referred to as *viral load* or *viral burden.* Viral load is representative of actively replicating HIV virus. It does not measure nonreplicating virus; in other words, virus that is in body reservoirs such as macrophages, follicular dendritic cells, and the central nervous system. Thus, PCR does not measure total body burden of HIV. A negative or undetectable plasma RNA does not mean that there is no HIV in the body but it does mean that the amount of virus in plasma is below the threshold of detection of the test.

Viral Load Tests

PCR involves target amplification of a specific segment of HIV viral RNA. It causes it to multiply to the point where there is enough RNA to be detected readily. This is done by DNA hybridization. bDNA involves signal amplification. bDNA attaches a large, branched segment of complementary DNA to a specific segment of HIV viral RNA. Both tests give comparable results. It is best to use the same method each time on any one given patient. Both PCR and bDNA are quite expensive, but use of viral load and CD4+ cell counts are well justified because the information can be used to assess antiretroviral activity and to initiate changes in therapy before clinical failure develops, both of which are also expensive.[49]

Reporting of Viral Load Levels

Viral load levels are reported in copies/ml. They can be described as very high, moderately high, low, and undetectable or too low to detect. The relationship between these descriptive terms and the absolute number of viral copies/ml is displayed in Table 2.2.

Uses of Viral Load

Plasma levels of viral RNA are useful to monitor HIV disease progression, determine prognosis, and measure effectiveness of antiretroviral therapy.[50] Plasma RNA measurement is also used to diagnose patients with end-stage disease who may have false-negative EIAs and Western blots because of severe immunodeficiency, as well as early diagnosis of infants born to HIV-infected mothers.[48] Within 6 months after seroconversion, the patient's viral load levels out to a so-called *setpoint*, which determines the rate of progression of disease, as displayed in Table 2.3. (see Chapter 1.)

Considered in combination with the CD4+ count, the viral load is useful in predicting progression of HIV toward AIDS. However, viral load and

Table 2.2 Viral Load (VL) Setpoints After Acute HIV Infection and Prognosis

Setpoint of VL	Absolute VL (copies/ml)	Progression Rate	Approximate 5-Year Risk of AIDS
High	$>10^5$	Rapid	60%
Medium	10^4–10^5	Intermediate	25–50%
Low	$<10^4$	Slow	8%

(Adapted from Ho DD. Viral counts count in HIV infection. *Science.* 1996;272:1124–1125.)

Table 2.3 Relationship between Viral Load Description and Levels

Description	Absolute No. of Viral Copies/ml
Very high	100,000
Moderately high	10,000
Low	1,000
Undetectable	<200

(From Fischer, Evelyn. Medical College of Virginia/Virginia Commonwealth University, February 1997.)

CD4+ count have a different significance. An analogy of this relationship is offered by John Coffin,[51] in which viral load is similar to the speed of a train moving along a track (HIV infection) moving toward a cliff (AIDS), and the CD4+ count is the current distance that the train has to travel to get to the cliff (Figure 1.7 on p. 18).

Using Viral Load

The goal of antiretroviral therapy (ART) is to reduce the viral load at least threefold or by one third, and preferably reduce it to undetectable levels for as long as possible.[49] *Undetectable levels* means that the levels are below the limit of detection by the assay, not the absence of HIV. Patients and the public are frequently misinformed about the meaning of an undetectable viral load and assume they are no longer infected. Patients must understand that they are still capable of transmitting the HIV infection when the viral load level is undetectable.

Each patient needs to be assessed individually regarding (1) baseline viral load, (2) CD4+ count, (3) previous ART regimen, (4) initial response to treatment, (5) commitment to ART, and (6) adherence to the regimen.[49] Guidelines for using viral load measures are as follows.[49,52,53]

1. A significant change in viral load is a threefold change. This means that viral load must either fall to a level that is one third the prior level or rise to a level that is three times higher than the prior level for the change to be meaningful.
2. If the ideal goal of ART is achieving undetectable levels, then sufficient time must be allowed before obtaining viral load. It may take 12 to 16 weeks after initial rapid decrease in the first 7 to 14 days.
3. To estimate prognosis or guide treatment decisions, the history and physical examination plus CD4+ count must also be considered.
4. Viral load should not be obtained within 1 month after an acute illness or any vaccination because it may rise transiently.
5. No clinical decision should be based on a single viral load test.
6. Ideally, two baseline viral loads should be obtained because of variability of the results. A 2- to 4-week interval is suggested.
7. Viral load should be checked every 3 to 4 months in patients who are stable to detect a rise in viral load that indicates the need for treatment (if not on ART) or the need to change ART if treatment is already underway. Viral load may need to be checked more fre-

quently in a patient nearing a treatment decision point, such as when viral load is rising.

8. HIV therapy changes should be considered if viral load does not fall by at least threefold (0.5 log) within 4 to 6 weeks of starting or changing HIV treatment.
9. A rise in viral load to within 0.5 log of baseline (or threefold less than baseline) in patients on HIV therapy suggests probable treatment failure and the need to change HIV therapy.
10. Viral load specimens must be processed properly to avoid results that are falsely low.
11. Consistent use of either acid citrate dextran (ACD; "yellow top") or ethylenediaminetetraacetic acid (EDTA, "purple top") tubes should be ensured. Heparinized ("green top") tubes should not be used because HIV RNA is less stable in heparin.

HIV Culture

HIV culture, when used to diagnose HIV infection, is highly specific but relatively insensitive. It involves culture of HIV viral cocultivation of the patient's peripheral blood mononuclear cells (PBMCs) with stimulated PBMCs from uninfected donors. This in vitro culture system causes explosive viral infection, resulting in production of millions of virions. Test results are read as positive by detecting RT or p24 antigen in the virus culture supernatant.[54] HIV culture is technically difficult and expensive. Varying degrees of viremia at different stages of HIV infection plus the difficulties of correct collection and transportation lead to variation in the success of HIV cultures.

Following diagnosis, managing symptoms and accessing appropriate services are major challenges in providing health care. Management of these clinical problems is discussed in Unit Two.

References

1. American Health Consultants. *AIDS Alert.* Atlanta, GA; American Health Consultants 1996;12:133–144.
2. World Health Organization. *Current and future dimensions of the HIV/AIDS pandemic: a capsule summary.* Presented at the World Health Organization Global Programme on AIDS. Geneva, Switzerland. April, 1991.

3. Centers for Disease Control. HIV prevalence estimates and AIDS case projections for the United States: report based upon a workshop. *MMWR*. 1990; 39(suppl RR-16):1–31.
4. O'Brien TR, George JR, Holmberg SD. Human immunodeficiency virus type 2 infection in the United States. *JAMA*. 1992;267:2775–2779.
5. Markovitz DM. Infection with the human immunodeficiency virus type 2. *Ann Intern Med*. 1993;118:211–218.
6. De Cock KM, Adjorlolo G, Ekpini E, et al. Epidemiology and transmission of HIV-2. *JAMA*. 1993;270:2083–2086.
7. Centers for Disease Control and Prevention. Update: acquired immunodeficiency syndrome—United States, 1994. *MMWR*. 1995;44:64–67.
8. Centers for Disease Control and Prevention. *HIV/AIDS Surveillance Report*. Atlanta, GA; U.S. Department of Health and Human Services, CDC, Center for Infectious Diseases, Division of HIV/AIDS 1995;7:1–34.
9. Centers for Disease Control and Prevention. 1993 Revised classification system of HIV infection and expanded surveillance of definition for AIDS among adolescents and adults. *MMWR*. 1992;41(suppl RR-17):1–19.
10. Clottey C, Dallabetta G. Sexually transmitted disease and human immunodeficiency virus, epidemiologic synergy? *Infect Dis Clin North Am*. 1993;7:753–770.
11. Laga M, Manoka A, Kivuvu M, et al. Non-ulcerative sexually transmitted diseases as risk factors for HIV-1 transmission in women: results from a cohort study. *AIDS*. 1993;7:95–102.
12. Saag MS. Natural history of HIV-1 disease. In: Broder S, Merigan TC, Bolognesi D, eds. *Textbook of AIDS Medicine*. Baltimore: Williams & Wilkens; 1994:45–53.
13. American College of Physicians. *Medical Knowledge Self-Assessment Program 10 (MKSAP 10)*. Part A, Book 1, HIV disease. Philadelphia: American College of Physicians; 1994:6.
14. Busch MP. HIV and blood transfusion: focus on seroconversion. *Vox Sang*. 1994;67(suppl 3):13–18.
15. Meyohas MC, Morand-Joubert L, Van de Weil P. Time to seroconversion after needlestick injury. *Lancet*. 1995;345:1634–1635.
16. Saag MS, Hammer SM, Lange JMA. Pathogenicity and diversity of HIV and implication for clinical management: a review. *J Acquir Immune Defic Syndr Hum Retrovirol*. 1994;7(suppl 2):S2–S11.
17. Valanis B. *Epidemiology in Nursing and Health Care*. 2nd ed. Norwalk, CT: Appleton & Lange; 1992.
18. Castro KG, Valdiserri RO, Curran JW. Perspectives on HIV/AIDS epidemiology and prevention from the Eighth International Conference on AIDS. *Am J Public Health*. 1992;82:1465–1470.
19. Rosenberg PS, Goedert JJ, Biggar RJ. Effect of age at seroconversion on the natural AIDS incubation distribution. *AIDS*. 1994;8:803–809.
20. Gauvreau K, Degruttola V, Pagano M, et al. Markers and incubation times the

effect of covariates on the induction time of AIDS using improved imputation of exact seroconversion times. *Stat Med.* 1994;13:2021–2030.

21. Clark SJ, Shaw GM. The acute retroviral syndrome and the pathogenesis of HIV-1 infection. *Semin Immunol.* 1993;5:149–155.
22. Clark SJ, Saag MS, Decker WD, et al. High titers of cytopathic virus in plasma of patients with symptomatic primary HIV-1. *N Engl J Med.* 1991;324:954–960.
23. Phillips AN, Pezzotti P, Lepri AC, et al. CD4+ lymphocyte count as a determinant of the time from HIV seroconversion to AIDS and death from AIDS: evidence from the Italian seroconversion study. *AIDS.* 1994;8(9):1299–1305.
24. Fauci AS, Rosenberg ZF. Immunopathogenesis. In: Broder S, Merigan TC, Bolognesi D, eds. *Textbook of AIDS Medicine.* Baltimore: Williams & Wilkins; 1994: 55–75.
25. Pederson C, Lindhardt BO, Jensen BL, et al. Clinical course of primary HIV infection. *BMJ.* 1989;299:154–157.
26. Saag MS. Evolving understanding of the immunopathogenesis of HIV. *AIDS Res Hum Retroviruses.* 1994;10:887–891.
27. Deeks SG, Smith M, Holodniy M, Kahn JO. HIV-1 protease inhibitors. *JAMA.* 1997;277:145–153.
28. Koot M, Keet IPM, Vos AHV, et al. Prognostic value of HIV-1 syncytium-inducing phenotype for rate of CD4+ cell depletion and progression to AIDS. *Ann Intern Med.* 1993;118:681–688.
29. UNAIDS, World Health Organization. The HIV/AIDS situation in mid 1996. In: *WHO Fact Sheet (#1): Global and Regional Highlights.* Geneva; July 1996.
30. World Health Organization. *The HIV/AIDS Pandemic; 1993 Overview.* Geneva: World Health Organization; 1993.
31. Centers for Disease Control and Prevention. *HIV/AIDS Surveillance Report.* 1994;6:1–39.
32. Osmond DH. Trends in HIV survival time. In: Cohen PT, Sande MA, Volberding PA, eds. *The AIDS Knowledge Base.* 2nd ed. Boston: Little, Brown; 1994:1.3–1.3-7.
33. Centers for Disease Control and Prevention. Trends in AIDS incidence, deaths, and prevalence—United States, 1996. *Morbidity & Mortality Weekly Report.* Atlanta, GA; U.S. Department of Health Education and Welfare, Public Health Service, Center for Disease Control 1997;46:165–173.
34. Lam NS, Liu K. Spread of AIDS in rural America. *J Acquir Immune Defic Syndr Hum Retrovirol.* 1994;7:485–490.
35. Centers for Disease Control and Prevention. *HIV/AIDS Surveillance Report.* 1996;8:1–33.
36. Centers for Disease Control and Prevention. Update: mortality attributable to HIV infection among persons aged 25–44 years—United States, 1994. *MMWR.* 1996;45:121–125.
37. Schleupner CJ. In: Mandell GL, ed. 103. Detection of HIV-1 Infection. *In Princi-*

ples and Practice of Infectious Diseases. 4th ed. New York: Churchill Livingstone; 1995:1253–67.
38. Fahey JL, Flemming DS. *AIDS;HIV: Reference Guide for Medical Professionals.* 4th ed. Baltimore: Williams & Wilkins; 1997.
39. Gaedeke MK. *Laboratory and Diagnostic Test Handbook.* Menlo Park, CA: Addison-Wesley; 1996.
40. Centers for Disease Control and Prevention. U.S. Public Health Service guidelines for testing and counseling blood and plasma donors for human immunodeficiency virus type 1 antigen. *MMWR.* Atlanta, GA; U.S. Department of Health, Education and Welfare, Public Health Service, Center for Disease Control 1996; 45(suppl RR-2):1–9.
41. Busch MP, Satten GA. *Am J Med.* 1997;102:117.
42. Fletcher RH, Fletcher SW, Wagner EH. *Clinical Epidemiology: The Essentials.* 3rd ed. Baltimore: Williams & Wilkins; 1996.
43. Treseler KM. *Clinical Laboratory and Diagnostic Tests Significance and Nursing Implications.* 3rd ed. Norwalk, CT: Appleton & Lange; 1995.
44. Fischbach F. *A Manual of Laboratory and Diagnostic Tests.* Philadelphia: Lippincott-Raven; 1996.
45. Tamashiro H, Constantine NT. Serological diagnosis of HIV infection using oral fluid samples. *Bull World Health Organ.* 1994;72:135–143.
46. Berrios DC, Avins AL, Haynes-Sanstad K, et al. Screening for human immunodeficiency virus antibody in urine. *Arch Pathol Lab Med.* 1995;119:139–141.
47. Centers for Disease Control and Prevention. Interpretation and use of the western blot assay for serodiagnosis of human immunodeficiency virus type 1 infections. *MMWR.* 1989;38(S7):1.
48. Diagnostic Tests for HIV. *Med Lett Drugs Therapeutics.* 1997;39(1008):81–83.
49. Saag MS. Use of HIV viral load in clinical practice: back to the future. *Ann Intern Med.* 1997;126(12):983–985.
50. O'Brien WA, et al. Changes in plasma HIV RNA levels and CD4+ lymphocyte counts predict both response to antiretroviral therapy and therapeutic failure. *Ann Intern Med.* 1997;126(12):939–945.
51. Coffin JM. HIV viral dynamics. *AIDS.* 1996;10(suppl 3):S75–S84.
52. Mellors JW, et al. Plasma viral load and CD4+ lymphocytes as prognostic markers of HIV-1 infection. *Ann Intern Med.* 1997;126:946–954.
53. Saag MS, et al. HIV viral load markers in clinical practice. *Nat Med.* 1996;2(6): 625–629.
54. Mandell GL, Mildvan D, eds. *Atlas of Infectious Diseases. Volume 1: AIDS.* 2nd ed. Philadelphia: Churchill Livingstone; 1997.

CHAPTER 3

Pharmacological Issues in HIV Treatment

Gail Wilkes, RNC, MS, AOCN
Ann Williams, Ed.D., RN, RN-C, FAAN

Chapter Preview

- Antiretroviral Therapy (ART) for HIV Infection
- Polypharmacy

Antiretroviral Therapy (ART) for HIV Infection

Background

Primary management of HIV infection involves the use of drugs designed to interfere with the life cycle of HIV, preventing viral replication and reducing the quantity of virus in the body. HIV is a retrovirus with RNA in its genetic material and it requires RT to synthesize viral DNA and use the host cell effectively to produce new virions. The two classes of agents currently available (Table 3.1) act at different points in the viral life cycle (Figure 3.1).

Today's therapeutic strategies are shaped by new insights into the dynamics of viral replication and the development of antiretroviral resistance. Current concepts emphasize that there is no latency period following initial HIV infection and seroconversion. Rather, there is consistent, high-level, viral replication throughout the continuum of HIV infection.[1,2] Reducing

Table 3.1 Classification of Antiretroviral Agents for HIV[a]

Class of Agent	Antiretroviral Agent
Reverse transcriptase inhibitors	NUCLEOSIDE REVERSE TRANSCRIPTASE INHIBITORS
	Zidovudine, AZT, ZDV (Retrovir™)
	Didanosine, ddI (Videx™)
	Zalcitabine, ddC (Hivid™)
	Stavudine, d4T (Zerit™)
	Lamivudine, 3TC (Epivir™)
	Abacavir[b]
	NONNUCLEOSIDE REVERSE TRANSCRIPTASE INHIBITORS
	Delavirdine (Rescriptor™)
	Nevirapine (Viramune™)
	Efavirenz[b] (Sustiva™)
Protease inhibitors	Indinavir (Crixivan™)
	Nelfinavir (Viracept™)
	Ritonavir (Norvir™)
	Saquinavir (Invirase™) (Fortovase™)

[a]Brand name appears in parentheses.
[b]Investigational agent, not yet approved.

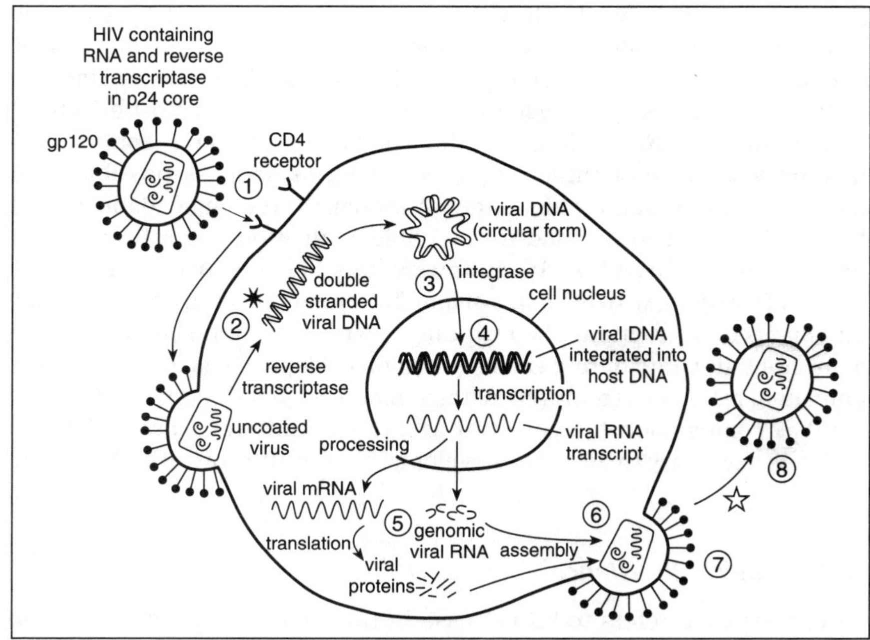

Figure 3.1 HIV Life Cycle: 1) Virus attaches to cell wall via gp120. 2) Virus uncoats, releasing viral RNA into cell cytoplasm; reverse transcriptase transcribes viral RNA to DNA. 3) Viral DNA is transported into cell nucleus. 4) Viral DNA is integrated into cellular DNA. 5) Cell produces viral RNA and proteins. 6) New virions are assembled. 7) Immature, noninfectious virions are released from cell. 8) Protease processes polyproteins into structural proteins/enzymes, forming mature virions. *Reverse transcriptase inhibitors work here (step 2). ☆Protease inhibitors work here (between steps 7 and 8).

this replication lowers the total viral burden and is associated with a better clinical outcome.

The lymph system is the primary site of HIV replication, and as normal, uninfected CD4 lymphocytes migrate through the lymph nodes, they become infected.[2] Production of CD4 cells by the immune system to fight HIV infection parallels viral replication, and is again fueled by the continual destruction of CD4 cells by HIV. Wei et al[3] and Ho et al[4] showed separately that approximately 2 billion CD4 cells are produced and destroyed daily in an HIV-infected person. The regenerative ability of the immune system is impressive, but eventually CD4 production is outpaced by CD4 cell destruction as a result of viral replication. As immune function diminishes, lymph nodes lose functional integrity and more free HIV is released into the serum.[2] To halt this cycle aggressive, early intervention is most effective.[5]

Current recommendations for ART emphasize the use of combination therapy with at least three drugs, beginning as soon as possible after infection and continuing indefinitely.[6] Although the recommendations must be individualized to respond to the clinical situation and reflect patient preferences, the trend is clearly toward this highly active antiretroviral therapy (HAART), with the goals of limiting viral replication and preventing immune cell destruction. The high rate of viral replication combined with a high mutation rate during each replication cycle explains the rapid development of resistance to antiretroviral monotherapy, and supports the premise that combination therapy with agents with different mechanisms of action is necessary to delay the development of antiretroviral resistance.[7–9]

Antiretroviral Resistance

Drug resistance refers to an increase in the amount of drug required to inhibit viral growth. Resistance can be analyzed either phenotypically or genotypically. In phenotypic analysis, virus from an HIV-infected person is isolated and grown in the presence of various concentrations of the drug. To say that a virus is phenotypically resistant to a drug means that the virus is able to grow in the presence of the drug. This ability to continue to grow, or *phenotypic resistance*, is the result of specific mutations in the genes for viral enzymes, which are the targets of antiretroviral drugs. The mutations associated with phenotypic resistance to individual drugs can be identified with gene sequencing techniques; this process is *genotypic analysis* of resistance.

Drugs do not induce resistance; rather, preexisting drug-resistant virus emerges under selective pressure, sometimes as rapidly as within 2 to 4 weeks of beginning drug therapy.[3] Some genetic mutations confer phenotypic resistance to more than one drug, leading to cross-resistance. For example, the mutations that emerge under the selective pressure exerted by indinavir allow those strains of virus to grow in the presence of both indinavir and ritonavir. The potential for cross-resistance is a serious concern for patients and clinicians when considering initial and subsequent choices of antiretroviral agents.

Available Agents

As of mid 1997, 11 antiretroviral agents were available on the US market for treatment of HIV infection (Table 3.2). Strategies for selection of initial and subsequent combination regimens continue to evolve, with today's standard practice outdated tomorrow. The rapid evolution of HAART offers great hope and substantial challenges to HIV-infected patients and health care professionals.

Monitoring Therapy

Because studies demonstrated a direct correlation of increasing viral replication and viral load with disease progression, the development of technologies that provide an accurate measure of HIV replication was a significant advance in HIV clinical care. Quantitative measures of viral load provide a direct assessment of both the risk of development of significant illness in the future, or prognosis, and the effects of specific treatment interventions for individual patients.

Two common methods for measuring viral burden are PCR and bDNA. Both allow the detection of minute quantities of HIV RNA in the plasma through the amplification of genetic fragments of HIV. Test results are expressed as the number of copies of HIV RNA per milliliter of blood plasma.

Interpretation of viral load assays should be guided by the following facts.

1. Viral quantitation tests are best used to measure changes in viral load over time. A single test result should be interpreted with caution.
2. Because results are not comparable between test methods, the same method should be used each time for an individual patient.
3. The tests can be affected by intercurrent infections, especially viral infections, and immunizations. In these instances, a sharp, temporary rise in viral load has been noted. The clinical significance of these rises is not known.
4. No information is available yet about the impact of alcohol or other drugs on viral load.

As a general principle, higher levels of plasma HIV RNA (viral load) are correlated with greater risk for HIV progression. However, there is no lower limit; that is, even patients with very low levels of plasma HIV RNA demonstrate some risk of clinical progression.[6] Thus, the goal of ART is to reduce plasma HIV RNA to undetectable levels for as long as possible.

Table 3.2 Antiretroviral Agents in Clinical Practice

Drug; Adult Dose	Common Side Effects	Comments	Patient Information
A. NUCLEOSIDE REVERSE TRANSCRIPTASE INHIBITORS			
Zidovudine (Retrovir, AZT, ZDV) 200 mg tid or 300 mg bid; higher doses if HIV-related neurological disease is suspected	*Early:* Headache, nausea, vomiting, insomnia, fatigue, malaise, myalgias	Treat early side effects symptomatically; usually resolve after first 4–6 weeks	Take with meals to decrease nausea
	Later: Bone marrow suppression	Monitor blood counts every 3 months; monthly if advanced HIV disease	Important to keep appointments for blood draws to monitor blood counts
	Anemia	Treat with recombinant human erythropoietin if necessary to maintain hemoglobin and hematocrit	
	Neutropenia	Treat with granulocyte colony stimulating factor to maintain absolute neutrophil count above 500 cells/mm^3	
	Long term: Nail pigmentation, myopathy	Check creatinine phosphokinase levels after 10–12 months of therapy	Report new onset of muscle weakness and myalgias

Didanosine (Videx, ddI); two formulations: tablet and powder; bid oral dose by weight: >60 kg 2–100-mg tablets or 250 mg powder; <60 kg, 125 mg in two tablets or 167 mg powder		Formulated with a buffer to ensure adequate bioavailability	Always take both tablets or all the powder to be sure the correct amount of buffer is obtained Take on an empty stomach one-half hour before or 1–2 hours after a meal; take with at least 120 ml of water; apple juice or ice water may improve the taste; do not take at the same time as dapsone or ketoconazole
	Pancreatitis (7–9%)	Increased risk with advanced HIV, previous pancreatitis, and alcoholism; monitor amylase, lipase, and triglycerides	Stop medication and report abdominal pain, nausea, and vomiting; avoid alcohol
	Peripheral neuropathy (9–13%)	Monitor for symptoms	Stop medication and report numbness, tingling, and burning in soles of feet
	Dry mouth, altered tase		No treatment necessary
	Diarrhea	Primarily a problem with the powder formulation	Treat symptomatically

(continued)

Table 3.2 *Continued*

Drug; Adult Dose	Common Side Effects	Comments	Patient Information
Zalcitabine (Hivid, ddC) 0.75 mg tid	Peripheral neuropathy (10–25%)	Monitor for symptoms	Stop medication and report numbness, tingling, and burning in soles of feet
	Pancreatitis (<1%)	Increased risk with advanced HIV, previous pancreatitis, and alcoholism; monitor amylase, lipase, and triglycerides	Stop medication and report abdominal pain, nausea, and vomiting; avoid alcohol
	Rash, fever, aphthous ulcers	Most common in first 4 weeks of therapy; may resolve without treatment	—
Stavudine (Zerit, d4T); dose by weight: >60 kg, 40 mg bid; <60 kg, 30 mg bid	Peripheral neuropathy (15–20%), dose related, reversible	Monitor for symptoms	Stop medication and report numbness, tingling, and burning in soles of feet
	Pancreatitis (<1%)	Increased risk with advanced HIV, previous pancreatitis, and alcoholism; monitor amylase, lipase, and triglycerides	Stop medication and report abdominal pain, nausea, and vomiting; avoid alcohol

Lamivudine (Epivir, 3TC) 150 mg bid	Data available only for combined therapy with zidovudine; slightly increased incidence of headache, nausea, neutropenia; rare reports of central nervous system events (mania, confusion, psychosis) have been reported to the company	Resistance develops rapidly with monotherapy; should be used only in combination regimens	—
Abacavir (1592U89) 300 mg bid	Nausea, vomiting, headache, dizziness, insomnia, asthenia, and hypersensitivity	Investigational agent available only through clinical trials or compassionate use as of 1/1/98	Stop medication and contact health care provider at once if high fever or severe rash develop
B. NONNUCLEOSIDE REVERSE TRANSCRIPTASE INHIBITORS			
Delavirdine (Rescriptor) 400 mg tid	Rash, potentially serious	—	Stop medication and contact health care provider immediately if rash or sore throat, fever, and myalgias occur
	Elevated hepatic enzymes	Monitor liver function tests	—

(continued)

Table 3.2 *Continued*

Drug; Adult Dose	Common Side Effects	Comments	Patient Information
Efavirenz (Sustiva) 600 mg qD	Lightheadedness, difficulty concentrating, anxiety, dysphoria, and rash	Usually resolve within a few weeks; investigated agent available only through compassionate use program as of 1/1/98	Take at bedtime
C. PROTEASE INHIBITORS			
Indinavir (Crixivan) 800 mg tid **q8h**	Nephrolithiasis in 4% of patients; dose-related, asymptomatic hyperbilirubinemia in 15% of patients; abdominal pain, nausea, and diarrhea also possible	Kidney stones are composed of precipitated drug; kidney function appears to be unaffected	Take on empty stomach or with light, nonfat, meal; drink at least 1½ liters of water daily; report any back or flank pain, or blood in urine at once; always keep enough medication on hand so that you do not run out; if you miss a dose, do not double up on the next
Nelfinavir (Viracept) 750 mg tid	Diarrhea; elevated liver function tests	Diarrhea is most often mild and can be managed symptomatically	Take with food; always keep enough on hand so that you do not run out; if you miss a dose, do not double up on the next

Ritonavir (Norvir) 600 mg bid in oral solution or 100 mg capsules	Nausea and gastrointestinal (GI) distress; dose escalation over 5 days may decrease GI symptoms; tingling in hands, feet, and lips	Requires 12 caps/day; cross-resistant with indinavir; many drug interactions; *contraindicated* with more than 25 analgesics, antiarrhythmics, antihistamines, and sedative hypnotics	Store capsules in refrigerator; take with food, preferably a high-fat meal; mix solution with chocolate milk, Ensure, or Advera to improve taste; always keep enough on hand so that you do not run out; if you miss a dose, do not double up on the next
Saquinavir (Invirase) 600 mg tid or (Fortovase) 1200 mg in six capsules tid	Mild GI discomfort; current formulation is well tolerated	Tolerability likely due to poor bioavailability and low plasma levels; new, better absorbed formulations will be available	Take within 2 hours of a full meal; always keep enough on hand so that you do not run out; if you miss a dose, do not double up on the next

Polypharmacy

A major issue in the management of HIV-infected patients at some time during the course of disease is polypharmacy. Polypharmacy, or *multiple drug therapy,* is accompanied by threats of drug-drug interactions or drug-food interactions that may increase or decrease effectiveness of one or both of the drugs and may then be accompanied by severe or even life-threatening side effects. Polypharmacy is a challenge for both nurse and patient. Nurses must keep up with the rapidly expanding pharmacological data base, not only about indications and dosages, but also drug-drug interactions as patients receive upward of 10 or more drugs to prevent or treat HIV and opportunistic infections (OIs). Patients must learn about self-care strategies, including self-administration of medications, drug-drug interactions, and food-drug interactions. Patients may have multiple providers, and one provider may be unaware of the drugs prescribed by the other provider. In addition, patients may not report to their provider all the medications they are receiving, and over-the-counter medications may not be reported because they are not perceived as medications requiring a prescription.

Patient noncompliance or inability to take prescribed medications can be related to many factors, including forgetting to take medication (for example, when away from home), side effects experienced or toxicity, believing the medication is not effective, substance abuse, mood changes, running out of medication, finding the self-administration schedule too difficult to follow, cognitive problems, and inability to purchase medications due to cost or copayment charges that prevent filling the prescription.

Nurses play a critical role in coordinating patient education, individualizing approaches to each patient and promoting readiness to learn, providing ongoing reinforcement and support, and managing symptoms as patients experience difficulties in taking the large number of medications and experience drug side effects and interactions. Patients should be instructed to bring *all* medications, including over-the-counter and complementary therapies, when they meet with their health care professional so that an up-to-date listing of medications can be made. Patients should ask their provider every time they receive a new prescription whether it will cause any problems with the medications they are currently taking. In addition, nurses themselves, or with the assistance of social services, can help patients find resources to purchase or receive prescribed medications.

Pharmacological Principles Underlying Drug Interactions

Drug interactions are classified as pharmacokinetic or pharmacodynamic interactions.[10] Many drug-drug interactions are possible, but not all result in adverse outcomes. In fact, some are advantageous and are used that way. However, there are a number of significant interactions possible, depending on the combination of HIV-related medications. Although it is impossible to remember them all, it is important to understand the general principles and resources so that each drug can be reviewed prior to their administration or education of the patient. Table 3.3 illustrates notable drug-drug interactions of drugs used in HIV therapy.

Pharmacokinetic Interactions

Pharmacokinetic interactions occur when the absorption, distribution, metabolism, or excretion of one drug is affected by another drug (drug-drug), by food (drug-food), or by disease (drug-disease).

Altered Absorption

An example of altered absorption is when ketoconazole, an antifungal medication, is administered with an antacid or with a histamine (H_2) antagonist. Ketoconazole requires an acidic environment for absorption. When combined with an antacid, which raises the pH of gastric contents, drug absorption is reduced by 40%.[11] Therefore, ketoconazole must be administered at least 2 hours after or before the antacid dose. In addition, if the individual is achlorhydric (little or no acidity in the stomach), a common condition in HIV infection, the individual can dissolve each 200-mg tablet in 60 ml of orange juice or 200 ml of 0.1 N hydrochloric acid.[12]

Altered Distribution

Altered distribution can occur when two drugs compete for binding sites on plasma proteins or tissues. This type of interaction is not usually significant unless one of the drugs is highly protein or tissue bound and has limited distribution.[10] The drug with the greatest affinity for the binding site displaces the other drug, resulting in increased unbound or free serum concentrations of one drug, resulting theoretically in increased drug action. For instance, when fluconazole is taken in combination with phenytoin, the interaction may result in increased levels of phenytoin, necessitating more frequent monitoring of phenytoin levels.[13]

Table 3.3 Potential Drug Interactions for Selected Drugs Used to Treat HIV

Drug	Interacting Drug	Documentation	Significance	Management
A. Antiviral Drugs				
Acyclovir	Narcotics	Johnson[18]	Possible meperidine toxicity related to decreased renal excretion	Monitor patient closely; consider same effect with other narcotics
Acyclovir	Probenecid	American Society of Hospital Pharmacists (ASHP)[12(p 430)]	Probenecid blocks acyclovir excretion, may increase mean plasma half-life, and may decrease renal clearance and urinary elimination of acyclovir; this may increase acyclovir toxicity	If used concomitantly, monitor closely for acyclovir toxicity, and reduce acyclovir dosage as necessary
Acyclovir	Zidovudine	Bach,[19] ASHP[12(p 430)]	Synergism; rarely, dramatic lethargy and fatigue may occur, especially when IV acyclovir is given	Observe for increased lethargy and decreased alertness; if this occurs, give oral acyclovir or may need to decrease drug
Foscarnet sodium	Pentamidine	Youle et al[20]	Reported severe hypocalcemia and potentially fatal seizures	Avoid concurrent use; monitor serum calcium; monitor for perioral tingling, paresthesias
Ganciclovir	Amphotericin B and other nephrotoxic drugs	ASHP[12(p 460)]	Potential for increased renal compromise	Monitor serum creatinine closely when drugs used concomitantly

Ganciclovir	Didanosine	Porche,[21] ASHP[12(p 460)]	Some studies show in vitro antagonism; others show increased steady state of didanosine	Assess efficacy and toxicity of didanosine; discuss didanosine dose modification with physician
Ganciclovir	Foscarnet	ASHP[12(p 460)]	Additive or synergistic antiviral activity against CMV and herpes simplex virus type 2	Useful combination for treatment of patients who failed either treatment alone; monitor for increased toxicity
Ganciclovir	Imipenem and cilastatin sodium	ASHP[12(p 460)]	Generalized seizures reported in patient receiving combined therapy	Avoid combined use; if necessary and benefits are greater than risks, monitor closely and discontinue either or both drugs as needed
Ganciclovir	Zidovudine	ASHP,[12(p 460)] Porche[21]	Decreases ganciclovir steady state, but increases zidovudine steady state	Discuss reducing or holding zidovudine dose during ganciclovir induction period with physician
Ganciclovir	Drugs with antiproliferative side effects (e.g., antineoplastic agents, dapsone, cotrimoxazole, flucytosine, pentamidine, pyrimethamine	ASHP[12(p 460)]	Possible overlapping toxicity in normal, rapidly dividing cell populations (bone marrow, gonads, GI mucosa, skin)	Monitor patient closely for signs and symptoms of increased toxicity: bone marrow suppression, stomatitis, diarrhea, loss of skin germinal layers, azospermia

Table 3.3 *Continued*

Drug	Interacting Drug	Documentation	Significance	Management
Ganciclovir	Immunosuppressive drugs (e.g., corticosteroids, antineoplastic agents)	ASHP[12(p 460)]	Additive immunosuppressive and bone marrow suppressive effects	Monitor effects and decrease dose or discontinue drug during treatment with ganciclovir
Ganciclovir	Food	Porche[21]	Increase time to peak serum concentration	Teach patient to take ganciclovir capsules with food
Interferon (alfa and beta)	Ganciclovir	ASHP[12(p 460)]	Synergistic antiviral activity	Studies under way
Interferon	Theophylline	Williams[22]	Possible theophylline toxicity due to decreased excretion	Monitor theophylline levels
Ribavarin	Didanosine, zidovudine, zalcitabine	ASHP[12(p 469)]	In vitro studies show potentiation of didanosine antiretroviral activity antagonism of zidovudine and zalcitabine activity against HIV	Unclear; further studies should be conducted
B. NUCLEOSIDE ANALOG ANTIRETROVIRAL REVERSE TRANSCRIPTASE INHIBITORS				
Didanosine (ddI, Videx)	Alpha interferon	Vogt and Hirsch[23]	Therapeutic synergism	—
Didanosine	Antacids	ASHP[12(p 444)]	Increases bioavailability of didanosine	Tablets are buffered to take advantage of this; oral solution is reconstituted with water and oral antacid

Didanosine	Cimetidine, ranitidine	ASHP[12(p 444)]	Increase in gastric pH theoretically increases bioavailability of didanosine	May increase risk of pancreatitis; monitor patient carefully if drugs used concurrently
Didanosine	Ciprofloxacin and other quinolone antibiotics	ASHP[12(p 444)]	Decreases oral absorption of antibiotic in presence of antacids	Administer at least 2 hours apart when didanosine preparation is buffered or admixed with antacids (suspension)
Didanosine	Dapsone	Jacobus Pharmaceutical Co.[24]	Didanosine buffer neutralizes gastric acidity, which decreases the gastric absorption of dapsone	Administer dapsone at least 2 hours from didanosine administration or avoid concurrent use
Didanosine	Ganciclovir	ASHP,[12(p 444)] Porche[21]	Some studies show antagonism; others show increased didanosine steady-state concentrations	Assess for didanosine effectiveness and toxicity; discuss didanosine dose modification
Didanosine	Itraconazole	ASHP[12(p 444)]	Decreases serum concentration of iatraconazole	Avoid concurrent drug administration; if used together, give itraconazole 2 hours prior to didanosine
Didanosine	Ketoconazole	ASHP[12(p 444)]	Ketoconazole requires acidic pH for absorption	Administer ketoconazole more than 2 hours prior to didanosine

Table 3.3 *Continued*

Drug	Interacting Drug	Documentation	Significance	Management
Didanosine	Pentamidine	Cooley et al,[25] ASHP[12(p 444)]	Increases risk of pancreatitis	Hold didanosine if administering IV pentamidine; consider resuming didanosine 1 week after IV pentamidine completed
Didanosine	Ribavarin	ASHP[12(p 444)]	Ribavarin may potentiate antiretroviral activity of didanosine in vitro	Observe for enhanced antiretroviral effects
Didanosine	Tetracycline	ASHP[12(p 444)]	Tetracycline chelates cations	Administer didanosine 1–2 hours before or after tetracycline dose
Didanosine	Vincristine	Cooley et al[25]	Increases risk of peripheral neuropathy	Monitor patient closely for signs or symptoms of peripheral neuropathy
Didanosine	Zalcitabine	ASHP[12(p 445)]	Overlapping peripheral neurotoxicity	Do not administer concomitantly
Didanosine	Zidovudine	ASHP[12(p 445)]	Synergistic antiretroviral effect	Used together for advantage
Didanosine	Drugs that are potentially toxic to the pancreas (IV pentamidine, co-trimoxazole)	ASHP[12(p 444)]	Theoretically, concomitant use may increase risk of pancreatitis	Consider holding didanosine during treatment with other drug and resume didanosine 1 week later

Didanosine	Food	Amodio-Groton and Currier[26]	Food decreases absorption of drug and decreases serum concentration by 50%	Didanosine should be taken on an empty stomach
Lamivudine (3TC, Epivir)	Trimethoprim/ sulfamethoxazole	Glaxo-Wellcome[27]	Possible increase in serum lamivudine concentration	When used concomitantly, monitor for lamivudine toxicity
Lamivudine	Zidovudine	Glaxo-Wellcome[27]	Synergistic antiretroviral activity	Use together to advantage
Lamivudine	Drugs that are toxic to the pancreas	Glaxo-Wellcome[27]	Adults, pancreatitis is rare (<0.5%); children, incidence may be as high as 15%	Adults, use together cautiously, monitor for signs or symptoms of pancreatitis and serum amylase; children, *do not* use combination lamivudine and zidovudine in children with history of pancreatitis or who are at high risk unless benefit outweighs risk; discontinue drug if signs or symptoms of pancreatitis or lab abnormalities occur
Lamivudine	Other drugs that are peripherally neurotoxic	Glaxo-Wellcome[27]	Twelve percent incidence in combination treatment with zidovudine; 13% in pediatric trial; risk of overlapping toxicity	Avoid concomitant use; assess for peripheral neuropathy

Table 3.3 *Continued*

Drug	Interacting Drug	Documentation	Significance	Management
Stavudine (d4T, Zerit)	Didanosine	Bristol-Myers-Squibb Immunology[28]	Didanosine provides additive antiretroviral effects	—
Stavudine	Zidovudine	AIDS Clinical Trials Group (ACTG) Study[29]	Possible antagonistic effect	Combinations not recommended at this time
Stavudine	Other drugs causing hepatic dysfunction	Bristol-Meyers-Squibb Immunology[28]	Stavudine may cause clinically significant increases in serum hepatic transaminase concentrations when used alone	Monitor liver function studies closely during treatment; use drugs together with caution, if at all
Stavudine	Other drugs that are peripherally neurotoxic	Bristol-Meyers-Squibb Immunology[28]	Overlapping peripheral neurotoxicity	Avoid concomitant use; assess for peripheral neuropathy
Stavudine	Other drugs that are toxic to the pancreas	ASHP[12(pp 472–473)]	Pancreatitis, including fatal pancreatitis, occurs rarely when drug used alone	Monitor patient closely for signs or symptoms of pancreatitis (abdominal pain, nausea, vomiting); monitor serum amylase
Zalcitabine (ddC, Hivid)	Antacids (e.g., Maalox)	ASHP[12(p 481)]	Magnesium- and aluminum-containing antacids decrease the bioavailability of zalcitabine by 25%	Avoid simultaneous administration; administer at least 2 hours apart

Zalcitabine	Cimetidine	ASHP[12(p 481)]	May reduce renal elimination of zalcitabine by 23% thus increasing serum concentration by up to 36%	Monitor for signs or symptoms of zalcitabine toxicity
Zalcitabine	Interferon alfa	ASHP[12(p 481)]	In vitro studies suggest synergisic antiretroviral effect	Unclear
Zalcitabine	Metoclopramide	ASHP[12(p 481)]	May decrease bioavailability by 10%	Monitor for decreased zalcitabine effect
Zalcitabine	Ribavarin	ASHP[12(p 481)]	May antagonize zalcitabine's antiretroviral action	Use together cautiously and monitor for decreased effectiveness of zalcitabine
Zalcitabine	Zidovudine	ASHP[12(p 481)]	Additive or synergistic effects	Use together to advantage
Zalcitabine	Other drugs toxic to the pancreas (e.g., pentamidine)	ASHP[12(p 481)]	Overlapping pancreatic toxicity can be fatal	*Do not use* concomitantly; hold zalcitabine during and for 1–2 weeks after pentamidine treatment (long half-life of pentamidine)
Zalcitabine	Other drugs causing peripheral neurotoxicity (e.g., chloramphenicol, dapsone, didanosine, ethionamide, hydralazine, isoniazid, metronidazole, phenytoin, ribavarin, vincristine)	ASHP[12(p 481)]	Overlapping peripheral neurotoxicity	Avoid concomitant use; monitor patients who have developed peripheral neuropathy on didanosine or zalcitabine who are then switched to the other drug

Table 3.3 *Continued*

Drug	Interacting Drug	Documentation	Significance	Management
Zalcitabine	Other drugs causing renal toxicity (e.g., aminoglycosides, amphotericin B, foscarnet)	ASHP[12(p 481)]	May decrease renal clearance of zalcitabine thus increasing risk of toxicity	Monitor patient closely for peripheral neuropathy, other toxicity; monitor BUN/creatinine; reduce zalcitabine dose as necessary
Zalcitabine	Food	ASHP[12(p 481)]	May decrease rate and extent of drug absorption but impact is unclear	Some clinicians may tell patients to take drug on empty stomach
Zidovudine (AZT, Retrovir)	Acetaminophen or ASA	Glaxo-Wellcome[30]	May competitively inhibit AZT metabolism, toxicity (granulocytopenia)	Monitor WBC; may be rare; Sattler et al[31] found no increase in hematologic toxicity
Zidovudine	Acyclovir	Bach[19]	Synergism; dramatic lethargy and fatigue, especially when IV acyclovir is given	Observe for increased lethargy and decreased alertness; if this occurs, give oral acyclovir or may need to decrease drug dosage
Zidovudine	Adriamycin, vinblastine	Holmes et al[32]	Possible increased risk of AZT toxicity, especially bone marrow suppression	Monitor labs closely
Zidovudine	Amphotericin B	Holmes et al[32]	Possible increased risk of AZT toxicity, especially bone marrow suppression	Monitor labs closely

Zidovudine	Dapsone	Holmes et al,[32] Glaxo-Wellcome[30]	May increase risk of AZT toxicity; additive bone marrow suppression	Monitor closely if used concurrently; otherwise avoid concurrent use
Zidovudine	Didanosine	ASHP[12(p 495)]	Synergistic antiretroviral activity against HIV-1	Use to advantage
Zidovudine	Fluconazole	ASHP[12(p 495)]	Decreases zidovudine metabolism and clearance with resulting higher, prolonged circulating serum levels	Monitor for increased zidovudine toxicity and reduce dose as needed
Zidovudine	Foscarnet	Krown[33]	Therapeutic additive or synergistic effect	—
Zidovudine	Ganciclovir	ASHP[12(p 495)]	Antagonizes antiretroviral activity of zidovudine in vitro; synergistic cytotoxicity	Avoid concurrent administration; if benefits greater than risks, monitor hematologic toxicity carefully and adjust doses of both drugs as needed; if treating for CMV retinitis, consider intravitreal ganciclovir or substitution of didanosine for zidovudine
Zidovudine	Interferon alfa	Krown[33]	Synergism with enhancement of HIV inhibition by zidovudine	Monitor closely for enhanced toxicity, granulocytopenia; modify drug dose as needed

Table 3.3 *Continued*

Drug	Interacting Drug	Documentation	Significance	Management
Zidovudine	Indomethacin	Burroughs Wellcome[34]	May increase zidovudine or indomethacin toxicity because it competitively inhibits glucuronidation	Monitor closely if used concurrently; otherwise, avoid concurrent use
Zidovudine	Methadone	Holmes et al[32]	May increase AZT concentrations with possible increased toxicity	Monitor closely
Zidovudine	Pentamidine	Holmes et al[32]	May increase risk of AZT toxicity due to inhibition of glucuronidation or decreased renal excretion	Monitor closely
Zidovudine	Phenytoin	Holmes et al[32]	Alterations in phenytoin levels may occur (may be decreased or increased)	Carefully monitor phenytoin levels
Zidovudine	Probenecid	ASHP[12(p 495)]	May inhibit metabolism and/or decrease renal excretion of zidovudine, resulting in higher and prolonged serum drug levels	Use together with caution; monitor for zidovudine toxicity and decrease dose as needed; observe for flulike symptoms within 1–2 weeks of combined therapy (e.g., myalgia, malaise, fever, rash) and decrease probenecid
Zidovudine	Pyrimethamine	ASHP[12(p 496)]	May decrease pyrimethamine activity against *Toxoplasma gondii*	Monitor for pyrimethamine effectiveness

Zidovudine	Ribavarin	Holmes et al[32]	Antagonistic antiviral effect	*Do not* use concurrently
Zidovudine	Stavudine (d4T)	ACTG[29]	Possible antagonism	*Do not* use concurrently
Zidovudine	Zalcitabine	ASHP[12(p 481)]	Additive or synergistic effects	Use together to advantage
Zidovudine	Antituberculous drugs (e.g., isoniazid, rifampin, ethambutol, pyrazinamide)	ASHP[12(p 495)]	May result in mild to moderate decrease in leukocyte count	Importance unclear; monitor patient's WBC
Zidovudine	Myelosuppressive drugs (e.g., vinblastine, doxorubicin)	ASHP[12(p 495)]	Overlapping myelosuppression possible	Monitor CBC, absolute neutrophil count closely
Zidovudine	Drugs that may cause renal toxicity (e.g., amphotericin B, dapsone)	ASHP[12(p 495)]	May reduce drug clearance and increase toxicity	Use together cautiously; monitor for increased zidovudine toxicity
C. NONNUCLEOSIDE REVERSE TRANSRIPTASE INHIBITORS				
Delavirdine (Rescriptor)	Antacids	Project Inform[35]	Reduces absorption when taken together, with resulting decrease in delavirdine levels	Take 1 hour apart
Delavirdine	Astemizole, diltiazem, midazolam, nifedipine, quinidine, terfenadine, triazolam	Project Inform[35]	Delavirdine may decrease metabolism of other drugs with increased serum levels and toxicity of these drugs	Do not use together; if no alternatives, use cautiously if at all
Delavirdine	Didanosine	Project Inform[35]	Increased activity in combination (in vitro); decreased absorption when taken together	Take drugs 1 hour apart

Table 3.3 *Continued*

Drug	Interacting Drug	Documentation	Significance	Management
Delavirdine	Erythromycin, clarithromycin	Project Inform[35]	May increase delavirdine levels	Monitor for increased toxicity when used in combination
Delavirdine	Itraconazole	Project Inform[35]	May increase both drug levels	Monitor for increased efficacy and toxicity
Delavirdine	Phenytoin, carbamazepine	Project Inform[35]	May decrease delavirdine levels	Avoid concurrent use
Delavirdine	Prednisone	Project Inform[35]	May increase prednisone and delavirdine levels	Monitor for increased toxicity
Delavirdine	Ritonavir, indinavir	Project Inform,[35] Pharmacia Upjohn[36]	Probably increases serum levels of protease inhibitors; may affect delavirdine level	Monitor for drug effectiveness and toxicity
Delavirdine	Rifabutin	Project Inform[35]	Decreases delavirdine levels	Avoid concurrent use
Delavirdine	Rifampin	Project Inform[35]	Delavirdine serum levels significantly decreased if taken separately	Take both medications at the same time
Delavirdine	Saquinavir	Cooley et al,[25] Pharmacia Upjohn[36]	Saquinavir serum levels increased five times	Consider dose modifications; monitor for saquinavir toxicity
Delavirdine	Testosterone, warfarin	Porject Inform[35]	Testosterone or warfarin serum levels may be increased	Monitor patients receiving warfarin closely and decrease dose as needed

Nevirapine (Viramune)	Amoxicillin, ticarcillin	Roxanne Pharmaceuticals,[37] ASHP,[12(pp 6–10)] Project Inform[35]	May increase the risk of rashes and Stevens-Johnson syndrome	Monitor patient very carefully for rashes, itching, desquamation, and if present stop drug immediately
Nevirapine	Astemizole, clarithromycin, dapsone, itraconazole, ketoconazole, prednisone, rifabutin, rifampin, terfenadine, trimetrexate	Roxanne Pharmaceuticals,[37] ASHP,[12(pp 6–10)] Project Inform[35]	May affect serum levels of interacting drug and/or nevirapine	Avoid concurrent use if possible; otherwise, monitor for drug effectiveness and toxicity; new data should be forthcoming
Nevirapine	Cimetidine	Project Inform,[35] Roxanne Pharmaceuticals[37]	Combination may decrease nevirapine serum levels	Do not administer together
Nevirapine	Clavulonic acid, Bactrim (TMP/SMX)	Project Inform,[35] Roxanne Pharmaceuticals[37]	May increase toxicity	Do not give either drug with nevirapine for first 6 weeks of taking nevirapine
Nevirapine	Didanosine, zidovudine	Project Inform,[35] Roxanne Pharmaceuticals[37]	Increased antiviral activity in vitro	Use together to advantage; await clinical study data
Nevirapine	Dicumarol, warfarin	Project Inform,[35] Roxanne Pharmaceuticals[37]	Dicumarol or warfarin serum levels may be increased	Do not use together
Nevirapine	Erythromycin	Project Inform,[35] Roxanne Pharmaceuticals[37]	May increase risk of hepatic toxicity	Do not use together
Nevirapine	Glucocorticoids (systemic)	Project Inform,[35] Roxanne Pharmaceuticals[37]	May increase rate of metabolism of glucocorticoids	Monitor for effectiveness of glucocorticoids and increase dose as needed

Table 3.3 *Continued*

Drug	Interacting Drug	Documentation	Significance	Management
Nevirapine	Indinavir, ritonavir, saquinavir	Project Inform,[35] Roxanne Pharmaceuticals[37]	May affect indinavir or ritonavir levels and/or nevirapine levels; decreases saquinavir levels	Await new clinical data on effect on protease inhibitor levels; do not use with saquinavir
Nevirapine	Oral contraceptives	Project Inform,[35] Roxanne Pharmaceuticals[37]	May decrease effectiveness of contraception	Teach patient to use barrier protection as well, or alternative contraception methods
Nevirapine	Phenytoin	Project Inform,[35] Roxanne Pharmaceuticals[37]	May increase rate of phenytoin metabolism with decreased serum levels; may decrease nevirapine serum level	Use together cautiously, if at all, and monitor for nevirapine and phenytoin effectiveness
Nevirapine	Tolbutamide	Project Inform,[35] Roxanne Pharmaceuticals[37]	Risk of increased toxicity when given in combination	Do not give concurrently
D. ANTIRETROVIRAL PROTEINASE INHIBITORS				
Indinavir (Crixivan)	Astemizole, terfenadine; cisapride, triazolam, midazolam	Merck[38]	Has affinity for cytochrome P450 isoenzymes in the hepatic metabolic pathway thus potentially increasing these serum drug levels and causing high risk for toxicity	Contraindicated; do not give together; substitute alternative medications

Indinavir	Didanosine	Merck[38]	Altered absorption when given together	Administer on an empty stomach 1 hour apart from ddI
Indinavir	Ketoconazole	Merck[38]	Increases indinovir levels	Consider decreasing dose to 600 mg every 8 hours
Indinavir	Rifabutin	Merck[38]	Rifabutin concentrations are increased	Decrease rifabutin dose by 50%
Indinavir	Rifampin	Merck[38]	Indinovir levels are significantly lowered	Do not give together
Indinavir	Food	Merck[38]	Interferes with absorption	Teach patients to take drug on empty stomach 1 hour before or 2 hours after food
Nelfinavir (Viracept)	Astemizole, cisapride, midazolam, rifampin, terfenadine, triazolam	Agouron Pharmaceuticals[39]	Nelfinavir selectively inhibits P450 (CYP3A) enzyme system; may result in increase in interacting drug doses and serious life-threatening arrhythmias	Do not use together; use alternative agents
Nelfinavir	Carbamazepine, phenobarbital, phenytoin	Agouron Pharmaceuticals[39]	May decrease nelfinavir serum drug levels	Monitor for drug ineffectiveness and consider using alternative anticonvulsant
Nelfinavir	Didanosine	Agouron Pharmaceuticals[39]	Increases absorption with food whereas didanosine absorption is decreased when administered with food	Administer nelfinavir 1 hour after or 2 hours before didanosine

Table 3.3 *Continued*

Drug	Interacting Drug	Documentation	Significance	Management
Nelfinavir	Protease inhibiting agents (indinavir, ritonavir)	Agouron Pharmaceuticals[39]	May increase nelfinavir plasma concentrations; may permit decreased doses or dosing frequency when given in combination	Significance in clinical practice currently being studied
Nelfinavir	Nevirapine	Agouron Pharmaceuticals[39]	Probably decreases nelfinavir concentrations	May require dosage adjustment
Nelfinavir	Oral contraceptives (ethinyl estradiol, norethindrone)	Agouron Pharmaceuticals[39]	Oral contraceptive plasma concentration may be decreased by 50%	Teach patient to use barrier contraception in addition to birth control pills; use alternative contraceptive methods
Nelfinavir	Reverse transcriptase inhibitors	Agouron Pharmaceuticals[39]	Additive to synergistic effects	Use together to advantage
Nelfinavir	Rifabutin	Agouron Pharmaceuticals[39]	Combination results in decreased metabolism and 200% increase in rifabutin serum levels	Reduce rifabutin dose by 50%
Nelfinavir	Saquinavir	Agouron Pharmaceuticals[39]	Increases saquinavir level by 400% and nelfinavir by 20%	Observe for toxicity; consider dose reduction and/or decrease in frequency of dosing
Nelfinavir	Food	Agouron Pharmaceuticals[39]	Oral absorption >70%, and is two to three times higher when ingested with food	Teach patient to take medication with food

Saquinavir Mesylate (Invirase)	Astemizole, terfenadine, disapride, triazolam, midazolam	Hoffman LaRoche[40]	Saquinavir mildly inhibits P450 cytochrome pathway (hepatic metabolism) thus potentially increasing these drug serum levels, which may cause cardiac arrhythmias (prolonged QT intervals) and, rarely, death	Do not use in combination; substitute other drugs for terfenadine or astemizole
Saquinavir mesylate	Calcium channel blocking agents, clindamycin, dapsone, quinidine, triazolam	Hoffman LaRoche[40]	Serum concentration of these drugs may be increased when given with saquinavir, as they are substrates of CYP3A4 pathways	Contraindicated; use alternative agents; if cannot use alternatives, closely monitor for side effects of these drugs
Saquinavir mesylate	Phenobarbital, phenytoin, dexamethasone, carbamazepine	Hoffman LaRoche[40]	Induces hepatic enzyme system (CYP3A4) and may decrease plasma saquinavir levels	Consider alternative medications; do not use concurrently if possible
Saquinavir mesylate	Rifabutin	Hoffman LaRoche[40]	Reduces plasma concentration by 40%	Do not give concomitantly
Saquinavir mesylate	Rifampin	Hoffman LaRoche[40]	Reduces plasma concentration of saquinavir by 80%	Do not give concomitantly
Saquinavir mesylate	Zalcitabine, zidovudine	Hoffman LaRoche[40]	Combination therapy with saquinavir showed no change in absorption, metabolism, or elimination of any of the drugs	Use together to advantage; saquinavir is FDA labeled for use with zalcitabine or zidovudine

Table 3.3 *Continued*

Drug	Interacting Drug	Documentation	Significance	Management
Saquinavir mesylate	High-fat foods	Hoffman LaRoche[40]	Doubles serum concentrations of saquinavir; food effect lasts 2 hours	Teach patient to take drug within 2 hours of full meal, preferably high-fat meal
Ritonavir (Norvir)	Alprazolam, clorazepate, diazepam, estozalam, flurazepam, midazolam, triazolam, zolpidem	Abbott Laboratories[41]	Metabolism of these drugs decreased; may cause severe sedation and respiratory depression due to large increases in serum levels	Do not administer concurrently; consider alternatives such as temazepam or lorazepam
Ritonavir	Amiodarone, astemizole, bepridil, bupropion, cisapride, clorozepate, clozapine, encainide, flecanide, meperidine, piroxicam, propafenone, propoxyphene, quinidine, rifabutin, terfenadine	Abbott Laboratories[41]	Ritonavir has affinity for cytochrome P450 isoenzymes in the hepatic metabolic pathway thus potentially increasing these drug serum levels, which may cause cardiac arrhythmias (prolonged QT intervals) and, rarely, death	Concurrent use with ritonavir is contraindicated; substitute other drugs; see accompanying drug information on ritonavir for recommended alternative medications
Ritonavir	Clarithromycin	Abbott Laboratories[41]	Increase in serum levels of clarithromycin; significant in patients with renal dysfunction	No significance in patients with normal renal function; reduce dose for creatinine clearance less than 50% (see package insert)

Ritonavir	Desipramine	Abbott Laboratories[41]	145% increase in desipramine serum levels	Dose reduction of desipramine recommended
Ritonavir	Ethinyl estradiol	Abbott Laboratories[41]	40% decrease in ethinyl estradiol serum levels	Increase dose of ethinyl estradiol or change to another contraceptive
Ritonavir	Theophylline	Abbott Laboratories[41]	43% decrease in theophylline serum level	May need to increase theophylline dose
E. ANTIFUNGAL DRUGS				
Amphotericin B	Corticosteroids	ASHP[12(p 76)]	May increase potassium excretion	Avoid concurrent administration if possible; closely monitor serum electrolytes, cardiac function
Amphotericin B	Dapsone, flucytosine, trimethoprim-sulfamethoxazole, zidovudine	ASHP[12(p 76)] Geletko and Dudley[42]	Increases risk of anemia when used in combination	Monitor hgb/hct and patient symptoms; transfuse as needed
Amphotericin B	Flucytosine	ASHP[12(p 76)]	Synergism with increased flucytosine toxicity related to decreased elimination or increased cellular uptake	Avoid; if concurrent use, closely monitor CBC and patient symptoms; monitor flucytosine serum concentration levels and decrease dose as needed
Amphotericin B	Mechlorethamine	ASHP[12(p 77)]	May enhance renal toxicity and cause bronchospasm and hypotension	Avoid concurrent use; if used together, monitor patient closely

Table 3.3 *Continued*

Drug	Interacting Drug	Documentation	Significance	Management
Amphotericin B	Neuromuscular blocking agents, cardiac glycosides (e.g., digoxin)	Miller and Bates,[43] ASHP[12(p 76)]	Increased neuromuscular blockade due to low K+	Monitor K+ level and neuromuscular status; monitor digoxin level
Amphotericin B	Other drugs causing renal toxicity (e.g., aminoglycoside antibiotics, pentamidine)	ASHP[12(p 77)]	Potential overlapping of renal toxicity	Closely monitor BUN, creatinine; avoid concurrent administration if possible
Fluconazole	Anticoagulants, oral	Pfizer/Roerig[44]	Increased prothrombin time after warfarin administration	Monitor prothrombin time carefully
Fluconazole	Astemizole, terfenadine	Pfizer/Roerig[44]	Potent inhibitor of cytochrome P4503A metabolic pathway, which may cause increased plasma concentration of terfenadine or astemizole, leading to prolonged QT intervals and cardiac arrhythmias, which have been fatal	Concomitant use contraindicated
Fluconazole	Cyclosporine	ASHP[12(p 85)]	May have increased cyclosporine levels	Monitor levels
Fluconazole	Methylprednisolone	Glynn and Brunner[45]	Fluconazole may inhibit hepatic metabolism of methylprednisolone, and may enhance toxicity and cortisol suppressive effects	Monitor for adverse effects of methylprednisolone; may need to reduce dose of steroid by 50%

Fluconazole	Phenytoin	Pfizer/Roerig[44]	Increases plasma concentrations of phenytoin	Monitor phenytoin levels closely
Fluconazole	Rifampin	Pfizer/Roerig[44]	Rifampin enhances fluconazole metabolism	May need to increase dose of fluconazole
Fluconazole	Sulfonylurea oral hypoglycemic agents (e.g., tolbutamide, glyburide, glipizide)	Pfizer/Roerig[44]	Increased plasma levels of hypoglycemics may occur due to decreased metabolism	Monitor blood sugar and adjust oral hypoglycemic dose accordingly
Fluconazole	Zidovudine	ASHP[12(p 84)]	May decrease metabolism and clearance of zidovudine; single study showed increased zidovudine serum levels	Monitor for increased zidovudine toxicity and reduce dose accordingly
Itraconazole	Astemizole, terfenadine	ASHP[12(p 93)]	Potent inhibitor of cytochrome P4503A metabolic pathway, which may cause increased plasma concentration of terfenadine or astemizole, leading to prolonged QT intervals and cardiac arrhythmias, which have been fatal	Concomitant administration contraindicated
Itraconazole	Cisapride (Propulcid)	ASHP[12(p 2147)]	Increases risk of serious and potentially fatal cardiac arrhythmias	Concomitant administration contraindicated
Ketoconazole	Alcohol	ASHP[12(p 98)]	Disulfiram reaction may occur rarely (e.g., flush, rash, peripheral edema, nausea, headache)	Teach patient to avoid alcohol during and for 48 hours after ketoconazole discontinued

Table 3.3 *Continued*

Drug	Interacting Drug	Documentation	Significance	Management
Ketoconazole	Antacids, aluminum hydroxide, magnesium hydroxide, histamine (H_2) blockers	Carlson et al[46]	Ketoconazole requires acidic environment; antacids and H_2-receptor antagonists increase intragastric pH but decrease ketoconazole absorption by as much as 40%	Administer antacids and H_2 blockers at least 2 hours apart from ketoconazole dose; avoid H_2 blockers
Ketoconazole	Anticoagulants	Smith[47]	Increased anticoagulant effect	Monitor prothrombin time
Ketoconazole	Astemizole, terfenadine	ASHP[12(p 98)]	Potent inhibitor of cytochrome P4503A metabolic pathway, which may cause increased plasma concentration of terfenadine or astemizole, leading to prolonged QT intervals and cardiac arrhythmias, which have been fatal	Concomitant use contraindicated
Ketoconazole	Cimetidine, ranitidine, sucralfate	Van der Meer et al,[11] ASHP[12(p 98)]	Decreases ketoconazole effect due to decreased absorption	Give sucralfate or antacids 2 hours before or after ketoconazole dose; avoid H_2 blockers
Ketoconazole	Cisapride (Propulcid)	ASHP[12(p 2147)]	Increases risk of serious and potentially fatal cardiac arrhythmias	Concomitant administration contraindicated

Ketoconazole	Corticosteroids (methylprednisolone or prednisolone)	ASHP[12(p 98)]	May decrease clearance resulting in increased plasma concentrations of corticosteroid; may increase adrenal suppression	Assess patient and decrease corticosteroid dose as needed
Ketoconazole	Cyclosporine	Shepard et al[48]	Possible increase in renal toxicity	Avoid concomitant use if possible; monitor renal function
Ketoconazole	Isoniazid, rifampin	Engelhard and Meunier,[49] ASHP[12(p 98)]	Rifampin may increase metabolism of ketoconazole, resulting in decreased ketoconazole serum levels; also may reduce rifampin levels; isoniazid and rifampin additively reduce serum ketoconazole levels	Monitor for drug effectiveness; increase dosage of ketoconazole as needed if drugs used together
Ketoconazole	Paclitaxel (Taxol)	ASHP[12(p 98)]	May inhibit paclitaxel metabolism with increased toxicity	Avoid concurrent use
Ketoconazole	Phenytoin	Physician's Desk Reference[50(p 1299)]	Alterations in metabolism and drug effects	Monitor phenytoin and ketoconazole levels
Ketoconazole	Theophylline (oral)	ASHP[12(p 98)]	May decrease serum theophylline levels	Monitor patient and serum theophylline levels, especially when beginning or ending ketoconazole treatment

Table 3.3 *Continued*

Drug	Interacting Drug	Documentation	Significance	Management
Ketoconazole	Triazolam	ASHP[12(p 98)]	Increased peak serum concentration, prolonged half-life, and decreased drug clearance can occur	Avoid concomitant drug administration
Ketoconazole	Drugs causing hepatotoxicity	ASHP[12(p 98)]	Possible overlapping hepatotoxicity	Monitor liver function studies closely
Miconazole	Anticoagulants	Smith[47]	Increased anticoagulant effect	Monitor prothrombin time
Miconazole	Oral sulfonylurea hypoglycemic agents	ASHP[12((p 101)]	Severe hypoglycemia may occur	Avoid concurrent use
F. ANTITUBERCULOUS DRUGS				
Ethambutol	Aluminum hydroxide	Mattila et al[51]	Gastric absorption may be reduced	Administer at least 1 hour apart
Isoniazid	Aluminum hydroxide	Hurwitz and Sclozman[52]	Large doses of antacid may reduce peak serum levels; high levels are important for antituberculous effect	Administer isoniazid at least 1 hour before antacid
Isoniazid	Alcohol	Kopanoff et al.[53]	Increased risk for hepatitis	Have patients avoid alcohol
Isoniazid		—		
Isoniazid	Rifampin	Lal and Coakley[54]	Hepatotoxicity risk may be increased	Assess for hepatotoxicity
Rifampin	Aminosalicylic acid	Berman[55]	Decreased absorption of rifampin	Give at least 8 hours apart

Rifampin	Anticoagulants, oral	Geletko and Dudley[42]	Decreased anticoagulant serum levels	Increase anticoagulant dose as necessary
Rifampin	Antacids	Geletko and Dudley[42]	May alter absorption	Teach patient to give 2 hours apart
Rifampin	Atovaquone	Physician's Desk Reference[50(p 1137)]	Combination significantly reduces atovaquone concentrations	Use alternative antituberculin therapy; avoid both rifampin and rifabutin
Rifampin	Chloramphenicol	Prober[56]	Rifampin increases hepatic metabolism of chloramphenicol	Monitor effect of chloramphenicol because dose may have to be increased
Rifampin	Contraceptives, oral	Breckinridge et al[57]	Increased incidence of menstrual disorders; pregnancy has occurred	Monitor for breakthrough bleeding and spotting, and counsel regarding other forms of birth control
Rifampin	Dapsone	Geletko and Dudley[42]	Decreased serum concentrations possible	Assess efficacy in patients
Rifampin	Fluconazole	Geletko and Dudley[42]	May decrease fluconazole serum levels	May need to increase fluconazole dose; monitor signs and symptoms of infection
Rifampin	Methadone	Geletko and Dudley[42]	May decrease serum methadone levels	Increase methadone dose and control withdrawal symptoms
Rifampin	Nelfinavir, saquinavir	Agouron Pharmaceuticals[39]	May increase metabolism and decrease serum levels of protease inhibitors	Avoid concurrent use

Table 3.3 *Continued*

Drug	Interacting Drug	Documentation	Significance	Management
Rifampin	Sulfonylureas	Geletko and Dudley[42]	Decreases sulfonylurea serum levels	Increase sulfonylurea dose based on blood glucose; monitor blood glucose after rifampin decrease
Rifampin	Theophylline	Geletko and Dudley[42]	Decreases serum theophylline levels	Monitor serum theophylline levels; increase dose as needed
Rifabutin	Contraceptives, oral	ASHP[12(p 415)]	Decreases effectiveness of contraception; increases incidence of menstrual disorders	Discuss alternative nonhormonal types of contraception
Rifabutin	Dapsone	ASHP[12(p 415)]	Decreases dapsone serum level	Assess dapsone effectiveness and increase drug dose as needed
Rifabutin	Fluconazole	ASHP[12(p 416)]	At high doses of rifabutin, increased risk of uveitis	Avoid concurrent use; monitor patient closely for uveitis
Rifabutin	Ketoconazole	ASHP[12(p 415)]	Decreases serum ketoconazole level and increased risk of uveitis	Avoid concomitant use
Rifabutin	Methadone	ASHP[12(p 415)]	Decreases methadone serum levels	Increase methadone dose and control withdrawal symptoms
Rifabutin	Nelfinavir	Agouron Pharmaceuticals[39]	Increases rifabutin levels by 200%	Decrease rifabutin dose by 50%

Rifabutin	Zidovudine	ASHP[12(p 415)]	May decrease serum zidovudine level	Unclear, more studies needed; monitor patient response to zidovudine
Rifabutin	Myelosuppressive agents (e.g., vinblastine, doxorubicin)	ASHP[12(p 415)]	Possible overlapping myelosuppression	Monitor CBC, platelets, and absolute neutrophil count closely
G. Other Drugs				
Atovaquone (oral)	Fatty meals	Physician's Desk Reference[50(p 1137)]	Enhanced absorption	Teach patients to take with fatty meals
Ciprofloxacin	Aluminum hydroxide, magnesium hydroxide, calcium products, and iron	Schentag[58]	May result in decreased absorption of ciprofloxacin	Separate administration by at least 2 hours
Clarithramycin	Anticoagulants	ASHP[12(p 236)]	May potentiate anticoagulant	Adjust dose as needed
Clarithramycin	Cisapride, terfenadine	ASHP[12(p 236)]	Potent inhibitor of cytochrome P4503A metabolic pathway, which may cause increased plasma concentration of terfenadine or astemizole, leading to prolonged QT intervals and cardiac arrhythmias, which have been fatal	Concommitant administration contraindicated
Clarithramycin	Theophylline	ASHP[12(p 236)]	May increase serum theophylline concentration due to decreased clearance or metabolism	Monitor theophylline levels and modify dose accordingly

Table 3.3 *Continued*

Drug	Interacting Drug	Documentation	Significance	Management
Clarithramycin	Zidovudine	ASHP[12(p 236)]	Decreases serum concentration and prolongs time to peak level of zidovudine	Further study needed
Dapsone	Rifampin	Gazzard[59]	Rifampin may accelerate hepatic metabolism of dapsone	Monitor patient for diminished effect of dapsone; may need to increase dose
Bactrim (TMP/SMX, Septra)	Phenytoin	Covington et al[60]	May decrease hepatic clearance of phenytoin, prolonging drug's half-life	Monitor for increased phenytoin levels; may need to decrease dose or increase interval between doses

ASA = acetylsalicyclic acid; CMV = cytomegalovirus; CR = creatinine; ETOH = alcohol; FDA = Food and Drug Administration; GI = gastrointestinal; h/o = history of; n/v = nausea and vomiting; TMP/SMX = trimethoprim sulfamethoxazole; PCP = pneumocystis carinii pneumonia; PT = prothrombin time

Altered Metabolism

Altered metabolism can occur with either increased or decreased levels of drug when one drug stimulates or inhibits the metabolism of another. This is the most frequently significant drug-drug interaction possible. When one drug stimulates the metabolism of another, it usually does so by *inducing the enzymes* in the hepatic enzyme system. The reaction is usually gradual, over 1 to 2 weeks, with gradual dissipation. The time course depends on a number of factors, including the half-life of the drug. Rifampin, for example, has a fairly short half-life, so onset and offset is less gradual than for phenobarbital, which has a longer half-life.[10] Enzyme induction results in decreased serum concentration of one of the drugs. For example rifampin, when given in combination with saquinavir mesylate (a protease inhibitor), decreases saquinavir serum concentrations by 80% and therefore should not be given in combination.[14]

The second type of metabolic alteration is caused by *enzyme induction or inhibition*, and this is far more clinically significant. It is usually rapid, occurring within one to two doses of the drug causing induction or inhibition. Hepatic metabolism involves the cytochrome P450 hepatic mixed-function oxidase system, and it is here that most activity occurs. Certain drugs may "induce" the enzyme system, thus accelerating metabolism or another drug, and thus reducing plasma levels of that drug and decreasing the therapeutic effect. Conversely, coadministration of a drug that inhibits the enzyme system reduces the metabolism of another drug and results in an increased serum concentration of the drug with the inhibited metabolism. While the protease inhibitor antiretroviral agents hold great promise, the four FDA-approved agents inhibit some part of the P450 isoenzyme system to varying degrees. Saquinavir and nelfinavir are mildly and selectively inhibitory, while ritonavir has a greater inhibitory effect. This effect on the P450 cytochrome system has the potential to result in increased drug concentrations that can be dangerous. Because drugs with similar enzyme inhibition, such as ketoconazole, have caused significantly higher drug concentrations of astemizole, terfenadine, or cisapride when given in combination with resulting cardiac arrhythmias (torsades de pointes), and even cardiac arrest, these drugs are contraindicated in combination with the protease inhibitor antiretroviral agents. Inducers such as the anticonvulsants (e.g., carbamazepine, phenobarbital, and phenytoin) or the antitubucular agent rifampin increase the metabolism of the protease inhibitor nelfinavir, resulting in decreased serum concentrations of nelfinavir.

Altered Excretion

The last type of pharmacokinetic interaction is related to renal excretion, when one drug alters the renal excretion of another, resulting in increased or decreased serum levels. Most clinically important are those in which the decreased renal excretion of a drug results in higher serum levels. The mechanisms involved are (1) changing the urinary pH so that a drug normally excreted unchanged in the urine or as an active metabolite is now reabsorbed or excreted to a greater degree, (2) decreasing glomerular filtration rate so that less drug is filtered and excreted, and (3) decreasing the drugs actively secreted from the renal tubules if both drugs normally are actively secreted from the renal tubules and now one interferes with the secretion of the other, altering serum levels.[10,15] A therapeutic example of this interaction is probenecid, a uricosuric agent that blocks the secretion of penicillins and some cephalosporin antibiotics, resulting in increased antibiotic serum levels. When drugs that may cause renal toxicity are used concurrently, the risk of renal toxicity and drug-induced side effects increases as drug excretion decreases.

Pharmacodynamic Interactions

Pharmacodynamic mechanisms involve *additive or synergistic effects* (increased drug effect and/or toxicity), *antagonistic effects* (having opposite effects), *altered serum electrolyte levels* (which can affect drug distribution), and *dysfunction at receptor sites* (which results in decreased drug effectiveness and increased toxicity). The additive effect is illustrated by the therapeutic combination of acetaminophen with a narcotic analgesic, whereas the synergistic effect is illustrated by a number of combinations such as zidovudine with acyclovir, zidovudine and didanosine, and zidovudine and interferon. The therapeutic synergism of zidovudine and interferon are important effects, but the enhanced toxicity requires careful monitoring. The antagonistic effect is suspected when zidovudine and ribavarin are used in combination, or when zidovudine (AZT) and stavudine (d4T) are given concurrently. Because of the antagonism encountered, these drugs should not be given in combination. Altered serum electrolytes can occur with amphotericin B administration, which causes renal tubular acidosis and subsequent potassium and magnesium wasting in the urine. Hypokalemia then may potentiate the toxicity of other drugs, such as digoxin.[16] Dysfunction at receptor sites is less common, but is illustrated by the interaction of monamine oxidase inhibitors such as procarbazine and tyramine-containing foods. Monamine oxidase is an enzyme that breaks down catecholamines (e.g., epinephrine, norepinephrine), and, if inhibited, catecholamines will accumulate at receptor sites in adrenergic nerve endings. Tyramine is a pressor substance broken down by monamine oxidase and it is found in foods such as certain cheeses, beer, and pepperoni. If large amounts of these foods are ingested and monamine oxidase inhibitors are present, tyramine cannot be broken down, large amounts accumulate, and norepinephrine is released from adrenergic neurons, resulting in hypertension, flushing, and an Antabuselike effect if alcohol is ingested.[17]

Table 3.3 gives examples of commonly prescribed drugs and potential interactions, as well as management suggestions. This listing is not exhaustive and the reader is advised to review drug-prescribing information and other references for full descriptions of potential drug-drug interactions. As persons with HIV infection live longer with improved management strategies, medicines, and prophylaxis of OIs, polypharmacy will continue to be an important issue. Nurses must remain current with the literature, as well as with prescribing information and potential drug interactions. Today, in the electronic age, resources for both patients and nurses are available. For example, Project Inform's Drug Interaction Chart is available on the Internet at *http://www.thebody.com/pinf/interact.html*, and Pharmacia and Upjohn Pharmaceuticals offer an interactive reference tool for IBM-compatible computers entitled HIV Drug Interactions. Finally, as most drug interaction studies are restricted to only two medications, and most patients with HIV infection take upward of 5 to 10 medications, drug studies evaluating drug-drug interactions among various combinations must be conducted.

Assessment of Polypharmacy

Important points for nursing assessment are (1) history of drug allergies (distinguish between *allergy* [e.g., rash, pruritus, angioedema] and *adverse reaction* [e.g., nausea]); (2) medical diagnoses and treatment plan, including all medicines; and (3) risk assessment for potential drug toxicity/drug interactions. Risk assessment of host variables that may influence drug metabolism and distribution, and toxicity are age, organ function for drug metabolism/excretion (hepatic and renal function), and target organ systems such as bone marrow, GI, pulmonary, cardiac, neurologic (peripheral and CNS), and skin and mucous membranes. For example, a patient receiving ganciclovir for cytomegalovirus (CMV) retinitis is at risk for developing neutropenia.[61] Other drugs that suppress the bone marrow should be avoided, such as zidovudine, trimethoprim-sulfamethoxazole, pyrimethamine, and myelosuppressive chemotherapy.[42] It may be the nurse who reviews the patient's medication list and identifies potential drug interactions or the potential for enhanced toxicity. Drugs that cause overlapping toxicity in an organ system should not be used concommitantly, such as drugs that may cause pancreatitis (didanosine and pentamidine) or peripheral neuropathy (stavudine and vincristine).

It is important to anticipate potential drug interactions so that known adverse reactions can be avoided. Often there are appropriate, noninteracting alternative drugs that can be substituted, or the offending drug can be held until the second drug treatment is completed. However, when it is determined that the benefit outweighs the risk of drugs with a high likelihood of interaction given concommitantly, then close monitoring of drug serum levels is imperative, as well as close monitoring of target organ systems for drug toxicity. Once drug interactions are identified, the implicated drugs should be discontinued then added back to the treatment regime one at a time to assess tolerance.

Patient Education

Patient education is a very important dimension of nursing care for individuals infected with HIV. Many patients want to know everything they can about HIV infection, their specific OIs or malignancy, and their medicines, whereas others may have less interest or ability to assimilate detailed information due to a low literacy level, illicit drug use, or cultural differences and health beliefs. Teaching about medications is challenging, and teaching-learning strategies must be tailored to each patient based on (1) what the patient is ready and willing to learn; (2) relevance to the person's sociocultural background, attitudes, and motivation; (3) level of knowledge; (4) literacy level; and (5) intactness of senses (e.g., vision, hearing).

Assessment of readiness to learn should include baseline knowledge of HIV infection and the condition being treated; general condition and ability to receive information; usual self-care strategies; motivation; supports; substance abuse; concerns such as finances, insurance, and ability to pay for medicines; primary language, educational level, and ability to understand the learning material. A patient with HIV-related dementia requires different teaching strategies compared with a college-educated, motivated patient, and this differs from the teaching strategy for an IV drug user who is actively using drugs.

Chaisson[62] identified common mistakes in teaching patients that included *telling people* what they *should* know instead of what they are ready and willing to learn, and *lack of coordination of patient teaching efforts across the care continuum*. Many pharmaceutical companies offer prepared patient educational literature that is very helpful for some patients. Depending on the assessment of the patient's readiness to learn, this literature may need to be modified to be appropriate for a particular patient. For instance, for many patients who have a low reading level, an educational booklet must be written at the fifth-grade reading level. In addition to written brochures, audiotapes and videotapes are often available.

Resources

It is exciting that pharmacologic and clinical research continues to produce increasingly more effective medications for management of HIV and the prevention and treatment of OIs. However, the cost of many of these medications is quite high. For some patients who live in a large, urban community with a large HIV-infected population there are many resources for patient emotional support, education, and access to state-supported free drug programs for indigent patients. For others, this is not the case. Many of the pharmaceutical companies do offer drug assistance programs for patients without insurance. It is often the nurse in any of the care settings (inpatient, clinic, or community) who, as the patient advocate, involves the social worker in the case or who tries to locate community resources.

Access to clinical trials is important. The AIDS Clinical Trials Information Service (ACTIS) provides current information on nationwide clinical trials to health care providers, patients, and their families. Information about HIV treatment options is available from specially trained specialists who tailor their response to the caller's health status and understanding of HIV infection.[63] This is a public health service-sponsored program and can be accessed using a toll-free number (1-800-TRIALS-A or 1-800-874-2572) from any state in the United States, or Canada. In addition, there are new Web pages on the Internet that offer treatment data bases that can be downloaded, and other resources such as legal rights and social support. There are national newsletters, journals, and other publications that provide updates on new drugs, such as the protease inhibitors and clinical trial results. An example of this is the newsletter *Positively Aware*, published in Chicago, Illinois, by Test Positive Aware Network.

In summary the mainstay of HIV management is pharmacologic therapy to counter HIV infection and to prevent and treat OIs. Most patients receive multiple-drug therapy, and polypharmacy poses many challenges to patient, nurse, and physician. Understanding the pharmacologic principles underlying drug interactions is helpful in anticipating and avoiding significant drug interactions. Patient education is critical and must be timely and relevant, and the nurse must offer ongoing reinforcement. Resources are available to nurses and patients for information regarding drugs and clinical trials. Nurses continue to play a critical role in ensuring that patients have equal access to state-of-the-art care for HIV infection.

References

1. Saag MS. Evolving understanding of the immunopathogenesis of HIV. *AIDS Res Hum Retroviruses.* 1994;10(8):887–892.
2. Pantaleo G, Graziosi C, Demarest JF, et al. Role of lymphoid organs in the pathogenesis of human immunodeficiency virus infection, *Immunol Rev.* 1994; 140:104–130.
3. Wei X, Ghosh SK, Taylor ME, et al. Viral dynamics in human immunodeficiency virus type 1 infection. *Nature.* 1995;373:117–122.
4. Ho DD, Neumann AU, Perelson AS, et al. Rapid turnover of plasma virions and CD4 lymphocytes in HIV-1 infection. *Nature.* 1995;373:123–126.
5. Ho DD. Time to hit HIV, early and hard. *N Engl J Med.* 1995;333:450–451.
6. Carpenter CC, Fischl MA, Hammer SM, et al. Antiretroviral therapy for HIV infection in 1997. *JAMA.* 1997;277:1962–1969.
7. Tisdale M, Kemp SD, Parry NR, Larder BA. Rapid in vitro selection of human immunodeficiency virus type I resistant to 3′ thiacytidine inhibitors due to a mutation in the YMDD region of reverse transcriptase. *Proc Natl Acad Sci U S A.* 1993;90:5633–5656.
8. Condra JH, Schleif WA, Blahy OM, et al. Dynamics of acquired HIV-1 clinical resistance to the protease inhibitor MK-639. In: *4th International Workshop on HIV Drug Resistance*, abstract 72. 1995. Sardinia, Italy July 6–9, 1995.
9. Condra JH, Schleif WA, Blahy OM, et al. In vivo emergence of HIV-1 variants resistant to multiple protease inhibitors. *Nature.* 1995;374:569–571.

10. Koda-Kimble MA, Young LY, eds. *Applied Therapeutics: The Clinical Use of Drugs.* 5th ed. Vancouver, WA: Applied Therapeutics, Inc.; 1992.
11. Van der Meer JWM. The influence of gastric activity on the bioavailability of ketoconazole. *J Antimicrob Chemother.* 1980;6:552–554.
12. American Society of Hospital Pharmacists, eds. *AHFS Drug Information 96.* Bethesda, MD: American Society of Hospital Pharmacists, 1996.
13. Mitchell AS. Fluconazole and phenytoin, a predictable interaction. *BMJ.* 1989; 298:1315.
14. Roche. *Invirase* package insert. December 1995.
15. Dorr RT, Fritz WL. *Cancer Chemotherapy Handbook.* New York: Elsevier North Holland; 1980.
16. Gilman AG, Rall TW, Nies AS, et al, eds. *Goodman and Gilman's The Pharmacologic Basis of Therapeutics.* 8th ed. New York: Pergamon Press; 1990.
17. McCoy LK, Smith CH. *Food Medications Interactions.* 6th ed. Phoenix: Food Medication Interactions Inc.; 1988.
18. Johnson R. Adverse effects with acyclovir and meperidine. *Ann Intern Med.* 1985;103:962.
19. Bach MC. Possible drug interactions during treatment with azidothymidine and acyclovir for AIDS. *N Engl J Med.* 1987;316:547.
20. Youle MS, Clarbour J, Gazzard B, Chanas A. Severe hypocalcemia in AIDS patients treated with foscarnet and pentamidine. *Lancet.* 1988;i:1455–1456. Letter.
21. Porche D. Treatment review: cytovene IV and capsules. *JANAC.* 1996;7(1):50–55.
22. Williams SJ. Inhibition of theophylline metabolism by interferon. *Lancet.* 1987; ii:939.
23. Vogt MW, Hirsch MS. Treatment of human immunodeficiency virus infections. *Inf Dis Clin North Am.* 1988;1:323–339.
24. Jacobus Pharmaceutical Co. *Dapsone* package insert. September 1991.
25. Cooley TP, Kunches LM, Saunders CA, et al. Once daily administration of 2′,3′-dideoxyinosine (ddI) in patients with the acquired immunodeficiency syndrome or AIDS-related complex. *N Engl J Med.* 1990;322:1340–1345.
26. Amodio-Groton M, Currier J. HIV drug interactions. *AIDS Clin Care.* 1992;4(4): 1–5.
27. Glaxo-Wellcome. *Epivir* package insert. November 1995.
28. Bristol Myers Squibb Immunology. *Zerit* package insert. June 1994.
29. AIDS Clinical Trials Group (ACTG) Study. Memo to ACTG Principal Investigators, October 30, 1996.
30. Glaxo-Wellcome. *Retrovir* package insert. June 1995.
31. Sattler FR, Ko R, Antoniskis D, et al. Acetaminophen does not impair clearance of zidovudine. *Ann Int Med.* 1991;114:937–940.
32. Holmes MA, Kornhauser DM, Petty BG, et al. Probenecid inhibits the metabo-

lism and renal clearance of zidovudine (AZT) in human volunteers. *Pharm Res.* 1990;7:41.
33. Krown SE. Approaches to interferon combination therapy in the treatment of AIDS. *Semin Oncol.* 1990;17(1):38–41.
34. Burroughs Wellcome. *Zidovudine* package insert. 1990.
35. Project Inform. *The HIV Drug Book.* New York: Simon and Schuster; 1995.
36. Pharmacia Upjohn. *Rescriptor* package insert, April 1997.
37. Roxanne Pharmaceuticals. *Viramune* package insert, August 1996.
38. Merck. *Crixivan* package insert. 1996.
39. Agouron Pharmaceuticals. *Viracept* (nelfinavir mesylate) package insert. March 1997.
40. Hoffman LaRoche. *Saquinavir* package insert. June 1994.
41. Abbott Laboratories. *Norvir* drug package insert. February 1996.
42. Geletko SM, Dudley MN. Drug interactions of medications used to prevent and treat opportunistic infections. *Opportun Compl HIV.* 1995;4(3):54–66.
43. Miller MS, Bates JH. Amphotericin toxicity. *Ann Intern Med.* 1969;71:1089–1091.
44. Pfizer/Roerig. *Fluconazole* package insert. November 1994.
45. Glynn AM, Brunner E. Effects of ketoconazole on methylprednisolone pharmacokinetics and cortisol excretion. *Clin Pharmacol Ther.* 1986;39:654–659.
46. Carlson JA, Shepherd JM, Moller J. Effect of pH on disintegration and dissolution of ketoconazole tablets. *Am J Hosp Pharmacol.* 1983;40:1334–1336.
47. Smith AG. Potentiation of oral anticoagulants by ketoconazole. *BMJ.* 1984;288: 188–189.
48. Shephard JH, Sheehan M, Ho M. Cyclosporine-ketoconazole: a potentially dangerous drug-drug interaction. *Clin Pharmacol.* 1986;5:468–472.
49. Englehard D, Meunier F. Interaction of ketoconazole with rifampin and isoniazid. *N Engl J Med.* 1984;311:1681–1684.
50. Physician's Desk Reference, 50th edition, 1996, Montvale, NJ: Medical Economics.
51. Mattila MJ, Lotawongs P, Barone JA. Effect of aluminum hydroxide and glycopyrrhonium on the absorption of ethambutol and alcohol in man. *Br J Clin Pharmacol.* 1978;5:161–166.
52. Hurwitz A, Schlozman A. Effects of antacids on gastrointestinal absorption of isoniazid in rat and man. *Am Rev Respir Dis.* 1974;109:41–47.
53. Kopanoff DE, Ferguson RM, Romberg GP. Isoniazid-related hepatitis. *Am Rev Respir Dis.* 1982;117:991–994.
54. Lal S, Coakley CS. Effect of rifampin and isoniazid on liver function. *BMJ.* 1972;1:148–150.
55. Berman G. Drug interaction: decreased serum concentrations of rifampin when given with PAS. *Lancet.* 1971;i:800.

56. Prober CG. Effect of rifampin on chloramphenicol levels. *N Engl J Med.* 1987; 312:788-790.
57. Breckinridge AM, Ascione FJ, Morrelli HF. Interaction between oral contraceptives and other drugs. *Pharmacol Ther.* 1979;7:617–618.
58. Schentag JJ. Time-dependent interactions between antacids and quinolone antibiotics. *Clin Pharmacol Ther.* 1988;43:135.
59. Gazzard BG. Problems of chemotherapy in multiply infected AIDS patients. *Trans R Soc Trop Med Hyg.* 1990;84(suppl):25–33.
60. Covington TR, DiPalma JR, Hussar DA, et al. *Drug Facts and Comparisons.* St. Louis, MO: Lippincott; 1991.
61. Jacobson MA, O'Donnell JJ. Approaches to the treatment of cytomegalovirus retinitis: gancyclovir and foscarnet. *J Acquir Immune Defic Syndr.* 1994; 4(suppl 1):S11–S15.
62. Chaisson GM. Patient education: whose responsibility is it and who should be doing it? *Nurs Admin Q.* 1980;4:1–11.
63. Brown CJ. The AIDS clinical trials information service (ACTIS). *JANAC.* 1996; 7(1):37–45.

CHAPTER 4

Opportunistic Infections

Joan A. Piemme, RN, MNEd, FAAN

Chapter Preview

- Fungal Infections
- Mycobacterial Infections
- Viral Infections
- *Pneumocystis* Infection
- Protozoal Infections
- Bacterial Infections

Opportunistic infections (OIs) are the single most frequent cause of morbidity and mortality among people with HIV disease. An OI generally results from a pathogen found in the environment that rarely causes serious illness in the immunocompetent person, but can be life threatening in an immunocompromised person. OIs are usually a reactivation of a previous primary infection. Concurrent or consecutive infections with different organisms may occur because of the degree of immunosuppression. A listing of the more common pathogens identified in people with HIV and their related infections is presented in Table 4.1.

Virulence among the HIV-associated OIs varies widely. Vulnerability to these organisms is dependent in part on the extent of immunosuppression as indirectly reflected by the CD4+ lymphocyte count. Although the CD4+ count is only an indirect or surrogate measure of HIV activity, it is very useful in determining the risk of developing specific opportunistic infections.[1] Appendix A includes those infections that the CDC classifies as AIDS-defining infections. In HIV-infected adults and adolescents, serious OIs do not usually develop until the CD4+ count falls below 200 cells/mm^3.

Table 4.2 lists the CD4+ level at which the organisms lead to infection, along with their common manifestations. An organism may affect different organ systems or exhibit varying severity depending on the degree of immunosuppression. Many organisms disseminate to other areas of the body. For example, *Candida albicans* affects the oral cavity and vagina at a CD4+ count between 200 cells/mm^3, and 500 cells/mm^3, but does not generally involve the esophagus until the CD4+ count is <200 cells/mm^3, or become disseminated (rare with *C. albicans*) until late in the course of AIDS.

Fungal Infections

Candida albicans (Candidiasis)

Biologic Basis and Epidemiology

Candida infections are the most common of the OIs in patients with HIV disease, affecting virtually all patients at some time during their illness. While there are many species of *Candida*, the most common species seen in HIV disease is *C. albicans*. This organism is ubiquitous—found in soil, food, inanimate objects, and hospital environments. It is also a part of normal body flora, and therefore most of these infections are endogenous.

Table 4.1 HIV Opportunistic Infections

Organism by Type	Condition Name (abbreviation)
A. FUNGAL INFECTIONS	
Candida albicans	Candidiasis
Coccidioides immitis	Coccidioidomycosis
Cryptococcus neoformans	Cryptococcosis
Histoplasma capsulatum	Histoplasmosis
B. MYCOBACTERIAL INFECTIONS	
Mycobacterium tuberculosis	Tuberculosis (TB)
Mycobacterium avium intracellulare	MAI (MAC disease)
C. VIRAL INFECTIONS	
Cytomegalovirus	CMV infection (CMV)
Herpes simplex virus	HSV infection (HSV)
Varicella zoster virus	Herpes zoster (HZ)
JC virus	Progressive multifocal leukoencephalopathy
Human papilloma virus	HPV infection (HPV)
D. PNEUMOCYSTIS INFECTIONS	
Pneumocystis carinii	*P. carinii* pneumonia (PCP)
E. PROTOZOAL INFECTIONS	
Cryptosporidium parvum	Cryptosporidiosis
Toxoplasma gondii	Toxoplasmosis (Toxo)
Isospora belli	Isosporiasis
Microsporidia	Microsporidiosis
F. BACTERIAL INFECTIONS	
Streptococcus pneumoniae	—
Haemophilus influenzae	—
Pseudomonas aeruginosa	—
Salmonella species	—

Table 4.2 Commonly Occurring Opportunistic Infections Based on CD4+ Count

CD4+ cell count/mm³	Organism	Common Manifestations
<500	*Streptococcus pneumoniae* (B)	Community-acquired pneumonia
	Haemophilus influenzae (B)	Community-acquired pneumonia
	Mycobacterium tuberculosis (M)	Pulmonary tuberculosis
	Candida species (F)	Oropharyngeal and vaginal candidiasis
	Herpes simplex virus (V)	Orogenital herpes
	Varicella zoster virus (V)	Dermatomal zoster (shingles)
	Epstein-Barr virus (V)	Oral hairy leukoplakia
	Cryptosporidium parvum (P)	Self-limited diarrhea
<250	*Coccidioides immitis* (F)	Pneumonia
<200	*Pneumocystis carinii* (P)	Pneumonia
	Cryptosporidium parvum (P)	Chronic diarrhea
<100	*Toxoplasma gondii* (P)	Encephalitis
	Microsporidia (P)	Diarrhea
	Candida species (F)	Esophagitis
	Cryptococcus neoformans (F)	Meningitis
	Mycobacterium tuberculosis (M)	Disseminated or extrapulmonary tuberculosis
	Herpes simplex virus (V)	Disseminated or aggressive herpes
	Varicella zoster virus (V)	Disseminated herpes zoster
	Epstein-Barr virus (V)	Primary CNS lymphoma
	Histoplasma capsulatum (F)	Disseminated or pulmonary
<50	*Mycobacterium avium intracellulare*	Disseminated *M. avium* complex
	Cytomegalovirus (V)	Retinitis, GI disease, encephalitis
	JC virus (V)	Progressive multifocal leukoencephalopathy, dementia

B = bacterial; CNS = central nervous system; F = fungal; GI = gastrointestinal; M = mycobacterial; P = protozoal; V = viral.

Their occurrence is related to the interruption of normal host mechanisms including immunosuppression, altered skin and mucous membrane barriers, and drug therapy. Human-to-human transmission occurs with mother to child after vaginal delivery, balanitis in uncircumcised men who have sex without a condom, and nosocomial transmission in health care settings.

Oropharyngeal candidiasis is a common, early manifestation of HIV infection. This localized infection, occurring with a CD4+ count as high as 500/mm^3 or higher, is viewed as a predictor of disease progression, irrespective of the CD4+ count. Recurrent vaginal candidiasis, which also occurs with a high CD4+ count, is often the first and most common problem in HIV-infected women. Esophageal candidiasis occurs more frequently with increased immunosuppression (i.e., CD4+ count < 100/mm^3). Candidemia in persons with HIV infection is uncommon except in those with certain predisposing factors. These characteristics are the same that predispose other populations to candidemia: (1) presence of venous access devices, (2) prolonged hospitalization, and (3) therapy with broad-spectrum antibacterial agents.

Presentation and Assessment

PRESENTATION. Oropharyngeal candidiasis most commonly presents as pseudomembranous white patches, which are easily removed from the oral mucosa. It can also present in erythematous form with smooth red patches on the palate, buccal mucosa, or tongue; as angular cheilitis with cracks or fissures at the corners of the mouth; and as *Candida leukoplakia* with white lesions that cannot be removed, similar to oral hairy leukoplakia.[1] Vaginal candidiasis presents with intense pruritus and a curdlike vaginal discharge. It is frequently recurrent and refractory to treatment. Esophageal candidiasis presents as dysphagia or odynophagia.

DIAGNOSIS. Oropharyngeal or vaginal candidiasis is diagnosed by wet-mount and/or potassium hydroxide (KOH) smear showing pseudohyphae or budding yeast forms. Diagnosis by tissue culture is generally unreliable because of the difficulty distinguishing between infection and colonization. Diagnosis is often made presumptively by visual inspection. Esophageal diagnosis may also be made by endoscopy with a biopsy of the tissue.

Related Care and Common Clinical Problems

If a definitive diagnosis of HIV infection has not been made, oropharyngeal or vaginal candidiasis may be considered as sentinel disease, indicating the need for careful history and counseling for HIV testing. Patient teaching focuses on primary and secondary prevention measures of candidiasis, such as oral hygiene, skin care, hand washing, and self-monitoring by assessing skin folds and genital and perianal areas. Table 4.3 summarizes symptoms and common clinical problems relevant to candidiasis.

Coccidioides immitis (Coccidioidomycosis)

Biologic Basis and Epidemiology

C. immitis, found in the soil, is endemic in the southwestern United States. Outside endemic areas, the disease occurs in travelers to endemic areas, in former residents of endemic areas, and as infections acquired by inhalation of spore-laden dust. In endemic regions as many as one third of the residents have had a primary infection due to *C. immitis*. Coccidioidomycosis usually occurs in patients with a CD4+ count $<250/mm^3$.

Presentation and Assessment

PRESENTATION. Primary infection may be asymptomatic or involve nonspecific, progressive constitutional signs and symptoms of fever, malaise, weight loss, cough, and fatigue, resembling an acute influenzal illness. Reactivation may occur with immunosuppression. With severe immunosuppression, disseminated or extrapulmonary disease occurs.

DIAGNOSIS. The main obstacle to detection is low index of suspicion. Chest radiographs most often show diffuse interstitial or nodular infiltrates. Definitive diagnosis is by demonstrating the fungus on culture or by microscopic examination of sputum, pus, urine, or CSF.

Related Care and Common Clinical Problems

Primary prevention is to restrict travel to the southwest desert area. Obtain an accurate travel and residential history for secondary prevention. Because reactivation may occur with immunosuppression, those at risk should be taught the signs and symptoms of the disease. Table 4.3 summarizes symptoms and common clinical problems relevant to coccidioidomycosis.

Table 4.3 Common Clinical Problems Associated with Opportunistic Infections: Fungal and Mycobacterial Organisms

Clinical Problem	Fungal				Mycobacterial	
	Candida	*Coccidioides*	*Cryptococcus*	*Histoplasma*	TB	MAI
A. NEUROLOGICAL IMPAIRMENTS						
Confusion, delirium			√	√		
Memory loss, dementia			√	√		
Decreased concentration, alertness, and alterations in consciousness						
Impaired coordination, balance, mobility						
Seizures			√			
B. NUTRITION-RELATED CHANGES						
Anorexia, cachexia, wasting, malnutrition	√	√		√	√	√
Taste change	√					
Xerostomia						
Stomatitis, mucositis	√					
Nausea, vomiting, retching						
Constipation						
Diarrhea				√		√
Fluid, electrolyte imbalance						
Dysphagia (+)	√					
C. RESPIRATORY CHANGES						
Dyspnea			√		√	
Cough		√	√	√	√	

D. Changes in Host Defenses						
Thrombocytopenia				√		
Neutropenia				√		
E. Skin Problems						
Itching (pruritis)	√					
Dry skin						
Skin, nail lesions			√			
Rash						
F. Psychosocial Responses						
Anxiety	√	√	√	√	√	√
Depression					√	√
Psychosis, mania						
Grief, loss	√	√	√	√	√	√
G. Changes in Functional Capacity and Performance						
Fatigue		√		√	√	√
Sleep alterations	√					
Visual changes			√			
H. Discomfort						
Pain	√		√	√	√	√
Peripheral neuropathy						
Night sweats					√	√
Fever, chills, shivering		√	√	√	√	√

TB = tuberculosis; MAI = *Mycobacterium avium intracellulare*.

Cryptococcus neoformans (Cryptococcosis)

Biologic Basis and Epidemiology

This ubiquitous organism, found in dirt and soil contaminated by bird droppings, is aerosolized and inhaled. After being inhaled, the organism may become dormant in the lungs or may spread to other parts of the body, particularly the CNS. Reactivation occurs with immunosuppression. Cryptococcal meningitis, the most common OI of the CNS in HIV-infected patients with a CD4+ count of <100/mm^3, is the most life-threatening of the fungal infections. *C. neoformans* is the most common cause of fungal pneumonia in people with AIDS. Cutaneous lesions occur in 10 to 15% of patients with disseminated disease and may precede CNS symptoms.

Presentation and Assessment

PRESENTATION. Cryptococcal infection, particularly meningitis, may be elusive and subtle. Signs and symptoms of CNS infection include fever, malaise, stiff neck, memory loss, confusion, seizures, and photophobia, with or without headache. Pulmonary infection presents with fever, cough, dyspnea, and pleuritic chest pain. Cutaneous manifestation presents as painless lesions that mimic Kaposi's sarcoma and *molluscum contagiosum.*

DIAGNOSIS. Serum cryptococcal antigen is more than 99% indicative for cryptococcal disease but does not distinguish meningitis from cryptococcemia. If positive, a lumbar puncture should be performed for confirmation of meningitis. The CSF usually reveals increased opening pressure, low white blood cell count with a predominance of lymphocytes, elevated protein, and decreased glucose. Cultures of the organism from the CSF provide a definitive diagnosis and are positive in 80 to 90% of patients. India Ink, positive in 70 to 90% of patients, can make a diagnosis before antigen or culture results are available. A computed tomographic scan is often performed to rule out toxoplasmosis or lymphoma.

Related Care and Common Clinical Problems

Patient and family teaching focuses on self-monitoring and observation, especially to detect cognitive impairment and changes in personality or behavior. Emphasis is on lifelong suppressive therapy after an acute episode to prevent relapse. Table 4.3 summarizes symptoms and common clinical problems relevant to cryptococcosis.

Histoplasma capsulatum (Histoplasmosis)

Biologic Basis and Epidemiology

H. capsulatum exists as mold in soil contaminated by bird and bat droppings or other organic material. Five to ten percent of patients with HIV develop this infection when spores are inhaled. The majority live in or have traveled to endemic areas in the Midwest or south central United States, the Caribbean, and Central and South America. Patients with AIDS who have a CD4+ count <100/mm^3 and have lived in endemic areas are at risk for disseminated disease due to reactivation of a latent infection or reinfection from constant exposure. The relative infrequency of infection to date is due at least in part to the disparity between the primarily metropolitan geographic distribution of HIV disease and endemic areas for *H. capsulatum.*[2]

Presentation and Assessment

PRESENTATION. Cough accompanied by fever is the most common initial complaint. Presentation is often subacute and progressive, with most immunocompromised patients demonstrating disseminated disease rather than pneumonitis. Signs and symptoms of disseminated disease include fever, weight loss, night sweats, fatigue, abdominal pain, nausea, diarrhea, myelosuppression, and hepatosplenomegaly. Anywhere from 5 to 20% of patients will have CNS abnormalities, including encephalopathy, meningitis, and focal brain lesions. Although usually a subacute illness, approximately 10% of patients with disseminated disease present with a sepsis syndrome characterized by hypotension, disseminated intravascular coagulopathy (DIC), and multiorgan failure.

DIAGNOSIS. Chest radiographs in patients presenting with pneumonia demonstrate diffuse bilateral interstitial infiltrates. However, one third of patients with disseminated infection will have a normal chest radiograph. Diagnosis may also be impaired due to a low index of suspicion. Definitive diagnosis is made with cultures of fungus from blood, or identification in bone marrow, liver, or sputum. A small percentage of patients (5–10%) initially have cutaneous lesions from which *H. capsulatum* can be identified through biopsy and culture.

Related Care and Common Clinical Problems

Primary prevention emphasizes restriction of travel to endemic areas, whereas secondary prevention includes obtaining an accurate travel and residential history. People with HIV residing in endemic areas should be instructed to avoid high-risk activities and areas likely to be contaminated. Table 4.3 summarizes symptoms and common clinical problems relevant to histoplasmosis. Lifelong maintenance therapy is required after treatment for an acute illness.

Mycobacterial Infections

Mycobacterium tuberculosis (Tuberculosis)

Biologic Basis and Epidemiology

Until the mid 1980s, tuberculosis (TB) was a declining disease. Today, depending on the geographic location and demographic features of the patient population, 4 to 50% of those patients with TB are coinfected with HIV. TB is most common in racial and ethnic minorities, especially those living in poverty or crowded conditions. TB may be the initial presentation of HIV infection because it occurs at higher CD4+ levels (300/mm^3 or higher) than many other OIs. HIV-infected individuals have a 30 to 40% risk of developing active TB after close contact with an infected person.[3,4] Those with a latent infection have an increased risk of progression to active disease, most particularly injection drug users.

M. tuberculosis is an aerobic organism transmitted almost exclusively by aerosolized respiratory secretions. A person with a pulmonary lesion can aerosolize droplets by coughing, singing, or even talking. These droplets can remain airborne for up to 48 hours. Nosocomial outbreaks have occurred in health care settings and congregate facilities. Multidrug-resistant TB, resistant to at least two established pharmacological agents, has a much shorter interval between diagnosis and death than nondrug-resistant TB.

Presentation and Assessment

PRESENTATION. Signs and symptoms vary with the degree of immunosuppression. Pulmonary TB is most common with early HIV disease (CD4+ count between 300 and 500 cells/mm^3), presenting with cough, dyspnea, hemoptysis, lymphadenopathy, and chest pain. In patients with greater immunosuppression (CD4+ count < 200/mm^3) features of TB are more atypical. General manifestations include fever, night sweats, weight loss, and fatigue. With advanced HIV disease, miliary TB is more frequent, involving the lymphatic system, CNS (parenchymal and meningeal), soft tissue, bone marrow, liver, and other viscera.

DIAGNOSIS. In the HIV-infected individual, a positive purified protein derivative (PPD) is defined as >5 mm of induration at 48 to 72 hours using the Mantoux intradermal method. Because anergy frequently occurs in late HIV infection, a negative PPD does not exclude the possibility of TB. Chest radiographs show findings typical of apical and cavitary infiltrates in patients with mild to moderate immunosuppression. With AIDS, findings may also be atypical and demonstrate intrathoracic adenopathy, extrapulmonary or disseminated disease, and bacteremia.[5] Diagnosis is confirmed by sputum for acid-fast bacilli (AFB) stain and culture repeated three times. Initial isolates should undergo drug susceptibility testing. Because of the high incidence of bacteremia, blood cultures for AFB should be obtained.[1] Diagnosis of miliary TB may require cultures of specimens from bone marrow, lymph nodes, brain tissue, CSF, urine, or stool.

Related Care and Common Clinical Problems

Individuals who are HIV-infected should be advised to have an initial screening for TB. PPD testing is strongly urged for those family and health care workers who may have had contact with people with TB or who could be infected, such as workers in correctional institutions and homeless shelters. Patients who are actively coughing and whose TB status is not known should be tested. These patients should wear a mask whenever outside an isolation unit until results are known. Due to nosocomial transmission, HIV-infected patients and health care workers need to be protected by the implementation of infection control measures, including (1) active patient finding and surveillance, (2) use of fitted respiratory masks and use of isolation rooms with 6-hour air exchanges, and (3) proper isolation signage.[6] Respiratory isolation should be continued for 2 weeks after initiation of therapy. Table 4.3 summarizes symptoms and common clinical problems relevant to pulmonary tuberculosis.

Mycobacterium avium intracellulare (MAI; MAC Disease)

Biologic Basis and Epidemiology

MAC is composed of two closely related species: *M. avium* and *M. intracellulare*. Before the era of AIDS, non-TB mycobacteria rarely caused serious illness, but now they are the most common cause of systemic bacterial infection in AIDS, affecting 15 to 40% of patients.[7] MAC is ubiquitous, found in water, soil, food, and animal sources. However, it is unclear which environmental sources are responsible for human infection. The incidence of MAC infection is increasing due to the extended survival of immunosuppressed patients. The most important risk factor is profound immune suppression with a CD4+ count of <50/mm³. Disseminated MAC is thought to follow primary infection rather than a reactivation of latent disease.

Presentation and Assessment

PRESENTATION. In patients with AIDS, MAC bacteremia is the most common syndrome. The most frequent signs and symptoms are multiple and nonspecific: fever, fatigue, weight loss, anorexia, nausea and vomiting, night sweats, diarrhea, abdominal pain, hepatosplenomegaly, and lymphadenopathy. Unlike *Mycobacterium tuberculosis*, respiratory symptoms are uncommon with MAC.

DIAGNOSIS. Positive blood cultures are explicitly diagnostic of invasive disease. Diagnosis is also confirmed by biopsy with AFB stain. Because the respiratory and gastrointestinal tracts are frequently colonized with MAC before dissemination occurs, cultures of sputum and stool are not diagnostic when used alone.[7] Culture of normally sterile sites such as the bone marrow, liver, or lymph nodes may reveal disseminated MAC prior to blood cultures. Laboratory studies usually demonstrate anemia and elevated alkaline phosphatase.

Related Management and Common Clinical Problems

Because chemoprophylaxis is an established method of prevention, patients need to understand the importance of prophylaxis or long-term maintenance therapy after treatment for active disease.[8] Table 4.3 summarizes symptoms and common clinical problems relevant to MAC disease.

Viral Infections

Cytomegalovirus (CMV, CMV Infection)

Biologic Basis and Epidemiology

CMV, a herpes virus, is the most common cause of serious opportunistic viral disease in people with AIDS. Reactivation of infection or superinfection with new CMV strains occurs in more than 40% of people with advanced HIV disease (CD4+ count < 50/mm³). Forty to sixty percent of the US population has antibodies to CMV, having contracted primary infection during childhood through a variety of routes or during young adulthood through sexual transmission. A distinction must be made between the presence of CMV and CMV disease because CMV is shed in blood, urine, semen, and cervical secretions, and is a nonspecific finding. It may be found in as many as 50% of patients with advanced HIV disease in the absence of signs and symptoms of active infection. Greater than 90% of homosexual men in the United States are CMV positive.[9] In CMV-infected AIDS patients, the virus may reactivate and cause retinitis, colitis, esophagitis, and wasting syndrome. CMV is found at autopsy in almost all patients who have died of advanced disease.[9]

Presentation and Assessment

PRESENTATION. Clinical presentation varies depending on the organ system involved. CMV retinitis is the most common clinical form (25%). Depending on the location of the retinal lesions, ocular disease may be asymptomatic or present with painless loss of visual acuity and symptoms of "floaters" or visual field deficits. Left untreated, blindness may occur in a matter of months. The gastrointestinal tract, involving the esophagus or colon, is the second most common site of involvement. Symptoms associated with CMV esophagitis are fever, odynophagia, dysphagia, and substernal or abdominal pain, in contrast to fever, bloody diarrhea, and abdominal pain with CMV colitis.

DIAGNOSIS. CMV retinitis, on ophthalmoscopic examination, is characterized by creamy yellow-white exudates with retinal hemorrhage. Gastrointestinal disease is diagnosed by endoscopic examination showing ulceration, and tissue biopsy demonstrating CMV inclusions. CMV encephalitis is presumed based on periventricular changes on magnetic resonance imaging (MRI) brain scan rather than a brain biopsy. CMV serologies may not determine primary CMV infection because the disease almost always represents a reactivation of latent virus. Theoretically, immunoglobulin (Ig) M antibody develops only during primary CMV infection, but it may reappear during CMV reactivation.[10]

Related Care and Common Clinical Problems

Instruct patients about early detection of visual changes. A visual grid may be helpful for those at high risk for infection. Primary prevention includes consistent, safer sexual practices for HIV-infected persons, and child care providers need to practice meticulous hand washing after contact with body fluids. Patients infected with HIV who are CMV antibody negative should receive only CMV-negative or leukocyte-depleted blood products, to reduce the chance of acquiring CMV.[11] Most adults have been infected with CMV and have antibodies to CMV. Those coinfected with HIV who do not have evidence of disease due to CMV do not require any specific treatment, although prophylactic regimens are being studied. Table 4.4 summarizes symptoms and common clinical problems relevant to CMV. Educate the patient about chronic maintenance and suppressive therapy after induction therapy for acute illness.

Table 4.4 Common Clinical Problems Associated with Opportunistic Infections: Viral Organisms

Clinical Problem	CMV	HSV	HZ	PML	HPV
A. NEUROLOGICAL IMPAIRMENTS					
Confusion, delirium				√	
Memory loss, dementia	√			√	
Decreased concentration, alertness, and alterations in consciousness	√			√	
Impaired coordination, balance, mobility				√	
B. NUTRITION-RELATED CHANGES					
Anorexia, cachexia, wasting, malnutrition					
Taste change					
Xerostomia					
Stomatitis, mucositis					
Nausea, vomiting, retching					
Constipation					
Diarrhea					
Fluid, electrolyte imbalance					
Dysphagia	√	√			
C. RESPIRATORY CHANGES					
Dyspnea					
Cough					

Table 4.4 *Continued*

Clinical Problem	CMV	HSV	HZ	PML	HPV
D. SEXUALITY CHANGES					
Decreased interest, impaired performance/activity		√			
Altered body image		√	√		
E. CHANGES IN HOST DEFENSES					
Thrombocytopenia					
Neutropenia					
F. SKIN PROBLEMS					
Itching (pruritus)					
Dry skin					
Skin, nail lesions			√		
Rash			√		√
G. PSYCHOSOCIAL RESPONSES					
Anxiety	√	√	√	√	
Depression	√	√	√		
Psychosis, mania					
Grief, loss	√	√	√	√	
H. CHANGES IN FUNCTIONAL CAPACITY AND PERFORMANCE					
Fatigue					√
Sleep alterations					
Visual changes	√				
I. DISCOMFORT					
Pain	√				
Peripheral neuropathy					
Night sweats					
Fever, chills, shivering	√				

CMV = cytomegalovirus; HSV = herpes simplex virus; HZ = herpes zoster; PML = progressive multifocal leukoencephalopathy; HPV = human papilloma virus.

Herpes Simplex Virus (HSV, HSV Infection)

Biologic Basis and Epidemiology

HSV is a herpes virus. Despite the close relationship of the two types of virus, HSV-1 and HSV-2, they display different epidemiological patterns and routes of transmission. HSV-1 is transmitted primarily by contact with oral mucous membranes and salivary secretions. HSV-2 spreads primarily by sexual transmission, most commonly associated with anogenital lesions. Following primary infection, HSV becomes latent in the neurons of sensory nerve ganglia. Individuals with HIV infection are at risk for HSV infection. The CD4+ count is generally $<100/mm^3$. Transmission may occur from those who are asymptomatic excretors as well as those who are actively infected.

Presentation and Assessment

PRESENTATION. Cutaneous ulcerative lesions may appear on any part of the body, but facial, genital, and perianal lesions are most common. Orolabial infection may be mild or may involve painful vesicular lesions on the lips, tongue, or buccal mucosa. Genital lesions begin as small papules and progress to painful vesicles. Orolabial lesions can progress to severe oral stomatitis, and anogenital lesions may progress to large sloughing ulcers with fissures and fistulas. Persistent shedding can last for weeks. HSV is a common cause of anorectal proctitis. Recurrent lesions usually occur in the same region as the primary infection, often with burning, tingling, or itching before the vesicular eruption. HSV may also cause esophagitis with dysphagia and odynophagia. HSV esophageal disease must be distinguished from the more common opportunistic pathogens, CMV and *Candida.* Late-stage AIDS patients may have systemic HSV infections.

DIAGNOSIS. HIV infection is suggested by visual inspection, with confirmation by viral swab culture, Tzanck smear, biopsy, or direct fluorescent antibody stain. Serological tests for HSV are not helpful because HSV antibody prevalence rates are high in HIV-positive patients.

Related Care and Common Clinical Problems

An accurate history of prior HSV infections is essential to determine the potential for recurrence. Patient teaching includes safer sexual practices with infected partners. Asymptomatic excretors (those with a history of HSV infection) may also be infectious. Meticulous hand washing is necessary to prevent autoinoculation and secondary infection. Health care providers need to use barrier precautions when examining oral, genital, or anal lesions to prevent nosocomial transmission. Table 4.4 summarizes symptoms and common clinical problems relevant to HSV.

Varicella Zoster Virus (VZV, VZ Infection [Shingles], Zoster)

Biologic Basis and Epidemiology

Infection with VZV, also a herpes virus, may be the initial presentation of HIV infection and therefore could suggest the need for HIV testing in an otherwise healthy person.[1] VZV usually remains dermatomal with higher CD4+ counts. Recurrent or disseminated involvement is more common in advanced HIV disease with a CD4+ count of $<100/mm^3$. Primary VZV infection is chicken pox, becoming latent in dorsal root ganglia and reactivating at the cutaneous surface innervated by the ganglion.

Presentation and Assessment

PRESENTATION. Radicular pain, a localized burning, is the most common symptom, followed or accompanied by localized or segmented rash, then progressing to maculopapules along one to three dermatomes. If not treated, lesions may progress to fluid-filled contiguous vesicles. Many patients experience a painful postherpetic neuralgia for one or more months after the lesions have healed. Visceral dissemination to lung, liver, or CNS may be life threatening.

DIAGNOSIS. The clinical appearance of shingles is usually diagnostic.[9] Scrapings of cutaneous lesions can be stained with specific fluorescein-conjugated monoclonal antibodies to confirm the presence of VZV antigens.

Related Care and Common Clinical Problems

Instruct patients with AIDS who are varicella naive that infection can result from exposure to chicken pox, with the rash appearing about 14 days after exposure. If exposed to chicken pox or herpes zoster, give VZIG within 96 hours. For VZV primary prevention, avoid any contact with varicella. Infected patients need instructions regarding wound care, the need for isolation, and pain management as secondary prevention measures. Chronic suppressive therapy may be indicated for prevention of recurrence. Table 4.4 summarizes symptoms and common clinical problems relevant to VZV.

Progressive Multifocal Leukoencephalopathy (PML, JC Viral Infection)

Biologic Basis and Epidemiology

PML is caused by the JC virus, a human papovavirus, causing rapidly progressive demyelination in the CNS. Only severely immunosuppressed patients with a CD4+ count of <50/mm³ are likely to develop PML. Rates are estimated at approximately 5% of patients with advanced HIV disease.

Presentation and Assessment

PRESENTATION. Patients demonstrate diverse focal neurological signs including selective intellectual deficits, cranial nerve palsies, hemiparesis, weakness, and gait abnormalities. Altered mental status and personality changes increase rapidly to progressive dementia, encephalopathy, and coma leading to death, generally within 6 months.

DIAGNOSIS. Head CT with contrast or a brain MRI shows single or multiple enhancing, infiltrative, gray-white to white matter lesions, particularly in the parieto-occipital region. Serum and CSF serology are nondiagnostic because of the high prevalence of JC virus in the general population. Brain biopsy and tissue in situ hybridization studies may be necessary to confirm the diagnosis.

Related Care and Common Clinical Problems

Family members or care givers of patients with advanced HIV disease need to be instructed about the signs and symptoms of PML. Table 4.4 summarizes symptoms and common clinical problems relevant to PML.

Human Papilloma Virus (HPV, HPV Infection)

Biologic Basis and Epidemiology

Infection with HPV is the most prevalent sexually transmitted disease in North America. HPV (genital warts) occurs with increased frequency in immunosuppressed patients. HIV infection in women increases the risk of developing HPV-induced cervical neoplasia (see Chapters 6 and 25).

Presentation and Assessment

PRESENTATION. External genital warts in women and perirectal warts in homosexual or bisexual men are usually indicative of the presence of internal warts.

DIAGNOSIS. Cytological dysplasia is evident on smears from the anal area or uterine cervix. Condylomata may also be biopsied for confirmation.

Related Care and Common Clinical Problems

Patient teaching for HIV-infected women includes advocating an annual pelvic examination, PAP smear, and colposcopy for women. Anoscopy with swabs should be encouraged for HIV-infected men. Primary prevention stresses safer sexual practices for men and women. Table 4.4 summarizes symptoms and common clinical problems relevant to HPV.

Pneumocystis Infections

Pneumocystis carinii (PCP, P. carinii *pneumonia)*

Biologic Basis and Epidemiology

PCP is one of the most common HIV-associated OIs and is the most common cause of pulmonary disease in AIDS. In the past, PCP was diagnosed in 50 to 80% of patients with AIDS, but with primary and secondary prophylaxis, the incidence is substantially reduced. Approximately one half of cases of PCP occur in the presence of previously undiagnosed HIV infection. Without prophylaxis, PCP most commonly presents when the CD4+ count is less than 200/mm^3. The transmission of *P. carinii* is thought to be airborne, but the source and mechanism of infection are unknown. Because of the high prevalence of *P. carinii* antibodies in children and adults, PCP in the immunocompromised person is thought to be a reactivation of latent infection.

Presentation and Assessment

PRESENTATION. The most common symptoms are fever, dyspnea, and a nonproductive cough. Presentation is often insidious and in some instances the initial presentation is asymptomatic. Pneumothorax has been reported in 2% of patients. Because PCP is the most common disease associated with pneumothorax in patients with HIV disease, any AIDS patient with a spontaneous pneumothorax should be considered to have PCP until it is ruled out.[12]

DIAGNOSIS. Confirmatory procedures include sputum induction, bronchoalveolar lavage and transbronchial biopsy. Although the chest X-ray may be normal, when it is abnormal the most common findings are diffuse bilateral interstitial infiltrates. Arterial blood gases reveal hypoxemia—a low oxygen (O_2) saturation or desaturation with exercise is especially noteworthy. Serum lactate dehydrogenase (LDH) is usually elevated. It increases with the onset of infection and decreases with recovery. Gallium scanning may be indicated when the chest radiograph and arterial blood gases are normal. Pulmonary function tests demonstrate a decrease in vital capacity, total lung capacity, and diffusion capacity for carbon monoxide.

Related Care and Common Clinical Problems

When patients comply with primary and secondary prophylaxis, PCP is now largely preventable.[1] Table 4.5 summarizes symptoms and common clinical problems relevant to PCP.

Table 4.5 Common Clinical Problems Associated with Opportunistic Infections: Protozoal Organisms

Clinical Problem	PCP	Cryptosp	Toxo	Isosp	Microsp
A. NEUROLOGICAL IMPAIRMENTS					
Confusion, delirium					
Memory loss, dementia					
Decreased concentration, alertness, and alterations in consciousness					
Impaired coordination, balance, mobility					
B. NUTRITION-RELATED CHANGES					
Anorexia, cachexia, wasting, malnutrition	√	√		√	√
Taste change					
Xerostomia					
Stomatitis, mucositis					
Nausea, vomiting, retching		√			√
Constipation					
Diarrhea		√		√	√
Fluid, electrolyte imbalance		√		√	√
Dysphagia (+)					

Table 4.5 *Continued*

Clinical Problem	PCP	Cryptosp	Toxo	Isosp	Microsp
C. RESPIRATORY CHANGES					
Dyspnea	√				
Cough	√				
D. CHANGES IN HOST DEFENSES					
Thrombocytopenia					
Neutropenia					
E. SKIN PROBLEMS					
Itching (pruritus)					
Dry skin					
Skin, nail lesions					
Rash					
F. PSYCHOSOCIAL RESPONSES					
Anxiety	√	√		√	√
Depression		√		√	√
Psychosis, mania					
Grief, loss	√	√		√	√
G. CHANGES IN FUNCTIONAL CAPACITY AND PERFORMANCE					
Fatigue					
Sleep alterations					
Visual changes					
H. DISCOMFORT					
Pain	√		√	√	√
Peripheral neuropathy					
Night sweats					
Fever, chills, shivering	√				

PCP = *Pneumocystis carinii* pneumonia; Cryptosp = cryptosporidiosis; Toxo = toxoplasmosis; Isosp = isosporiasis; Microsp = microsporidiosis.

Protozoal Infections

Cryptosporidium parvum (Cryptosporidiosis)

Biologic Basis and Epidemiology

C. parvum, the only species of *Cryptosporidium* pathogenic for humans, is transmitted through fecally contaminated water used for drinking, recreational purposes, or food. It is a major cause of diarrhea in patients whose CD4+ counts are 200/mm^3 or less. The organism has an autoinfective capacity, which means it can complete its life cycle development within a single host. This autoinfective capacity may contribute to the refractory nature of the infection.[12] Oocysts can remain infective outside the body for 2 to 6 months and, when excreted, are immediately infective to the same host and to others.

Presentation and Assessment

PRESENTATION. The most common symptoms are profuse, watery diarrhea; severe, crampy abdominal pain; nausea; flatulence; and weight loss; which may lead to malabsorption, malnutrition, and wasting syndrome. Patients tend to have a protracted illness that increases in severity as immunosuppression increases.

DIAGNOSIS. Diagnosis is confirmed by modified acid-fast or fluorescent antibody stain of stool specimens or duodenal fluid. The organism may also be found by a small-bowel biopsy.

Related Care and Common Clinical Problems

Patient teaching for suspected infection includes infection control measures, including (1) enteric precautions; (2) precautions for feces, vomitus, and contaminated clothing/linens; and (3) meticulous hand washing to prevent person-to-person and fomite transmission. Preventive practices include drinking bottled water and safer sexual practices. When swimming, avoid swallowing water and avoid swimming in water that could be contaminated. During community outbreaks of cryptosporidiosis, boil tap water for 1 minute because chemical disinfectants are not effective against *C. parvum* oocysts.

During an acute diarrheal episode, parenteral hydration may be necessary to maintain fluid and electrolyte balance, and additional nutritional support (enteral or parenteral) may be indicated. A diet that is low lactose, low fat, and high protein is desirable. Table 4.5 summarizes symptoms and common clinical problems relevant to cryptosporidiosis.

Toxoplasma gondii (Toxoplasmosis)

Biologic Basis and Epidemiology

Toxoplasmosis is now a major cause of neurological morbidity and mortality with advanced HIV disease. Patients with CD4+ counts of <100/mm^3 are susceptible to toxoplasmosis, which infects through ingestion of oocysts from contact with cat feces or ingestion of rare or uncooked meat, vegetables, and unpasteurized dairy products. Most involve reactivation of a latent infection. It is the most common cause of CNS mass lesions in patients with AIDS[1]; however, it may also effect the heart, lungs, eyes, prostate, testes, and peritoneum.

Presentation and Assessment

PRESENTATION. Toxoplasmosis encephalitis, the most common clinical manifestation, has signs and symptoms of fever, headache, altered mental status, focal neurological deficits, and seizures. Neurological findings include hemiparesis; altered speech, vision or gait; cranial nerve palsies; and cerebellar dysfunction.

DIAGNOSIS. Laboratory studies are nonspecific. CT with contrast or brain MRI shows multiple bilateral enhancing mass lesions with edema. Examination of CSF is not usually helpful.[14] Diagnosis is established by a positive *T. gondii* titer with clinical and radiographic evidence of response to empiric therapy. Definitive diagnosis requires a brain biopsy.

Related Care and Common Clinical Problems

After a person is known to be HIV infected, testing for IgG antibody to *T. gondii* is recommended to detect latent infection, in addition to obtaining a serum toxoplasmosis titer. CSF titers are less sensitive, being positive in only 30 to 60% of patients with CNS toxoplasmosis.[14] Table 4.5 summarizes symptoms and common clinical problems relevant to toxoplasmosis. Patient teaching focuses on primary prevention (e.g., cooking meat until it is well done, washing fruits and vegetables, and wearing gloves when gardening). All HIV-infected people should be told to avoid direct contact with cat feces. Litter boxes should be cleaned daily using gloves. HIV-infected individuals do not need to give up their pets.

Isospora belli (Isosporiasis)

Biologic Basis and Epidemiology

Infection with *I. belli* is most common in the tropics and endemic in Africa, South America, and Asia. Approximately 1 to 3% of patients with AIDS in the United States are infected. Transmission of *I. belli* is not fully understood, but contaminated water, and transmission from infected animals to man and from person to person in a manner similar to other coccidia is most likely.[13]

Presentation and Assessment

PRESENTATION. The signs and symptoms of isosporiasis are similar to cryptosporidiosis with severe, profuse, watery diarrhea; severe, crampy abdominal pain; and weight loss. Charcot-Leyden crystals are often present in the stool, and peripheral eosinophilia may occur.

DIAGNOSIS. The presence of the oocyst in the stool is determined by a modified acid-fast stain or small-bowel biopsy. It should be differentiated from *Cryptosporidium.*

Related Care and Common Clinical Problems

Although nosocomial transmission has not been reported, transmission patterns suggest it is possible.[15] Preventive practices include drinking bottled water, and washing fresh fruits and vegetables thoroughly. Table 4.5 summarizes symptoms and common clinical problems relevant to isosporiasis.

Microsporidia (Microsporidiosis)

Biologic Basis and Epidemiology

Microsporidia includes multiple species, of which several are pathogenic to humans. *Enterocytozoon bieneusi* is the most common species detected in patients with chronic diarrhea and wasting. *Encephalitozoon hellum* has been found in the corneal epithelium of AIDS patients, and *Encephalitozoon intestinalis* (formerly *Septata intestinalis*) is associated with chronic diarrhea and disseminated disease.[13] *Microsporidia* has worldwide distribution but is reported most frequently in the tropics. The organism has been found in as many as 50% of patients with diarrhea, especially in those with CD4+ counts of <100/mm³. The mode of transmission is not known. Fecal oral transmission is most probable by ingestion of material contaminated with spores that can live outside the body for up to 4 months. The presence of spores in urine and respiratory secretions suggests possible human-to-human transmission.

Presentation and Assessment

PRESENTATION. The most common symptoms are profuse, watery diarrhea with crampy, abdominal pain; malabsorption; weight loss; and wasting similar to cryptosporidiosis. Generally patients present without a fever unless cholangitis has developed.[16]

DIAGNOSIS. Due to the small size of the organism and poor staining qualities, detection is more difficult than with cryptosporidiosis. Detection usually requires endoscopy with small-bowel biopsy. Electron microscopic examination of tissue makes a definitive diagnosis. Methylene blue-modified trichrome-, or Giemsa-stained stool specimens are currently used.[17]

Related Care and Common Clinical Problems

Hand washing and good personal hygiene are the best primary preventive measures. Drinking bottled water, especially when traveling, is essential. Table 4.5 summarizes symptoms and common clinical problems relevant to microsporidiosis.

Bacterial Infections

Streptococcus pneumoniae (Community-Acquired Pneumonia, Bacterial Pneumonia)

Biologic Basis and Epidemiology

S. pneumoniae is the most common cause of bacterial pneumonia in HIV-infected patients, with IV drug users at highest risk.[18] Because severe immunosuppression is not necessary for infection, streptococcal pneumonia may be an early manifestation of HIV infection. HIV-infected individuals with higher CD4+ counts (500 cells/mm^3) are at greatest risk of infection due to community-acquired pathogens (CAPs) such as *S. pneumoniae.* Transmission is by inhalation of droplets, with increased risk in crowded conditions.

Presentation and Assessment

PRESENTATION. An acute onset of the following signs and symptoms, similar to the general population, is common: fever, chills, dyspnea, productive purulent cough, and pleuritic chest pain. This may progress to bacteremia. The incidence of pneumococcal bacteremia in patients with AIDS is almost 100 times greater than in healthy age-matched populations.[19]

DIAGNOSIS. Chest radiographs usually demonstrate segmented, lobar, or multilobar consolidation, although diffuse bilateral interstitial infiltrates have been seen. Bacterial cultures of blood are very specific, whereas sputum cultures are less definitive because the organism can be part of normal oropharyngeal flora. Gram's stain of the sputum is helpful to establish a presumptive diagnosis.

Related Care and Common Clinical Problems

Because streptococcal infection may be an early manifestation of HIV infection in an undiagnosed person, HIV testing should be recommended, especially if the person has recurrent episodes of streptococcal infection. Pneumococcal vaccine is also recommended as early in the course of HIV infection as possible to produce antibodies before advanced HIV disease,[20,21] although controversy continues regarding the effectiveness of vaccination. Instruct HIV-infected persons to avoid crowds, especially during seasonal peaks in fall, winter, and spring. Table 4.6 summarizes symptoms and common clinical problems relevant to bacterial pneumonia.

Haemophilus influenzae (Community-Acquired Pneumonia, Bacterial Pneumonia)

Biologic Basis and Epidemiology

H. influenzae is a frequently encountered CAP that, like *S. pneumoniae,* can occur without severe immunosuppression and cause pneumonia in an HIV-infected person. Transmission is by inhalation of airborne droplets or by direct contagion with secretions.

Table 4.6 Common Clinical Problems Associated with Opportunistic Infections: Bacterial Organisms

Clinical Problem	S. pneu	H. flu	Pseud	Salm	Staph
A. NEUROLOGICAL IMPAIRMENTS					
Confusion, delirium					
Memory loss, dementia					
Decreased concentration, alertness and alterations in consciousness					
Impaired coordination, balance, mobility					
B. NUTRITION-RELATED CHANGES					
Anorexia, cachexia, wasting, malnutrition				√	
Taste change					
Xerostomia					
Stomatitis, mucositis					
Nausea, vomiting, retching					
Constipation					
Diarrhea				√	
Fluid, electrolyte imbalance					
Dysphagia (+)					
C. RESPIRATORY CHANGES					
Dyspnea	√	√	√		
Cough	√	√	√		
D. CHANGES IN HOST DEFENSES					
Thrombocytopenia					
Neutropenia					
E. SKIN PROBLEMS					
Itching (pruritus)					
Dry skin					
Skin, nail lesions					
Rash			√		√

(continued)

Table 4.6 *Continued*

Clinical Problem	S. pneu	H. flu	Pseud	Salm	Staph
F. Psychosocial Responses					
Anxiety	√	√	√	√	√
Depression					
Psychosis, mania					
Grief, loss	√	√	√	√	√
G. Changes in Functional Capacity and Performance					
Fatigue					
Sleep alterations					
Visual changes					
H. Discomfort					
Pain	√	√	√		√
Peripheral neuropathy					
Night sweats					
Fever, chills, shivering	√	√	√	√	

S. pneu = *Streptococcus pneumoniae;* H. flu = *Haemophilus influenzae;* Pseud = *Pseudomonas aeruginosa;* Salm = *Salmonella* species; Staph = *Staphylococcus aureus.*

Presentation and Assessment

PRESENTATION. *H. influenzae* usually has a rapid onset with the following symptoms: fever, productive purulent cough, dyspnea, and chest pain. While *H. influenzae* most commonly presents as pneumonia, it can present as sinusitis characterized by coryza, headache, and cough. Either presentation may progress to bacteremia.

DIAGNOSIS. Chest radiographs usually demonstrate lobar or segmental infiltrates, however bilateral interstitial infiltrates characteristic of PCP may also be seen. Blood and sputum should be cultured.

Related Care and Common Clinical Problems

HIV testing is important because *H. influenzae* pneumonia occurs prior to marked immunosuppression (CD4+ count >300/mm^3). Influenza type

B vaccine (Hib) is not strongly advocated at present.[21, 22] Instruct HIV-infected individuals to avoid crowds, especially during seasonal peaks of infection. Table 4.6 summarizes symptoms and common clinical problems relevant to bacterial pneumonia.

Pseudomonas aeruginosa (*Pseudomonas* Infection)

Biologic Basis and Epidemiology

P. aeruginosa is an important pathogen in late HIV disease. The organism is isolated from soil, water, plants, and animals. This is most frequently a hospital-acquired nosocomial pulmonary or cutaneous infection; however indolent, community-acquired forms have been described. While this infection occurs less frequently than *S. pneumoniae* and *H. influenzae*, it is associated with a high rate of relapse in patients who survive the initial infection.

Presentation and Assessment

PRESENTATION. In addition to the pulmonary symptoms of fever, productive cough, dyspnea, and chest pain, sinusitis is a common presenting problem. Recurrent cellulitis is found as well.

DIAGNOSIS. Blood cultures and sputum cultures should be obtained. Culture any suspected skin lesions or wounds. Focal X-ray findings are similar to other bacterial pneumonias.

Related Care and Common Clinical Problems

Rigorous attention to infective control measures for hospitalized and ambulatory patients are essential. Patients with central venous access devices should be instructed regarding proper care, with return demonstration for competency. Table 4.6 summarizes symptoms and common clinical problems relevant to *Pseudomonas* infection.

Salmonella Species (*Salmonella* Infection)

Biologic Basis and Epidemiology

The relative risk in HIV-infected patients is far greater than in the HIV-negative population. Transmission is usually by ingestion of contaminated food or water. Food sources of *Salmonella* include unpasteurized milk, raw eggs, meat, and other unprocessed foods or animal by-products. Nonfood sources include pet turtles and contaminated marijuana.[23]

Presentation and Assessment

PRESENTATION. Fever, chills, anorexia, and diarrhea are symptoms of *Salmonella* infection in immunocompromised persons as compared with nausea, vomiting, and diarrhea in the immunocompetent person. Abdominal cramping, headache, and myalgias may or may not be present. Bacteremia, with or without diarrhea, is much more common in patients with AIDS.

DIAGNOSIS. *Salmonella* infection can be suspected after obtaining a history of food intake for the previous 48 hours. Stool cultures for enteric pathogens should be obtained but may be negative initially. Thereafter, anoscopy or sigmoid examination for direct culture may be performed.

Related Care and Common Clinical Problems

Patient teaching for primary prevention includes (1) using bottled liquids when traveling; (2) avoiding fast-food restaurants and other eateries where many people handle food; (3) washing all fresh food before eating or cooking; (4) cooking meat, poultry, and fish well; (5) eliminating raw fish or meat from the diet; (6) using pasteurized dairy products; and (7) restricting consumption to fully cooked eggs, with no partially cooked or raw eggs as in egg nog, Caesar salad, and meringues. Meticulous hand washing and thorough cleaning of food preparation areas is imperative. Contact with turtles, iguanas, chicks, and ducklings should be avoided. Table 4.6 summarizes symptoms and common clinical problems relevant to *Salmonella* infection.

References

1. Gallant JE. Infectious complications of HIV disease. *Emerg Med Clin North Am.* 1995;13:73–104.
2. Lee BL, Tauber MG. Histoplasmosis. In: Cohen PT, Sande MA, Volberding PA, eds. *The AIDS Knowledge Base.* 2nd ed. Boston: Little, Brown; 1994:6.9–12.
3. Barnes PF, Block AB, Davidson PT, et al. Tuberculosis in patients with human immunodeficiency virus infection. *N Engl J Med.* 1991;324:1644–1650.

4. Hamburg MA, Freidens TR. Tuberculosis transmission in the 1990's. *N Engl J Med.* 1994;330:1750–1751.
5. Shafer RW, Kim DS, Weiss JP, et al. Extrapulmonary tuberculosis in patients with human immunodeficiency virus infection. *Medicine.* 1991;70:384–397.
6. Centers for Disease Control. Guidelines for preventing the transmission of *Mycobacterium tuberculosis* in health care facilities. *MMWR.* 1994;43:1–132.
7. French AL, Benator DA, Gordin FM. Nontuberculosis mycobacterial infections. *Med Clin North Am.* 1997;81:361–362.
8. Eccles E, Ptak J. *Micobacterium avium* complex infection in AIDS: clinical features, treatment and prevention. *J Assoc Nurses AIDS Care.* 1995;6:37–47.
9. Cavert W. Viral infections in human immunodeficiency virus disease. *Med Clin North Am.* 1997;81:411–426.
10. Drew WL, Jacobson MA. Cytomegalovirus. In: Cohen PT, Sande MA, Volberding PA, eds. *The AIDS Knowledge Base.* 2nd ed. Boston: Little, Brown; 1994: 6.13–6.136.
11. Scaglia M, Atzon C, Marchetti G, et al. Effectiveness of aminosidine (paramycin) sulfate in chronic *Cryptosporidium* diarrhea in AIDS patients: an open, uncontrolled, prospective trial. *J Infect Dis.* 1994;170:1349–1350.
12. Santamauro JT, Stover DE. *Pneumocystis carinii* pneumonia. *Med Clin North Am.* 1997;81:229–318.
13. Framm SR, Soave R. Agents of diarrhea. *Med Clin North Am.* 1997;81.2:433.
14. Lingappa JR, Sande MA. Toxoplasmosis. In: Cohen PT, Sande MA, Volberding PA, eds. *The AIDS Knowledge Base.* 2nd ed. Boston: Little, Brown; 1994; 6.19–6.11.
15. Petersen C, Wofsy CB. Isosporiasis. In: Cohen PT, Sande MA, Volberding PA, eds. *The AIDS Knowledge Base.* 2nd ed. Boston: Little, Brown; 1994;6.20–6.24.
16. Casey KM, Cohen F, Hughes A, eds. *ANAC'S Core Curriculum for HIV/AIDS Nursing.* Philadelphia: Nursecom; 1996:123–124.
17. Weber R, Bryan RT, Owen RL, et al. Improved light-microscopial detection of microsporidia spores in stool and duodenal aspirates. *N Engl J Med.* 1992;326: 161–166.
18. Janoff EN, Breima RF, Daly CL. Pneumococcal disease during HIV infection. *Ann Intern Med.* 1992;117:314–324.
19. Daley CL. Infections with encapsulated bacteria. In: Cohen PT, Sande MA, Volberding PA, eds. *The AIDS Knowledge Base.* 2nd ed. Boston: Little, Brown; 1994:6.2–12.
20. Kaplan JE, Masur H, Holmes KK, et al. USPHS/IDSA guidelines for the prevention of opportunistic infections in persons infected with human immunodeficiency virus: an overview. *Clin Infect Dis.* 1995;21:S12–S31.
21. USPHS/IDSA Prevention of Opportunistic Infections Working Group. USPHS/ IDSA guidelines for the prevention of opportunistic infections in persons in-

fected with human immunodeficiency virus: disease-specific recommendations. *Clin Infect Dis.* 1995;21:S32–S43.
22. CDC. USPHS/IDSA guidelines for the prevention of opportunistic infections in persons infected with human immunodeficiency virus: a summary. *MMWR.* 1995;44:1–34.
23. Panther LA, Sande MA. *Salmonella.* In: Cohen PT, Sande MA, Volberding PA, eds. *The AIDS Knowledge Base.* 2nd ed. Boston: Little, Brown; 1994:6.1–8.

CHAPTER 5

Pharmacological Treatment of Opportunistic Infections

Vivian L. Bruzzese, MD • Lisa G. Kaplowitz, MD

Chapter Preview

- Acute Therapy
- Maintenance Therapy
- Prevention
- Fungal Infections
- Mycobacterial Infections
- Viral Infections
- *Pneumocystis carinii* Infection
- Protozoal Infections
- Bacterial Infections

In persons infected with HIV, opportunistic pathogens generally cause opportunistic infection (OI) after significant destruction of the immune system has occurred, usually when the CD4+ cell count is <200 cells/mm^3. (See Chapter 4 for details related to OI epidemiology, clinical presentation, diagnosis, and intervention.) This chapter summarizes the common pharmacological treatments of these OIs, including acute therapy, maintenance therapy, and prophylactic therapy.

Acute Therapy

Once an OI is diagnosed, initial treatment, *acute therapy* (also called *induction therapy*) should be given. *First-line therapy* is preferred over *second-line therapy* based on greater efficacy, lower cost, lower rate of adverse effects, or a combination of these factors. The therapy chosen, when more than one first-line agent is available, is dependent on provider preference and individual patient characteristics. *Second-line therapy* must be used when a patient is intolerant of or unresponsive to the first-line therapies. In addition to these specific therapies, highly active antiretroviral therapies (HAARTs), are combinations of antiretroviral agents usually containing a protease inhibitor. (See Chapter 3 for details of ART.) HAART have been shown to be effective in treating some OIs that have been poorly responsive to available treatments, such as PML,[1] *molluscum contagiosum*,[2] cryptosporidiosis, and microsporidiosis.[3,4]

Maintenance Therapy

After the successful treatment of the acute infection, most OIs require the continued use of suppressive medications (i.e., *maintenance therapy*) to prevent recurrence of the illness. Infections that are exceptions to this rule and thus do not require maintenance therapy include TB, bacterial respiratory infections, syphilis, gonorrhea, chlamydial genital infections, HZ infection, and giardiasis.

Prevention

Because many of these OIs are common in the person with HIV and cause significant morbidity, prevention of the infections is preferable to the strategy of prescribing medications after infections occur. One reason for encouraging HIV antibody testing in certain populations is that optimal prevention of OIs requires the early identification of persons at risk for these infections. HAART may prove to be effective in preventing OIs by maintaining and restoring immune function in persons diagnosed with HIV infection. OI prevention measures include not only the use of prophylactic medications and antiretroviral treatment, but also limiting exposure to organisms through lifestyle changes or avoiding regions of the world where certain infections are endemic (see Chapter 4). The use of prophylactic agents is beneficial in patients who have a high risk of certain OIs and when medications are available that can significantly decrease this risk without causing unacceptable toxicity. For example, prolonged survival has been demonstrated for HIV-infected populations who received prophylaxis for *Pneumocystis carinii*.[5] However, prophylactic agents are not 100% effective in preventing infections and can even modify the presentation of illness, making diagnosis of the OI difficult. Another limitation to the effectiveness of prophylactic agents is the possibility of the emergence of resistance of certain pathogens to medications after widespread use. For example, clinical and laboratory resistance of mucosal candidiasis to azoles can occur in patients previously treated with these agents.[6,7]

Fungal Infections

Candida albicans (Candidiasis)

Treatment of *C. albicans* infection in the mouth (oropharyngeal candidiasis or thrush), esophagus (esophageal candidiasis), or vagina (vaginal candidiasis) in persons with HIV infection is listed below.

Medications for Thrush (Oropharyngeal Candidiasis)

- **Acute treatment, first line**

  Clotrimazole troches 10 mg dissolved in mouth qid until resolved

  or

  Nystatin 100,000 U swish-and-swallow five times per day until resolved

  or

  Amphotericin B oral suspension 100 mg swish-and-swallow qid until resolved

(continued)

- **Acute treatment, second line**
  Ketoconazole 200 mg PO qd until resolved
  or
  Fluconazole 100 mg PO qd until resolved
  or
  Itraconazole suspension 200 mg PO qd until resolved

Medications for Esophageal Candidiasis

- **Acute treatment, first line**
  Ketoconazole 200 mg PO qd for 7 to 21 days
  or
  Fluconazole 100 to 200 mg PO qd for 7 to 21 days
  or
  Itraconazole suspension 200 mg PO qd for 14 to 21 days
- **Acute treatment, second line**
  Amphotericin B 0.3 to 0.5 mg/kg/day IV until able to swallow
  then
  Oral agent as listed in first-line therapy

Medications for Vaginal Candidiasis

- **Acute treatment**
  Clotrimazole 1% cream qhs for 7 nights
  or
  Clotrimazole vaginal tablet qhs for 7 nights
  or
  Nystatin 100,000 U vaginal tablet qhs for 14 nights
  or
  Terconazole cream intravaginally qhs (40 mg for 3 nights or 20 mg for 7 nights)
  or
  Fluconazole 150 mg PO for 1 day
- **Prophylaxis**
  Fluconazole 200 mg PO once weekly[8]

Other *candida* species that can cause infections at these sites are generally also responsive to the medications listed. Itraconazole and ketoconazole are not useful if the person is also taking antacids, H_2 blockers, omeprazole, or rifampin.

Parenteral amphotericin B is an antifungal agent that is effective therapy for most systemic fungal infections, including candidal infections resistant to therapy with the azoles (clotrimazole, ketoconazole, fluconazole, and itraconazole). Intravenous amphotericin B is infrequently used for mucosal candidiasis because it has significant toxicities. New parenteral formulations of amphotericin B complexed with lipids in beads or ribbons have become available and may have fewer toxicities than conventional amphotericin.[9] An oral suspension of amphotericin B that is not systemically absorbed is now available for the treatment of thrush and is the agent of choice for mucosal candidiasis resistant to all azoles. Itraconazole suspension has been reported to be effective in treating some cases of fluconazole-resistant oropharyngeal or esophageal candidiasis.[10,11]

Coccidioides immitis (Coccidioidomycosis)

The treatment of coccidioidomycosis in persons with HIV infection differs from that of other populations in several regards. All patients coinfected with HIV and *Coccidioides* should receive acute and then lifelong maintenance therapy as listed below.

Medications for Coccidioides immitis

- **Acute treatment**
  Itraconazole 200 mg PO q12h
  or
  Fluconazole 400 to 800 mg PO qd
  or
  Amphotericin B IV
- **Maintenance therapy (lifelong), first line**
  Fluconazole 400 to 600 mg PO qd
  or
  Itraconazole 200 mg PO q12h
- **Maintenance therapy (lifelong), second line**
  Amphotericin B 1 mg/kg IV weekly

Immunocompetent persons with this infection usually do not require lifelong suppressive therapy and some do not require acute treatment.

Ketoconazole is not effective for the treatment or prevention of coccidioidomycosis in persons with HIV.[12] Primary prophylaxis for coccidioidomycosis with 200 mg PO qd of fluconazole or itraconazole can be considered for patients living in endemic areas who have a CD4+ count <50 cells/mm^3.[13]

Cryptococcus neoformans (Cryptococcosis)

As with coccidioidomycosis, the treatment of cryptococcosis in persons with HIV infection differs from that of other populations. All patients coinfected with HIV and *Cryptococcus* should receive both acute and then lifelong maintenance therapy as listed below.

Medications for Cryptococcus neoformans

- **Acute treatment**
  Amphotericin B 0.7 to 0.8 mg/kg/day IV ± 5-FC 100 mg/kg/day divided qid for 14 days
  or
  Fluconazole 400 PO qd for 2 months (for mild nonmeningeal disease)
- **Maintenance therapy (lifelong), first line**
  Fluconazole 200 to 400 mg PO qd
  or
  Itraconazole 200 mg PO q12h
- **Maintenance therapy (lifelong), second line**
  Amphotericin B 1 mg/kg IV one to three times per week

Ketoconazole is not effective for the treatment of cryptococcosis in persons with HIV. Flucytosine should not be used alone for any infection because organisms become quickly resistant to this agent. Itraconazole at a dose of 200 mg PO daily has proved to be ineffective in preventing relapse of cryptococcal meningitis.[12]

Management of cryptococcal meningitis includes monitoring intracranial pressure, which can be done by measuring the opening pressure at a lumbar puncture. An elevated pressure, >25 cm H_2O, necessitates drainage of CSF to normalize the pressure. Repeat the lumbar puncture within several days to verify continued normal pressure. Some patients require daily to weekly lumbar punctures or surgical placement of a lumbar or ventricular drain[12] to prevent the complications of elevated intracranial pressure, which includes blindness, deafness, and death.

Histoplasma capsulatum (Histoplasmosis)

As with coccidioidomycosis and cryptococcosis, the treatment of histoplasmosis in persons with HIV infection differs from that of other populations. All patients coinfected with HIV and *Histoplasma* should receive acute and then lifelong maintenance therapy as listed below.

Medications for Histoplasma capsulatum

- **Acute treatment**
  Amphotericin B (for serious illness)[12] 0.5 to 1 mg/kg/day for 14 days
  or
  Itraconazole (for mild disease)[12] 200 mg PO q12h
  or
  Fluconazole (unable to tolerate or absorb itraconazole)[12] 1,600 mg Day 1 then 800 mg PO qd to complete 12 weeks
- **Maintenance therapy (lifelong), first line**
  Itraconazole 200 mg PO q12h
  or
  Fluconazole 400 mg PO qd
- **Maintenance therapy (lifelong), second line**
  Amphotericin B 0.5 to 0.8 mg/kg IV every week

Immunocompetent persons usually do not require suppressive therapy and most do not require acute treatment. Ketoconazole is not effective for the treatment of histoplasmosis in persons with HIV.[12] Prophylaxis for histoplasmosis with 200 mg PO qd of itraconazole or fluconazole can be considered for patients who have resided in endemic areas and who have <50 CD4+ cells/mm^3.[13]

Mycobacterial Infections

Mycobacterium tuberculosis (TB)

Patients coinfected with HIV and sensitive isolates of *Mycobacterium tuberculosis* can be cured of TB if given appropriate treatment. Early diagnosis and compliance with treatment are essential to prevent TB drug resistance. A variety of regimens using the agents listed here have proved to be effective treatment of TB in persons coinfected with HIV.

Medications for Mycobacterium tuberculosis

- **Acute treatment**
  Isoniazid 300 mg/day for ≥6 months
  and
  Vitamin B6 50 mg/day for ≥6 months
  and
  Rifampin 600 mg/day *or* rifabutin 150 to 300 mg/day for ≥6 months
  and
  Pyrazinamide 20 to 30 mg/kg/day for 2 months
  and
  Ethambutol 15 mg/kg/day for 2 months
- **Prophylaxis**
  Isoniazid 300 mg PO qd plus vitamin B6 50 mg PO qd for 12 months
  or
  Isoniazid 900 mg PO twice weekly plus vitamin B6 100 mg PO twice weekly for 12 months
  or
  Rifampin 600 mg PO qd plus pyrazinamide 25 mg/kg PO qd for 2 months (for isoniazid intolerance)

Other regimens include giving medications three times weekly instead of daily, and therapy for 6 months instead of 12 months,[14] although treatment for 9 months rather than 6 months improves relapse-free survival.[15]

Pills combining some of the medications commonly used to treat TB are available and include Rifater (isoniazid 50 mg, rifampin 120 mg, and pyrazinamide 300 mg) and Rifamate (isoniazid 150 mg and rifampin 300 mg). These combination pills are more expensive than the individual medications but could improve compliance in some patients.[16] Patients who cannot tolerate both isoniazid and rifampin require at least 18 months of therapy with isoniazid or rifampin plus ethambutol and pyrazinamide. It is recommended that all patients beginning treatment for TB be started on four antituberculous drugs and that patients complete treatment with at least two agents to which the organism is susceptible. Those patients exposed to TB in areas with a high incidence of resistance or who are suspected of having resistant TB can be given more than four medications. Other agents that are useful in the treatment of persons with known or suspected resistant TB or in persons intolerant to a first-line agent include fluoroquinolones (ciprofloxacin or ofloxacin), aminoglycosides (amikacin, kanamycin, streptomycin, or capreomycin), or cycloserine.[17] Persons infected with TB resistant to one or more antituberculous drugs are more difficult to treat and require more prolonged therapy (up to 24 months after the sputum culture is negative for TB).[17]

TB Treatment and Protease Inhibitors

Due to the interactions between the rifamycins (rifampin and rifabutin) and the HIV protease inhibitors, the CDC has issued recommendations regarding treating persons with concurrent HIV and TB. Rifamycins increase the metabolism of protease inhibitors, resulting in subtherapeutic levels of these medications. The protease inhibitors, especially ritonavir and saquinavir, inhibit the metabolism of rifamycins, resulting in increased serum levels of rifamycins. The options for treating patients with HIV and TB include (1) discontinue or delay institution of the protease inhibitor while treating TB according to the standard recommendations; (2) discontinue or delay institution of the protease inhibitor while using a short course of a rifampin-containing regimen until a bacteriologic response is achieved (for at least 2 months) and sensitivity is verified, then reinstitute or start therapy with a protease inhibitor while continuing the TB treatment with 16 months of isoniazid (15 mg/kg) and ethambutol (50 mg/kg) two times per week; and (3) continue or start the protease inhibitor treatment as indinavir (800 mg PO tid) and use rifabutin (150 mg/day) instead of rifampin in the TB treatment regimen.[18] Rifabutin at a daily dose of 150 mg has been shown to be at least as effective as rifampin in the treatment of TB.[19]

TB Prophylaxis

Prophylaxis for TB should be provided to any person with a positive skin test (PPD ≥ 5 mm of induration) without current active TB infection or prior treatment, and those known to have been exposed to an active case of pulmonary TB.[17] Prophylaxis should be considered in persons who are anergic to skin testing, especially in populations with a high incidence of TB.

Mycobacterium avium-intracellulare Complex (MAC Disease)

In contradistinction to TB, disseminated MAC infection in persons with HIV infection is not curable, thus treatment listed as follows must be continued indefinitely.

Medications for Mycobacterium avium-intracellulare Complex

- **Acute treatment, first line**
  Macrolide (clarithromycin 500 mg q12h *or* azithromycin 500 mg qd)
  and
  Rifabutin 300 to 600 mg qd
  and
  Ethambutol 800 to 1,200 mg/day
- **Acute treatment, second line**
  Macrolide (as listed in first-line acute treatment)
  and
  One or more of the following:
    - Rifabutin 300 to 600 mg/day
    - Ethambutol 800 to 1,200 mg/day
    - Ciprofloxacin 750 mg PO q12h
    - Amikacin 7.5 to 15 mg/kg IV qd
- **Prophylaxis**
  Rifabutin 300 mg PO qd
  or
  Clarithromycin 500 mg PO q12h
  or
  Azithromycin 500 mg PO three times per week
  or
  Azithromycin 1,200 mg PO once per week [20]

The treatment of MAC results in clinical improvement that is maintained for a variable time period. Monotherapy (use of a single agent at any one time) cannot be used in the treatment of MAC because the organism becomes quickly resistant to a single agent, usually with associated clinical deterioration.[21] Drug intolerance is common so that regimens may require frequent modification.

MAC prophylaxis with rifabutin, clarithromycin, or azithromycin should be considered for patients with CD4 cell counts of <75 to 100 cells/mm^3 only after evidence of active MAC or TB infection is excluded.[13] Rifabutin prophylaxis has been shown to prevent deaths[22] and hospitalizations.[23] Some clinicians are reluctant to use the macrolides for MAC prophylaxis because the organisms that do infect persons taking these agents could be resistant to these macrolides, which are necessary for effective treatment of MAC infection.[24] Rifabutin cannot be used in patients taking ritonavir or saquinavir due to potential drug interactions. Patients taking indinavir can be given rifabutin at a daily dose of 150 mg instead of 300 mg.[18]

Viral Infections

Cytomegalovirus (CMV Infection)

The treatment of CMV infection involving the eyes, known as *CMV retinitis*, requires lifelong therapy (see Chapter 18). All of the systemic antiviral agents listed here require dosage adjustment in patients with impaired creatinine clearance (≤1.6 ml/min/kg).

Medications for Cytomegalovirus

- **Acute treatment**

  Ganciclovir 5 mg/kg IV q12h for 14 days

  or

  Ganciclovir via implant (intraocular) 1–2 micrograms/hour sustained release

  or

  Foscarnet IV 60 mg/kg q8h or 90 mg/kg q12h for 14 days

  or

  Foscarnet 90 mg/kg IV q12h + ganciclovir 5 mg/kg/d IV for 14 days

  or

  Foscarnet 90 mg/kg IV + ganciclovir 5 mg/kg/d IV q12h for 14 days

  or

  Cidofovir 5 mg/kg each week for 2 weeks *(continued)*

- **Maintenance therapy**
  Ganciclovir 5 mg/kg IV qd or 1 g PO q8h
  or
  Foscarnet 120 mg/kg IV qd
  or
  Combination of ganciclovir 5 mg/kg/day IV plus foscarnet 90 mg/kg/day IV
  or
  Cidofovir 3 to 5 mg/kg IV every other week

Cidofovir should not be used in persons with renal dysfunction (serum creatinine > 1.5 mg/dl, creatinine clearance ≤ 55 ml/min, or proteinuria ≥ 100 mg/dl).[25] Patients with CMV retinitis in a single eye and no evidence of systemic disease have been treated successfully with ganciclovir eye implants[26] or intravitreal cidofovir 20 μg.[27] Persons with retinitis that respond to the initial 2- to 3-week induction course of IV ganciclovir and do not have sight-threatening infection can be given suppressive oral, rather than IV, ganciclovir.[28] It is not known whether oral ganciclovir will be of any benefit in the treatment or suppression of CMV disease other than retinitis. The optimal duration of therapy or suppressive regimen for infection in extraophthalmologic sites is not known. Both IV cidofovir and foscarnet can be nephrotoxic and must be given with adequate hydration. Persons taking IV cidofovir must take oral probenecid (2 g 3 hours prior to infusion, 1 g 2 hours after infusion, and 1 g 8 hours after infusion) to prevent nephrotoxicity.[25] Patients taking foscarnet often require supplemental calcium, magnesium, and phosphorous.[29]

Herpes Simplex Virus (HSV Infection)

The agents used in the treatment of HSV infection are listed below.

Medication for HSV

- **Acute treatment, acyclovir sensitive**
  Acyclovir 200 mg PO five times per day for 7 to 10 days
  or
  Acyclovir 5 mg/kg IV q8h for 7 to 10 days
  or

Valacyclovir 500 mg PO q12h for 5 days
or
Famciclovir 125 mg PO q12h for 5 days

- **Acute treatment, acyclovir resistant**
  Foscarnet 40 mg/kg IV q8h
  or
  Cidofovir IV if being used for CMV disease
  and/or
  Topical trifluorothymidine, foscarnet, or cidofovir
- **Maintenance therapy (to prevent reactivation), acyclovir sensitive**
  Acyclovir 400 mg PO every 8 to 12 hours
  or
  Famciclovir 125 to 250 mg PO q12h
  or
  Ganciclovir PO or IV if being used to treat or prevent CMV disease
- **Maintenance therapy (to prevent reactivation), acyclovir resistant**
  Foscarnet or cidofovir IV if being used to treat CMV

Isolates of HSV resistant to acyclovir, and thus resistant to ganciclovir, do exist. Several studies have reported that patients taking acyclovir[30] or acyclovir with zidovudine[31,32] have prolonged survival. Regimens proven to be effective for prevention of HSV reactivation are acyclovir 400 mg PO bid or 200 mg PO tid[29] or any of the medications listed in the previous section for treatment or maintenance of CMV infection.

Varicella-zoster Virus (Herpes Zoster)

Higher doses of acyclovir, famciclovir, or valacyclovir are required to treat VZV infection than are required for the treatment of HSV. The agents used in the treatment of VZV infection are listed below.

Medications for VZV

- **Acute treatment**
  Acyclovir 800 mg PO five times daily or 10 mg/kg IV q8h for 7 to 10 days
  or

(continued)

Famciclovir 500 mg PO q8h for 7 days
or
Valacyclovir 1 g q8h for 7 to 14 days
or
Ganciclovir 5 mg/kg IV q12h
or
Foscarnet 40 mg/kg IV q8h

JC Virus (Progressive Multifocal Leukoencephalopathy)

Some patients with PML reportedly have been treated successfully with intrathecal or IV cytarabine (Ara-C),[33] although a recent study showed no benefit with these treatments.[34] Several cases of improvement in PML infection after institution of ART[1,35] or alpha-interferon[36] have been reported.

Human Papilloma Virus (HPV infection)

The treatment of HPV infection depends on the site of infection and whether anogenital or cervical neoplasia has developed. The treatment of neoplastic lesions is surgical removal, as indicated in Chapter 6. *Condyloma acuminata* can be treated with topical agents as listed here, but the lesions often recur. Extensive disease involving the anus or cervix can be surgically excised.[37]

Medications for HPV

- **Acute treatment, first line**

  Trichloroacetic acid 50% applied topically every week
  or
  Podophyllin 25% applied topically every week
  or
  Podofilox applied topically every week
  or
  5-fluorouracil cream applied topically every week
  or

(continued)

Imiquimod 5% cream applied topically qhs three times per week for up to 16 weeks
or
Liquid nitrogen applied topically every week
- **Acute treatment, second line**
Cidofovir gel applied topically qd for 5 to 10 days
or
Interferon α-2B 0.1 ml of 10 million U/ml injected into each lesion three times per week for 3 weeks
or
Electrosurgery
or
Surgical excision

Pneumocystis carinii Infection

P. carinii infection usually involves the lungs but may also infect extrapulmonary tissues. The regimens listed here are effective for the treatment of pulmonary and extrapulmonary disease.

Medications for P. carinii, Acute Pulmonary, or Extrapulmonary Infection
- **First line**
Trimethoprim-sulfamethoxazole 5 mg/kg of the trimethoprim component every 6 to 8 hours PO or IV for 21 days
or
Dapsone 100 mg PO qd with trimethoprim 5 mg/kg PO every 6 to 8 hours for 21 days
- **Second line**
Pentamidine 4 mg/kg IV qd for 21 days
or
Clindamycin 450 to 600 mg PO *or* IV q6h plus primaquine 15 to 30 mg PO qd for 21 days
or
Atovaquone 750 mg suspension PO q12h for 21 days
or

(continued)

Trimetrexate 45 mg/M² qd for 21 days plus leucovorin (folinic acid) 20 mg/m² q6h IV or PO to complete 24 days of therapy (or 3 days after trimetrexate has been stopped)
Adjunctive corticosteroids for moderate to severe infection (in addition to one of the above antipneumocystis regimens):
Adjunctive corticosteriods (for moderate to severe infection): prednisone or prednisolone 40 mg q12h for 5 days, then 40 mg qd for 5 days, then 20 mg qd for the remaining 11 days of therapy

Trimethoprim-sulfamethoxazole, either IV or PO, or oral trimethoprim with dapsone should be used in all patients able to tolerate these regimens. All other agents are considered to be second-line treatments.[38] Adjunctive steroids should be used in any patient with hypoxia demonstrated on initial room air-blood gas (PO_2 < 70 torr or A-a gradient > 35 torr) because the addition of steroids to the anti-*Pneumocystis* regimen has been shown to reduce mortality in this group of patients.[38] Treatment for *Pneumocystis* infection should be given for 21 days followed by maintenance therapy to prevent recurrence.

Prophylaxis to prevent *P. carinii* infections should be instituted when the patient's CD4+ count has fallen below 200 cells/mm³ (or 15%) or when the patient develops symptoms related to HIV infection such as thrush or unexplained fever for 2 weeks or more. Maintenance therapy to prevent recurrence of *P. carinii* infection after successful treatment should be given to all patients with prior *Pneumocystis* infection regardless of CD4+ count.[13,39] The regimens used for prophylaxis and maintenance therapy are identical and are listed below.

Prophylaxis and maintenance therapy of P. carinii

- **First line**
  Trimethoprim-sulfamethoxazole DS PO three to seven times per week
- **Second line**
  Dapsone 100 mg PO two to seven times per week (if sulfa-allergic)
  or
  Pentamidine 300 mg via nebulizer every month (if allergic to sulfa and dapsone)

Protozoal Infections

Cryptosporidium parvum (Cryptosporidiosis)

HAART has led to resolution of cryptosporidial infection in some patients.[3,4] Cryptosporidiosis is otherwise poorly responsive to therapy in persons with advanced HIV disease so that chronic treatment is often required. Paromomycin[40,41] or azithromycin, as listed here, have proved to be somewhat beneficial in the treatment of infections due to cryptosporidiosis; however, a recent placebo-controlled study showed no benefit with the use of paromomycin for cryptosporidial infection.[42]

Medications for Cryptosporidium

- **Acute treatment**

  ART

  and

  Paromomycin 1,500 to 3,000 mg PO divided every 6 to 8 hours

  or

  Azithromycin 900 to 1,200 mg qd

Symptomatic therapy with fiber, opiates, or octreotide[43] have some effectiveness in the treatment of cryptosporidiosis. The starting dose of octreotide for treatment of diarrhea is 50 μg SC tid and may be increased up to 500 μg SC tid.[43] Nitazoxanide is available under a compassionate access program from Unimed Pharmaceuticals (1-800-864-6330, ext. 3032).[44]

Toxoplasma gondii (Toxoplasmosis, Toxo)

Patients with indication of past *Toxoplasma* infection (IgG antibodies to *Toxoplasma*) and <100 CD4+ cells/mm^3 should receive lifelong prophylaxis to prevent reactivation infection. Recommended regimens are trimethoprim-sulfamethoxazole as given for PCP prophylaxis or weekly pyrimethamine 50 mg with 25 mg leucovorin and daily dapsone 50 mg for those unable to tolerate sulfa medications.[13] Regimens for acute and maintenance treatment of toxoplasmosis are listed on the following page.

Medications for Toxoplasma gondii

- **Acute treatment**
  Pyrimethamine 200-mg PO load then 50 to 75 mg PO qd
  and
  Folinic acid 10 mg PO or IV qd
  and
  One of the following first-line or second-line agents:
- **First line**
  Sulfadiazine 1 g PO q6h
  or
  A second-line agent
- **Second line**
  Clindamycin 600 mg IV or PO q6h
  or
  Atovaquone 750 mg PO q6h
  or
  Clarithromycin 1 g PO q12h
  or
  Azithromycin 1,200 to 1,500 mg PO qd
  or
  Dapsone 100 mg PO qd
- **Maintenance (lifelong) treatment**
  Pyrimethamine 25 to 50 mg PO qd
  and
  Folinic acid 10 mg PO qd
  and
  One of the following:
  Sulfadiazine 1 g PO q6h
  or
  Clindamycin 600 mg PO q6h
  or
  Atovaquone 750 mg PO q6h
  or
  Azithromycin 1,200 to 1,500 mg PO qd
  or
  Dapsone 100 mg PO two to seven times per week

Isospora belli (Isosporiasis)

The following describes the agents used for acute and maintenance therapy of *Isospora* infection:

Medications for I. belli

- **Acute treatment**
  Trimethoprim 160 mg plus sulfamethoxazole 800 mg PO (Bactrim DS) q6h for 10 days
  or
  Pyrimethamine 50 to 75 mg PO qd (if sulfa-allergic) with folinic acid 5 mg PO qd for 10 days
- **Maintenance treatment**
  Trimethoprim 160 mg plus sulfamethoxazole 800 mg PO three times per week
  or
  Pyrimethamine 25 mg PO qd plus folinic acid 5 mg PO qd

Microsporidia (Microsporidiosis)

Albendazole 400 to 1,600 mg PO q12h has proven to be beneficial in the treatment of infections due to microsporidiosis. HAART has led to resolution of chronic microsporidial infections in some patients.[3,4] In general, microsporidiosis (except infections caused by *Septata intestinalis*[45]) is poorly responsive to therapy, so treatment is often required indefinitely. Octreotide, a nonspecific antidiarrheal agent, is successful occasionally in the treatment of microsporidial infections involving massive diarrhea. The starting dose of octreotide for treatment of diarrhea is 50 μg SC tid and may be increased up to 500 μg SC tid.[43]

Bacterial Infections

The treatment of bacterial infections in patients with HIV infection is similar to that in immunocompetent patients in that antimicrobial therapy should be based on culture and sensitivity testing. As in patients without HIV infection, empiric antibacterials should be administered to persons with HIV infection and life-threatening bacterial infections until culture results are available.

Streptococcus pneumoniae

Most respiratory infections in patients with HIV and recurrent bronchitis are caused by *S. pneumoniae*, *H. influenzae*, or *P. aeruginosa*.[46] Low-dose trimethoprim-sulfamethoxazole (one double strength three to seven times per week)[13] has been used successfully as secondary prophylaxis for sinopulmonary infections in patients not already taking this medication for PCP prophylaxis. Clarithromycin or azithromycin,[20] at doses used to treat or prevent MAC infection, may be beneficial as well. Other modalities that might decrease the recurrence of these infections include smoking cessation; improved nutrition; use of inhaled bronchodilators; use of orally or nasally inhaled steroids; and immunization with pneumococcal, hemophilus, and influenza vaccines. All HIV-infected persons should be immunized with 23-valent polysaccharide pneumococcal vaccine once.[13,39] Vaccination with *H. influenzae* type b vaccine should be considered[39] in persons with HIV infection. HIV-infected patients with neutropenia may benefit from treatment with granulocyte stimulating factors[13] or discontinuation of bone marrow-suppressing medications, if other interventions are not successful in reducing the recurrence of these infections. In adults with HIV infection, IV Ig at a dose of 200 to 400 mg/kg every 21 days has been shown to reduce infections and hospitalizations.[47]

Haemophilus influenzae

Most respiratory infections in patients with recurrent bronchitis are caused by *H. influenzae*, *S. pneumoniae*, or *P. aeruginosa*.[46] Low-dose trimethoprim-sulfamethoxazole, clarithromycin, or azithromycin may be effective secondary prophylaxis for sinopulmonary infections. The measures listed in the section on *S. pneumoniae* that may decrease the risk of sinopulmonary infection (such as improved nutrition and smoking cessation) should be undertaken to prevent *H. influenzae* infections as well. Vaccination with the *H. influenzae* type b vaccine should be considered[39] in persons with HIV infection. HIV-infected patients with neutropenia may benefit from treatment with granulocyte stimulating factors[13] or discontinuation of bone marrow-suppressing medications.

Pseudomonas aeruginosa

P. aeruginosa can be a cause of recurrent bronchitis[46] and is more resistant to therapy than either *H. influenzae* or *S. pneumoniae*. Because agents used for prophylaxis of PCP or MAC infections are not effective in the prevention of *Pseudomonas* infections, preventive efforts must be focused on optimizing immunologic status and reducing risks for *Pseudomonas* infection when possible. Modalities that might decrease the recurrence of these infections include (1) decrease in days of hospitalization; (2) smoking cessation; (3) attention to nutrition; (4) use of inhaled bronchodilators; (5) use of orally or nasally inhaled steroids; and (6) immunization with pneumococcal, hemophilus, and influenza vaccines to prevent sinopulmonary infections that can become secondarily infected with *Pseudomonas*. Patients with neutropenia may benefit from treatment with granulocyte stimulating factors[13] or discontinuation of bone marrow-suppressing medications. The treatment of *Pseudomonas* infections generally requires two or more antipseudomonal agents.

Salmonella

Salmonella infection tends to recur in persons with HIV infection, especially in those with advanced disease. For this reason, maintenance therapy as listed here may be necessary to prevent a relapse of *Salmonella* infection.[39]

Medications for Salmonella

- **Acute treatment**

  Ampicillin 8 to 12 g/day IV divided q6h for 1 to 4 weeks *then* amoxicillin 500 mg PO q8h to complete 2- to 4-week course (if sensitive)

  or

  Fluoroquinolone IV or PO for 2 to 4 weeks

  or

  Ciprofloxacin 500 to 750 mg PO q12h for 2 to 4 weeks (other fluoroquinolone)

(continued)

or
Cefotaxime 1 to 2 g IV q6h for 2 to 4 weeks
or
Ceftriaxone 0.5 to 1 g IV qd for 2 to 4 weeks
or
Trimethoprim-sulfamethoxazole 5 to 10 mg/kg/day of the trimethoprim component IV or PO for 2 to 4 weeks

- **Maintenance treatment**
  Trimethoprim-sulfamethoxazole DS PO q12h
  or
  Amoxicillin 250 mg PO q12h (if sensitive)
  or
  Ciprofloxacin 500 mg PO every 12 to 24 hours

References

1. Henry K, Worley J, Sullivan C, Stawarz K, McCabe K. Documented improvement in late stage manifestations of AIDS after starting ritonavir in combination with two reverse transcriptase inhibitors. Abstract 356. Presented at the Fourth Conference on Retroviruses and Opportunistic Infections. Washington, DC. January 22–27, 1997.
2. Hicks CB, Myers SA, Giner J. Resolution of intractable *molluscum contagiosum* in a human immunodeficiency virus-infected patient after institution of antiretroviral therapy with ritonavir. *Clin Infect Dis.* 1997;24:1023–1025.
3. Benhamou Y, Bochet MV, Carriere J, et al. Effects of triple antiretroviral therapies including an HIV protease inhibitor on chronic intestinal cryptosporidiosis and microsporidiosis in HIV-infected patients. Abstract 357. Presented at the Fourth Conference on Retroviruses and Opportunistic Infections. Washington, DC. January 22–27, 1997.
4. Carr A, Foudraine N, Reiss P, Marriott D, Lange J, Cooper D. Resolution of antibiotic-resistant *Cryptosporidium* (C) and microsporidiosis (M) with potent combination antiretroviral therapy. Abstract 688. Presented at the Fourth Conference on Retroviruses and Opportunistic Infections. Washington, DC. January 22–27, 1997.
5. Osmond D, Charlebois E, Lang W, Shiboski S, Moss A. Changes in AIDS survival time in two San Francisco cohorts of homosexual men, 1983 to 1993. *JAMA.* 1994;271:1083–1087.

6. Sangeorzan JA, Bradley SF, He X, et al. Epidemiology of oral candidiasis in HIV-infected patients: colonization, infection, treatment, and emergence of fluconazole resistance. *Am J Med.* 1994;97:339–346.
7. Espinel-Ingroff A, Quart A, Steele-Moore L, et al. Molecular karyotyping of multiple yeast species isolated from nine patients with AIDS during prolonged fluconazole therapy. *J Med Vet Mycol.* 1996;34:111–116.
8. Schuman P, Capps L, Peng G, et al. Weekly fluconazole for the prevention of mucosal candidiasis in women with HIV infection: a randomized, double-blind, placebo-controlled trial. *Ann Intern Med.* 1997;126:689–696.
9. Ng TT, Denning DW. Liposomal amphotericin B (AmBisome) therapy in invasive fungal infections. Evaluation of United Kingdom compassionate use data. *Arch Intern Med.* 1995;155:1093–1098.
10. Phillips P, Zemecov J, Mahmood W, et al. Itraconazole cyclodextrin solution for fluconazole-refractory oropharyngeal candidiasis in AIDS: correlation of clinical response with in vitro susceptibility. *AIDS.* 1996;10:1369–1376.
11. Fessel WJ, Merrill KW, Ward D, et al. Itraconazole oral solution (IS) for the treatment of fluconazole-refractory oropharyngeal candidiasis (OC) in HIV-positive patients. Abstract 327. Presented at the Fourth Conference on Retroviruses and Opportunistic Infections. Washington, DC. January 22–27, 1997.
12. Saag MS. Cryptococcosis and other fungal infections (histoplasmosis, coccidioidomycosis). In: Sande MA, Volberding PA, eds. *The Medical Management of AIDS.* 4th ed. Philadelphia: WB Saunders; 1995:437–459.
13. Kaplan JE, Masur H, Homes KK, et al. USPHS/IDSA guidelines for the prevention of opportunistic infections in person infected with human immunodeficiency virus: an overview. *Clin Infect Dis.* 1995;21(suppl 1):S12–S31.
14. Perriens JH, St. Lous ME, Mukadi YB, et al. Pulmonary tuberculosis in HIV-infected patients in Zaire: a controlled trial of treatment for either 6 or 12 months. *N Engl J Med.* 1995;332:779–784.
15. Pulido F, Pena JM, Rubio R, et al. Relapse of tuberculosis after treatment in human immunodeficiency virus-infected patients. *Arch Intern Med.* 1997;157: 227–232.
16. Drugs for tuberculosis. In: Abramowicz M, ed. *The Medical Letter.* New Rochelle, NY: Medical Letter, Inc. 1995:67–70.
17. Hopewell PC. Tuberculosis in persons with HIV infection. In: Sande MA, Volberding PA, eds. *The Medical Management of AIDS.* 4th ed. Philadelphia: WB Saunders; 1995:416–436.
18. Villarino E. Clinical update: impact of HIV protease inhibitors on the treatment of HIV-infected tuberculosis patients with rifampin. *MMWR.* 1996;45:921–925.
19. Grassi C, Peona V. Use of rifabutin in the treatment of pulmonary tuberculosis. *Clin Infect Dis.* 1996;22(suppl):S50–S54.
20. Havlir DV, Dube MP, Sattler FR, et al. Prophylaxis against disseminated *Myco-*

bacterium avium complex with weekly azithromycin, daily rifabutin, or both. *N Engl J Med.* 1996;335:392–398.

21. Shafran SD, Singer J, Zarowny DP, et al. A comparison of two regimens for the treatment of *Mycobacterium avium* complex bacteremia in AIDS: rifabutin, ethambutol, and clarithromycin versus rifampin, ethambutol, clofazamine, and ciprofloxacin. *N Engl J Med.* 1996;335:377–383.
22. Moore RD, Chaisson RE. Survival analysis of two controlled trials of rifabutin prophylaxis against *Mycobacterium avium* complex in AIDS. In: *Abstracts of the 35th Interscience Conference on Antimicrobial Agents and Chemotherapy.* Abstract I204. San Francisco: American Society for Microbiology; 1995:242 (addendum).
23. Nightingale SD, Cameron W, Gordin F, et al. Two controlled trials of rifabutin prophylaxis against *Mycobacterium avium* complex infection in AIDS. *N Engl J Med.* 1993;329:828–833.
24. Ostroff SM, Spiegel RA, Feinberg J, Benson CA, Horsburgh CR. Preventing disseminated *Mycobacterium avium* complex disease in patients infected with human immunodeficiency virus. *Clin Infect Dis.* 1995;21(suppl 1):S72–S76.
25. Stagg RJ, Gathe J, Lieberman RM, et al. The Vistide (cidofovir injection) treatment IND for relapsing CMV (CMV-R). Abstract Presented at the Fourth Conference on Retroviruses and Opportunistic Infections. Washington, DC. January 22–27, 1997.
26. Martin DF, Parks DJ, Mellow SD, et al. Treatment of cytomegalovirus retinitis with an intraocular sustained-release ganciclovir implant: a randomized controlled clinical trial. *Arch Ophthalmol.* 1994;112:1531–1539.
27. Kirsch LS, Arevalo JF, de la Paz EC, Munguia D, de Clercq E, Freeman WR. Intravitreal cidofovir (HPMPC) treatment of cytomegalovirus retinitis in patients with acquired immunodeficiency syndrome. *Ophthalmology.* 1995;102: 533–542.
28. Drew WL, Ives D, Lalezari JP, et al. Oral ganciclovir as maintenance treatment for cytomegalovirus retinitis in patients with AIDS. *N Engl J Med.* 1995;333: 615–620.
29. Drew WL, Buhles W, Erlich KS. Management of herpes virus infections (CMV, HSV, VZV). In: Sande MA, Volberding PA, eds. *The Medical Management of AIDS.* 4th ed. Philadelphia: WB Saunders; 1995:512–536.
30. Youle MS, Gazzard BG, Johnson MA, Cooper DA for the European-Australian Acyclovir Study Group. Effects of high-dose oral acyclovir on herpes virus disease and survival in patients with advanced HIV disease: a double-blind, placebo-controlled study. *AIDS.* 1994;8:641–649.
31. Stien DC, Graham NM, Park LP, et al. The effect of the interaction of acyclovir with zidovudine on progression to AIDS and survival: analysis of data in the Multicenter AIDS Cohort Study. *Ann Intern Med.* 1994;121:100–108.

32. Cooper DA, Pehrson O, Pederson C, et al. The efficacy and safety of zidovudine alone or as cotherapy with acyclovir in the treatment of patients with AIDS and AIDS-related complex: a double-blind, randomized trial. *AIDS.* 1993;7: 197–207.
33. Portegies P, Algra PR, Hollak CE, et al. Response to cytarabine in progressive multifocal leucoencephalopathy in AIDS. *Lancet.* 1991;337:680–681 (letter).
34. Hall C, Timpone J, Davni I, et al. Ara-C treatment of PML in AIDS patients. Abstract 8. Presented at the Fourth Conference on Retroviruses and Opportunistic Infections. Washington, DC. January 22–27, 1997.
35. Singer EL, Stoner GL, Singer P, et al. AIDS presenting as progressive multifocal leukoencephalopathy with clinical response to zidovudine. *Acta Neurol Scand.* 1994;90:443–447.
36. Huang S, Skolasky R, Dal Pan G, Royal W, McArthur J. Survival prolongation and symptom palliation in HIV-seropositive patients with PML treated with alpha-interferon. Abstract 341. Presented at the Fourth Conference on Retroviruses and Opportunistic Infections. Washington, DC. January 22–27, 1997.
37. Oriel D. Genital human papillomavirus infection. In: Holmes KK, Mardh P, Sparling PF, Wiesner PJ, eds. *Sexually transmitted diseases.* 2nd ed. New York: McGraw-Hill; 1990:433–441.
38. Hopewell PC, Masur H. *Pneumocystis carinii* pneumonia: current concepts. In: Sande MA, Volberding PA, eds. *The Medical Management of AIDS.* 4th ed. Philadelphia: WB Saunders; 1995:367–401.
39. Kaplan JE, Masur H, Homes KK, et al. USPHS/IDSA guidelines for the prevention of opportunistic infections in person infected with human immunodeficiency virus: disease-specific recommendations. *Clin Infect Dis.* 1995;21(suppl 1): S32–S43.
40. White AC Jr, Chappell DL, Hayat CS, Kimball KT, Flanigan TP, Goodgame RW. Paromomycin for cryptosporidiosis in AIDS: a prospective, double-blind trial. *J Infect Dis.* 1994;170:419–424.
41. Scaglia M, Atzori C, Marchetti G, et al. Effectiveness of aminosidine (paromomycin) sulfate in chronic *Cryptosporidium* diarrhea in AIDS patients: an open, uncontrolled, prospective clinical trial. *J Infect Dis.* 1994;170:1349–1350.
42. Hewitt RG, Yiannoutsos CT, Carey J, et al. A double-blind, placebo-controlled trial of paromomycin (Par) for the treatment of cryptosporidiosis (CS) in patients with advanced HIV disease and CD4 counts under 150 (ACTG 192). Abstract 4. Presented at the Fourth Conference on Retroviruses and Opportunistic Infections. Washington, DC. January 22–27, 1997.
43. Cello JP, Grendell JH, Basuk P, et al. Effect of octreotide on refractory AIDS-associated diarrhea: a prospective, multicenter clinical trial. *Ann Intern Med.* 1991;115:705–710.
44. Feregrino GM, et al. Extraordinary potency of nitazoxanide, a new antiparasi-

tary, against *Cryptosporidium parvum* infections in advanced AIDS. Abstract B4213. Presented at the Eleventh International Conference on AIDS. Vancouver, BC, Canada. 1996.

45. Asmuth DM, DeGirolani PC, Federman M, et al. Clinical features of microsporidiosis in patients with AIDS. *Clin Infect Dis.* 1994;18:819–825.
46. Verghese A, Al-Samman M, Nabhan D, Naylor AD, Rivera M. Bacterial bronchitis and bronchiectasis in human immunodeficiency virus infection. *Arch Intern Med.* 1994;154:2086–2091.
47. Kiehl MG, Stoll R, Broder M, Mueller C, Foerster E, Domschke W. A controlled trial of intravenous immune globulin for the prevention of serious infections in adults with advanced human immunodeficiency virus infection. *Arch Intern Med* 1996;156:2545–2550.

Chapter 6

Opportunistic Malignancies

Mary Beth Tombes, RN, MN, OCN
C. Fay Parpart, RN, MS, ANP, OCN

Chapter Preview

- Lymphoma
- Kaposi's Sarcoma
- Cervical Cancer

Almost half of all HIV-infected persons develop cancer during the course of their disease.[1,2] These cancers, which develop in the HIV-mediated immunosuppressed state, are called *opportunistic malignancies* and include the AIDS-defining conditions Kaposi's sarcoma (KS), non-Hodgkin's lymphoma (NHL), and invasive cervical cancer.[3] Other cancers that are sometimes seen in HIV-infected persons include Hodgkin's disease, multiple myeloma, testicular cancer, anogenital cancer, basal cell carcinoma, lung cancer, malignant melanoma, and leukemia.[4–7] However, this latter group of cancers are not considered "AIDS-defining malignancies" and there is still considerable debate about the role of HIV-mediated carcinogenesis in these malignancies.[5]

According to Krown, "there is realistic concern that cancers will grow in importance as survival with severe immunosuppression is prolonged."[6(p 441)] The incidence of opportunistic malgnancies will likely continue to increase.[1,4,8–11]

Although HIV-associated malignancies are similar to cancers seen in other immunosuppressed persons (organ transplant recipients, persons with congenital immunodeficiencies), immunosuppression alone does not explain the development of opportunistic malignancies.[12] Whether HIV itself is carcinogenic, or whether it provides a milieu ideal for carcinogenesis via immunosuppression or through cofactors (environmental or viral), is an area of intense investigation.[5]

Opportunistic cancers are atypical in their presentation, natural history, and response to therapy.[12,13] They tend to be more disseminated at diagnosis, more aggressive, and less responsive to therapy.[9,14–17] Treatment is made more complicated by virtue of the already immunocompromised state of the host. Patients with HIV-associated cancer are faced with the dual crises of cancer and HIV/AIDS. Sensitivity to the patient's situation is critical, as is an understanding of the underlying pathology, natural history, and medical management of cancer in the HIV/AIDS patient.[18]

Lymphoma

Malignant lymphomas are a group of cancers caused by uncontrolled proliferation of lymphatic tissue, usually arising in the lymph nodes, bone marrow, spleen, and liver. In HIV-infected persons, NHLs occur in uncharacteristically high numbers in extralymphatic organs, arising from the CNS, bone marrow, GI tract, and liver.

Definition

NHL typically originates in B or T lymphocytes, but most HIV-associated NHLs are intermediate or high-grade B-cell lymphomas, pathologically classified according to the working formulation based on morphology, aggressiveness, and median survival (Table 6.1).[19] Rarely, low-grade B-cell lymphoma, multiple myeloma, T-cell lymphoma, or T-cell leukemia are seen, but these are not considered AIDS-defining diagnoses.[3] Anatomic staging of NHL is accomplished using the Ann Arbor Staging System (Table 6.2), which is identical to that used for non-HIV-related NHL.[19]

Biologic Basis and Epidemiology

Epidemiology

Overall, the rate of NHL in the HIV-infected population is 73 times higher than in the general population.[20] The risk of developing NHL, specifically primary CNS lymphoma, appears to be highest in those persons with a CD4 count of <50/mm^3,[16] and in older white males.[21,22] Persons with HIV who develop NHL are typically younger compared with those in the general population, with a median age at diagnosis of 38 years vs. 56 years.[16,17]

Table 6.1 Working Formulation of Non-Hodgkin's Lymphomas

Grade	Description
Low	Small lymphocytic cell Follicular, predominantly small cleaved cell Follicular, mixed small cleaved, and large cell
Intermediate	Follicular, predominantly large cell Diffuse, small cleaved cell Diffuse, mixed small and large cell Diffuse, large cell, cleaved or noncleaved
High	Diffuse large cell, immunoblastic Lymphoblastic (convoluted or nonconvoluted) Small, noncleaved cell (Burkitt's or non-Burkitt's)

Used with the permission of the American Joint Committee on Cancer (AJCC®), Chicago, Illinois. The original source for this material is the AJCC® Manual for Staging of Cancer, 3rd edition (1988) published by Lippincott-Raven Publishers, Philadelphia.

Table 6.2 The Ann Arbor Staging Classification for Non-Hodgkin's Lymphomas

Stage	Description
I	Involvement of a single lymph node region (I) or localized involvement of a single extralymphatic organ or site (IE)
II	Involvement of two or more lymph node regions on the same side of the diaphragm (II) or localized involvement of an extralymphatic organ or site and its regional nodes on the same side of the diaphragm (IIE)
III	Involvement of lymph node regions on both sides of the diaphragm (III), which also may be accompanied by localized involvement of an extranodal organ, or side (IIIE), or spleen (IIIS), or both (IIISE)
IV	Multifocal or disseminated involvement of one or more distant extralymphatic organs with or without associated lymph node involvement, or isolated extralymphatic organ involvement with distant (nonregional) nodal involvement

Used with the permission of the American Joint Committee on Cancer (AJCC®), Chicago, Illinois. The original source for this material is the AJCC® Manual for Staging of Cancer, 3rd edition (1988) published by Lippincott-Raven Publishers, Philadelphia.

CNS involvement is unusually high in HIV-infected persons with NHL.[23] Primary CNS lymphoma may be the only site of lymphoma in 20 to 30% of HIV-infected persons diagnosed with NHL.[9,24]

Biologic Basis

Although the exact etiology of NHL in HIV-infected individuals is unknown, complex interactions between multiple factors may affect its development.[12,25] Immunosuppression, especially impaired cell-mediated immunity (such as that which results in organ transplant recipients and HIV infection), predisposes people to the risk of cancer, particularly lymphomas.[12]

Chronic antigenic stimulation and cytokine overproduction along with HIV-mediated T-cell suppression permits B-cell hyperactivation and overproliferation.[26] This leads first to benign nodal hyperplasia and then to PGL, which is associated with increased risk of lymphoma in HIV-infected persons.[9] Epstein-Barr virus (EBV) can also stimulate B-cell proliferation, and in the presence of T-cell dysfunction, EBV may be a cofactor in the development of HIV-related lymphoma.[7,9,23,26] Chromosomal abnormalities seem to predispose to lymphoma development in the setting of HIV infection, probably via oncogene activation and/or disabling of tumor suppressor genes.[9,12,26,27]

Presentation and Assessment

Extranodal or advanced disease (stage III or IV) or the presence of B symptoms (i.e., unexplained fever, night sweats, unintentional loss of >10% of body weight, and diarrhea persisting for more than 2 weeks) are common findings at diagnosis in HIV-infected persons.[12,17] In addition to stage, several other prognostic factors must be considered including (1) CD4 count (reflective of underlying immune deficiency), (2) presence or history of OIs, and (3) performance status (indicative of the person's ability to perform activities of daily living [ADLs] independently). These characteristics affect both prognosis and treatment selection.[28]

Though both are lymphomas, primary CNS lymphoma and systemic NHL must be clearly differentiated from each other in persons with HIV because they are managed differently and have different prognoses.[12] Clinical evaluation of HIV-infected persons includes a thorough assessment with an eye toward subtle changes that signal the onset of systemic NHL or primary CNS lymphoma (Table 6.3). Delineating such changes from those caused by other HIV-related problems, such as OIs or AIDS-related dementia, is an important challenge because it has implications for prognosis, treatment, and outcomes.[9,18,29,30]

Presenting symptoms of primary CNS lymphoma include headache, seizures, or focal neurological abnormalities.[9,30] Subtle personality or behavior changes may be the only warning signs that a neurological evaluation should be initiated.[24] Systemic NHL most commonly presents as obstruction of the GI tract, infection or bleeding due to bone marrow infiltration, or enlarged lymph nodes. Any body site may serve as the tissue of origin of systemic NHL.[24]

Tissue biopsy is required to diagnose any AIDS-related NHL because tumor cell type has implications for prognosis and treatment. For primary CNS lymphoma, pathological diagnosis is necessary to rule out other AIDS-related CNS diseases, such as toxoplasmosis, encephalitis, tuberculosis, cryptococcal infections, or bacterial abscesses.[24] CT, MRI, bone marrow aspiration and biopsy, or lumbar puncture may be used to determine the nature and extent of HIV-related NHL.

Table 6.3 Assessment of AIDS-Related Malignancies[a]

Type of Malignancy System or Site	NHL	PCNSL	KS	Cervical Cancer
A. NONSPECIFIC				
Constitutional symptoms: fever, weight loss (>10% body weight), night sweats, anorexia	√			
Generalized or localized lymphadenopathy	√	√		
Obstructive lymphedema	√	√		
Pruritus	√			
B. HEMATOLOGIC/IMMUNOLOGIC				
CD4 count <500 cells/mm^3	√	√	√	√
C. SKIN				
Painless, nonpruritic linear lesions, especially on the face, tips of nose or ears, trunk, posterior pharynx, glans penis, thigh, and sole of foot			√	
D. EYES				
Conjunctival lesions; may look like hemorrhage		√		
Periocular skin lesions			√	
Visual field deficits	√	√		
E. ORAL MUCOSA				
Mucosal nodules or lesions, especially gingival surfaces, palate, and peritonsillar areas			√	
F. RESPIRATORY				
SOB/dyspnea			√	
Dry cough exacerbated by deep inspiration			√	

Type of Malignancy System or Site	NHL	PCNSL	KS	Cervical Cancer
G. Gastrointestinal				
Abdominal pain	√			
Dysphagia			√	
Esophagitis			√	
Splenomegaly	√			
Hepatomegaly	√		√	
Pain, constipation, nausea, or vomiting due to bowel obstruction by tumor or lymphadenopathy	√		√	
Changes in bowel habits	√		√	
Ulceration	√		√	
Perirectal pain due to abscess	√		√	
H. Neurological				
Focal deficits: hemiparesis, aphasia, seizures, cranial nerve palsies		√		
Confusion, lethargy, memory loss		√		
Headache		√		
Subtle alterations in mental status		√		
I. Genitourinary				
Foul-smelling discharge				√
Watery discharge				√
Painful intercourse				√
Bleeding during or after intercourse, or between periods				√
HPV anogenital warts				√

[a]Data culled from various sources.[15,29–33]
NHL = non-Hodgkin's lymphoma; PCNSL = primary central nervous system lymphoma; KS = Kaposi's sarcoma; SOB = shortness of breath; HPV = human papilloma virus.

Medical Management

Radiation therapy is the treatment of choice for primary CNS lymphoma[14] (see Chapter 8). Even with a complete response rate of 20 to 50%, median survival is only 2 to 5 months.[24,27] Survival is longer for patients with better performance status (independence in most ADLs) and no history of OIs.

In patients with primary CNS lymphoma, cognitive and functional symptoms range from those that are annoying (such as headaches or subtle memory lapses) to those that are debilitating (such as severe cognitive, motor, or sensory dysfunction). Although response duration is short, radiation therapy does decrease symptoms and improve quality of life in >75% of patients, thus it is a reasonable option for palliation of symptoms despite the dismal survival statistics.[14,16,24,27]

Systemic NHL must be treated with systemic chemotherapy. Initially, HIV-infected persons with NHL were treated with regimens identical to those used for NHL in the non-HIV-infected population, but standard doses of chemotherapeutic agents proved too toxic in the chronically immunosuppressed HIV population.[9] Regimens using lower total doses have proven useful because they are associated with less morbidity and mortality related to infection. Unfortunately these regimens also have less antineoplastic efficacy. It has become more common to utilize standard-dose antineoplastic regimens accompanied by hematopoietic growth factors to overcome myelosuppressive effects of chemotherapy.[9] Lower dose regimens may still be useful for those persons who are severely immunocompromised (CD4 < 100 cells/mm^3) and have a recent history of multiple OIs.[16]

Common Clinical Problems and Related Care

Refer to Table 6.4 and other chapters in Unit Two for guidelines about the prevention, assessment, and management of common clinical problems that can be associated with HIV-related NHL and primary CNS lymphoma.

Kaposi's Sarcoma

Definition

HIV-related KS is referred to as *epidemic KS* to distinguish it from several other forms of KS that occur in non-HIV-positive persons (classic, African,

Table 6.4 Common Clinical Problems Associated with Opportunistic Malignancies

Clinical Problem	NHL	PCNSL	KS	Cervical Cancer
A. NEUROLOGICAL IMPAIRMENT				
Confusion and delirium		√		
Memory loss and dementia		√		
Decreased concentration, alterations in conciousness and alertness		√		
Impaired coordination, balance, and mobility		√		
Seizures		√		
B. NUTRITION-RELATED CHANGES				
Anorexia, cachexia, wasting, malnutrition	√	√	√	√
Taste changes	√tx	√tx	√tx	√tx
Xerostomia	√tx	√tx	√tx	
Stomatitis and mucositis	√tx	√tx	√tx	√tx
Nausea, vomiting, retching	√tx	√tx	√tx	√tx
Constipation				
Diarrhea	√tx	√tx	√tx	
C. RESPIRATORY CHANGES				
Dyspnea	√	√		
Cough	√	√		
D. CHANGES IN HOST DEFENSES				
Thrombocytopenia	√tx	√tx	√tx	√tx
Neutropenia	√tx	√tx	√tx	√tx
E. SEXUALITY CHANGES				
Decreased interest; impaired performance/activity	√	√	√	
Altered body image	√	√	√	√

Table 6.4 *Continued*

Clinical Problem	NHL	PCNSL	KS	Cervical Cancer
F. SKIN PROBLEMS				
Itching (pruritus)	√			
Dry skin				
Skin and nail lesions		√		
Rash				
G. PSYCHOSOCIAL RESPONSES				
Anxiety	√	√	√	√
Depression and suicidal tendencies	√			
Psychosis and mania	√			
Grief and loss	√	√	√	√
H. CHANGES IN FUNCTIONAL CAPACITY AND PERFORMANCE				
Fatigue	√	√	√tx	√
Sleep alterations		√		
Visual changes	√	√	√	
I. DISCOMFORT				
Pain	√	√	√	√
Peripheral neuropathy	√tx	√tx	√tx	√tx
Night sweats	√	√		
Fever, chills, shivering	√	√		

NHL = non-Hodgkin's lymphoma; PCNSL = primary central nervous system lymphoma; KS = Kaposi's sarcoma; tx = the clinical problem is associated more with treatment of the malignancy (by chemotherapy, radiotherapy, or biologic therapy) than with the cancer itself.

immunosuppressive treatment-related, and nonepidemic homosexual-related KS). KS is a soft-tissue vascular cancer that arises from the mid-dermis and is characterized by uncontrolled growth of spindle-shaped reticuloendothelial cells. These lymphatic endothelial cells are found throughout the body, so KS can arise in virtually any organ or tissue.[31] Pathologically, epidemic KS and other types of KS are identical, but their clinical presentation and natural history differ significantly.[34]

Biologic Basis and Epidemiology

Epidemiology

Originally described as a rare, unusual, and indolent neoplasm affecting mostly older men of Mediterranean or Jewish ancestry, classic KS differs significantly from HIV-related KS.[12] Epidemic KS is the most common HIV-associated malignancy, but it occurs in particularly high frequency in men who have sex with men.[34] In some cohorts of men who have sex with men and who have AIDS, the lifetime risk of KS approaches 50%. Surveillance data indicate that KS is roughly 20 times more likely to develop in men with AIDS compared with men who are HIV negative, and that the risk of KS is associated with specific sexual practices and geographic locations.[35] Similar forms of KS do occur in men who have sex with men but who are not HIV infected.[35] Following widespread institution of "safer sex" behaviors among men who have sex with men, the incidence of AIDS-related KS has declined.[17,22]

Biologic Basis

Even before the identification of HIV/AIDS, KS was known to be related to disruption of cellular immunity on the basis of findings in persons with other immunodeficiency syndromes. In the HIV-infected population, HIV-mediated T-cell suppression clearly serves as the biologic basis for the development of KS.

Presentation and Assessment

Clinical assessment can reveal manifestations of KS in virtually any tissue (see Table 6.3),[30,31] but it is most often found in the GI tract, mucous membranes, lymph nodes, and skin.[9,30,31] KS lesions are classified as patch, plaque, and/or nodular lesions.[9] Skin lesions may be any color, size, or configuration and are usually seen on the trunk, arms, head, or neck.

Histological examination of a tissue biopsy is necessary to confirm a diagnosis of KS.

KS lesions of the GI tract are often found initially in the oral cavity. Lesions throughout the GI tract may be associated with bleeding, pain, weight loss, or diarrhea. Because mucosal lesions are flat and are not well visualized by barium studies, they are best evaluated endoscopically.[31] Lymph node involvement is usually a late-stage manifestation of KS and commonly results in lymphedema due to a local inflammatory response to cytokine release from KS cells rather than to compression of lymphatics.[31] Pulmonary KS occurs in 20 to 50% of patients with KS and may mimic pneumonia.[9] Symptoms include fever, shortness of breath, wheezing, or cough. Pulmonary KS is easily diagnosed with bronchoscopy but has a poor prognosis, with a median survival of less than 3 months.[36] The presence of B symptoms described earlier (p. 175), a CD4 count of <300 cells/mm^3, or any history of OIs is associated with a worse prognosis in HIV-related KS.[31]

Medical Management

A proposed staging classification system for HIV-related KS incorporates not only tumor bulk, but also immune function and concomitant systemic illness or symptoms (Table 6.5).[27] Treatment is generally based on immunologic status, the involved organ system (i.e., skin, lymphatics, or viscera), and the presence or absence of B symptoms (p. 175).

Treatment for HIV-related KS focuses on the goal of reducing "tumor-related signs and symptoms through methods that can be integrated with the individual patient's need for anti-retroviral therapy, treatment and prophylaxis of opportunistic infections, and overall performance status."[31(p 236)] Three basic principles guide the treatment of HIV-related KS[9,31]:

1. Long-term survival is possible after minimal treatment.
2. Malignant KS is inherently disseminated at presentation.
3. No therapy is considered curative.

Important considerations in treatment choice include both the status of the patient's KS and the status of the patient's HIV disease.[31] In general, minimal, asymptomatic disease dictates minimal therapy, whereas more extensive, cosmetically unacceptable, or symptomatic lesions require more aggressive therapy. In any case, the CD4 count also impacts choice of

Table 6.5 Proposed Staging Classification for Kaposi's Sarcoma

Good Risk: All of the Following	Poor Risk: Any of the Following
A. TUMOR	
Confined to skin and/or lymph nodes and/or minimal oral disease (e.g., non-nodular oral KS confined to the palate)	Tumor-associated edema or ulceration Extensive oral KS lesions Gastrointestinal KS lesions KS lesions in other non-nodal viscera
B. IMMUNE SYSTEM	
CD4+ cells ≥ 200/mm³	CD4+ cells < 200/mm³
C. SYSTEMIC ILLNESS	
No history of OIs or thrush No B symptoms[a] Karnofsky performance status ≥ 70	History of OI and/or thrush B symptoms present[a] Karnofsky performance status < 70 Other HIV-related illness (e.g., neurological disease, lymphoma)

[a]B symptoms are unexplained fever, night sweats, >10% involuntary weight loss, or diarrhea persisting for more than 2 weeks.
KS = Kaposi's sarcoma; OI = opportunistic infection.
Adapted from Kaplan L, Northfelt D. Malignancies associated with ADIS. In: Sande MV, Volberding PA, eds. *The Medical Management of AIDS.* 4th ed. Philadelphia: WB Sauders; 1995:568.

therapy. Due to the highly variable nature of KS the disease can follow an aggressive or indolent course; thus *observation* or *watchful waiting* is a reasonable course of action in patients in whom KS appears indolent.[31] Active treatment modalities for KS include localized or systemic therapy.

Localized Therapy

KS lesions are highly radiosensitive, with radiation therapy yielding complete response rates of 20 to 85%.[9,27,31] Radiation therapy is used most often to palliate painful lesions or to relieve edema due to bulky lymphadenopathy.[31] KS tumors involving the face or eyelid with periorbital swelling are particularly well suited for radiotherapy because it can help both cosmetically and functionally by alleviating visual problems.[31]

The use of local excision to treat KS has been limited in the past due to the poor health of the patient, the location of the lesion, and the presumed systemic nature of KS. Patients who present with isolated KS lesions are excellent candidates for local therapy with liquid nitrogen cryosurgery or laser excision.[31] Cryotherapy and laser surgery are used most often to resect lesions that interfere with function or cosmesis, such as lesions in the upper aerodigestive tract or the skin of the head, neck, and upper extremities. Cryotherapy (freezing the lesion with liquid nitrogen) must be used with caution in dark-skinned individuals because melanocytes are sensitive to freezing, and hypopigmentation may result, negating any cosmetic benefit of lesion removal in these persons.[31] Intralesional injections of chemotherapy (primarily the vinca alkaloids) have been useful in the local control of small intraoral or cutaneous KS lesions[9,31] (see Chapter 7).

Systemic Therapy

Single-agent IM or subcutaneous interferon alpha (IFN-α; a potent cytokine inhibitor) yields response rates of 30%.[31] Combinations of IFN-α and antiretroviral agents, such as the RT inhibitor zidovudine, yield greater benefit than IFN-α alone.[31] IFN-α combined with chemotherapy has been tried with minimal success in KS. Such regimens do not confer any increased efficacy over IFN alone and are associated with excessive toxicity.[31] Side effects of systemic IFN-α include flulike symptoms such as fever, weight loss, fatigue, chills, anorexia, nausea, and diarrhea. These must be managed symptomatically and differentiated from possible OIs.[9,31] These "constitutional" side effects can adversely affect functional status, having important implications for compliance with treatment and the patient's quality of life. Antipyretics and nonsteroidal anti-inflammatory drugs (NSAIDs) may be used prophylactically or as needed to manage these effects. Patients will often experience *tachyphylaxis* or adaptation to these biologic side effects, with the symptoms lessening over a period of 3 to 6 weeks. Even so, patients must be encouraged to stick with the treatment plan long enough to see if tachyphylaxis will occur.

Single-agent or combination chemotherapy may be used to treat KS. Single-agent response rates vary between 30 to 70%.[9] Combination chemotherapy regimens have shown greater success (80–90% response rates), but these more myelosuppressive regimens are complicated by precipitation of OIs in this already immunocompromised population.[9]

Common Clinical Problems and Related Care

Refer to Table 6.4 and other chapters in Unit Two for guidelines about the prevention, assessment, and management of common clinical problems associated with HIV-related KS.

Cervical Cancer

Invasive cancer of the cervix in HIV-infected females became an AIDS-defining condition according to the January 1993 revision of the CDC Classification System and Expanded Case Definition.[3,37] Both invasive cervical cancer and a continuum of preinvasive precursor lesions called *cervical intraepithelial neoplasia* (CIN) occur more often in HIV-infected women than in noninfected women.[38–41] Some clinicians are adamant that the incidence of HIV in women with cervical cancer is still severely underestimated.[42]

Cervical cancer in non-HIV-infected women is highly curable when detected early, but in women with HIV infection, cervical cancer (like NHL) tends to be more aggressive, more advanced at diagnosis, and less responsive to definitive treatment.[43,44] Although there may be pathophysiologic mechanisms for these differences in natural history, access to care also affects these characteristics, prompting recent social and political interventions to encourage cervical cancer screening among vulnerable populations.[32]

Definition

Cervical cancer arises primarily from cells in the transformational zone of the cervix, where columnar epithelium and squamous epithelium converge in a zone of squamous metaplasia. This transformational zone is characterized by a high cell turnover rate and is thus susceptible to carcinogenesis.[32] Cervical smear cytology, used to classify cervical abnormalities on a continuum between dysplasia and invasive cancer, is shown in Table 6.6. CIN in HIV-infected women behaves in a more aggressive manner than in the general population, with rapid progression of disease, poorer response to therapy, and increased risk of relapse.[9]

Table 6.6 Cervical Smear Classification

Class	Description	Dysplasia Level
I	Normal smear; no abnormal cells	—
II	Atypical cells present below the level of cervical neoplasia	—
III	Smear contains abnormal cells consistent with dysplasia	Mild dysplasia = CIN 1; moderate dysplasia = CIN 2
IV	Smear contains abnormal cells consistent with carcinoma in situ	Severe dysplasia and carcinoma in situ = CIN 3
V	Smear contains abnormal cells consistent with carcinoma of squamous cell origin	—

CIN = cervical intraepithelial neoplasia.
Adapted from Nelson J, Averette H, Richart R. Cervical intraepithelial neoplasia (dysplasia and carcinoma in situ) and early invasive cervical carcinoma. *CA Cancer J Clin.* 1989;39:157–178.

Biologic Basis and Epidemiology

Epidemiology

HIV-infected women have a 7 to 10 times greater risk of developing precancerous or cancerous cervical lesions than noninfected women.[32] Furthermore, HIV-infected women have a significantly higher rate of recurrence of CIN following local excision or cervical cancer according to standard curative therapy, as compared with non-HIV-infected women. Risk of recurrence increases as the CD4 count drops.[45] The association of these squamous cell carcinomas with human papilloma virus (HPV) infection has been well documented, with predominant implication of HPV types 16, 18, 31, 33, and 35.[6]

Biologic Basis

Sexually transmitted cofactors are thought to play a significant role in the development of CIN and invasive cervical cancer regardless of HIV status. The HPVs are a family of more than 66 viruses, several of which have been implicated in the development of CIN and cervical cancer.[6] Although data about the exact nature of the relationship between HIV and HPV are conflicting, it is suggested that a state of HIV-mediated immunosuppression permits HPV infection and proliferation, and thus an increased risk of cervical dysplasia.[32,40,46,47]

Presentation and Assessment

Due to the aggressive and recurrent nature of cervical abnormalities in HIV-infected women, many HIV centers encourage these women to have screening Papanicolaou (Pap) smears as often as every 6 months.[47,48] Clinical practice guidelines for the evaluation and management of early HIV infection recommend Pap smears be performed twice in the first year following diagnosis of HIV infection, then annually provided the initial Pap smears were normal. If there is a history of HPV infection, previous abnormal Pap smears, or symptomatic HIV infection, then Pap smears are recommended every 6 months.[49] Additionally, because of the more aggressive natural history of cervical cancer in women with HIV infection, Maiman et al.[43] suggest that HIV screening be done in all women less than 50 years old who are also found to have invasive cervical cancer.

Early invasive cervical cancer can be "silent," regardless of HIV status. Gynecologic evaluation should be initiated when any woman reports any of the following: painful intercourse; postcoital, coital, or intermenstrual bleeding; or a foul-smelling or watery discharge (see Table 6.3).

Women with abnormal Pap smears usually undergo colposcopy, which is a means of visualizing the cervical canal and identifying abnormalities for biopsy. In some cases, a cone biopsy or *conization* (resection of a cone-shaped portion of cervical tissue) is performed to obtain adequate tissue for diagnosis of CIN or invasive cancer. The outpatient loop electrosurgical excision procedure (LEEP) is an alternative to conization.[50,51]

Some practitioners have suggested that the need for increased screening vigilance in HIV-infected women necessitates that screening colposcopy be used as a routine adjunct to the Pap smear because of concerns about false-negative Pap smears in HIV-infected females.[9,52] However, Wright et al[38] report that the Pap smear false-negative rate in HIV-infected women is similar to that in the general population. Nonetheless, "liberal colposcopic biopsy" is recommended to assess for recurrent CIN in HIV-infected women.[45]

Minority women scheduled to undergo colposcopy have been found to have inadequate information about the test and its implications.[53] Such knowledge deficits can create a potential for noncompliance with screening and diagnostic testing. Because of their higher risk associated with a cancer diagnosis, compliance with surveillance testing is even more critical for HIV-infected women than the general population.

Medical Management

Regardless of HIV status, choice of therapy is dictated by the stage of disease (Table 6.7) and the degree of cervical abnormality.[54] In general, more extensive disease requires more invasive treatment. Treatment options for preinvasive disease include cryotherapy, laser surgery, therapeutic conization, or LEEP. Because of the high risk of recurrence, the optimal treatment for noninvasive disease (CIN) in HIV-infected women has not yet been defined. Maiman et al[45] have suggested that cryotherapy alone for CIN in HIV-infected women be used with caution, as it may prove to be less than optimal in this high-risk subset of women with CIN.

Currently, HIV-infected women with invasive cervical cancer are being medically managed in the same way as those without HIV, although controlled studies comparing outcomes in these two populations are lacking.[43] Surgery, consisting of total abdominal or radical hysterectomy, depending on the depth of invasion, with or without oophorectomy, is standard for invasive disease, with no apparent differences reported in immediate postsurgical outcomes between HIV-infected and non-infected women.[43]

Similarly, women who would be suitable candidates for radiation or chemotherapy were they not HIV infected may still be appropriate candidates for such therapy as long as special attention is paid to managing local and hematologic sequelae of treatment (see Chapters 7 and 8). Less myelotoxic chemotherapy may be given combined with zidovudine therapy.[43] For patients in whom local therapy is preferable, local treatment with 5-fluorouracil cream or IFN-α therapy may be useful.[43]

Common Clinical Problems and Related Care

Refer to Table 6.4 and other chapters in Unit Two for guidelines about the prevention, assessment, and management of common clinical problems that can be associated with HIV-related cervical cancer.

Table 6.7 Clinical Staging of Cervical Cancer

Stage	Description
0	Carcinoma in situ, intraepithelial carcinoma
I	Carcinoma strictly confined to the cervix (extension to the corpus disregarded)
IA	Preclinical carcinoma of the cervix (i.e., those diagnosed by microscopy)
IA1	Minimal microscopically evident stromal invasion
IA2	Microscopic lesions that are measurable; upper limit of measurement should not show depth of invasion of >5 mm from the base of the epithelium, either surface or glandular, from which it originated, and a second dimension (the horizontal spread) must not exceed 7 mm; larger lesions should be staged as IB
IB	Lesions of greater dimension than stage IA2 whether seen clinically or not; preformed space involvement should not alter the staging, but should be specifically recorded to determine whether it should affect treatment decisions in the future
II	Carcinoma extends beyond the cervix, but not to the pelvic wall; involves the vagina, but not as far as the lower third
IIA	No obvious parametrial involvement
IIB	Obvious parametrial involvement
III	Carcinoma extends to the pelvic wall; on rectal exam, no cancer-free space between the tumor and pelvic wall; tumor involves the lower third of the vagina; all patients with hydronephrosis or nonfunctioning kidney are included
IIIA	No extension to the pelvic wall, but tumor involves lower third of vagina
IIIB	Extension to the pelvic wall and/or hydronephrosis or nonfunctioning kidney
IV	Carcinoma extends beyond the true pelvis or clinically involves the mucosa of the bladder or rectum; a bullous edema as such does not permit a patient to be assigned to stage IV
IVA	Spread of the tumor to adjacent organs
IVB	Spread to distant organs

Adapted from Nelson J, Averette H, Richart R. Cervical intraepithelial neoplasia (dysplasia and carcinoma in situ) and early invasive cervical carcinoma. *CA Cancer J Clin.* 1989;39:159.

Summary

Familiarity with resources is critical, both because of the multiplicity of information available and because of the rapid changes in the field of HIV care. Resources abound about cancer and HIV (e.g., books, journals, pamphlets, the Internet, people within the community). Free cancer care resources are available from the National Cancer Information Service (1-800-4-CANCER). Providers unfamiliar with HIV care can access the National AIDS Information Clearinghouse for reference assistance and publications (1-800-458-5231). A network of 15 centers in the country have been funded by Health Resource Services (HRS) to provide HIV training to health care providers. Regional AIDS education and training centers may be accessed by calling the National HIV/AIDS Education and Training Centers Program at 301-443-6364. There are numerous ways to access cancer and AIDS information on the Internet as well.

Assessment of HIV-infected persons with or at risk for opportunistic malignancies requires an awareness of both the nature of HIV disease and associated neoplastic complications. Table 6.3 lists assessment indicators for common clinical manifestations of opportunistic malignancies in the HIV-infected person according to the type of opportunistic malignancy. The importance of differentiating between signs and symptoms of cancer and those of other HIV-related problems cannot be overemphasized.

The following are some special considerations to keep in mind when caring for HIV-infected persons with opportunistic malignancies:

- Sequelae of radiation therapy, chemotherapy, or biologic response modifier therapy can range from troublesome to debilitating depending on the patient's overall health and aggressiveness of treatment. Proactive patient teaching and interventions to prevent or minimize common side effects are described in Unit Two.
- Psychosocial well-being may be at risk in the patient trying to deal with the "double whammy" of AIDS and cancer. Open discussion of coping strategies and support services will serve the patient and significant others well.
- Body image issues may be new for the patient diagnosed with new, visible lesions; lymphedema; or lymphadenopathy from KS or NHL, or the sequelae of treatment. Persons who have not had to deal with outward manifestations of HIV infection previously may have to adjust to a new phase of their illness.

References

1. Peters B, Beck E, Coleman D. Changing disease patterns in patients with AIDS in a referral centre in the United Kingdom: the changing face of AIDS. *BMJ.* 1991;302(6770):203–207.
2. Hoover D, Saah A, Bacellar H, et al. Clinical manifestations of AIDS in the era of pneumocystis prophylaxis. Multicenter AIDS cohort study. *N Eng J Med.* 1993;329:1922–1926.
3. CDC. 1993 revised classification system for HIV infection and expanded surveillance case definition for AIDS among adolescents and adults. *MMWR.* 1992; 41(RR–17).
4. Conant M. Management of human immunodeficiency virus-associated malignancies. *Recent Results Cancer Res.* 1995;139:423–432.
5. Lyter D, Bryant J, Thackeray R, Rinaldo C, Kingsley L. Incidence of human immunodeficiency virus-related and nonrelated malignancies in a large cohort of homosexual men. *J Clin Oncol.* 1995;13(10):2540–2546.
6. Krown S. AIDS-associated malignancies. In: Pinedo H, Longo D, Chabner B, eds. *Cancer Chemotherapy and Biological Response Modifiers Annual 16.* Amsterdam: Elsevier Science; 1996:441–461.
7. Schulz T, Boshoff C, Weiss R. HIV infection and neoplasia. *Lancet.* 1996;348: 587–591.
8. Gail M, Pluda J, Rabkin C, et al. Projections of the incidence of non-Hodgkin's lymphoma related to acquired immunodeficiency syndrome. *J Natl Cancer Inst.* 1991;83(10):695–701.
9. Levine A. AIDS-related malignancies: the emerging epidemic. *J Natl Cancer Inst.* 1993;85(17):1382–1396.
10. Pluda J, Yarchoan R, Jaffe E, et al. Development of non-Hodgkin's lymphoma in a cohort of patients with severe human immunodeficiency virus (HIV) infections on long-term antiretroviral therapy. *Ann Intern Med.* 1990;113(4):276–282.
11. Straus D. Human immunodeficiency virus-associated lymphomas. *Med Clin North Am.* 1997;81(23):495–510.
12. Biggar R. Cancer in acquired immunodeficiency syndrome: an epidemiological assessment. *Semin Oncol.* 1990;17(3):251–260.
13. Bernstein L, Hamilton A. The epidemiology of AIDS-related malignancies. *Curr Opin Oncol.* 1993;5(5):822–830.
14. NCI. AIDS-related lymphoma. In: *National Cancer Institute (NCI) Physicians Data Query (PDQ) Statement.* 1996.
15. Stanley H, Fluetsch-Bloom M, Bunce-Clyma M. HIV-related non-Hodgkin's lymphoma. *Oncol Nurs Forum.* 1991;18(5):875–880.
16. Pluda J, Venzon D, Tosato G, et al. Parameters affecting the development of non-Hodgkin's lymphoma in patients with severe human immunodeficiency

virus infection receiving antiretroviral therapy. *J Clin Oncol.* 1993;11(6): 1099–1107.
17. Safai B, Diaz B, Schwartz J. Malignant neoplasms associated with human immunodeficiency virus infection. *CA Cancer J Clin.* 1992;42(2):74–95.
18. Ungvarski P. Nursing management of the adult client. In: Flaskerud J, Ungvarski P, eds. *HIV/AIDS: A Guide to Nursing Care.* 3rd ed. Philadelphia: WB Saunders; 1995:146–151.
19. American Joint Committee on Cancer. *American Joint Committee on Cancer: Manual for Staging of Cancer.* 3rd ed. Philadelphia: JB Lippincott; 1988.
20. Lyter D, Bryant J, Thackeray R, Zhao P, Rinaldo C, Kingsley L. (Abstract) Incidence of Kaposi's sarcoma (KS), non-Hodgkin's lymphoma (NHL), and other malignancies in a cohort of gay men with human immunodeficiency virus (HIV) infection. *Proc Annu Meet Am Soc Clin Oncol.* 1994;13(A2).
21. Biggar R, Rabkin C. The epidemiology of acquired immunodeficiency syndrome-related lymphomas. *Curr Opin Oncol.* 1992;4(5):883–893.
22. Biggar R, Rosenberg P, Cote T. Kaposi's sarcoma and non-Hodgkin's lymphoma following the diagnosis of AIDS. Multistate AIDS/Cancer Match Study Group. *Int J Cancer.* 1996;68(6):754–758.
23. Flinn I, Amdinder R. AIDS primary central nervous system lymphoma. *Curr Opin Oncol.* 1996;8(5):373–376.
24. Levine A. AIDS-associated malignant lymphoma. *Med Clin North Am.* 1992; 76(1):253–268.
25. Armenian H, Hoover D, Rubb S, et al. Risk factors for non-Hodgkin's lymphomas in acquired immunodeficiency syndrome (AIDS). *Am J Epidemiol.* 1996;143(4): 374–379.
26. Knowles D. Etiology and pathogenesis of AIDS-related non-Hodgkin's lymphoma. *Hematol Oncol Clin North Am.* 1996;10(5):1081–1109.
27. Kaplan L, Northfelt D. Malignancies associated with AIDS. In: Sande MV, Volberding PA, eds. *The Medical Management of AIDS.* 4th ed. Philadelphia: WB Saunders; 1995:568.
28. Levine A, Sullivan-Halley J, Pike M, et al. Human immunodeficiency virus-related lymphoma: prognostic factors predictive of survival. *Cancer.* 1991; 68(11):2466–2472.
29. Cohen F. The clinical spectrum of HIV infection and its treatment. In: Durham J, Cohen F, eds. *The Person with AIDS: Nursing Perspectives.* 2nd ed. New York: Springer Publishing; 1991:135–192.
30. Ungvarski P. Clinical manifestations of AIDS. In: Flaskerud J, Ungvarski P, eds. *HIV/AIDS: A Guide to Nursing Care.* 3rd ed. Philadelphia: WB Saunders; 1995: 54–127.
31. Krown S, Myskowski P, Pareded J. Kaposi's sarcoma. *Med Clin North Am.* 1992;76(1):235–268.
32. Lovejoy N, Anastasi J. Squamous cell cervical lesions in women with and

without AIDS: biochemical risk factors, prevention and policy. *Cancer Nurs.* 1994;17(4):294–307.
33. Levine A. AIDS-related malignancies. *Curr Opin Oncol.* 1994;6(5):489–491.
34. Krown S. Acquired immunodeficiency syndrome-associated Kaposi's sarcoma: biology and management. *Med Clin North Am.* 1997;81(2):471–494.
35. Moore P, Chang Y. Detection of herpes virus-like DNA sequences in Kaposi's sarcoma in patients with and those without HIV infection. *N Engl J Med.* 1995; 332(18):1181–1185.
36. Levine A, Gill P, Salahuddin S. Neoplastic complications of HIV infection. In: Wormser G, ed. *AIDS and Other Manifestations of HIV Infection.* 2nd ed. New York: Raven Press; 1992:443–452.
37. Stratton P, Ciacco K. Cervical neoplasia in the patient with HIV infection. *Curr Opin Obstet Gynecol.* 1994;6(1):86–91.
38. Wright T, Ellerbrock T, Chiasson M, Van Devanter N, Sun X. Cervical intraepithelial neoplasia in women infected with human immunodeficiency virus: prevalence, risk factors, and validity of Papanicolaou smears. *Obstet Gynecol.* 1994; 84(4-1):591–597.
39. Vermund S, Kelley K, Klein R, et al. High risk of human papillomavirus infection and cervical squamous intraepithelial lesions among women with symptomatic human immunodeficiency virus infection. *Am J Obstet Gynecol.* 1991;165(2): 392–400.
40. Shafer A, Friedmann W, Mielke M, Schwartlander B, Koch M. The increased frequency of cervical dysplasia-neoplasia in women infected with the human immunodeficiency virus is related to the degree of immunosuppression. *Am J Obstet Gynecol.* 1991;164:593–599.
41. Feingold A, Vermund S, Burk R, et al. Cervical cytologic abnormalities and papillomavirus in women infected with human immunodeficiency virus. *J Acquir Immune Defic Syndr.* 1990;3(9):896–903.
42. Mascolini M. Oncologists scout new directions for KS and lymphoma therapies. *J Int Assoc Phys AIDS Care.* 1995;6/95:10–14.
43. Maiman M, Fruchter R, Guy L, Cuthill S, Levine P, Serur E. Human immunodeficiency virus infection and invasive cervical carcinoma. *Cancer.* 1993; 71(2): 402–406.
44. Stratton P, Ciacco K. Cervical neoplasia in the patient with HIV infection. *Curr Opin Obstet Gynecol.* 1994;6(1):86–91.
45. Maiman M, Fruchter R, Serur E, Levine P, Arrastia C, Sedlis A. Recurrent cervical intraepithelial neoplasia in human immunodeficiency virus-seropositive women. *Obstet Gynecol.* 1993;82(2):170–174.
46. Maiman M, Tarricone N, Vieira J, Suarex J, Serur E, Boyce J. Colposcopic evaluation of human immunodeficiency virus-seropositive women. *Obstet Gynecol.* 1991;78(1):84–88.
47. Mandelblatt J, Fahs M, Garibaldi K, Senie R, Peterson H. Association between

HIV infection and cervical neoplasia: implications for clinical care of women at risk for both conditions. *AIDS* 1992;6:173–178.
48. Maiman M. Cervical neoplasia in women with HIV infection. *Oncology (Huntingt).* 1994;8(8):83–89.
49. Agency for Health Care and Policy Research (AHCPR). *Clinical Practice Guidelines, Evaluation and Management of Early HIV Infection.* Washington, DC: U.S. Department of Health and Human Services, Public Health Service; 1994. Report no.: AHCPR publication no. 94-0572.
50. Bloss J. The use of electrosurgical techniques in the management of premalignant diseases of the vulva, vagina, and cervix: an excisional rather than an ablative approach. *Am J Obstet Gynecol.* 1993;169(5):1081–1085.
51. Naumann R, Bell M, Alvarez R, et al. LLETZ is an acceptable alternative to diagnostic cold-knife conization. *Gynecol Oncol.* 1994;55(2):224–228.
52. Hankins C, Lamond J, Handley M. Cervicovaginal screening in women with HIV infection: a need for increased vigilance? *Can Med Assoc J.* 1994;150(5):681–686.
53. Tomaino-Brunner C, Freda M, Runowicz C. "I hope I don't have cancer": colposcopy and minority women. *Oncol Nurs Forum.* 1996;23(1):39–44.
54. Nelson J, Averette H, Richart R. Cervical intraepithelial neoplasia (dysplasia and carcinoma in situ) and early invasive cervical carcinoma. *CA Cancer J Clin.* 1989;39:157–178.

CHAPTER 7

Treatment of Opportunistic Malignancies: Chemotherapy

Kathleen M. Doherty, RN, MS, OCN

Chapter Preview

- Goals of Treatment
- Cellular Replication of Cancer Cells
- Classification of Chemotherapeutic Agents
- Administration of Chemotherapeutic Agents
- Application of Chemotherapy to AIDS-Related Malignancies
- Nursing Care of Patients Receiving Chemotherapy for AIDS-Related Malignancies

Goals of Treatment

Chemotherapy is used with one of four possible goals: cure, control, palliation, or prevention of recurrence. When utilized with the intention of cure, chemotherapy is employed because the anticancer agents have been shown to cause total eradication of tumor cells. When used to control malignancy, chemotherapy is implemented even though the tumor burden is thought or known to be greater than the agents' ability to destroy it. The goal is to control further progression of the disease and to provide an optimal quality of life. Chemotherapy is used for palliation even when particular tumors rarely or minimally respond to the treatment. The goal of palliative treatment is to provide temporary improvement and control of symptoms related to the tumor. Adjuvant chemotherapy is therapy given in the absence of any documented disease in an attempt to prevent recurrence. It is also given to patients to augment other forms of therapy, such as surgery or radiation, when the patient is thought to be at high risk for micrometastases or recurrence.[1]

Some malignancies are potentially curable by chemotherapy in the absence of HIV disease. When treating malignancies related to HIV disease, most often chemotherapy is used in an attempt to control or palliate the diseases. Cure is rare, if not impossible, when the disease occurs in a person also living with HIV disease.[2] Cure is difficult in the setting of HIV disease because the standard doses of chemotherapy required to eradicate the malignancy cannot be tolerated by an already compromised immune system. Patients with HIV disease are more prone to life-threatening complications of infection when traditional chemotherapy dosages are employed because chemotherapy routinely causes severe bone marrow toxicity.[2] Persons with AIDS have limited bone marrow reserve even before encountering chemotherapy. Control and palliation of malignancies associated with HIV infection are by in large the overall goals of the administration of chemotherapy.

Cellular Replication of Cancer Cells

All cells in the body go through a DNA-driven replication process called the *cell cycle*, which is similar for both normal and malignant cells and ultimately results in the formation of two cells from one. Several substances such as DNA, RNA, enzymes, and proteins are necessary for cell replication. DNA is often referred to as the genetic makeup of all cells, and its role is control of the cellular activities and functions in the body. DNA consists of two single chains of nitrogenous bases (adenine, cytosine, guanine, and thymine) that are connected by hydrogen bonds. The structure of DNA is the double-helix form shown in Figure 7.1. Bonding between the specific nitrogenous bases is very selective and can only occur such that adenine bonds only with thymine and cytosine bonds only with guanine.[1]

As the cell undergoes replication, the double strand of DNA separates, bearing exposed nitrogenous bases. These nitrogenous bases can again reconnect only with supplementary bases. Therefore, in cellular replication each single strand of nitrogenous bases couples with a new single strand of nitrogenous bases, resulting in two identical, double-stranded chains of DNA. Another important component of cellular replication is RNA. RNA is a chemical substance that transfers DNA from the nucleus of the cell to the cytoplasm, where protein synthesis takes place.

In the cell cycle (Figure 7.2), it is essential that duplication of DNA occur by the final stages. There are five phases of the cell cycle, and during all except the G0 phase the cell is either actively preparing for division or it is actually dividing.[3] The phases of the cell cycle are

- G0 This is the resting phase, when the cell is not in the process of undergoing replication. The cell, while in this phase, is out of the cycle temporarily, but it is able to be recruited to replicate if stimulated.
- G1 This is the first active phase of the cell cycle leading to replication. While in this phase the cell is preparing for the synthesis of DNA by making the necessary cellular RNA and protein enzymes.
- S During this phase of cellular replication, DNA is synthesized/duplicated.
- G2 The cell in this phase of the cycle is synthesizing RNA and proteins, along with producing the mitotic spindle apparatus.
- M This phase is when mitosis actually occurs. Mitosis is the physical process of cellular division, where one cell splits to form two complete, new cells. This phase consists of the subphases of prophase, metaphase, anaphase, and telophase, which describe the actual separating activities of cellular replication.[3]

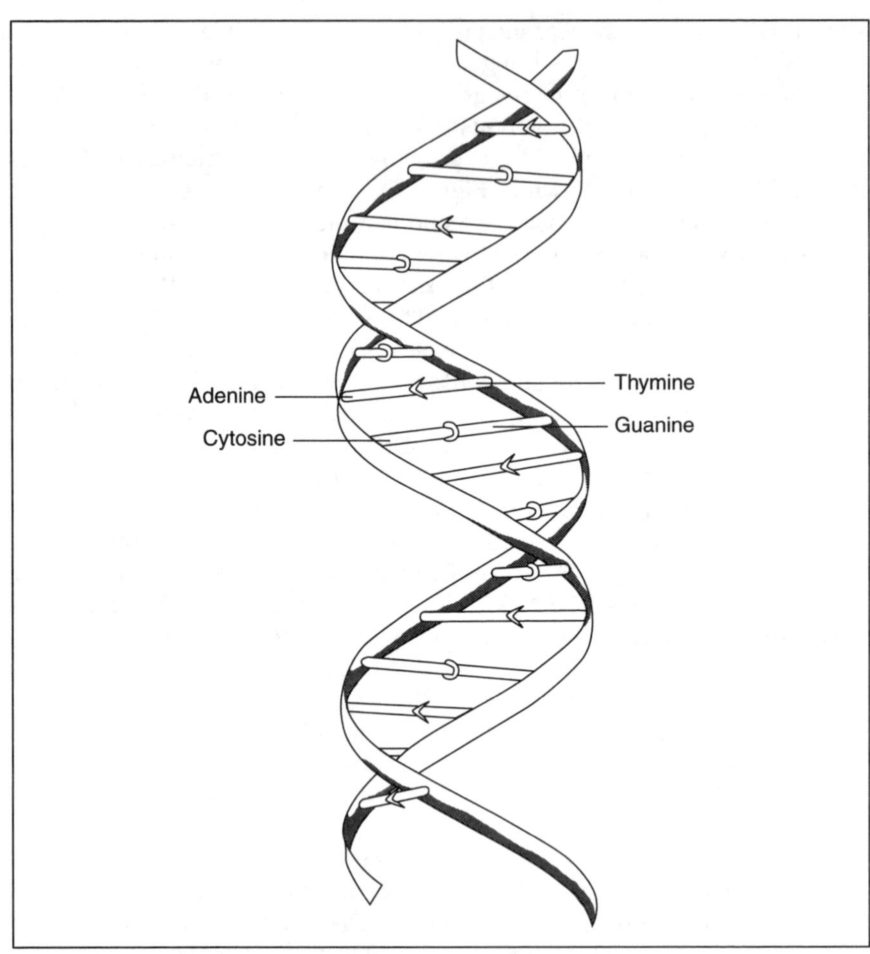

Figure 7.1 DNA, Deoxyribonucleic Acid, in the Double Helix Formation. (From Bender CM. In Ziegfeld CR, ed. *Core Curriculum for Oncology Nursing.* Philadelphia: WB Saunders; 1987. Reprinted with permission.)

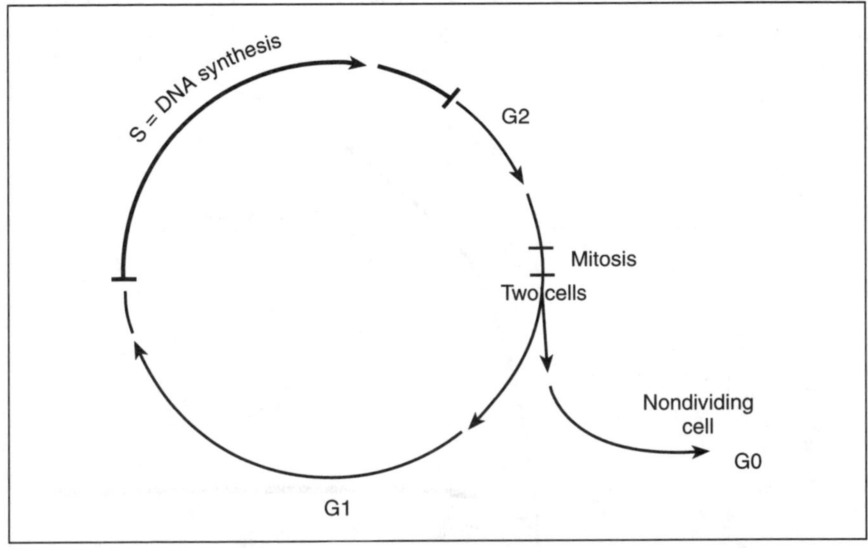

Figure 7.2 Schematic Diagram of the Cell Life Cycle. After mitosis the sibling cells have two options: (1) they may continue to divide, going through the cell cycle phases, G1, S, G2, back to mitosis; or (2) they may leave the cell cycle to become nondividing cells, a state sometimes called *G0.* Some nondividing G0 cells can reenter the cell cycle if an appropriate stimulus is applied. Others (terminally differentiated cells) are destined to die without dividing again. (From Calabretta B, Baserga R. Control of cell growth and differentiation. In: Hoffman R, et al, eds. *Hematology Basic Principles and Practice.* New York: Churchill Livingstone; 1991.)

A review of the accepted theories related to cancer cell growth is needed to appreciate how chemotherapeutic treatment strategies are employed against malignant diseases.

Gompertzian Model of Growth

While there are many similarities between normal and malignant cells, there are some essential differences. The Gompertzian model of tumor cell growth illustrates one of these essential differences (Figure 7.3). This model shows that in normal, healthy cell replication, the number of cells

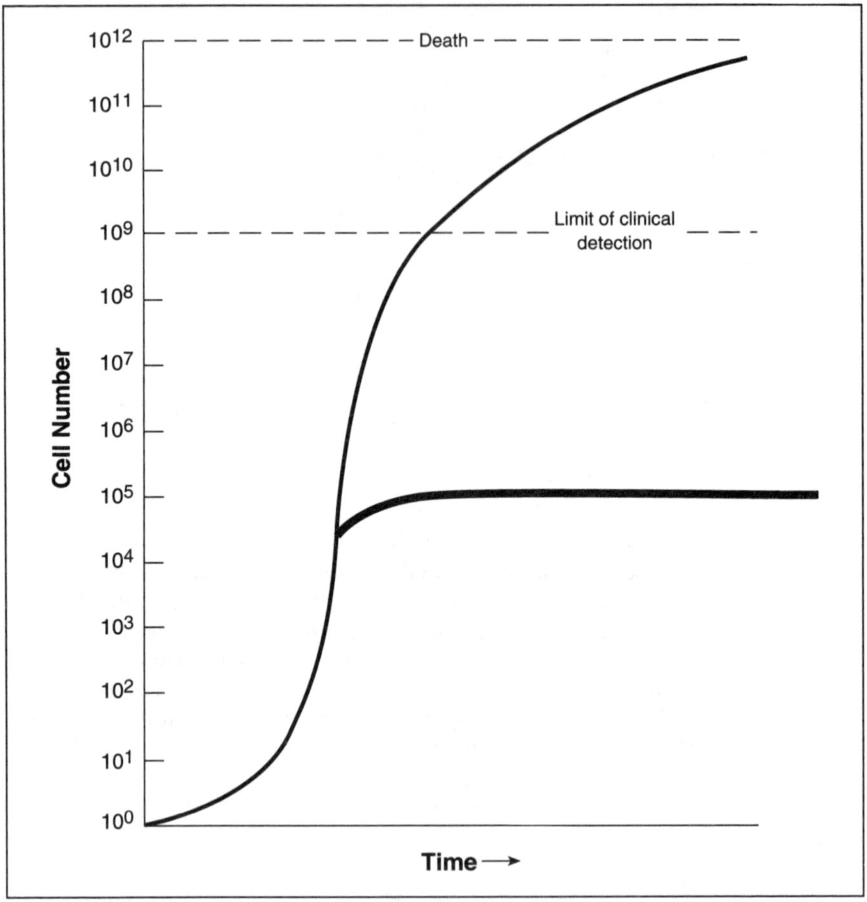

Figure 7.3 The Gompertzian Model of Growth. During the early stages of its development, a tumor's growth is exponential. As a tumor enlarges, the growth slows. By the time a tumor becomes large enough to cause symptoms and be clinically detectable, the majority of its growth has already occurred and is no longer exponential. In nonmalignant cell growth, cell birth equals cell death, providing a constant mass of cells. (Reprinted by the permission of the American Cancer Society, Inc.)

produced equals the approximate number of cells that die; thus a steady total mass of cells exists. In tumors, however, this is not true. When a tumor is small and begins to develop, the cellular replication is exponentially fast. With increasing size, however, the cellular replication continues, but at a much slower rate than previously experienced.[4]

From the knowledge obtained regarding the four active phases of the cell life cycle (G1, S, G2, and M) and the nonactive or resting phase of the cycle (G0), one can deduce that in small tumors the majority of cells are in the active phases of the cell life cycle. Alternately, in large, bulky tumors, a higher percentage of the tumor cells are in the resting or inactive phase of the cell life cycle.[4]

Drug Specificity in the Cell Cycle

When looking at the multiple chemotherapeutic drugs available to combat malignancy, the practitioner utilizes the Gompertzian model of growth to guide the choice of drugs utilized. While there are similarities between groups or classes of drugs, there are also differences. One very important difference between available drugs is related to how and when they damage the cells. Two fundamental types of agents are known: cell cycle-specific agents and cell cycle-nonspecific agents.[1,4]

Cell cycle-specific agents work to damage the cells during a specific, active phase of the cell cycle. Cell cycle-specific agents cannot exert much effect unless the cell is in one of the active phases of the cell cycle (G1, S, G2, or M). In other words, cell cycle-specific agents have little impact on cells that are in the resting phase (the G0 phase).[1,4,5] Accordingly, if a patient presents with a small tumor that requires chemotherapy, the practitioner would expect that based on the Gompertzian model of growth, exponential cellular replication would be occurring in the tumor and that a large percentage of cells would be in the active phases of the cell cycle. The use of cell cycle-specific agents as the cornerstone of treatment would be strongly considered.

Cell cycle-nonspecific agents, however, have a cytotoxic effect while the cell is in any phase of the cell cycle, including the resting phase. If a patient presents with a large, bulky tumor, the practitioner would assume that although cellular replication is continuing, it is occurring at a much slower rate than would have been encountered previously. Accordingly, a greater percentage of cells would be found in the resting phase of the cell life cycle, requiring the use of cell-cycle nonspecific agents.[1,4,5]

While these principles continue to direct practitioners, it has also been established that chemotherapeutic regimens are able to provide better responses when a combination of various drugs are utilized as opposed to single-agent therapy. In reviewing the many chemotherapeutic drugs chosen to treat various malignancies, there is almost always a mixture of cell cycle-specific and cell cycle-nonspecific agents.

Cell Kill Hypothesis

Another theory to understand regarding the impact of chemotherapy on cancer cells is the *cell kill hypothesis*. This hypothesis claims that every time a person with a malignancy is given a consistent dosage of chemotherapy, a constant percentage of cancer cells will die.[3–5] In following this theory, if repeated doses of chemotherapy were administered to a tumor over time, the tumor burden would decrease at a steady rate, however chemotherapy would never be able to eradicate totally all of the cancer cells, only a fixed percentage of cells. Appropriately, then, the hypothesis further theorizes that once the number of cancer cells is reduced to a small enough number, the immune system takes over to eliminate the few remaining cancer cells.

In selected non-AIDS related cancers this is thought to happen, providing the patient with cure. When dealing with AIDS-related malignancies (ARM), difficulty in obtaining cure arises when either one of two situations occurs. When treating AIDS-related malignancies, suboptimal doses of chemotherapy may be required to minimize life-threatening side effects to healthy tissues, specifically bone marrow cells. In delivering suboptimal doses of drug, the tumor may not regress adequately due to only a small percentage of cell death, or it may even develop chemotherapy drug resistance and continue to grow.[2]

If, however, ideal dosages of drugs are utilized and desired regression of tumor cells is accomplished, an additional challenge presents itself. Persons with HIV disease have damaged immune systems which may be inadequate to complete the process of "mopping up" the few remaining cancer cells which is required according to the cell kill hypothesis. The few remaining cells which escape immunosurveillance often proliferate and eventually cause a recurrence.

Classification of Chemotherapeutic Agents

Today more than 100 anticancer agents are being utilized and researched in an attempt to improve long-term survival of persons dealing with a diagnosis of cancer.[6] Eight major categories of anticancer drugs have been identified, based on their mechanism of action: alkylating agents, antimetabolites, anthracenediones, anti-tumor antibiotics, nitrosureas, podophyllum derivatives, plant/vinca alkaloids, and hormonal agents. There are also a number of drugs which are classified as miscellaneous agents as their mechanism of action does not closely resemble that of the eight previously mentioned classes. Among the several classes of drugs there is variation as to how each class of drug exerts its effect on both the malignant and healthy cells to cause eventual cell death (1). Some agents directly kill the cells and are called cytocidal agents. Other drugs prevent the duplication of the cell by changing the environment in which the cell lives and are therefore called *cytostatic agents*. Table 7.1 lists currently available chemotherapeutic agents used to treat AIDS-related malignancies. Drug information is presented by class along with data on dosage, schedule, routes, and possible and probable side effects.

Administration of Chemotherapeutic Agents

Traditionally, chemotherapy has been delivered via oral, IV, IM, and subcutaneous routes.[6,7] As these drugs are absorbed they provide bodywide or systemic treatment to malignant cells throughout the body. While systemic IV administration continues to be the principal route of delivery, alternative routes of delivery are used to provide local control of individual areas of disease.[7] In many tumors drugs may be delivered directly into the CSF via intrathecal injection, into a malignant lesion by intralesional administration, into the peritoneal space by intraperitoneal administration, and into body cavities such as the lung or bladder via the intrapleural or intravesicular routes.[7] In the treatment of AIDS-related malignancies the majority of tumors are treated by either oral, IV, intrathecal, and intralesional routes. Regardless of the route chosen, it is crucial that chemotherapeutic agents be administered safely and are accompanied by relevant patient and family education.

Table 7.1 Chemotherapy Drugs to Treat AIDS-Related Malignancies (ARM)

Agents	ARM	Class	Dosage	Side Effects[a]
Bleomycin	KS, NHL	Antitumor, antibiotic	10–15 U/m^2; maximum lifetime dose of 400 U	Anaphylaxis, fevers *(p)*, chills *(p)*, pulmonary fibrosis
Cisplatin	Cervical	Miscellaneous	50–100 mg/m^2	Myelosuppression *(p)*, severe nausea and vomiting *(p)*, renal toxicity, *(p)*, ototoxicity *(p)*, alopecia *(p)*
Cyclophosphamide	NHL	Alkylating agent	300–600 mg/m^2	Myelosuppression *(p)*, hemorrhagic cystitis *(p)*, nausea and vomiting *(p)*, alopecia *(p)*
Dexamethasone	NHL	Steroidal hormone	10–20 mg	Depressed cellular immunity *(p)*, mood swings *(p)*, insomnia *(p)*
Doxorubicin (vesicant)	KS, NHL	Antitumor antibiotic	20–50 mg/m^2; maximum lifetime dose of 500–550 mg/m^2 (400–450 mg/m^2 if previous XRT to chest)	Myelosuppression *(p)*, cardiotoxicity, alopecia *(p)*, nausea and vomiting *(p)*, red urine *(p)*, stomatitis
Doxorubicin liposomal	KS	Antitumor antibiotic	20–50 mg/m^2	Myelosuppression *(p)*, alopecia *(p)*, nausea and vomiting
Etoposide	KS	Podophyllotoxin	150 mg/m^2 IV, 50 mg PO qd	Myelosuppression *(p)*, nausea and vomiting, alopecia *(p)*, hypotension, bronchospasm

5-Fluorouracil	Cervical	Antimetabolite	300–600 mg/m^2	Myelosuppression *(p)*, stomatitis *(p)*, diarrhea *(p)*, nausea and vomiting
Ifosfamide with Mesna	Cervical	Alkylating agent	Ifosfamide, 700–1,000 mg/m^2 qd for 3–5 days; Mesna, 700–1,000 mg/m^2 qd for 4 days	Myelosuppression *(p)*, hemorrhagic cystitis *(p)*, nausea and vomiting *(p)*
Methotrexate	NHL	Antimetabolite	25–50 mg/m^2	Myelosuppression *(p)*, diarrhea *(p)*, stomatitis *(p)*, nausea and vomiting
Prednisone	NHL	Steroidal hormone	10–50 mg/day	Depressed cellular immunity *(p)*, GI upset *(p)*, depressed adrenal function *(p)*, mood swings *(p)*
Taxol	Cervical	Miscellaneous	125–150 mg/m^2	Myelosuppression *(p)*, hypersensitivity, peripheral neuropathies *(p)*
Vinblastine (vesicant)	KS, NHL	Vinca alkaloid	4–20 mg/m^2	Constipation *(p)*, peripheral neuropathies *(p)*, myelosuppression *(p)*
Vincristine (vesicant)	KS, NHL	Vinca alkaloid	1.4 mg/m^2	Constipation *(p)*, peripheral neuropathies *(p)*

(p) = probable side effect.
KS = Kaposi's sarcoma; NHL = non-Hodgkin's lymphoma; XRT = radiation therapy; GI = gastrointestinal.

Application of Chemotherapy to AIDS-Related Malignancies

The three most frequently occurring malignancies that occur in persons with HIV infection are non-Hodgkin's lymphoma, Kaposi's sarcoma, and cervical cancer. Each of these neoplasms presents new challenges to practitioners in determining the best treatment strategy.[2,8–10]

AIDS-Related NHL

The two most common presentations of NHL are a lymphatic, systemic presentation and a CNS presentation. Treatment of the two presentations differs dramatically.[18,19]

Systemic NHL

Systemic presentations of AIDS-related NHL tend to be intermediate or high-grade lymphomas.[18,19] Grading of the lymphoma describes the aggressiveness of the tumor growth. Higher grade lymphomas require more expedient intervention with chemotherapy. Prior to initiation of chemotherapy, tissue confirmation of the diagnosis and staging of the disease is essential. Systemic chemotherapy is generally required in the treatment of AIDS-related NHL.[20,21] Many chemotherapeutic drugs are active against NHLs—the most active agent being cyclophosphamide. The choice of drugs utilized to halt the lymphoma include a combination approach utilizing cyclophosphamide with a mixture of doxorubicin, vincristine, vinblastine, methotrexate, prednisone, dexamethasone, and bleomycin. Although several different combinations are utilized, no superior regimen exists. Studies have shown that the higher the dose of cyclophosphamide used, the worse the patient outcome. This is related to marrow toxicity and the ensuing life-threatening OIs. The standard dosage of cyclophosphamide for treating AIDS-related NHLs is now between 400 to 600 mg/m^2.[21,22]

Because myelosuppression is expected along with the potential for OIs, patients receiving chemotherapy for AIDS-related NHL are commonly treated with colony stimulating factors to minimize the degree of marrow suppression and shorten the period of time during which the patient is at high risk for infection. Granulocyte colony stimulating factor (G-CSF) stimulates the bone marrow stem cells to produce granulocytes, especially neutrophils, which are a person's first line of defense against infection.[12]

A common complication related to initiation of therapy aimed at high-grade lymphomas is the development of a syndrome identified as *tumor lysis syndrome.* Tumor lysis syndrome is a predictable complication in the treatment of high-grade lymphomas, especially in patients with a large tumor burden. The syndrome occurs when chemotherapy lyses, or kills, the cancer cells. The intracellular components spill into the bloodstream. Intracellular ions that flood into the bloodstream include phosphorus, potassium, and uric acid; thus, hyperphosphatemia, hyperkalemia, and hyperuricemia are exhibited. As serum phosphorous levels increase, an inverse decrease in serum calcium is seen. With the overload of phosphate, uric acid, and potassium, there is an increased excretory demand placed on the kidneys. To complicate the syndrome further, the high amounts of uric acid tend to crystallize in an acidic environment, such as urine, and have the potential to cause acute renal failure. If the kidneys are not able to maintain rapid excretion of potassium, phosphorus, or uric acid, complications will be evident as seen in any person experiencing hyperkalemia, hyperphosphatemia, and hyperuricemia.

Because this syndrome is predictable, it is important that the nurse and physician identify patients at risk and initiate interventions to minimize complications. Strategies to prevent the complications of tumor lysis syndrome include beginning allopurinol, ideally 24 hours before commencing chemotherapy. Aggressive hydration and diuresis is essential and often includes addition of sodium bicarbonate in an effort to alkalinize the urine. Frequent monitoring of laboratory values is standard to identify early indicators of renal injury and potential renal failure.

AIDS-Related CNS Lymphoma

Primary CNS lymphoma is a rare and unique presentation of NHL. The connection of this malignancy to HIV disease appears to be strongly correlated to immunosuppressed conditions.[23,24] While the pathogenesis is similar to systemic lymphatic NHL, CNS lymphoma is different in that it is considered multicentric. Again, as in KS this implies that each individual brain lesion identified is a new primary cancer, and multiple lesions are not metastatic disease but separate areas of new primary cancers. Workup of this malignancy includes lumbar puncture with large-volume (10–12 cc) taps of CSF. Despite these efforts, reports of CSF cytology are often nonspecific, with some studies reporting only 25 to 50% positive cytology readings, despite a true presence of CNS lymphoma. The potential morbidity and mortality associated with brain biopsies in this population is frequently a deterrent. Therefore the treatment of AIDS-related CNS lymphoma is occasionally initiated without confirmed tissue diagnosis.[23,24]

Radiation therapy along with intrathecal chemotherapy provide some response and are the treatment of choice in traditional non-AIDS-related CNS lymphoma. In AIDS-related CNS lymphoma, radiation continues to be employed, however the use of chemotherapy is primarily palliative for two reasons. First, systemic chemotherapy is not able to cross the protective blood-brain barrier adequately to reach the malignant cells effectively. Secondly, it is not possible to deliver high enough doses of chemotherapy intrathecally to eradicate the CNS lymphoma without the development of arachnoiditis or other complications. When intrathecal chemotherapy is utilized for palliation of CNS lymphomatous symptoms, the drugs applied are most often cytosine arabinoside and methotrexate. The majority of patients receiving intrathecal chemotherapy obtain an improvement in neurological symptoms, albeit very short lived.[23,24]

AIDS-Related KS

The use of chemotherapy to treat KS is based on the presentation and aggressiveness demonstrated by the tumor. Traditional non-AIDS-related KS most commonly presents as a single cutaneous lesion on the extremities or face and has a low potential for dissemination. In the setting of HIV disease, however, KS can present either locally or in a disseminated fashion.[11] Most commonly, patients with AIDS-related KS present with *multicentric skin lesions*, which means that each individual skin lesion is a new primary tumor and that multiple lesions are not metastatic disease but separate areas of new primary cancers. Thus, localized therapy such as surgery does not play a role in the treatment of this type of malignancy. To prevent the development of new primary lesions, the practitioner must depend on systemic treatment such as chemotherapy.[12,13] Additionally the use of systemic chemotherapy is further supported, as the literature states that by the time someone has lesions on their skin, upward of 35% of patients will have some degree of pulmonary involvement with KS.[14,15]

In addition to the more common presentation of cutaneous KS, an increasing number of persons with AIDS will present with KS in the oral mucosa or visceral organs such as the lungs and GI tract. Often the diagnosis of pulmonary KS is difficult to make because one must also consider the possibility of one of the many pulmonary OIs causing the clinical symptoms of nonproductive cough, fever, and dyspnea. Pulmonary KS generally tends to be a more aggressive, virulent form of the disease, and some studies show that without chemotherapy, average survival may be as little as 4 to 5 months. However, with systemic treatment, survival with pulmonary KS may be prolonged to upward of an average of 8 to 10 months.[11,14,15]

When considering survival outcomes utilizing chemotherapy in either cutaneous KS or pulmonary KS, several factors are taken into consideration. Good prognostic factors include helper/suppressor ratios of >0.5 cells/μl and CD4 counts of >300 cells/μl. Another important prognostic indicator is the presence or absence of two of the following three B symptoms: fever of unknown origin, night sweats, and >10% unintentional weight loss. The absence of B symptoms and lack of previous OIs are good prognostic factors.[11–13]

Use of chemotherapy for treating AIDS-related KS depends on multiple variables, most importantly presentation of disease, CD4 counts, bone marrow reserve, presence of neutrophil function, and patient functional status.[16] Single-agent chemotherapy includes the use of IV vincristine, vinblastine, doxorubicin, liposomal doxorubicin, and oral etoposide. Additionally intralesional vincristine is used to control individual cutaneous KS lesions.[17] For more aggressive forms of KS (as seen in pulmonary presentation), a combination of drugs is used.[11,14,15] Drug selection varies and is based on the patient's baseline status. Therapy most often includes combinations of IV doxorubicin, bleomycin, and vincristine.[11,14]

When using chemotherapy to treat AIDS-related malignancies it is essential that blood counts be monitored regularly to assess the degree of suppression of neutrophils related to therapy. Additionally if the patient experiences neutropenia with associated fever and infection, one may consider chemotherapy dosage reductions to minimize complications related to future treatments. If neutropenia is profound after chemotherapy, future treatments may be altered to include only those drugs that do not have myelosuppression as a side effect, such as vincristine and/or bleomycin.

An additional treatment option for persons with AIDS-related KS is the use of biologic response modifiers such as IFN. IFN-α is the only biologic therapy presently approved for the treatment of KS. Response rates to IFN-α are associated with patients who have CD4 counts of >400 cells/μl.[16] The ideal IFN dose of KS treatment remains unclear, however many studies are investigating the use of doses >10 MU/m²/day. The dose-limiting toxicity is a flulike syndrome characterized by low-grade fever, chills, myalgia, and fatigue.[16]

AIDS-Related Cervical Cancer

AIDS-related cervical cancer is the most recently recognized malignancy that establishes an index diagnosis of AIDS.[8] The goal of treatment in AIDS-related cervical malignancies is the detection of preinvasive disease followed by surgical intervention.[25] It is known that there is a high prevalence of CIN and carcinoma in situ in women who are HIV positive. Pap smear screening of cervical cells is routinely done every 6 months in HIV-positive women in an effort to detect precancerous conditions and ultimately to curtail the progression of these lesions into frankly invasive cervical cancer.[26,27]

When invasive cervical cancer is diagnosed, treatment options are limited. Cryosurgery provides a poor outcome because multiple recurrences are common. Radiation therapy and chemotherapy are standards of treatment.[25] It is unclear which chemotherapeutic agents are most effective in treating AIDS-related cervical cancer, and at present outcomes are poor. Some believe that chemotherapy may have a limited effect if the patient has had multiple previous surgeries, as there may be a limited vascular supply to carry the anticancerous drugs to the malignant cells.[8,25] A variety of drugs are administered systemically in an effort to halt the progression of cervical cancer cell proliferation. Systemic 5-fluorouracil is one of the main drugs chosen in treating AIDS-related cervical cancer, and is often combined with other drugs such as cisplatin, doxorubicin, taxol, ifosfamide, and cyclophosphamide. Modest success has been achieved in the topical application of chemotherapeutic drugs, such as 5-fluorouracil, in the treatment of AIDS-related cervical cancer.[25] With topical application of chemotherapy, systemic side effects such as myelosuppression, mucositis, alopecia, and GI distress are almost nonexistent. If tumor responses from topical application of drugs prove to be equal or better than systemic delivery of drugs, topical application may be considered a more acceptable method of drug delivery in treating this malignancy.

Nursing Care of Patients Receiving Chemotherapy for AIDS-Related Malignancies

The nurse caring for a patient receiving chemotherapy for an AIDS-related malignancy has special opportunities that affect patient and family outcomes. The nurse is able to provide support and education to the patient and family while using expert assessment and intervention skills to minimize side effects and to assist the patient in obtaining the best quality of life possible. As most persons have some misconceptions of what chemotherapeutic treatments entail, education about the realities of chemotherapy and management of side effects is essential. Before teaching about disease and treatment, it is critical that the nurse determine the knowledge base from which both the patient and family are operating. Education is an ongoing process that should begin before chemotherapy treatments are started. The approach to educating patients and families must be individualized and continue throughout the cancer trajectory. It is common for the patient and family to be overwhelmed by the enormous amount of information they must retain and use, along with the realization that the cancer diagnosis in the setting of AIDS may significantly reduce the patient's life expectancy. Ultimately the education of the patient and family should be presented not only verbally but also in written form for later reference. In addition to treatment schedules and understanding how chemotherapy acts to eliminate malignancy, patients are concerned with how chemotherapy will affect their quality of life and what side effects they will encounter. Although it is important for the patient to be prepared for the realities of treatment, it is also essential that the nurse educate the patient and family about methods that will be applied to minimize complications, and self-care management techniques that can be utilized to provide an optimal quality of life during treatment. Common complications related to chemotherapeutic treatment of AIDS-related malignancies include myelosuppression, GI distress, mucosal toxicity, diarrhea, alopecia, photosensitivity, extravasation, and organ toxicity. Often it is difficult to determine the etiology of many symptoms because they may be related to the chemotherapy, HIV disease, or OIs.[1,5,6,28]

Myelosuppression

Bone marrow suppression is most often the dose-limiting toxicity of many chemotherapeutic drugs.[1,5] While some anticancer drugs are nonmarrow toxic, the majority of chemotherapeutic drugs cause significant marrow suppression, peaking approximately 10 to 14 days posttreatment.[1,5] There is, however, some variation in the timing of myelosuppression among individual drugs. Chemotherapy-induced myelosuppression is displayed as neutropenia, thrombocytopenia, and anemia. Neutropenia and the potential subsequent infections are the most critical aspect of bone marrow suppression. In the setting of AIDS, when patients already have altered immune function, the potentially severe neutropenia associated with chemotherapeutic treatments increases the risk for life-threatening infections.

Strategies to minimize the complications related to neutropenia include the use of G-CSF after chemotherapy to stimulate bone marrow production of neutrophils. With the production of neutrophils provided by G-CSF, the degree and duration of neutropenia is decreased and likewise the risk of infection is minimized. Because of the severe toxicity to the bone marrow caused by chemotherapy, another strategy is to reduce the dosages of marrow-toxic drugs. This, although necessary at times, is not ideal because it may result in suboptimal response rates.

Thrombocytopenia related to chemotherapy may be asymptomatic or may present with classical symptoms of petechiae, bruising, or bleeding. The risk for bleeding is increased when platelet counts are <50,000 cells/mm^3, and the risk for spontaneous bleeding is increased with platelet counts <20,000 cells/mm^3.[1,5] Spontaneous bleeding occurs without previous trauma. Although bleeding can occur from any site, most often bleeding related to thrombocytopenia occurs from mucous membranes, into the skin, into the CNS, or at sites of previous trauma. Platelet transfusions are the primary strategy for management of bleeding in the thrombocytopenic patient. Platelet transfusions are available as random platelets, single-donor platelets, and human leukocyte antigen (HLA)-compatible platelets, with increasing compatibility between the donor and patient.

Anemia is also common as a result of chemotherapy-induced marrow toxicity. Anemia may develop gradually, leading to symptoms after several cycles of chemotherapy. Anemia may also be intensified in the setting of AIDS because many patients receiving chemotherapy are also receiving antiretroviral drugs such as AZT, which are associated with profound anemia. Symptoms of anemia related to chemotherapy are classic of most anemias and include dyspnea, fatigue, weakness, and shortness of breath. In patients with good cardiovascular function, symptoms of anemia usually do not appear until the hemoglobin reaches approximately 8.5 g/dl and the hematocrit lowers to approximately 25 to 30%. Two major treatment options exist for managing anemia related to chemotherapy. Administration of erythropoietin, a colony stimulating factor that stimulates the production of red blood cells, is frequently used to treat anemia related to both chemotherapy and ART. Erythropoietin is most effectively used as a prophylactic treatment against anemia. For treatment of acute anemia, the backbone of treatment continues to be red blood cell transfusion.

GI Side Effects

Consistently, patients are most aware and concerned about the side effects of nausea and vomiting related to chemotherapy. Nausea and vomiting related to chemotherapy can present in one of three forms: acute nausea and vomiting, delayed nausea and vomiting, or anticipatory nausea and vomiting.[1,5] Acute nausea and vomiting occurs within 24 hours after chemotherapy administration, whereas delayed nausea and vomiting occurs between 1 and 5 days postchemotherapy. Anticipatory nausea and vomiting occurs in the absence of chemotherapy but is related to factors associated with chemotherapy.[1,5] Examples of factors triggering anticipatory nausea include entry into the clinic where previous chemotherapeutic treatments occurred, smells, and even just the thought of returning for further chemotherapy. Anticipatory nausea is a real phenomenon that is well documented in recent literature and may raise one of the greatest challenges related to symptom management.

Nausea is defined as an unpleasant sensory experience with the propensity to vomit, whereas vomiting is the physical act of expelling GI contents via the oral cavity. The two symptoms are distinct but often occur together as a physical syndrome and may be associated with eventual dehydration, dizziness, and compromised renal function. Many chemotherapeutic agents, with some exceptions, have the potential to cause some degree of nausea and vomiting, ranging from mild to severe. Oftentimes the severity of nausea and vomiting experienced by the patient is related to: (1) stimulation of the chemoreceptor trigger zone in the medulla oblongata via bloodborne exposure to chemotherapeutic agents, (2) direct irritation of the GI mucosa provided by chemotherapeutic agents, (3) dosage of drugs administered, (4) multiplicative effects of other medications with emetogenic potential, (5) presence of increased intracranial pressure, and (6) any combination of these factors.

There are additional risk factors for nausea and vomiting specific to persons with AIDS who are receiving chemotherapy for treatment of malignancy. Polypharmacy, or the administration of a large number of drugs, can intensify the emetogenic potential of chemotherapy. Additionally, when dealing with diseases such as AIDS-related CNS lymphoma, an increase in intracranial pressure can potentiate increased levels of nausea and vomiting than ordinarily experienced based solely on chemotherapeutic agents.[23]

Although nausea and vomiting from chemotherapy can be a very intense and distressing side effect, it is important that the nurse caring for patients receiving such therapy understand that prophylactic and regular use of antiemetics are very effective at ameliorating such symptoms. A wide variety of antiemetics are available to aid in reducing the intensity of nausea and vomiting. These antiemetics work in a variety of ways but most often block the effect of chemotherapy drugs on the chemoreceptor trigger zone. Table 7.2 lists antiemetics currently available for management of chemotherapy-induced nausea and vomiting.

The serotonin antagonists ondansetron and granisetron have revolutionized the treatment of nausea related to severely emetogenic chemotherapeutic agents. When utilized prophylactically these agents decrease the incidence and severity of nausea and vomiting dramatically. For most patients the side effects of serotonin antagonists are limited; the most common is headache.

Additional antiemetics are also available to assist in the management of chemotherapy-induced nausea and vomiting. High-dose IV metoclopramide (2–3 mg/kg) has been used successfully in the management of nausea and vomiting related to highly emetogenic drugs. However, a relatively high incidence of extrapyramidal symptoms is associated with high-dose metoclopramide usage. Benzodiazepines, such as lorazepam, are also utilized, with the side effects of sedation, increased risk of falls, and amnesia.

Table 7.2 Antiemetics Utilized to Manage Chemotherapy-Induced Nausea and Vomiting[a]

Generic Name	Brand Name	Standard Dosage
Ondansetron	Zofran	32 mg IV qd
Granisetron	Kytril	10 μg/kg IV qd
Metoclopramide hydrochloride	Reglan	2–3 mg/kg IV for cisplatin; 10–20 mg PO IV for noncisplatin chemotherapy
Prochlorperazine	Compazine	5 to 10 mg IV PO every 4–6 hours, 25 mg PR q6h
Lorazepam	Ativan	0.5–2.0 mg PO, SL, IV every 4 to 6 hours
Diphenhydramine	Benadryl	25–50 mg PO IV every 4 to 6 hours
Butyrophenone	Droperidol	0.5–2.0 mg IV every 4 to 6 hours
Dexamethasone	Decadron	10–20 mg PO IV daily
Dronabinol (delta-9-tetrahydrocannabinol)	Marinol	2.5–10 mg PO q8h
Haloperidol	Haldol	1–2 mg PO every 6 to 8 hours IM
Dimenhydrinate	Dramamine	50 mg PO q8h
Chlorpromazine	Thorazine	10–25 mg PO IM every 4 to 6 hours

[a]Dosages vary based on patient condition. This table is only a guideline to the typical doses encountered.
IM = intramuscularly; PR = per rectum; SL = sublingual.

Another agent used is delta-9-tetrahydrocannabinol (THC). This is the active ingredient in marijuana, which has had some success in patients in whom conventional approaches to managing nausea and vomiting have been unsuccessful.

Chosen agents should be administered prophylactically and on a regular schedule because nausea and vomiting are much more difficult to manage once they begin. Because response to antiemetics is very individualized, the nurse must assure the patient that if the first antiemetics are unsuccessful, other agents will be used. Likewise, patients should be encouraged to use antiemetics liberally to manage delayed nausea and vomiting. It should be reinforced to patients, families, and other health care providers that prevention of nausea and vomiting is key to success.

Mucosal Toxicity

Because chemotherapy affects cells with rapid rates of proliferation, the mucous membranes are particularly vulnerable to damage from exposure to chemotherapy. Mucous membranes line the GI tract, thus side effects of stomatitis, mucositis, and diarrhea are common complications of chemotherapy. The classes of chemotherapeutic agents that are most likely to cause these complications include the antimetabolites and antitumor antibiotics.

Stomatitis is the breakdown of mucous membranes located in the oral mucosa. Early signs of stomatitis include redness and ulceration of the mucosa, often accompanied by varying degrees of pain, bleeding, and infection. The potential for oral infections within the area of breakdown is compounded by the fact that most chemotherapeutic drugs also cause bone marrow suppression. The most common oral infection continues to be *Candida albicans*, which is a yeast that appears as a pearly white coating of the mucous membranes and/or tongue. HSV is another common culprit for oral infections in persons receiving chemotherapy. Nursing management of mucositis should be directed toward frequent, thorough cleansing of the oral cavity with noncaustic rinses such as normal saline or dilute sodium bicarbonate. Both full-strength or dilute hydrogen peroxide should be avoided unless visible crust and debris are evident, because this appears to damage recovering epithelial cells that are being produced in an attempt at healing. Pain associated with stomatitis may be managed temporarily with local anesthetics such as viscous lidocaine and diclonine hydrochloride. If stomatitis and pain are excruciating, it is not uncommon to utilize systemic narcotics during the recovery period.

Diarrhea

Mucositis, or damage to mucous membranes, can occur throughout the GI tract.[1,5,6,21] Ulceration, bleeding, infection, and pain can occur in the esophagus, gut, colon, and/or rectum, although this may not be evident on visual inspection. Exacerbations of mucositis in the small and large intestines often causes problems with fluid and electrolyte absorption, resulting in severe diarrhea. In the setting of AIDS this can intensify preexisting diarrhea and dehydration. When diarrhea occurs in a person receiving chemotherapy for an AIDS-related malignancy, it is imperative that the practitioner does not assume that the chemotherapeutic agent is automatically the cause. These patients are also at risk for diarrhea directly from the impact of HIV disease in the gut, along with multiple OIs that cause severe diarrhea. OIs must be ruled out as the etiology of diarrhea, especially when the diarrhea is coupled with myelosuppression. If OIs are ruled out, treatment of severe diarrhea routinely includes fluid replacement; drugs to slow down gut motility, such as Imodium; and in extreme cases narcotics such as tincture of opium. The nurse plays a critical role in educating the patient about management of diarrhea, including the need for scrupulous perianal care to prevent anal-rectal abscess formation.

Alopecia

Second only to the side effects of nausea and vomiting, patients are acutely aware of the potential for hair loss associated with chemotherapy. Alopecia is a common side effect of chemotherapy because hair follicular cells are some of the fastest replicating cells in the body and are thus prone to damage by chemotherapy. Most chemotherapeutic agents, although not all, cause alopecia. Approximately 3 to 5 weeks after initial chemotherapeutic treatments, patients often experience hair thinning, followed by total hair loss. Hair returns once treatments are stopped, however texture, wave, and pattern may be altered. Techniques to minimize hair loss include scalp tourniquets and scalp hypothermia. By causing constriction of blood vessels in the scalp, these techniques minimize the delivery of drugs to the scalp, and thus minimize damage of the hair follicular cells. These strategies may be appropriate when chemotherapy is used to palliate the disease. It is not, however, appropriate to use these techniques when CNS or brain involvement is present. Use of these techniques requires a physician order and must be implemented at least 15 minutes before, during, and for 15 minutes after completion of the chemotherapeutic treatment for optimal outcome.

Photosensitivity

Photosensitivity can occur with administration of many selected agents. Patients should be instructed to limit time in direct sunlight; to use protective clothing, which includes a wide-brim hat and cotton clothing; and to utilize sunscreen liberally. Sunscreen used should have an SPF of 15 or greater to ensure the greatest sun protection.

Extravasation

Desquamation and necrosis of cutaneous tissue may result if infiltration of selected chemotherapeutic agents occurs.[29] Those agents that have the potential to cause ulceration of healthy tissue if extravasation occurs are called *vesicant agents.* Procedures used to minimize the likelihood of extravasation include (1) thorough education of nurses administering such drugs, including an intensive skill component; (2) continual observation of the administration site; (3) frequent blood-return confirmations; (4) dilution of such drugs with normal saline using the intravenous side-arm (IVSA) technique; and (5) interruption of any infusion at the first sign of discomfort, altered flow rate of diluent, or any local reaction.[28,29] Additionally, the use of a vascular access device greatly decreases the risk of extravasation.

The administration of chemotherapy is a specialized area of care requiring knowledgeable, professional practice. Over the years the responsibility for administration of therapy and management of symptoms related to chemotherapy has shifted from being exclusively in the domain of physician practice to currently being the responsibility of qualified nurses. To ensure optimal quality of care and patient outcomes, the Oncology Nursing Society (ONS), the professional organization of oncology nurses, has recommended that only adequately prepared professional, registered nurses who are skillful in chemotherapy administration assume the responsibility for actual drug delivery. It is imperative that the practitioner who administers chemotherapy has a thorough understanding of the drugs being administered, including metabolism, elimination, side effects, techniques for symptom management, the precise skill of venipuncture, and the necessary components of patient and family education.

Organ Toxicity

Extended administration of chemotherapeutic agents may damage either temporarily or permanently healthy organs, most commonly the kidneys, liver, and lungs. The majority of chemotherapeutic agents depend on the effective functioning of the liver for drug breakdown and the kidneys for efficient elimination of drugs from the body. As increasing demands are placed on these organs by the administration of chemotherapeutic agents, the potential for organ toxicity increases. Early signs of organ toxicity can be identified by assessment of serial laboratory tests that measure liver and kidney function. In addition to liver and kidney toxicity, select agents have organ-specific toxicities. Adriamycin is associated with cumulative cardiac toxicity that may cause congestive heart failure. Cardiac toxicity increases tremendously after maximum lifetime dosages of 500 to 550 mg/m^2 adriamycin. Serial multigated acquisition (MUGA) scans and electrocardiograms may be used to highlight cardiac dysfunction in symptomatic and asymptomatic patients. Additionally, select agents such as bleomycin and BCNU have pulmonary toxicity as an unfavorable outcome. Symptoms of lung toxicity may include shortness of breath, dyspnea, and difficulty in completing routine activities. Pulmonary toxicity is commonly confirmed with pulmonary function tests.[1,5,6]

In summary, chemotherapy provides some level of control of selected AIDS-related malignancies, however this does not occur without producing toxicity and anxiety for the patient. Because treatment with chemotherapy does not usually provide a cure, it is imperative that the patient and family understand the goals of treatment. Patients must weigh carefully the potential toxicities and risks of aggressive treatment against the potential benefits. The nurse plays a crucial role in assisting the patient to make important treatment decisions through education and support. Once treatment is initiated, it is essential that the nurse, along with the physician, provide continued support and education, while utilizing expert assessments and interventions to alleviate or minimize the symptoms and toxicities associated with therapy.

While the outcome for patients diagnosed with AIDS-related malignancies is less than ideal, there is reason to be optimistic about the future. Research continues to identify better techniques to minimize toxicities that will hopefully provide continued improvement in the quality of life of persons receiving chemotherapy. Additionally, research continues to identify more effective delivery methods and treatment plans. As the incidence of AIDS-related malignancies increases, it is imperative that support for such research continue in the hope of obtaining better responses and ultimately improved quality of life for persons dealing with a diagnosis of AIDS-related malignancy.

References

1. Bender CM. Chemotherapy. In: Ziegfeld CR, ed. *Core Curriculum for Oncology Nursing*. Philadelphia: WB Saunders; 1987:225–236.

2. Moran TA. Cancers in HIV infection. In: Gee G, Moran TA, eds. *AIDS Concepts in Nursing Practice.* Baltimore: Williams and Wilkins; 1988:123–140.
3. Calabretta B, Baserga R. Control of cell growth and differentiation. In: Hoffman R, Benz EJ, Shattil SJ, et al, eds. *Hematology Basic Principles and Practice.* New York: Churchill Livingstone; 1991:51–71.
4. Cooper MR, Cooper MR. Principles of medical oncology. In: Holleb AI, Fink DJ, Murphy GP, eds. *American Cancer Society Textbook of Clinical Oncology.* Atlanta: American Cancer Society; 1991.
5. Hubbard SM, Galassi A. Chemotherapy. In: Gross J, Libbey Johnson B, eds. *Handbook of Oncology Nursing.* 2nd ed. Boston: Jones and Bartlett; 1994:55–94.
6. Holmes BC. Administration of cancer chemotherapy agents. In: Dorr RT, Von Hoff DD, eds. *Cancer Chemotherapy Handbook.* 2nd ed. Norwalk, CT: Appleton and Lange; 1994:57–94.
7. Koeller JM, Fields S. Alternative routes of chemotherapy administration. In: Dorr RT, Von Hoff DD, eds. *Cancer Chemotherapy Handbook.* 2nd ed. Norwalk, CT: Appleton and Lange; 1994:95–108.
8. Kaplan LD, Northfelt DW. Malignancies associated with AIDS. In: Sander ME, Volberding PA, eds. *The Medical Management of AIDS.* 4th ed. Boston: WB Saunders; 1995:555–590.
9. Volm MD, Von Roenn JH. Treatment strategies for epidemic Kaposi's sarcoma. *Curr Opin Oncol.* 1995;7:429–436.
10. Northfelt D, Kahn J, Volberding P. Treatment of AIDS-related Kaposi's sarcoma. *Hematol Oncol Clin North Am.* 1991;5:297–310.
11. Gill P, Akil B, Colletti P, et al. Pulmonary Kaposi's sarcoma: clinical findings and results of therapy. *Am J Med.* 1989;87:57–61.
12. Gill PS, Bernstein-Singer M, Espina BM, et al. Adriamycin, bleomycin and vincristine chemotherapy with recombinant granulocyte-macrophage colony-stimulating factor in the treatment of AIDS-related Kaposi's sarcoma. *AIDS.* 1992;6:1477–1481.
13. Gill PS, Rarick MU, Espina B, et al. Advanced acquired immune deficiency syndrome-related Kaposi's sarcoma: results of pilot studies using combination chemotherapy. *Cancer.* 1990;65:1074–1078.
14. Irwin D, Kaplan L. Pulmonary manifestations of acquired immunodeficiency syndrome-associated malignancies. *Semin Resp Infect.* 1993;8(2):139–143.
15. Kaplan LD, Hopewell PC, Jaffe H, et al. Kaposi's sarcoma involving the lung in patients with the acquired immunodeficiency syndrome. *J Acquir Immune Defic Syndr.* 1988;1:23–30.
16. Mauss S, Jablonowski H. Efficacy, safety, and tolerance of low-dose, long-term interferon-alpha 2b and zidovudine in early-stage AIDS-associated Kaposi's sarcoma. *J Acquir Immune Defic Syndr Hum Retrovirol.* 1995;10:157–162.
17. Lipman MC, Swaden LS, Sabin CA, et al. Kaposi's sarcoma in HIV infection treated with vincristine and bleomycin. *AIDS.* 1993;7:592–593.

18. Gail MH, Pluda JM, Rabkin CS, et al. Projections of the incidence of non-Hodgkin's lymphoma related to acquired immunodeficiency syndrome. *J Natl Cancer Inst.* 1991;83:695–701.
19. Kaplan LD, Abrans DI, Feigel E, et al. AIDS-associated non-Hodgkin's lymphoma in San Francisco. *JAMA.* 1989;261:719–724.
20. DeVita V, Hubbard S, Young R, et al. The role of chemotherapy in diffuse aggressive lymphomas. *Semin Hematol.* 1988;25(suppl 2):2–10.
21. Gisselbrecht C, Oksenhendler E, Tirelli U, et al. High-dose chemotherapy for HIV-associated non-Hodgkin's lymphoma. *Am J Med.* 1993;95:188–196.
22. Errante D, Tierelli U, Olesenhelder E, et al. Prospective study with combined low-dose chemotherapy and zidovudine for 37 patients with poor prognosis HIV-related non-Hodgkin's lymphoma. *Proceedings of the American Society of Clinical Oncology.* 1992:11. Abstract.
23. DeAngelis L, Yahalom J, Rosenblum M, et al. Primary CNS lymphoma: managing patients with spontaneous and AIDS related disease. *Oncology.* 1987;1(16): 52–62.
24. Formenti SC , Gill PS, Rarick M, et al. Primary central nervous system lymphoma in AIDS: results of radiation therapy. *Cancer.* 1989;63:1101–1107.
25. Maiman M, Fructer RG, Guy L, et al. Human immunodeficiency virus infection and invasive cervical carcinoma. *Cancer.* 1993;1:402–406.
26. Maiman M, Fruchter R, Serur E, et al. Recurrent cervical intraepithelial neoplasm in human immunodeficiency virus-seropositive women. *Obstet Gynecol.* 1993;82(2):170–174.
27. Adachi A, Fleming I, Burk R, et al. Women with human immunodeficiency virus infection and abnormal Papanicolaou smears: a prospective study of colposcopy and clinical outcome. *Obstet Gynecol.* 1993;81(3):372–377.
28. Miller SA. Legal implications for the nurse involved in the administration of cytotoxic agents. In: Dorr RT, Von Hoff DD, eds. *Cancer Chemotherapy Handbook.* 2nd ed. Norwalk, CT: Appleton and Lange; 1994:119–128.
29. Dorr RT. Pharmacologic management of vesicant chemotherapy extravasation. In: Dorr RT, Van Hoff DD, eds. *Cancer Chemotherapy Handbook.* 2nd ed. Norwalk, CT: Appleton and Lange; 1994:109–118.

CHAPTER 8

Treatment of Opportunistic Malignancies: Radiation Therapy

Roberta Anne Strohl, RN, MN, AOCN

Chapter Preview

- Radiation Therapy
- Opportunistic Malignancies

Radiation Therapy

Radiation therapy is a local treatment for cancer in which ionizing radiation is directed to a particular tumor site. The energy imparted by radiation is sufficient enough to break the covalent bonds that link the strands of DNA, yielding single- and double-strand breaks. The net result is the inability of the cell to survive mitosis (cell division). The effect of radiation therapy is thus linked mitotically and is expressed as a cell's attempt to divide. The degree of damage is determined by the mitotic activity of the cell. Radiosensitive tumors are those that are derived from actively dividing cell lines such as lymphomas, leukemias, and seminomas. Radioresistant tumors are those in which the cells do not divide as rapidly, such as rhabdomyosarcoma, a tumor derived from muscle. Table 8.1 identifies the relative radiosensitivity of a variety of cancers.[1,2]

Side Effects

Normal cells within the field of radiation are also affected. The same principle of sensitivity applies to normal tissue—tissues that divide rapidly respond more quickly and exhibit early damage. Compared with damaged cancer cells, normal cells have a better ability to recover from radiative damage, although permanent changes do occur. For each normal cell line there is a maximal amount of radiation that can be tolerated (Table 8.2). Higher doses increase the potential for irreversible damage, and meticulous

Table 8.1 Radiosensitivity of Tumors

Tumor	Radiosensitivity
Lymphoma, leukemia, seminoma, dysgerminoma, Kaposi's sarcoma	High
Squamous cell, oropharyngeal, esophageal, bladder, skin, and cervical epithelial cancer	Fairly high
Vascular and connective tissue of all tumors, astrocytomas	Medium
Adenocarcinoma of the breast, renal epithelia, pancreatic epithelia, thyroid and colon epithelia	Fairly low
Rhabdomyosarcoma, leiomyosarcoma	Low

Table 8.2 Complications of Radiation Therapy[a]

Organ	Response	Dose	Time to Onset
Skin	Erythema	3,000–4,000 cGy	Early, 2–3 weeks
	Moist desquamation	4,500–6,000 cGy	5–6 weeks or within 6 weeks of the end of therapy
	Telangiectasis	4,500–6,000 cGy	Late, months to years
Hair	Loss within treatment area	300–400 cGy	Early, few weeks
Teeth	Caries	4,000 cGy	Late, months to years
Mouth/tongue	Mucositis	3,000 cGy	Early, 2.5–3 weeks
	Xerostomia, changes in taste	3,000–4,000 cGy	
Larynx	Edema	5,000–6,000 cGy	Late, months or years
	Necrosis of cartilage	6,500+ cGy	
Thyroid	Hypothyroidism	3,500–4,000 cGy	Late, years
Lung	Pneumonitis	2,500–3,000 cGy whole lung	Early, 6–8 weeks after treatment
		4,000 cGy one lobe	Late, 6 months
GI tract	Posttreatment nausea and vomiting	125+ cGy+	Early, 1–2 hours after treatment

Small intestine	Cramps, diarrhea	2,000–3,000 cGy	Early, 2–3 weeks
	Malabsorption, ulceration	3,000–4,000 cGy whole abd.	Late, months to years
	Strictures, necrosis	6,000–7,000 cGy small areas	
Urinary/bladder	Cystitis	3,000 cGy	Early, few weeks
	Contracted bladder	6,500–7,000 cGy	Late, months to years
Ovary	Sterility	500–1,000 cGy	Late
Uterus	Necrosis	20,000+ cGy	Late
Brain and spinal cord	Neurological deficits	5,000 cGy whole brain or cord	Late, months to 1 year
	Necrosis	6,500–7,000 cGy smaller areas	
Bone (child)	Arrested growth	2,000–3,000 cGy	Late, depends on area

[a]Data compiled from various sources.[1–3]
GI = gastrointestinal; abd. = abdomen.

care must be taken during treatment planning to calculate normal tissue doses and to prepare a treatment plan that delivers sufficient radiation to the tumor while minimizing normal tissue effects.[1,2] Acute reactions to radiation related to parenchymal damage occur in cell lines such as skin, mucous membranes, bone marrow cells, GI membranes, and hair follicles. Acute reactions occur during the course of treatment. Some, such as GI effects, occur as early as the first treatment. The majority of early effects begin within 2 to 3 weeks of therapy. Late effects of therapy are those that occur 6 months to years after the completion of treatment. These are primarily related to the effect of radiation on the vasculature. The narrowing of vessels results in further parenchymal damage. At the present time, useful predictors of late effects do not exist. The severity of acute reactions does not seem to determine the severity of late effects. Once again, treatment planning to minimize normal tissue dose is the most effective means of preventing late toxicities.[1–3]

Combined Modality Treatment

In patients in whom radiation therapy is administered in addition to other antineoplastic agents, side effects occur earlier and are more severe. Combined modality therapy requires patients to have an adequate immune status, since immunosuppression is a potential side effect. Each institution will have a standard of limits for counts. White cell counts $<2,000$ cells/mm^3 require daily monitoring, and treatment may be interrupted until counts increase. Systemic glutathione plays an important part in the cellular defense against the damaging effect of free radicals that are formed by radiation and that are responsible for radiation damage to DNA. HIV-infected individuals have lower levels of glutathione than noninfected persons. Cellular resistance to radiation is reduced when intracellular thiols such as glutathione are low. Although further work is needed in this area, guiding principles for the nurse caring for HIV-positive patients receiving combined modality therapy are as follows.[1–4]

- Expect normal tissue reactions to occur earlier than in other populations.
- Expect reactions to be more severe.
- Assess the patient daily from the start of treatment.
- Remember that this is a vulnerable host, so instruct the patient to avoid contact with individuals who have colds and infections.
- Instruct the patient and family to stress hand washing.

Opportunistic Malignancies

CNS Lymphomas

Forty percent of persons with AIDS develop CNS symptoms from infections and neoplasms. It is estimated that 1.9 to 6% of patients develop CNS lymphomas. The incidence is probably higher, but a histology-confirming diagnosis requires a biopsy. Therefore, differentiating infection from lymphoma can be difficult. Primary CNS lymphoma is the second most frequent CNS mass lesion in adults with AIDS, and the most frequent in children. Patients present with confusion, memory loss, lethargy, hemiparesis, dysphagia, seizures, and cranial nerve deficits. Lesions are usually multifocal and require whole-brain radiation. Doses are in the range of 4,000 cGy at 200 cGy per fraction. Lymphomas are extremely radiosensitive, and most patients will respond. In a study of patients who were able to complete 4,000 cGy of radiation, they had a median survival of 134 days, compared with 42 days in untreated patients.[17] Whole-brain radiation produces little morbidity (alopecia, skin reactions) and is well tolerated by even extremely ill individuals. The patient's status at the time of diagnosis should determine therapeutic decisions and goal setting.[17,18]

Kaposi's Sarcoma

KS typically presents as a rust-colored infiltrate. It occurs anywhere on the extremities—head and neck mucosa and conjunctiva are common sites. The lesions rapidly become red-purple plaques with nodules that can coalesce to become large lesions characterized by burning, itching, and pain. Untreated, the lesions ulcerate, hemorrhage, and progress to lymphadenopathy and visceral involvement.

KS and lymphomas are extremely sensitive to radiation, with low doses of radiation achieving adequate responses (see Table 8.1). Radiation may be used in the early phases of KS or used palliatively to relieve pain. Since the lesion is sensitive to radiotherapy, results can be achieved with a few treatments or even a single treatment depending on the site. Palliation of KS lesions on the soles of the feet has been achieved with a single treatment of radiation.[5,6]

Skin Lesions

Patients present with both early and extensive disease. Local field irradiation can encompass several lesions, and patients may identify lesions that are most problematic from a pain or cosmetic perspective. The lesions are treated with electron beam therapy, a superficial form of radiation that treats skin but does not deliver radiation to the critical structures under the skin. The treatment plan varies from 1,000 to 3,000 cGy in three to five treatments per week. Skin reactions are the major side effect. Disruption of lymphatic drainage may result in swelling of the hands and feet. Because of the superficial nature of the radiation, bone marrow effects are not seen.[5–7]

If patients present with extensive cutaneous lesions throughout the skin surface, extended field treatment may be recommended. The technique of total skin electron beam therapy is used primarily in patients with mycosis fungoides, a cutaneous T-cell lymphoma. This technique requires that the patient stand during treatment so that the electron beam can encompass the entire skin surface. Because the machine cannot create a large enough field when the patient is on the treatment table, the only means of achieving a field this size is to increase the distance between the patient and the source of radiation. Several fields are needed to treat the entire skin surface. Patients receive total skin treatment twice weekly to a dose of 2,400 cGy at 200 cGy per fraction. Boost treatments are given to areas that are not exposed while the patient is standing (e.g., the soles of the feet). Eyeshields are put in place to protect the eyes during therapy. The infection control office should be consulted about care of the eyeshields. The eyes are rinsed with saline after the shields are removed. Irritation of the eye may occur. Ophthalmologic consults are obtained, and antibiotic cream may be prescribed, which may be put on the eyeshield during treatment.[5,6]

The major problem in treating persons with HIV disease with total skin treatment is that many of these individuals are simply too ill to stand safely for the amount of time required for treatment (45 minutes to 1 hour, with breaks in between fields). Sometimes it is possible to extend treatment fields to treat larger areas with the patient sitting on the treatment table. If patients are unable to tolerate this technique, the most painful lesions may be treated with local field irradiation. Side effects include skin reactions and alopecia.[7,8]

Oral Cavity

Oral KS lesions are common, and occur most often on the palate, predominantly the hard palate and gingiva. Candidiasis and/or hairy leukoplakia often coexist with KS. Radiative doses of 800 to 1,800 cGy at 180 to

200 cGy/day are effective. Mucositis, xerostomia, and loss of taste are temporary side effects. Even with low doses (1,200 cGy) one may see skin reactions early in the treatment course.[9] Reactions occur on the skin as well as in the oral cavity. Watkins et al[10] observed severe reactions at 1,200 cGy unrelated to oral candidiasis and without a correlation to CD4 counts. Mucositis initially appeared 5 to 7 days after the start of therapy, with maximum signs and symptoms at day 10. Resolution occurred over the next 10 days. This is an enhanced time frame for mucositis, as it is commonly seen at 3,500 cGy when treating non-HIV-related squamous cell cancers of the oral cavity.[10]

Oral care during treatment consists of a mouthwash of 1 liter water with 1 tsp salt and 1 tsp bicarbonate of soda used two to three times daily from the first day of treatment and continued until symptoms subside. When mucositis begins, mouthwashes are prescribed according to institutional protocol and may include nystatin, hydrocortisone, tetracycline, and diphenhydramine. Oral narcotics and IV hydration may also be required.[10,11]

Ocular and Eyelid

Involvement of the eyelids or conjunctiva occurs in 20 to 24% of patients with KS. Lesions tend to be slow growing and may be asymptomatic. Treatment is initiated when the lesions cause discomfort, obstruct vision, or are cosmetically disturbing. Radiative doses may range from 800 to 3,600 cGy given in 1 to 20 fractions. Side effects include loss of cilia, conjunctivitis, hyperpigmentation, and edema. Intervention includes rinsing the eyes with a sterile saline solution to alleviate discomfort.[12,13]

Male Genitalia

KS involves the genitalia in 20% of patients. Lesions may be single or multiple. Patients present with pain, edema, swelling, irritative or obstructive voiding, and a palpable mass. Doses of radiation range from 600 to 3,000 cGy given in 1 to 20 fractions. Doses of 800 cGy in a single fraction may be used successfully for palliation in individuals with urinary obstruction and advanced disease. Skin reactions are the only reported side effect. Severe skin reactions are documented in individuals who have received prior bleomycin therapy. Nursing interventions include keeping the area clean and dry. Moist reactions should be treated with a topical hydroactive gel.[13,14]

Pulmonary

Involvement of the trachea, bronchi, lung, and pleura occur as late manifestations of KS. Severe dyspnea is the most common presenting symptom along with nonproductive cough, fever, hemoptysis, and chest pain. Whole-lung irradiation has been given in doses of 150 cGy per fraction to a total dose of 1,500 cGy. Cough, dyspnea, and hemoptysis improve in most patients, at least for a period of time. Short-term palliation with radiation may be a realistic goal, allowing the patient to return home and be more comfortable. Side effects of whole-lung irradiation include increased productive cough, which can be managed with a cough suppressant.[15]

Anal Cancer

An increase in the incidence of squamous cell cancer of the anus occurs in persons with AIDS. These lesions respond more slowly to radiation. Infection and cancer can often occur together in these patients. Patients treated with radiation receive a dose of 4,000 cGy to the pelvis, with a boost to the tumor of an additional 1,000 cGy. It is also possible to boost with local brachytherapy using a high-dose remote afterloader, allowing implants to be given on an outpatient basis. In this treatment, a source of radiation is delivered within a short period (usually about 10 minutes). The radiation is introduced into a catheter or device that is inserted into the rectum. Usually two to three treatments are given. Combined modality therapy may be given with inclusion of 5-fluorouracil and mitomycin-C. The response rates are comparable to the experience in non-HIV-infected patients, but toxicity is increased, particularly skin reactions and myelosuppression. Chadha et al[16] reports on patients who developed chronic diarrhea, and 2 patients with protracted skin morbidity with fistulas and local infection. The patient and significant others need to be taught local care, and the nurses involved must follow these individuals very closely. Daily inspection of the treatment site is necessary for quick identification and treatment of skin reactions. If the patients have diarrhea, the skin in the perianal region becomes sensitive and macerated, posing a risk of severe infection. The site must be observed at least daily and the patient taught to keep the area as clean as possible. Sitz baths with tepid water and topical anesthetics may be used.

Cervical Cancer

The incidence of CIN is increased in persons with HIV infection. There are reports of rapidly progressive cervical cancer in women with AIDS. Rellihan et al[19] describe a relapse at 2 months following radiation with disseminated carcinomatosis. This aggressive pattern is not the usual natural history of cervical carcinoma and may be related to immune deficiency and HPV proliferation. Patients with HIV disease and cervical cancer receive the conventional 4,000 to 45,000 rads to the pelvis followed by one to two brachytherapeutic implants. Reactions including diarrhea and response in the vaginal mucosa are enhanced. Diarrhetic episodes increase to 8 to 10 per day and may occur 2 weeks earlier than seen in women without HIV infection. The aggressive nature of this lesion challenges us to determine a follow-up schedule that takes into account the potential for rapid recurrence and dissemination. Patients should be seen monthly for the first year after diagnosis. Nursing interventions include increasing fluid intake and inspecting the treatment site for signs of mucosal damage. Warm sitz baths and hydroactive gel can be used.

In conclusion, radiation therapy is an effective treatment modality for many of the cancers that occur in persons with AIDS. The nurse caring for these individuals must remember that whenever any cancer occurs in a person with AIDS, effects of radiation may be enhanced and accelerated. The time frame and severity of effects does not follow previously determined patterns. Frequent assessment is critical because the potential for life-threatening side effects always exists.

References

1. Withers R II. Biologic basis of radiation therapy. In: Perez C, Brady L, eds. *Principles and Practice of Radiation Oncology.* 2nd ed. Philadelphia: JB Lippincott; 1992:64–97.
2. Fajardo L. Morphology of radiation effect on normal tissue. In: Perez C, Brady L, eds. *Principles and Practice of Radiation Oncology.* 2nd ed. Philadelphia: JB Lippincott; 1992:114–124.
3. Rubin P, Constine L, Nelson D. Late effects of cancer treatment: radiation and drug toxicities. In: Perez L, Brady L, eds. *Principles and Practice of Radiation Oncology.* 2nd ed. Philadelphia: JB Lippincott; 1992:124–162.

4. Vallis KA. Glutathione deficiency and radiosensitivity in AIDS patients. *Lancet.* 1991;337:918–919.
5. Stelzer K, Griffin T, Koh W. Radiation recall skin toxicity with bleomycin in a patient with Kaposi sarcoma related to acquired immune deficiency syndrome. *Cancer.* 1993;71:1322–1325.
6. Geara F, Piedbois P, Pavlovitch J, et al. Radiotherapy in the management of cutaneous epidemic Kaposi's sarcoma. *Int J Radiat Biol Phys.* 1991;21:1517–1522.
7. Chang L, Reddy S, Shidnia H. Comparison of radiation therapy of classic and epidemic Kaposi's sarcoma. *Am J Clin Oncol.* 1992;15:200–206.
8. Stelzer K, Griffin T. A randomized prospective trial of radiation therapy for AIDS-associated Kaposi's sarcoma. *Int J Radiat Oncol Biol Phys.* 1993;27:1057–1061.
9. Epstein J, Scully C. HIV infection: clinical features and treatment of thirty-three homosexual men with Kaposi's sarcoma. *Oral Surg Oral Med Oral Pathol.* 1991; 71:38–41.
10. Watkins EB, Findlay MD, Gelmann E, et al. Enhanced mucosal reactions in AIDS patients receiving oropharyngeal irradiation. *Int J Radiat Oncol Biol Phys.* 1987; 13:1403–1408.
11. Scully C, Laskaris G, Pindborg J, et al. Oral manifestations of HIV infection and their management. I—more common lesions. *Oral Surg Oral Med Oral Pathol.* 1991;71:158–166.
12. Ghabrial I, Quivey J, Dunn J, et al. Radiation therapy of acquired immunodeficiency syndrome-related Kaposi's sarcoma. *Arch Ophthalmol.* 1992;110: 1423–1426.
13. Bourgeois JP, Frikha H, Piedbo P, et al. Radiotherapy in the management of epidemic Kaposi's sarcoma of the oral cavity, the eyelid and the genitals. *Radiother Oncol.* 1994;30:263–266.
14. Vapnek J, Quivey J, Carroll P. Acquired immunodeficiency syndrome-related Kaposi's sarcoma of the male genitalia: management with radiation therapy. *J Urol.* 1991;146:333–336.
15. Meyer J. Whole-lung irradiation for Kaposi's sarcoma. *Am J Clin Oncol.* 1993;16: 372–376.
16. Chadha M, Rosenblatt E, Malamud S, et al. Squamous-cell carcinoma of the anus in HIV-positive patients. *Dis Colon Rectum.* 1994;37:861–865.
17. Baumgartner J, Rachlin J, Beckstead J, et al. Primary central nervous system lymphomas: natural history and response to radiation therapy in 55 patients with acquired immunodeficiency syndrome. *J Neurosurg.* 1990;73:206–211.
18. Goldstein J, Zeifer B, Chao C, et al. CT appearance of primary CNS lymphoma in patients with acquired immunodeficiency syndrome. *J Comput Assist Tomogr.* 1991;15:39–44.
19. Rellihan M, Dooley D, Burke T, et al. Rapidly progressing cervical cancer in a patient with human immunodeficiency virus infection. *Gynecol Oncol.* 1990;36: 435–438.

UNIT TWO

HIV Common Clinical Problems

CHAPTER 9

Neurological Manifestations

Kristin Ownby, PhDc, MPH, RN, OCN, ACRN
John Ownby, MD

Chapter Preview

- Confusion and Delirium
- Memory Loss and Dementia
- Alterations in Consciousness
- Impaired Coordination, Balance, and Mobility
- Seizures

The nervous system is a common target of HIV infection. Ten percent of patients will have a neurological manifestation as their initial clinical symptom of AIDS.[1] Approximately 40% of persons with AIDS will have neurological complications of AIDS, which are a frequent cause of mortality and morbidity. Seventy to 80% of adult AIDS patients will have neuropathological changes on autopsy.[1]

HIV and AIDS are complicated by a variety of CNS and peripheral nervous system disorders. HIV infection affects the nervous system through four processes: (1) primary diseases due to HIV within the nervous system, (2) opportunistic infections (OIs) due to the immunodeficiency of HIV infection (see Chapters 4 and 5), (3) opportunistic malignancies due to the immunodeficiency of HIV infection (see Chapter 6), and (4) diseases of unknown etiology that may be autoimmune in nature. Manifestations of nervous system invasion include focal neurological deficits, and alterations in memory and consciousness.

Confusion and Delirium

Definition

Confusion is a state in which there is a defect in attention, along with impaired capacity to think with usual speed and clarity, and a generalized reduction of mental activity.[2] *Delirium* is an acute confusional state characterized by a fluctuating state of altered consciousness and cognition. The fluctuating course is generally short in duration, ranging from a several hours to a few days, and is generally a complication of an underlying medical condition.[3]

Characteristics of Delirium

- **Diminished level of consciousness with inattention**
- **Cognitive disturbance**
  - Disorganized thinking
  - Disorientation
  - Perceptual disturbances (not due to preexisting dementia)
  - Memory disturbances
  - Psychomotor agitation or retardation
  - Language disturbance

(continued)

- **Acute in onset (hours to days), fluctuating course (within the course of a day)**
- **Consequence of an underlying medical condition, as discerned by**
  - History
  - Physical examination
  - Laboratory evaluation

Biological and Behavioral Basis

Delirium is a consequence of an underlying medical condition or toxic exposure causing a generalized disturbance in brain function. Patients with advanced AIDS are most at risk for states of delirium. Consciousness is invariably compromised, although the mechanism of this phenomenon is poorly understood.

Etiologies Related to HIV Infection and Its Medical Treatment

The etiologies of delirium are varied, and multiple etiologies frequently coexist in the same patient. Metabolic and toxic etiologies far exceed causes that are structural in nature in the AIDS patient, as well as the population at large. For example, the delirious hypoxemic patient with pneumocystis pneumonia may also have severe hyponatremia. The malnourished AIDS patient with cryptococcal meningitis may now be suffering delirium tremens from alcohol withdrawal. Competing etiologies should always be suspected in the delirious patient and may not necessarily be specific to their course of AIDS. The clinician will recognize the close parallel between the differing diagnoses of delirium and that of stupor and coma.

Causes of Delirium

Drugs and toxins

- Ethanol and methanol
- Anticholinergic agents
- Anticonvulsants
- Antihypertensive agents
- Antiparkinsonian agents
- Antipsychotic agents
- Amphetamines

(continued)

- Cardiac glycosides
- Cimetidine
- Clonidine
- Cocaine
- Disulfiram
- Insulin and oral hypoglycemic agents
- LSD
- Marijuana
- Opiates
- Phencyclidine
- Phenytoin
- Ranitidine
- Salicylates
- Sedatives and hypnotics
- Steroids
- Tricyclics

Withdrawal syndromes
- Ethanol
- Benzodiazepines

CNS disease
- Epilepsy
  - Partial complex status
  - Postictal states
- Brain trauma; concussion
- Infections
  - Meningitis
  - Encephalitis
  - Brain abscess
- Neoplasms
  - CNS lymphoma
  - Metastatic
  - Carcinomatosis meningitis
  - Paraneoplastic encephalopathy
- Vascular disorders
  - Vasculitis
  - Meningitis (any cause)
  - Immune mediated
  - Ischemic states (see above)

Infectious causes

- Remote effects of infection
  - Fevers
  - Sepsis syndromes
- Viral
  - Herpes simplex encephalitis
  - CMV
- Bacterial
  - *Haemophilus*, *Neisseria*, *Streptococcus*
  - Syphilis
- Mycobacterial
  - *Mycobacterium tuberculosis*
  - Atypical *Mycobacterium*
- Fungal
  - Cryptococcol meningitis

Metabolic complications of disease

- Cerebral hypoxia and hypercapnia
  - Cardiac failure
  - Hypotension
  - Pneumonitis
  - Pneumonia
- Inflammatory states
- Glucose, water, and electrolyte balance
  - Glucose, hyper- and hypoglycemia
  - Sodium, hyper- and hyponatremia
  - Water, dehydration or overload
  - Calcium, hyper- and hypocalcemia
  - Electrolyte shifts with dialysis
- Liver
  - hepatitis
- Gastrointestinal
  - Enteritis/colitis
  - Ischemic bowel
  - Bowel perforation/peritonitis
- Lung
  - Pneumonia
  - Acute respiratory distress syndrome

(continued)

- Renal; electrolyte disturbances
- Systemic disorders
  - Hypo- and hyperthermic states

Nutritional deficiency states
- Thiamin (Wernicke's encephalopathy)
- Nicotinic acid
- Vitamin B12
- Folate

Other important etiologies
- Postoperative states
- Postpartum
- Sleep deprivation/intensive care unit "psychosis"

Adverse effects of prescribed drugs, over-the-counter drugs, or illicit drugs are among the most common causes of delirium. Almost any agent may cause delirium in the patient with advanced AIDS.

Withdrawal syndromes must also be suspected and specifically assessed, even in the absence of confirmatory history. It is not uncommon for available historians such as spouses or family to have denied or been deceived regarding, for example, ongoing ethanol consumption. It is within the clinician's discretion to treat empirically for possible dangerous withdrawal syndromes in the questionable patient.

Metabolic complications of underlying medical disease are particularly common in the patient with advanced AIDS. Cardiovascular, pulmonary, renal, hepatic, and endocrine functions must be carefully assessed. This evaluation requires both a careful physical examination and appropriate laboratory analysis.

Nutritional deficiencies must be suspected in every patient with AIDS, especially if there are overt signs of malnutrition. Malabsorption syndromes may predispose the patient to nutritional and vitamin deficiencies.

OIs involving the CNS may give rise to meningitis and encephalitis (see Chapter 4). Examples include cryptococcal meningitis and herpes simplex encephalitis. Vasculitis of the CNS may be caused by meningitis or autoimmune disease, and may cause diffuse cerebral inflammation or ischemia. Systemic infections or infections remote from the CNS may predispose the AIDS patient with preexisting CNS disease (e.g., AIDS dementia complex [ADC]) to states of delirium.

Confusion may be an early conspicuous manifestation of ADC and should be distinguished from delirium. ADC will not manifest other characteristic features of delirium or psychosis. If the patient with ADC is found to suffer delirium, then other underlying etiologies must be sought.

Presentation and Assessment

Careful history, physical examination, and laboratory analysis are the cornerstones to diagnosis in the delirious patient. Confusion is not specific to delirium. Delirium should be differentiated from dementia and psychotic disorders based on clinical grounds (Table 9.1).

Subjective

An accurate history is generally not forthcoming from the delirious patient. Family members, friends, and emergency medical response personnel may provide the vital information needed. Review of systems may lend insight to the nature of the process, such as meningismus, headache, or focal neurologic deficits. The past health history, including CNS and other vital organ pathologies, is of particular importance.

Medication lists of prescribed, over-the-counter, and illicit drugs must be obtained. Ethanol history must be specifically investigated. Determine any possibility of medication overdose or toxic exposure, with or without suicidal intent.

Objective

PHYSICAL EXAMINATION. The physical examination must attend to the possibility of multiple etiologies in the delirious patient. The general physical exam is centered on evidence of organ dysfunction and OIs. Meningismus should be specifically assessed, but a generalized headache remains a much more sensitive clue to the presence of meningitis. The mental status examination characterizes the nature of altered mentation: Not all confusion is delirium. Differentiate carefully between aphasia (disturbance in language), dysarthria (disturbance in articulation of speech), and confusion. The remainder of the neurologic examination should reveal any focal neurologic deficits or unexpected asymmetry of neurologic function. Subtle neurologic findings may have dramatic clinical import.

LABORATORY EVALUATION. Laboratory studies may reveal the most compelling evidence for specific organ dysfunction giving rise to delirium.

Table 9.1 Differentiating the Nature of Altered Mentation

Parameter	Dementia	Delirium	Psychosis
Onset	Insidious	Acute	Established
Course	Stable	Fluctuating	Fluctuating or stable
Duration	Persistent	Limited	Persistent
Level of consciousness	Normal	Fluctuating	Normal
Attention	Poor, but unaffected	Distractible	Normal or diminished
Memory	Recent and remote impaired	Immediate and recent impaired	Intact
Hallucinations	None	Visual	Auditory
Sleep/wake cycle	Fragmented but generally consistent	Disrupted	Disrupted
Activity level	Normal or diminished	Hyper- or hypoactive	Hyper- or hypoactive

Evaluations should include blood cultures, sputum Gram stain, and cultures; and urinalysis, Gram stain, and cultures; and a complete blood count (CBC). Electrolytes, including calcium, and parameters of renal and hepatic function should be checked routinely in the delirious patient. Either a serum or urine screen of toxic compounds must be obtained. CSF should be obtained for analysis, unless specifically contraindicated. Supratentorial brain masses are not contraindications to lumbar puncture, unless increased intracranial pressure is specifically suspected.

DIAGNOSTIC TECHNIQUES. Neuroimaging techniques must be utilized in the patient with focal neurological deficits and may be advised in all delirious patients. Effective sedation must first be achieved in the delirious patient to afford a technically adequate study without motion artifact. Electroencephalography (EEG) generally reflects diffuse brain dysfunction, usually without affording the clinician insight as to the cause of the delirium.

Related Medical Management

Medical management is generally directed at the underlying cause of the delirium (as previously listed on pp. 235-238). However, empiric therapies are often utilized in most patients including (1) reversal of narcotic or benzodiazepine overdose; (2) thiamin, multivitamin, and glucose replenishment; and (3) the consideration of acyclovir for possible viral encephalitis. Definitive diagnosis of herpes encephalitis is almost always delayed, even though efficacy of acyclovir in the treatment of viral encephalitis is directly related to the promptness of administration. Given the low toxicity profile of acyclovir and the devastating effects of the disease, the clinician may be best advised to treat empirically unless a compelling alternate reason for the patient's delirium is known. Electrolyte imbalances should be appropriately corrected. The medical regimen in the delirious patient should be made as simple as possible, specifically avoiding medications that are known to cause altered mentation (such as cimetidine and anticholinergic medications). Medications should be discontinued that may be responsible for altered mentation. Anxiolytic or antipsychotic drugs may still be utilized to control the patient's behavior and afford a safe environment for the patient and health personnel.

Interventions

Nursing care is the cornerstone in the management of the delirious patient.

Acute

Maximizing the patient's level of function and preventing further deterioration are key goals when caring for the patient with an acute confusional episode. The nurse maintains a calm environment by providing normal levels of essential sensory and tactile stimulation while eliminating extraneous noise and stimuli. Orientation to the surroundings, staff, and activities is a continual process affected by both the health care team and the family/significant other. The nurse gives the patient simple directions and allows sufficient time for the patient to respond, communicate, and make decisions. Providing continuity of caregivers, maintaining routines in ADLs, and keeping the environment familiar reduces agitation associated with delirium.

The health care team assesses the patient's behavior for signs of restlessness and agitation. If signs of restlessness and agitation occur, then the patient is cautiously administered the appropriate psychotropic medication. The use of physical restraints may worsen agitation, so their use is contraindicated. Fatigue can worsen agitation. Providing undisturbed rest periods lessens the likelihood of agitation associated with confusion and dementia.

Chronic

Once the underlying cause of the delirium is identified, the health care team is instrumental in reevaluating for subtle changes indicating recurrence of acute confusion. Monitoring for conditions that could exacerbate delirium requires diligent evaluation by nurses, doctors, friends, and family.

Caregiver Information: Confusion

- Maintain a calm and quiet environment.
- Assign the same caregiver to the patient if at all possible.
- Keep ADLs (e.g., bathing, brushing teeth) on a regular schedule.
- Remove any sharp or dangerous objects from the patient's reach.
- Administer medicine for agitation as ordered.
- Make sure the patient gets adequate rest and keep the patient's bedtime on a set schedule.

Memory Loss and Dementia

Definition

Memory is the ability to retain or store thoughts and learned experiences, and to retrieve previously stored material. *Memory impairment* is characterized by a decline in problem-solving ability by (1) preventing the acquisition of new material, (2) interfering or interrupting the retrieval of previously stored material, or (3) actually destroying stored material. *Dementia* may be defined as a slowly evolving, progressive, global deterioration in which a panorama of mental dysfunction is prominent.[4] The diagnosis of dementia must include memory impairment, cognitive impairments other than memory, and impaired social or occupational functioning (Table 9.2). Dementia must be differentiated from altered levels of consciousness, psychiatric disorders, mood depression, and delirium (see Tables 9.1 and 9.2).

Biologic and Behavioral Basis

Dementia is always a complication of an underlying neuropathologic process. Dementias are differentiated as cortical or subcortical (Table 9.3).

Etiologies Related to HIV Infection and Its Medical Treatment

Neuropathological states underlying the clinical presentation of dementia are many and varied, treatable and untreatable. Probably 80 to 90% of all dementias are untreatable. However, a portion of disorders presenting with dementia are treatable, if not curable.[5]

The "Reversible" Dementias

- Depression
- Drugs
- Infectious encephalopathies
- Vasculopathies
- Neoplasms
- Alcohol
- Hepatic disorder
- B12 deficiency
- Other metabolic derangements
- Other causes

Table 9.2 DSM IV-R Criteria for Dementia

Diagnostic Criteria for Dementia	DSM IV-R
Impairment in short-term memory	Long-term memory may be defective in later stages
Cognitive impairments in at least one of the following areas:	
Abstract thinking	Faulty definitions or concepts
Judgment	Inability to plan for personal problems
Higher cortical dysfunction	Aphasia, apraxia, agnosia
Personality change	Accentuation of premorbid traits, uncharacteristic or inappropriate behavior
Disturbances significantly interfere with social and personal activities	
Delirium is not present	
Considerations as to cause	History, physical examination, or laboratory studies indicate specific organic factors related to the disturbances; an organic cause can be presumed, even in the absence of such evidence, if diffuse cognitive impairment is present and other conditions are excluded

DSM IV-R = Diagnostic and Statistical Manual of Mental Disorders
(Reprinted with permission from the Diagnostic and Statistical Manual of Mental Disorders, Fourth Edition. Copyright 1994 American Psychiatric Association)[6]

The clinician is therefore compelled to undertake the proper evaluation and diagnosis of every dementia, in every age group, with the intent of discerning any and all treatable causes or aspects of the disease.

The most common primary HIV infection of the neurological system presents as a progressive dementia called ADC. ADC presents generally as a subcortical dementia (Table 9.4).

CNS infections can manifest as an alteration in mental status. CMV encephalitis presents with nonspecific symptoms including altered mental status, sensory impairment, and meningismus. Personality changes may be noted. Herpes simplex causes encephalitis in the patient with AIDS.

Table 9.3 Clinical Features Differentiating Cortical and Subcortical Dementias

Parameter	Cortical Dementias	Subcortical Dementias
Neuroanatomic regions involved	Cerebral cortex	White matter and associated cortical fibers
Clinical features	Intellectual decline, memory impairment, aphasia, apraxia	Slowness of processing and execution of action
Examples	Alzheimer's disease	AIDS dementia complex; progressive multifocal leukoencephalopathy
Memory and cognition	Impaired	Relatively spared
Language	Impaired	Relatively spared; the patient may answer questions accurately, but there is often a long latency between the examiner's question and the reply, which is often of great frustration to the examiner
Visuospatial orientation	Impaired	Relatively spared
Motor function	Apraxias may present; the patient may not understand how to put his pants on (dressing apraxia)	Slowed, but accurate; apaxias generally not present; the patient dresses appropriately, but may take an extraordinarily long time to do so

Table 9.4 Clinical Presentation of the AIDS Dementia Complex

Signs and Symptoms	Early	Late
Cognition	Impaired concentration, forgetfulness, mental slowing, impaired attention, slowed information processing, sequencing problems	Worsening of cognitive symptoms
Behavior	Apathy, withdrawal; personality change; confusion; irritability; loss of interest in usual activities	Worsening of behavioral symptoms, disinhibition
Mental status	Psychomotor slowing, impaired serial sevens, impaired memory, impaired calculations	Global dementia, severe psychomotor slowing, reduced verbal output, unawareness of illness, confusion, disorientation

Adapted from Price RW, Brew BJ, Roke M. Central and peripheral nervous system complications of HIV-1 infection and AIDS. In: DeVita VT Jr, Hellman S, Rosenberg SA, eds. *AIDS: Etiology, Diagnosis, Treatment, and Prevention.* 3rd ed. Philadelphia: Lippincott; 1992: 237–257.

Herpetic encephalitis is associated with a necrotizing encephalitis that is seen in the temporal and inferior frontal lobes. The patient may present with mental status changes ranging from mild cognitive or behavioral dysfunction to profound coma.[7] In contrast to other forms of dementia in the patient with AIDS, infectious encephalopathies, especially due to herpes virus, pursue a subacute to acute course of deteriorating mentation and consciousness.

Progressive Multifocal Leukoencepholopathy (PML) is associated with a progressive demyelinating disease. PML may present with cognitive abnormalities manifested by decreased attention and memory, confusion, personality changes, and dementia[7,8] (see Chapter 4).

Primary CNS lymphoma presents with alterations in mental status manifested by confusion, lethargy, memory loss, and alterations in personality and behavior[8] (see Chapter 6).

Vitamin deficiencies giving rise to altered mentation are common and frequently treatable, if not reversible. Patients with AIDS are frequent victims of competing pathologies associated with vitamin deficiencies, such as alcoholism and malnutrition. Supplemental thiamin and folate should be administered appropriately.

Depression is common in the AIDS population and may present clinically with apathy, social withdrawal, psychomotor slowing, and apparent cognitive decline, thus termed *pseudodementia* (Table 9.5). (See Chapter 15 for depression.)

Presentation and Assessment

Subjective

Dementing disorders in the patient with AIDS may be insidious. Frequently, dementing disorders rob the patient of insight and judgment, such that he may not understand that he has lost cognitive milestones. Witnesses are often better sources for subjective data than the patient himself. The intellectual nature of the patient's career or day-to-day activities predicts

Table 9.5 Differentiating Dementia from Pseudodementia

Feature	Pseudodementia	Dementia
Onset	Depression precedes cognitive impairment	Cognitive impairment precedes mood depression
Past medical history of depression	Present	Less likely
Patient's description of cognitive loss	Accurate or exaggerated	Minimizes deficits, fails to show insight into his own cognitive impairment
Apathy vs. anomia reflected in conversation:		
Replies "I don't know"	Frequent	Variable
Makes paraphasic errors	Rare	Usual
Orientation	Normal	Impaired
Memory	Normal	Impaired
Physical exam	Normal	Occasionally abnormal
Electroencephalogram	Normal	Diffuse slowing
Reversibility	Reversible	Irreversible

how early in the disease course the dementia is detected. The examiner should elicit concrete landmarks that sketch the course of the dementing process.

Important Questions in the Patient with Possible Dementia

- Orientation
  - Recall of current, recent, and past events?
  - Orientation to time and date?
  - Forgetting important dates or appointments?
- Concentration and information processing
  - Able to remain attentive?
  - Leaving tasks incomplete?
  - Losing personal belongings?
- Business affairs
  - Who writes the checks, and when did the patient relinquish this responsibility?
  - Have mistakes or overdrafts been made?
  - Has the bank had to inform the patient of problems or inconsistencies?
- Reading and language skills
  - Does the patient still read the paper or write letters?
  - Have difficulty holding conversations on the phone? Avoid phone calls?
  - Become lost in conversation? Have word-finding difficulties?
- Visuospatial orientation
  - Does the patient still drive a car?
  - Become lost in familiar or unfamiliar surroundings?
  - Avoid going outside or to the mall?
- Behavior
  - Mood changes?
  - Apathetic? Is behavior appropriate?
  - General appearance?
- Drug abuse or interactions
  - Ethanol or illicit drugs?
  - Medication listing, including over-the-counter medications?
  - Anticholinergic or sedative medications?
- Past medical history
  - Preexisting medical or psychiatric conditions?
  - History of depression?

Objective

The Mini-Mental State Examination should be the first priority in the health assessment[9] (Figure 9.1). Many examiners move quickly to mental status assessment when they realize that cognitive difficulties compromise the quality of the subjective assessment. The distinction between dementia and depression is one of the most difficult challenges for the clinician, but is of paramount importance since pseudodementia is a treatable and potentially reversible disorder.

MEMORY. Memory disturbances are a consistent feature of dementing illnesses. The onset of mental change is so insidious that a precise date of onset is not possible to determine. An important clinical axiom is Ribot's law, which states that remote memories are preserved whereas recent ones are lost in dementing illnesses. However, Ribot's law may only be relatively true; memory loss usually extends to all decades of life.

LANGUAGE. Expressive difficulties manifest early as halting speech because of failure to recall the needed word. An analogous phenomenon can occur in the written word. Vocabulary becomes restricted and expressive language becomes stereotyped and inflexible. Eventually the search for words becomes a continual and increasingly arduous task, and the patient fails to speak in full sentences, resorting to phrases and words that only approximate intended meanings (paraphasic errors).

Comprehension difficulties for the spoken and written word may appear initially intact, inasmuch as the affected patient remains alert and responsive to simple conversation, and the patient may remain comfortable with familiar routines. However multiple-step commands frequently reveal severe deficits. The patient with advanced dementia may only repeat words spoken to them (echolalia).

CALCULATION. Calculation disturbances become apparent with advancing disease, and tasks requiring arithmetic calculation become increasingly difficult. The spouse or partner may assume responsibilities such as balancing the household budget or checkbook, even though the patient may have done so capably for many years. The difficulties in calculation may be in large part due to deficits in attention and memory registration in advanced disease.

ORIENTATION (Ask the following questions):	(Maximum score is 10)	
What is today's date?	Date (e.g., Jan 21)	1 ( )
What is the year?	Year	1 ( )
What is the month?	Month	1 ( )
What day of the week is today?	Day	1 ( )
Can you also tell me what season it is?	Season	1 ( )
Can you also tell me the name of this hospital (clinic)?	Hospital (*Clinic*)	1 ( )
What floor are we on?	Floor	1 ( )
What town or city are we in?	Town or City	1 ( )
What county are we in, or the county in which you live?	County	1 ( )
What state are we in?	State	1 ( )
IMMEDIATE RECALL	(Maximum score is 3)	
Ask the subject if you may test his/her memory. Then say **"ball," "flag," "tree"** clearly and slowly, about one second for each. After you have said all three words, ask him/her to repeat them. The first repetition determines his/her score (0–3), but keep saying them until s/he can repeat all three, up to six tries if s/he does not eventually learn all three, recall cannot be meaningfully tested.	"Ball" "Flag" "Tree" Number of Trials:	1 ( ) 1 ( ) 1 ( ) ( )
ATTENTION AND CALCULATION	(Maximum score is 5)	
Ask the subject to begin with 100 and count backwards by 7. Stop after five subtractions **(93, 86, 79, 72, 65).** Score the total number of correct answers. If the subject cannot or will not perform the "count backwards test" task, place a diagnonal line through this task and ask him/her to spell the word "world" backwards. The score is the number of letters in correct position. For example "dlrow" is 5, "dlorw" is 3, "lrowd" is 0.	"93" ( ) "D" ( ) "86" ( ) "L" ( ) "79" ( ) "R" ( ) "72" ( ) "O" ( ) "65" ( ) "W" ( )	1 ( ) 1 ( ) 1 ( ) 1 ( ) 1 ( )
RECALL (Maximum score is 3)	(Maximum score is 3)	
Ask the subject to recall the three words you previously asked him/her to remember.	"Ball" "Flag" "Tree"	1 ( ) 1 ( ) 1 ( )

Instructions	Item	Score
LANGUAGE (Maximum score is 9)	(Maximum score is 9)	
NAMING Show the subject a wrist watch and ask him/her what it is. Repeat for pencil.	Watch Pencil	1 ( ) 1 ( )
REPETITION Ask the subject to repeat **"No ifs, ands, or buts."**	Repetition	1 ( )
THREE-STAGE COMMAND Give the subject a piece of plain paper and say, **"Take the paper in your right hand, fold it in half, and place it on the floor."**	Takes paper in right hand Folds paper in half Places it on the floor	1 ( ) 1 ( ) 1 ( )
READING Hold up the card which reads, "Close your eyes," so the subject can see it clearly. Ask him/her to read it and do what it says. Score correctly only if he/she actually closes his/her eyes.	Closes eyes	1 ( )
WRITING Give the subject the blank piece of paper provided and ask him/her to write a sentence. It is to be written spontaneously. It must contain a subject and a verb, and be sensible. Correct grammar and punctuation are not necessary.	Writes sentence	1 ( )
COPYING On the page provided, ask the subject to draw intersecting pentagons (as shown) two must intersect to score one point. Tremor and rotation are ignored.	Draws pentagons	1 ( )
TOTAL SCORE Sum the number of correct replies to the test items. If item "world spelled backward" was used, add the number of correct letters given in proper position (one to five). The maximum score is 30 for this test.	TOTAL SCORE	(of)

Figure 9.1 The Mini-Mental State Examination (Reprinted from *Journal of Psychiatric Research,* 12:189–198, Folstein et al., Mini-mental state, 1975, with permission from Elsevier Science)

VISUOSPATIAL ORIENTATION. Visuospatial disturbances might manifest as difficulty (1) driving or parking a car, perhaps making a wrong turn and becoming lost; (2) giving or understanding directions; (3) finding the appropriate sleeves when putting on a garment; or (4) making up the bed. Clinically, visuospatial disturbances are reflected in the inability to copy a geometric pattern (e.g., intersecting pentagons).

IDEATIONAL AND IDEOMOTOR APRAXIA. Apraxia is defined as the inability to perform a task despite adequate strength and coordination. Difficulty with planning of complex activities, conceptualizing their final purpose, and continuously modifying the individual components of a motor sequence until the goal is achieved might manifest as the inability to apply the razor to the face correctly or to apply makeup, or to use eating utensils effectively.

BEHAVIORAL DISTURBANCES. Personality changes are among the most tragic effects of dementing illnesses that may be witnessed by families. The patient may become restless and easily agitated or frustrated. Judgment may be affected, such that the patient makes imprudent business deals or purchases. Sleeping habits are frequently disturbed, such that the task of a caretaker to render continuous care effectively to a patient, who may be awake at any hour of the day, becomes impossible.

MOTOR DISTURBANCES. Difficulty in locomotion with unsteadiness of gait, characterized by short steps, but with preservation of motor strength might be observed in advanced disease. Spasticity or extrapyramidal features may develop.

Related Medical Management

Persons with ADC who receive zidovudine show dramatic improvement in cognitive functions including memory, attention, and improvement in motor skills.[9] Clinical trials have demonstrated that zidovudine is associated with improvement in neuropsychological tests in a significant proportion of adults and children with established disease.[1] Progression of ADC may be slowed in some patients.

As ADC progresses and psychomotor retardation advances, the CNS stimulant methylphenidate (Ritalin) may be prescribed to improve motivation. CNS psychostimulants may improve the function of the remaining neurons through increased noradrenergic activity.[11]

Pharmacological therapies can be prescribed for behavioral problems associated with dementia. Neuroleptic drug therapy may assist specific behaviors including anxiety, hostility, hallucinations, excitement, and emotional lability.[11,12] Haloperidol, a neuroleptic agent, is a medication commonly prescribed for behavioral problems such as agitation, aggression, delusions, hallucinations, anxiety, or screaming.

CMV and herpetic encephalitis are treated with the appropriate antiviral agents (see Chapter 5). Currently there is no treatment available for PML. Primary CNS lymphoma is treated with cranial radiation or intrathecal methotrexate. The prognosis is poor and patients experience only a short improvement in their neurological function (see Chapter 6).

Interventions

Prevention

Zidovudine crosses the blood-brain barrier and has been shown to diminish the incidence of ADC. Health care providers provide education to ensure adherence with the prescribed therapy. (See Chapter 21.)

Acute Dementia

The patient who is newly diagnosed with mild ADC is faced with many concerns and decisions. The goals of care for the individual with mild to moderate dementia include (1) promote independence of the patient, (2) identify factors that contribute to sensoriperceptual alteration, (3) provide meaningful and sufficient sensory input, (4) minimize disorientation, (5) provide for safety, and (6) improve the individual's ability to cope with reality.[13,14]

Independence is maintained by always supplying information to the patient as to the purpose of activities, procedures, therapies, and goals. The caregiver considers the amount of information to present to the patient, the complexity of the information, and the rate at which the patient can process the information. The caregiver repeats information often to reinforce the patient's understanding and memory of activities. When providing information, the health care provider uses a low-pitched, calm voice and avoids the use of technical jargon. When asking questions, the patient is asked only one question at a time and the questions do not require decision making. Directions are simple and concise, and are given in a slow, clear manner.

Caregiver Information: Dementia

- Reduce stress by protecting the patient from the following potential sources of stress
  - A change in routine, caregiver, or environment
  - Fatigue
  - Overwhelming or competing stimuli
  - Excessive demands
- Keep the patient's daily routine stable
  - List the activities necessary for the patient's daily care
  - Establish bedtime rituals
  - Stick to the schedule as closely as possible so that the patient won't be surprised or have to make decisions
  - Keep a copy of the patient's schedule for other caregivers to follow
- Reality orientation should include orienting the patient as to the day of the week and the activity the patient will perform.
- Keep the patient's surroundings simple
  - Keep the noise level low
  - Avoid busy places such as shopping malls
  - Remove mirrors and photographs if the patient mistakes the images as real people
  - Provide cues in the environment, such as hanging a picture of a toilet on the bathroom door
- Help the patient avoid fatigue (See Chapter 16: Fatigue and Chapter 17: Sleep Alterations.)
  - Plan activities in the morning when the patient's functioning is best
  - Save less demanding activities for later in the day
  - Schedule breaks between activities
  - If the patient requires a nap during the day, use a reclining chair rather than a bed so the patient won't confuse day and night
- If the patient becomes restless or agitated, divert the patient's attention with appropriate activities. Repetitive activities, such as rocking in a rocking chair, do not require planning or concentration.
- Maintain safety
  - Remove potential safety hazards including knives, forks, scissors, and other sharp objects
  - Serve food on unbreakable dishes

- Taste food for temperature before serving it to the patient to prevent a burn
- Adjust the water heater to a lower temperature (approximately 110°F)
- Cover unused electrical outlets
- Remove throw rugs and cover slippery floors with large area rugs
- Keep floors and stairways clear of objects to prevent the patient from tripping
- Camouflage doors with murals so they don't look like an exit or install locks on the doors
- Barricade stairways with high gates
- Store all medications out of the patient's reach
- Remove all breakable pictures from the walls and attach curtains to the wall with Velcro fastening tape

- Install assistive devices
  - Pad sharp furniture corners with plastic covers
  - Provide a low bed for the patient and side rails if necessary
  - Keep the house well illuminated; have night lights for the bathroom
  - Attach safety rails in the bathtub, near the toilet, and on stairways
  - Place nonskid strips in the bathtub and in front of the toilet
  - Provide an identification bracelet for the patient with information such as the patient's name, address, and phone number
  - Give local police a photograph and description of the patient in case the patient is found wandering in the streets
  - Provide memory aids to help the patient remember to take medications

Patients with mild dementia are quickly frustrated. Suggestions for easy, practical methods for coping with minor memory and concentration problems can reduce the frustration. The health care team implements memory-retaining techniques, such as writing lists, memory cue games, mnemonic devices, and calendars. Compensation strategies are instituted to improve functional lifestyle. These strategies include (1) menu planning with a shopping list, (2) timely completion of tasks on a daily planner, and (3) checklists at the front door to ensure that electrical appliances and lights are off before leaving the house. Tasks can be broken into parts so that the patient is better able to concentrate, thus reducing frustration.

Caregiver/Patient Information: Memory Loss

- Establish a routine for daily activities
  - List the activities necessary for daily care
  - Write out the schedule for daily activities
  - Have the schedule available for other caregivers
  - Establish a routine bedtime ritual
  - Have the patient do one activity at a time
  - Keep activities simple
- Maintain a stress-free environment
  - Adhere to the schedule of daily activities; avoid changes in the routine
  - Prevent or reduce overwhelming or competing stimuli in the environment
  - Prevent fatigue by providing rest periods and maintaining a bedtime ritual
- Maintain orientation
  - Keep a calendar of activities visible on the wall and cross off days as they pass
  - Keep familiar objects nearby; encourage the presence of familiar people
  - Maintain a photo album with labeled pictures of family members, friends, and home
  - Keep daily activities on a set schedule
  - Help the patient identify memory aids to assist with activities of daily living

Keeping the environment consistent and the daily activities on a routine schedule assists the patient in maintaining independence. Family and friends are encouraged to make frequent contact to help orient the patient. Calendars, radios, clocks, and television are helpful to provide time orientation. Electronic medication boxes can be used to remind the patient when to take scheduled medications. Orientation is reinforced by having the patient's personal effects such as family photographs, books, pillow, or diary available.

Caregivers assist the patient in coping with functional limitations such as loss of driving privileges or inability to work. The patient is encouraged to make critical decisions he may not be able to make later on. The patient and family should discuss life support issues. The health care team can be instrumental in arranging a conference between the patient, family, and physician so that everyone involved in the patient's care will have a clear understanding of the patient's wishes. Legal discussions should also be made (see Chapter 24). Discuss with patient and family/significant other the importance of establishing advance directives such as a durable power of attorney. Encourage the patient to write both a will and a living will. Preparing ahead of time will ensure that the patient's wishes are observed and helps spare the family/significant other the pain of making difficult decisions.

Chronic Dementia

Behavioral problems associated with dementia include wandering, difficulty with personal care tasks, paranoia or suspiciousness, agitation, incontinence, and/or sleep disturbances.[15]

WANDERING. The behavior of wandering can be caused by stress, losing or misplacing objects or a person, boredom, needing to use the toilet, side effect of certain medications, or environmental stimuli such as exit signs. To prevent wandering, reduce excessive environmental stimuli. Keep frequently used, familiar objects nearby so patients can readily find the objects. Providing the patient with a safe area in which to wander and the opportunity for exercise, such as walking, helps to reduce restlessness. Instituting a toileting schedule decreases the patient's need to wander in response to the need to void or defecate.

SUSPICIOUSNESS. The person with dementia may demonstrate suspicious or paranoid behaviors. Potential causes of suspiciousness include forgetting where objects were placed, misinterpreting actions or words, misinterpreting people and their actions, or misinterpreting the environment. Strategies to prevent or decrease paranoid behavior include (1) offering to help find missing objects, (2) having more than one of the same object available when misplaced, and (3) learning where the patient's favorite hiding places are and searching these areas for missing objects. The caregiver practices patience and does not argue or try to reason with the severely demented patient. Trying to distract and draw on old memories can divert the patient's attention and may reduce the suspiciousness. A routine of care and activities provides continuity. Sensory impairments can cause demented patients to become suspicious since their environment is difficult to appraise. The caregiver assesses for sensory impairment, such as visual losses from CMV retinitis.

AGITATION. Agitation can occur due to many different etiologies including discomfort; pain; physical illness, such as cystitis; fatigue; overstimulation; overextending capabilities (frustrated because of failure); multiple questions that exceed abilities; side effects of medication; preventing a patient from enacting a desired activity; lowered stress threshold; or restlessness.

Assessing for and managing sources of pain and discomfort can reduce agitation. Eliminating caffeine and alcohol from the diet prevents agitation. Ensuring that the patient receives adequate rest reduces agitation. Environmental stimuli, such as television, are minimized. Calming music may diminish agitation. Overstimulation is avoided. The caregiver controls their own affect by remaining calm and talking to the patient in a low tone and at a slow rate. The caregiver avoids arguments and does not reprimand the patient. Keep tasks simple and do not put the patient into failure-oriented situations. Persistent testing of the patient's memory should be avoided. Ask only one question at a time and allow the patient ample time to respond. Questions that require abstract thought should be eliminated. The caregiver redirects energy to an activity similar to the one the patient wants to do if the initial activity is not warranted. Asking the patient to help with meaningful activities and assigning tasks that provide exercise reduces restlessness. The caregiver needs to be consistent, avoid changes or surprises, and make changes gradually. The caregiver should have diversionary tactics available for outbursts.

SAFETY CONSIDERATIONS. Safety is imperative because the patient has impaired judgment. The patient requires close supervision and should wear an identification bracelet. All medications including over-the-counter drugs are to be kept locked. The patient requires supervision in the kitchen and bathroom. Because wandering is a problem, exits should be kept locked or installed with alarms. Decrease the temperature to the hot-water heater (110°F) so that the patient is not burned.

CARE FOR THE CAREGIVER. Providing constant care for a person afflicted with dementia is physically and emotionally demanding. Health care providers constantly need to assess for caregiver burnout. Helping the caregiver access community supports such as respite care or adult day care can provide relief and prevent burnout.

Alterations in Consciousness

Altered consciousness in the patient with HIV presents an urgent need for rapid clinical evaluation, diagnosis, supportive care, and directed intervention.

Definition

Consciousness is the state of being awake and aware of one's environment. It may be described by one of four terms that have gained specific and well-recognized meaning in the medical literature: alertness, lethargy, stupor, and coma. *Alert* describes the patient who is awake without requiring continued stimulation and is readily interactive with their environment. *Lethargy* describes the patient who appears to be asleep, but with stimulation can be aroused to such a state as to be able to interact with their environment. *Stupor* describes the patient with a more profound deterioration of consciousness who appears to be asleep and cannot be aroused to a degree of wakefulness that would allow interaction with their environment. *Coma* is the extreme degree of depression of consciousness in which the patient appears to be in a sleeplike state and is unresponsive to environmental stimuli.

Biologic and Behavioral Basis

Consciousness is characterized by wakefulness and awareness, functionally subserved by the reticular activating system (RAS) and the cerebral cortex respectively. The RAS is a diffuse array of nuclei and tracts extending through the pons and midbrain of the brainstem to the thalamus, and is fundamentally responsible for states of arousal. Pathologic processes involving both cerebral hemispheres depress awareness independent of the RAS. Alterations in consciousness therefore reflect neuropathology localized to the cerebral hemispheres (bilaterally) or brainstem (the RAS). The rapidity of onset of coma and the clinical neurolocalization of the pathologic process dictate the differential diagnosis, and the urgency and nature of therapeutic interventions.

Etiologies Related to HIV Infection

Etiologies of coma can be classified as metabolic or structural. Structural causes of coma include space-occupying lesions such as tumors and hemorrhages. Certain OIs, if left untreated, may cause the patient to progress into a metabolic coma. Other metabolic etiologies of coma related to HIV are listed below.

Metabolic Etiologies of Coma

- **Hypoxia**
  - Hypoxemia
  - Anemia
- **Ischemia**
  - Cardiac arrest
  - Shock
  - Blood hyperviscosity
  - Disseminated intravascular coagulation (DIC)
- **Hypoglycemia**
- **Cofactor deficiency**
  - Thiamin
  - Niacin
  - Pyridoxine
  - Vitamin B12
  - Folate
- **Infections**
  - Meningitis
  - Encephalitis
  - Postinfectious demyelinating encephalomyelitis
  - Brain abscess
- **Systemic diseases**
  - Septicemia
  - Paraneoplastic syndromes
- **Exogenous toxins and drugs**
  - Benzodiazepines
  - Opiate analgesics
  - Barbiturates
  - Anticonvulsants
  - Salicylates

  - Ethanol
  - Tricyclic antidepressants
  - Anticholinergics
  - Phenothiazines
  - Amphetamines
  - Cocaine
  - Lithium
  - Monoamine oxidase inhibitors
  - Antihistamines
  - Lysergic acid diethylamide (LSD)
  - Penicillins
- **Fluid and electrolyte disorders**
  - Hyper-/hyponatremia
  - Hyper-/hypo-osmolality
  - Hyper-/hypocalcemia
  - Acid/base disorders
  - Magnesium
  - Phosphorus
- **Hepatic/renal failure**

Cryptococcus neoformans (See Chapters 4 and 5.) is a fungal agent that gains access through the respiratory tract and is the third leading cause of neurologic disease in AIDS patients.[16] Cryptococcal meningitis presents with fever, photophobia, neck stiffness, and in some instances hydrocephalus and increased intracranial pressure.[17] If not treated aggressively, cryptococcal meningitis will alter the patient's level of consciousness.

Viral encephalitis caused by CMV or herpes (see Chapters 4 and 5) can cause rapid changes in the level of consciousness. Mortality rates are extremely high—more than 70%—and less than 10% of patients with herpes simplex encephalitis ever return to a normal functioning life.[18] Both primary and recurrent herpes simplex infections can cause disease of the CNS. CMV encephalitis presents with altered mental status, sensory impairment, and meningismus, and can progress from stupor to coma.[1]

OIs affecting the pulmonary system (*Pneumocystis carinii*) can result in hypoxemia and subsequent alteration in consciousness. Alcohol abuse and withdrawal is another cause of altered consciousness.

Presentation and Assessment

The patient with HIV/AIDS presenting with stupor or coma should be considered a medical emergency. The initial clinical evaluation and treatment should be systematic and expeditious.

Subjective

Pertinent details from the history are listed below.

Historic Details of Interest

- CNS OIs
- CNS neoplasms
- CNS vasculitides
- Medications
- Trauma
- Seizure disorders
- Alcohol or other illicit drug usage
- Diabetes or other systemic disease
- Noncompliance with medications

Objective

The neurologic examination is directed at stratifying an intelligent differential diagnosis on which further diagnostic and therapeutic decisions can be based. Differential diagnosis depends most importantly on the localization of the lesion within the CNS. The neurologic examination affords the opportunity to assess the brainstem directly through a series of involuntary reflexes. No such reflexes exist at the level of the cerebral hemispheres. Therefore, if brainstem reflexes are compromised, pathology directly affecting the brainstem is implicated. If brainstem reflexes are found to be intact in the comatose patient, then pathology affecting the cerebral hemispheres is implicated. Health care providers know that either the brainstem or bilateral cerebral hemispheres must be compromised in the comatose patient. Pathology causing acute deterioration of consciousness localizing to the brainstem is usually structural or vascular in nature, such as acute hemorrhagic, tumoral, or hernial syndromes. However, pathology localizing to the cerebral hemispheres is usually "metabolic" in etiology, such as hypoglycemia, hypoxemia, or sepsis. Stupor or coma in the patient with HIV/AIDS is most often "metabolic" in origin.

The efficient neurologic examination of the comatose patient should allow rapid neurologic assessment of critical neurologic subsystems, including (1) the pattern of respiration, (2) pupillary size and reaction to light, (3) brainstem reflexes, and (4) posturing. The respiratory pattern provides important localizing information in patients with depressed levels of consciousness. Eye movements provide perhaps the most critical localizing information in the clinical evaluation of the comatose patient. Neurologic systems subserving eye movements extend from the vestibular nucleus (medulla) to the oculomotor nucleus (midbrain).

Related Medical Management

Cardiorespiratory assessment and stabilization of the patient receives first priority. The airway should be secured, and ventilatory and oxygenation status emergently accessed and supported. Rapid assessment of circulatory function, including blood pressure, heart rate, and rhythm, is paramount. Intravenous access should be established, providing the opportunity to draw blood quickly for several critical initial tests listed below.

Initial Blood Tests in the Comatose Patient

- **Chemistries**
  - Glucose
  - Electrolytes
  - Calcium
  - Blood urea nitrogen (BUN) and creatinine
  - Osmolality
  - Liver function tests
  - Creatinine kinase
- **CBC**
- **Coagulation studies** (prothrombin time (PT) and partial thromboplastin time (PTT)
- **Toxicology screen** (including ethanol)
- **Blood cultures**

Empiric initial therapies may provide rapid reversal of potentially serious processes, give insight to underlying disease processes, and should be administered without reservation or delay. Thiamin and glucose attenuate the risk for the development of Wernicke's encephalopathy. Naloxone and flumazenil reverse the toxic effects of narcotics and benzodiazepines respectively.

Meningitis and viral encephalitis must be ruled out rapidly in the comatose patient, especially in the febrile patient. It has been argued that the clinician should simply initiate empiric antibacterial, antifungal, and possibly antiviral therapy in the patient with HIV without the benefit of CSF examination. However, far more patients die from inadequately diagnosed meningitis than from a hernial syndrome that the clinician might precipitate by performing a diagnostic lumbar puncture. The diagnostic lumbar puncture should not be delayed except in suspected posterior fossa mass lesions or in clinical scenarios when the probable etiology is already known.

Interventions

Acute Alterations in Consciousness

During the initial diagnosis and management of a comatose patient, critical care is required. During this stage the patient is at great risk for rapid neurologic deterioration. Preventing secondary brain injury is a goal during the acute stage of coma and is dependent on the health care provider's ongoing assessment of the patient's neurologic status to detect decreases in the level of brain function and initiating the therapies prescribed by the physician. Diligent monitoring for cardiac arrhythmias, atelectasis, pulmonary edema, acid-base imbalance, temperature alterations, and fluid and electrolyte imbalance is crucial to prevent secondary brain injury.

Acute care of the patient in a coma includes preventing deconditioning and preventing infection. Interventions include activities to maintain or restore the skin, oral mucosa, and corneal integrity.

The health care provider talks to the patient and explains the plan of care even if the patient does not respond. Maintaining a calm, quiet environment reduces agitation. If agitation is not controlled through minimizing environmental stimuli, mild tranquilizers may be necessary.

Chronic Alterations in Consciousness

The primary goal of rehabilitation in a comatose patient is to increase the patient's level of responsiveness.[19] A coma stimulation program is initiated. The actual coma stimulation program considers the order of development of the CNS system. Sensory systems develop in the following order: tactile, vestibular, olfactory, gustatory, auditory, and visual systems.[20]

Impaired Coordination, Balance, and Mobility

Impaired coordination, balance, and mobility are common and important problems in the HIV patient with advancing disease. Proper diagnosis and appropriate intervention can alter morbidity, preserve mobility and dignity, and enhance quality of life. The causes of incoordination and immobility are legion, so this discussion centers on neurologic etiologies.

Definition

Coordination involves the complex interplay of musculoskeletal and neurological systems. Impairment of any one or several of these subsystems may give rise to problems in coordination and mobility. Careful clinical history and examination remains the most effective diagnostic tool. *Balance* refers to a harmonious performance of interactive functions commonly involved in the act of ambulating. This process involves the proper centering of one's weight against gravity over a stable base of support. Balance, therefore, has an integral role in mobility or the ability to move about freely.[19] *Immobility* is "a state in which the individual experiences a limitation of ability for independent physical mobility."[21] The ability to integrate these functions effectively for the smooth performance of motor tasks is termed *motor coordination.*

Biologic and Behavioral Basis

Ambulation involves the dynamic interaction of musculoskeletal and neurologic functions that enable the individual to maintain balance as he propels himself through space. The process of ambulation has been likened to a controlled fall. The center of gravity is displaced away from the base of support (the legs) in the direction of the intended movement, as the base of support is brought forth behind the center of gravity to reposition support as the body moves forward through space. Inability to ambulate effectively due to impaired balance compromises mobility and increases the chance of falling, thereby incurring injury. Several functional and anatomic substrates are required for the proper execution of the complicated dynamics of ambulation and mobility.

Functional Substrates for Coordination

- Neurological systems
  - Mentation/executive function (dementia, judgment, apraxia)
  - Vision (impaired vision, depth perception)
  - Muscle (impaired strength, tone, and bulk)
  - Sensation (impairments of proprioception and touch sensations)
  - Cerebellum
- Musculoskeletal systems
  - Muscle (muscle wasting and poor nutritional status)
  - Joint (limitations in range of motion, joint stability, or pain)
- Cardiovascular, perfusion
- Pulmonary, oxygenation and ventilation
- Hematologic, hemoglobin/oxygen transport

Etiologies Related to HIV Infection and Its Medical Treatment

Impairment of mobility can be caused by neurological, musculoskeletal, cardiovascular, respiratory, or hematologic disorders. Neurological problems that affect mobility in the person with HIV infection include CNS malignancies, OIs affecting the central or peripheral nervous system, cerebrovascular accidents, or ADC (Table 9.6.).[3,22,23] Physical immobility can be due to pathology affecting either the upper or lower extremities, and may be temporary or permanent depending on the underlying etiology. Pain is often a complicating feature of HIV disease, which is associated with limitations in mobility.[22] (See Chapter 19.)

Early ADC presents with motor changes such as psychomotor slowing, ataxia, tremor, hyperreflexia, and handwriting changes.[6,7,22] Late ADC manifests with incontinence, paraplegia, and marked generalized motor slowing.[6,7,22]

CNS malignancies commonly diagnosed in the patient with AIDS are NHL and primary CNS lymphoma (see Chapter 6). Motor deficits associated with AIDS-related lymphoma include paraplegia (midline masses) or hemiparesis (hemispheric masses).

Musculoskeletal complications of HIV include arthritis, particularly Reiter's syndrome.[22] Myositis and myopathy occur in HIV-infected patients as a result of the HIV-related inflammatory response or as a side effect of the antiretroviral agent Zidovudine.[24] Side effects from HIV-related pharmacologic agents including alcohol and isoniazide, chemotherapeutic agents

Table 9.6 Neuropathologic and Physical Assesment Correlates

Neurological System	Pathological Processes	Physical Assessment
Mentation	Dementia (HIV dementia), delirium (adverse drug effect), apraxia (HIV dementia)	Mental status testing, constructional testing
Vision		Visual field testing, retinal examination
Retina	CMV retinitis	
Optic nerve and radiations	Demyelinating diseases	
Optical cortex	CNS toxoplasma, cryptococcal meningitis	
Motor		Muscle tone, bulk, and strength; deep tendon reflexes
Upper motor neuron	Transverse myelitis	
Lower motor neuron	Guillian-Barré syndrome	
Neuromuscular junction	Myasthenic syndromes	Muscle fatigue that immediately recovers with rest
Muscle	Myositis	Muscular fibrillations, proximal muscle involvement
Sensory	Peripheral neuropathy	Light touch, pinprick, temperature, vibration, and proprioception
Cerebellum	CNS lymphoma	Rapid alternating movements, finger to nose, heel to shin

CMV = cytomegalovirus; CNS = central nervous system.

such as vincristine or velban, and antiretroviral agents such as ddI or ddC, may inhibit neurological or musculoskeletal function. KS lesions on the soles of the feet or on the lower legs can impair mobility. Fatigue caused by factors such as anemia or malnutrition can lead to impaired cardiovascular and respiratory function.

HIV-related processes that affect the peripheral nervous system and that can lead to impaired mobility include peripheral neuropathies, myopathy, and polyradiculopathy. Distal symmetrical peripheral neuropathy is the most common syndrome affecting the peripheral nervous system (see Chapter 19).[25,26] The patient may experience tingling and numbness in a stocking/glove distribution. Hyperesthesia and paresthesia can result in a sensory ataxia and weakness. Sensory ataxia describes an incoordination because one cannot sense where the limb or body part is in space.[26]

Inflammatory demyelinating polyradiculoneuropathy is a less frequent but more aggressive form of neuropathy. The disease process damages the fatty membrane covering the nerve fibers that allow nerve impulses to be transmitted smoothly.[23,24] Inflammatory demyelinating polyradiculopathy is recognized in an acute form, acute inflammatory demyelinating polyradiculopathy (AIDP, or Guillain-Barré syndrome) and a chronic form, chronic inflammatory demyelinating polyradiculoneuropathy (CIDP). CIDP is diagnosed commonly in the asymptomatic, chronic HIV-infected individual. AIDP is diagnosed at any time during the HIV disease continuum, and causes severe motor dysfunction with relative sparing of sensory modalities.[23,24] Both syndromes may result in paralysis and, if the diaphragmatic nerves are involved, high cervical spinal cord compression, and the patient may require mechanical ventilation for survival.

Presentation and Assessment

The patient who presents with complaints or complications of imbalance, incoordination, or impaired mobility warrants a careful history, review of systems, and physical examination to discern the true nature of the problem. The assessment should enable the examiner to identify clearly the organ or neurological systems involved.

Subjective

Questions asked to assess mobility, coordination, and balance include whether the patient experiences the following:

- Stiffness, pain, restrictive motion of joints; redness or swelling of joints?
- Dyspnea, wheezing, or cough; fatigue or malaise?
- Weakness, dizziness, or seizures?
- Abnormal sensation or coordination?
- Loss of memory?
- Past or current history of alcohol or illicit drug use? Tobacco use?
- Difficulty with vision (one or both eyes)?

- Bowel or bladder problems (e.g., incontinence)?
- Difficulty performing ADLs?

Objective

A complete physical examination is required. Blood pressure and pulse are hemodynamic measures, and should be recorded in supine and standing positions. Respiratory rate and depth are indirect indicators of respiratory function. Cardiac examination may yield evidence of myocardial, pericardial, or valvular disease that could impact hemodynamic function adversely. Pulmonary examination may yield evidence of pulmonary or further cardiac disease. Musculoskeletal examination should discern any limitation of joint mobility or weakness. Ear, nose, and throat examination may yield evidence of middle ear disease giving rise to disequilibrium syndromes.

THE NEUROLOGICAL EXAMINATION. The neurological examination should identify quickly and systematically any abnormalities giving rise to impaired muscular incoordination. The patient's level of consciousness and ability to mentate should be first assessed. These are discussed in other related sections of this chapter.

MENTATION. The Mini-Mental State Examination[9] is a brief but effective test of several important aspects of mental function, including orientation, immediate memory, attention, language, and construction (see Chapter 15). Impaired reasoning and judgment occurring in HIV-related dementing disorders are often a major risk for unsafe ambulation. The patient's ability to sequence movements effectively to perform tasks requires proper visuospatial perception. The inability to perform sequential motor tasks is termed *apraxia*, and may manifest as difficulty dressing (dressing apraxia) or drawing (constructional apraxia).

CRANIAL NERVES. Visual impairment is a common problem in the patient with AIDS (see Chapter 18) and can give rise to difficulty mobilizing in the immediate environment. Visual acuity and visual field testing with confrontation are bedside screening techniques for deficits of this nature. The retinal examination, especially the macula and optic disk, are of particular importance in the patient with AIDS who may suffer visual complications of CMV retinitis.

Gaze should be tested in all cardinal directions to discern any disconjugate movements. Disconjugate gaze may cause the patient to perceive double images. Ocular pursuits should be smooth to allow even tracking of elements in the environment.

MOTOR. Cardinal features of the motor examination include assessment of muscle tone, bulk, and strength. Neuroanatomic substrates subserving motor function include (in sequence) the upper motor neuron, the lower motor neuron, the neuromuscular junction, and muscle (Figure 9.2). Therefore pathology interrupting motor function may be localized to the cerebral

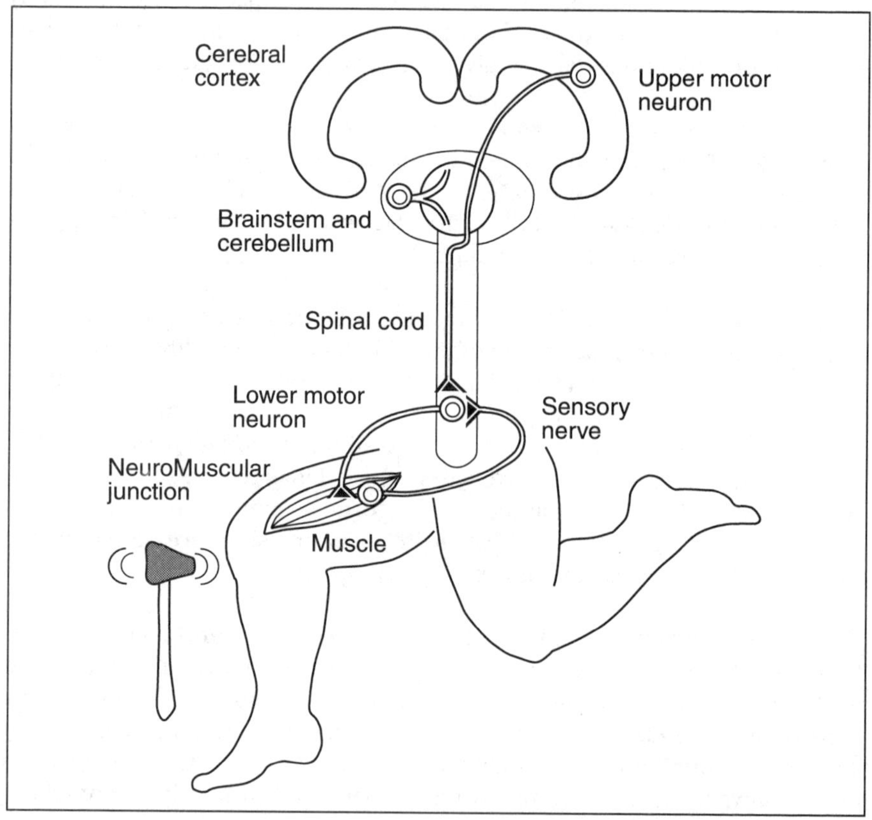

Figure 9.2 Neuroanatomy Involved in Motor Function. (Used with permission of J. Ownby.)

cortex, subcortex, brainstem, spinal cord, peripheral nerve, neuromuscular junction, or muscle. Localization of the pathology is essential to the differential diagnosis and may be assisted by associated important features found in the history and physical examination.

SENSORY. Peripheral neuropathy remains a leading cause of incoordination and impaired mobility in the patient with AIDS. Proprioceptive difficulties, or impaired positional sense, are largely to blame. The patient ambulates with a wide and cautious gait and with eyes wide open. He cannot judge the position or posture of his limbs and body within his environment without continuous visual surveillance. When such a patient closes his eyes or enters a dark room and becomes robbed of his visual cues, he may fall and incur injury. The key physical assessment maneuver to diagnose this common problem is the Romberg test. This condition is termed *sensory ataxia* and is diagnostic of proprioceptive loss. Sensory ataxia may be due to a severe peripheral neuropathy, but neurosyphilis and vitamin B12 deficiency must also be considered.

CEREBELLAR. The cerebellum coordinates movement functionally. Cerebellar dysfunction manifests clinically as irregularities in the rate, rhythm, force, and accuracy of movements. Clinical features of cerebellar dysfunction are listed in Table 9.7. Cerebellar difficulties may be most pronounced when the patient is required to extend his arm fully.

Table 9.7 Clinical Features of Cerebellar Dysfunction

Motor System Involved	Physical Findings
Eyes	Nystagmus, ocular dysmetria
Speech	Abnormalities in articulation and prosody ("scanning" or explosive speech, altered accent)
Limbs	Tremor on rest, sustained posture, and intention; hypotonia; asynergy of movement in finger-to-nose and heel-to-shin maneuvers (past pointing) or rapid alternating movements (irregularities of rate, range, force, and accuracy)
Gait	Broad base; tandem gait difficulty; postural instability, rag doll (flaccid) posture

The neurological examination should discern accurately any significant deficit in visual, motor, sensory, and cerebellar function that may impair coordinated movement. All incoordination is not cerebellar disease. Table 9.8 notes important clinical clues the examiner should note to distinguish motor deficits from cerebellar dysfunction. The Romberg test is designed to distinguish proprioceptive deficits from cerebellar dysfunction.

Table 9.8 Differentiating Motor Neuron from Cerebellar Dysfunction

Physical Examination	Motor Neuron	Cerebellar
Power	Impaired	Patient is strong but unable to coordinate his movements
Tone	Tone is increased in chronic upper motor neuron disorders (e.g., remote transverse myelitis) Tone is decreased in lower motor neuron disorders or acute upper motor neuron disorders	Tone is decreased
Bulk	Muscle bulk may be decreased in weakness due to any cause, but actual muscle atrophy may occur in disorders of the lower motor neuron	Muscle bulk is normal
Finger to nose	The arm may waver up and down as patient struggles against gravity, but the patient does not past point 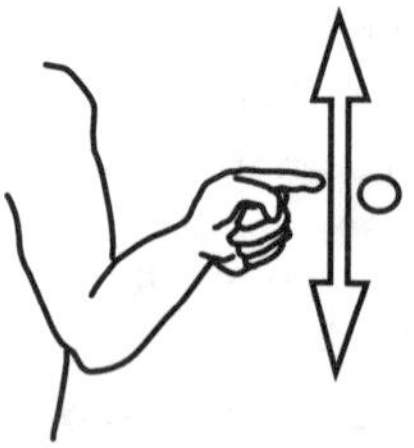	Patient is able to hold up his arm against gravity, but past pointing occurs as the patient moves past the target and back again 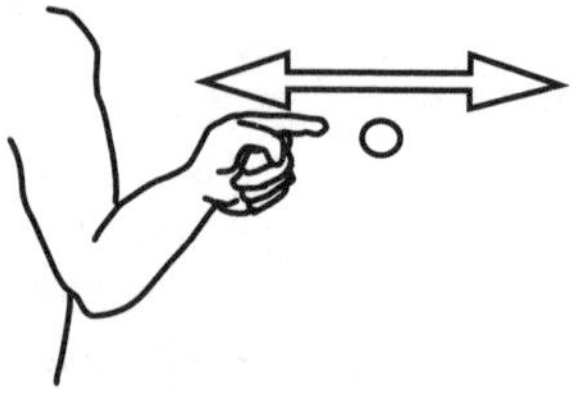

Figures used with permission of J. Ownby.

Related Medical Management

Treatment of underlying causes may prevent cerebellar dysfunction from occurring. Cerebellular problems may be related to side effects of certain medications. Changing the dose or the regimen may eliminate the side effects of the offending medication. Other medical problems associated with HIV may indirectly impact mobility. An example is fatigue caused by anemia can be treated with blood transfusions. Symptom management also includes administrating the appropriate medications to manage pain. (See Chapter 19.)

Arthritis may be treated with sulfasalazine, prednisone, or corticosteroid injections combined with joint immobilization using a splint. Physical therapy is imperative for the HIV patient with arthritis.[22]

For the patient suffering from myositis or myopathy who is receiving Zidovudine, the patient may switch from Zidovudine to another antiretroviral agent. In profoundly disabled individuals, prednisone may be initiated until improvement in muscle strength occurs.

Interventions

Prevention

Identifying the contributing factors affecting coordination, balance, and mobility allows early intervention to prevent or reverse the process. Thorough assessment may reveal subtle changes in the patient's motor function. Reviewing medications the patient is taking and knowing the potential side effects that could impair motor function is important. If side effects develop, share the information with the appropriate health care provider so medication doses or alternative treatment regimens can be started. A common side effect of the antimycobacterial agent isoniazid is peripheral neuropathy, which can be prevented by administrating pyridoxine (vitamin B6) with the agent.

Perceptual and/or cognitive impairment can be a causative factor leading to impaired motor function. Early identification and treatment can prevent or reduce these associative problems. Impaired vision from CMV retinitis is an example of a perceptual impairment that may affect mobility.

Encouraging mild exercise, such as walking, maintains strength, coordination, balance, muscle tone, and cardiovascular endurance. If the patient is unable to perform exercise, encourage range-of-motion (ROM) and strengthening exercises to maintain joint mobility and muscle tone.

Untreated pain can impair physical mobility. Adequate pain management may improve mobility for the individual (see Chapter 19). The administration of pain medications prior to activities may improve tolerance and endurance.

Impaired Mobility

Goals of care for the patient experiencing problems with mobility include (1) maintaining strength of nonaffected muscles; (2) moving joints freely; (3) regaining physical function if possible; (4) maintaining integrity of other body systems including the skin, pulmonary, and cardiovascular systems; (5) achieving maximal independence; and (6) maintaining safety to reduce or minimize potential for injury.[3] A multidisciplinary team approach is essential to the initial plan of care. An occupational therapist is consulted to evaluate the patient's ADL ability and need for equipment or environmental adaptations. A physical therapist is consulted for mobility training such as gait training, stair climbing, transfers, stretching and strengthening exercises, and balance activities. The physical therapist determines the ambulation aids required by the patient, such as various types of walkers, canes, and crutches that are individually fitted to the patient's height and mobility needs.

Patient Information: Impaired Mobility

- Administer pain medication prior to activities as needed
- Remove environmental hazards such as scatter or area rugs, and extension cords; place nonskid strips on tile floors, especially around the toilet and shower and/or bathtub
- Keep environment well lit
- Provide frequent rest time between activities
- Use assistive devices as taught when moving or walking
- Perform exercises as prescribed by the physical therapist
- If bed bound, deep breath and cough every 2 hours
- Drink at least eight glasses of water every day to ensure adequate urination
- Make sure diet is rich in fruits, vegetables, and grains to ensure adequate bowel movements
- Move your bowels whenever you feel the urge
- Urinate whenever you feel the urge
- Wear elastic stockings as prescribed

- Keep skin lubricated, clean, and dry
- Reposition yourself every 2 hours when in bed; reposition yourself every 30 minutes when sitting in a chair
- If you experience any of the following problems, call your health care provider
    - Temperature elevation lasting longer than 3 days
    - Skin breakdown
    - Productive cough of tan, yellow, or green sputum
    - Pain or swelling in any extremity
    - Chest pain
    - Pain in the small of the back
    - Frequency, urgency, or burning on urination
    - Cloudy, foul-smelling urine
    - Nausea and vomiting
    - Decreased movement of any joint

To ensure adequate joint mobility the health care provider teaches the patient about active or passive ROM exercises. Movements are carried out slowly and smoothly, and should not cause pain. The patient is encouraged to perform ROM exercises at least three times daily.

Impaired mobility ranges from complete inability to ambulate by oneself without aids or assistance to lesser degrees of dysfunction. Continuing to maintain an optimal level of functioning and preventing complications are imperative because immobility can have detrimental effects on the cardiovascular, respiratory, musculoskeletal, skin, GI, and urinary systems.

Seizures

Seizures in the patient with HIV are frequently sentinel events heralding underlying malignant complications of HIV infection.

Definition

A *seizure* is an abnormal, sudden, excessive discharge of electrical activity within the cerebral cortex of the brain, giving rise to distinctive changes in behavior and body function. *Epilepsy* is the propensity to suffer recurrent seizures. Seizures may be described as partial (focal) or generalized, primarily generalized (Figure 9.3) or secondarily generalized, and simple or complex. A generalized seizure involves the spread of epileptic discharge through both cerebral hemispheres and is therefore often associated with abnormal motor activity involving both sides of the body (e.g., tonic or tonic-clonic movements) and absolute loss of consciousness (see the section on loss of consciousness/coma). A partial seizure remains localized to one cerebral cortex (without secondary spread to the opposite cerebral cortex), giving rise to clinical manifestations focally involving the contralateral body (Figure 9.4). Although sometimes associated with confusion or

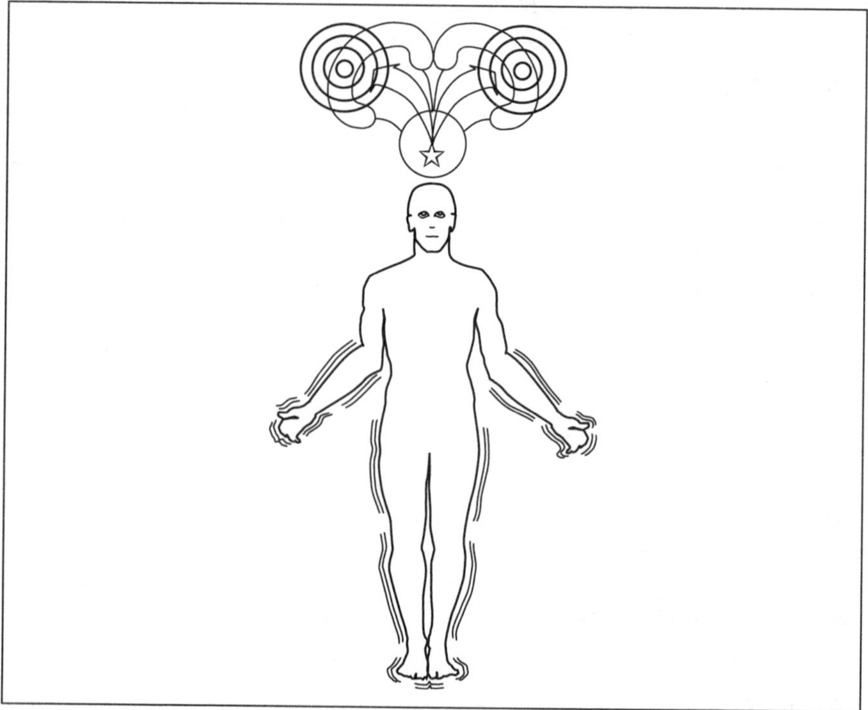

Figure 9.3 **Primary Generalized Seizure the Discharge Giving Rise to the Primary Generalized Seizure is Theorized to Originate in the Brainstem or Thalamus and Spreads Simultaneously to Both Cerebral Cortices.** (Used with permission of J. Ownby)

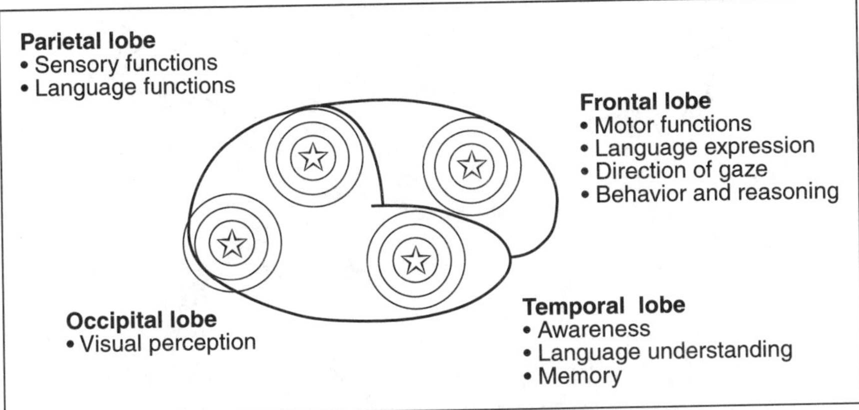

Figure 9.4 Regional Neurological Functions That Might be Expected to be Compromised When Abnormally Activated During the Course of Local Spread of Epileptic Discharges in Partial Seizures (Used with permission of J. Ownby.)

alterations in behavior involving the temporal or frontal lobe, partial seizure activity does not give rise characteristically to alterations of consciousness and the patient remains awake. A seizure may be partial in character during the initial aspect of the seizure, then become generalized as the discharge spreads over the remainder of the ipsilateral and contralateral cerebral cortices by mechanisms that are not fully understood at this time. This phenomenon is referred to as *secondary generalization* of a partial seizure (Figure 9.5). The term *simple* implies that consciousness was relatively preserved during the attack, as opposed to *complex*, which means that the consciousness was relatively compromised. Generalized seizures are necessarily complex because there is always a loss of consciousness as the discharge spreads to both hemispheres. Partial seizures may be complex or simple. *Ictus* refers to the seizure event, and the *postictus* or *postictal phase* refers to the period immediately following the seizure.

If the motor cortex of the frontal lobe is involved, then the patient may manifest tonic or tonic-clonic movements confined to that respective body region. The frontal eye fields are usually involved, causing the patient to gaze in the direction contralateral to the seizure activity (Figure 9.6).

These terms, though useful in the characterization of a seizure, are not mutually exclusive and a single seizure may have several different, appropriate descriptions. The classification of seizures is based primarily

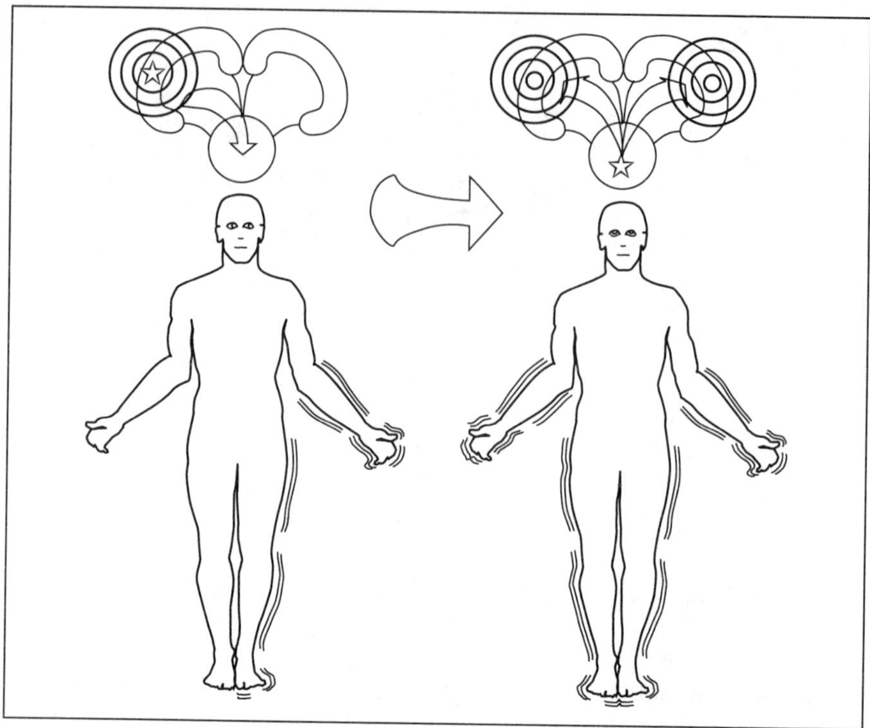

Figure 9.5 Focal Seizure with Secondary Generalization (Used with permission of J. Ownby.)

on the clinical manifestations of the spread of the epileptic discharge, and gives important insight as to the location and therefore differential etiology of the seizure. Several classification schemes exist, which may seem somewhat confused and redundant at first glance, but they emphasize the current understanding of pathophysiological principles underlying seizures. One classification system is displayed in Table 9.9.

Biologic and Behavioral Basis

Seizures are the clinical manifestations of abnormal waves of neuronal discharge of neurons in the cerebral cortex. The clinical manifestations of the seizure reflect the compromise of neurologic function that the involved cerebral cortex subserves.

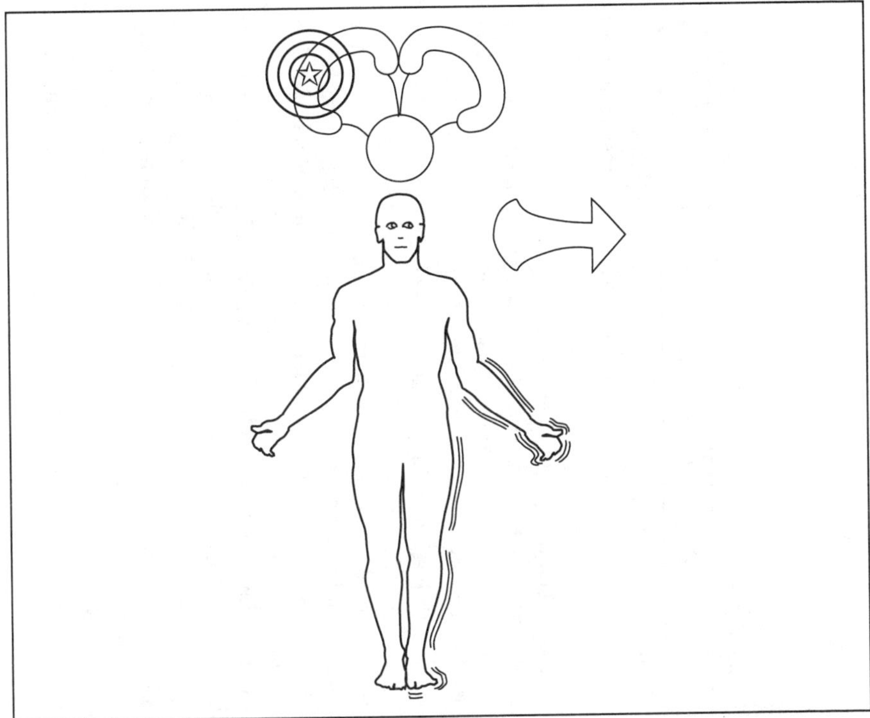

Figure 9.6 Focal Motor Seizure. A Focal Motor Seizure Involves the Motor Cortex, Giving Rise to Abnormal Motor Functions Contralateral to the Seizure Focus. Note That the Patient Will "Look Away" from Seizure Focus if the Frontal Eye Fields are Involved. (Used with permission of J. Ownby)

Etiologies Related to HIV Infection and Its Medical Treatment

The major clinical importance of a new-onset seizure in the patient with HIV is the underlying disease process that gives rise to the seizure. Primary generalized seizures are often precipitated by metabolic derangements such as drug withdrawal, electrolyte abnormalities, or hypoglycemia. A seizure of focal onset is suggestive of a focal brain lesion, such as toxoplasma, primary CNS lymphoma, or herpes encephalitis. Note that metabolic abnormalities lower the seizure threshold, causing an otherwise dormant epileptic focus due to a structural brain abnormality, which may give rise to a seizure. For example, CNS toxoplasma may be more likely

Table 9.9 A Classification and Description of Epileptic Seizures

Seizure	Description
Generalized (primary)	Involves the abnormal spread of the epileptic discharge over both hemispheres. Consciousness is always lost during the ictus (i.e., generalized seizures are always complex in nature).
Tonic/tonic-clonic	Primary motor areas (precentral gyri) are bilaterally involved. The muscles become generally contracted tonically. Often the tonic phase gives way to rapidly alternating phases of contraction and relaxation of the involved musculature, known as tonic-clonic movements. Grand mal seizures are generalized and tonic-clonic in nature.
Absence	Otherwise known as petit mal, these little seizures are characterized by brief lapses of awareness, lasting usually seconds, but may be frequently recurrent during the day. There is no apparent postictal phase. The patient is amnestic for the event (does not usually even realize that the event just occurred). Occurs usually in children, though may persist into young adulthood. A new-onset paroxysmal lapse of awareness in the adult HIV patient may be due to a seizure disorder and is most often a partial complex seizure (not absence in origin) originating in the temporal or frontal lobes. The EEG manifests a paroxysmal, regular 3-Hz spike-and-wave pattern, and is the diagnostic study for this disorder.
Myoclonic	Evidenced by repetitive jerking of the limbs, occurring in brief attacks lasting only a few seconds, but may be recurrent and frequent. The EEG typically manifests single or multiple spikes and waves in one or both cerebral cortices.
Atonic	Manifested as paroxysmal, momentary complete loss of muscle tone, causing the patient to fall or slump to the ground. Occurs in infants and children. No particular characteristic EEG pattern is recognized.

Partial	A focal abnormality of the cerebral cortex gives rise to a focal epileptic discharge that may spread locally.
Simple partial (motor, sensory, autonomic, psychic [behavioral])	The seizure involves only regional areas of cerebral cortex unilaterally, giving rise to respective regional neurological dysfunction without the loss of consciousness. The nature of the neurological abnormality reflects the function of the cerebral cortex involved, and may be motor, sensory, autonomic, or behavioral in nature.
Complex partial	The nature of the seizure may be as mentioned, but the patient's level of consciousness is compromised and usually implies involvement of the temporal or frontal lobes. This distinction may be of more theoretical than clinical utility, since the management strategies are similar.
Generalized (secondary)	The seizure begins focally, but then spreads bilaterally. Such a seizure may begin with an aura or focal area of tonic or tonic-clonic motor activity, with or without the loss of consciousness. However, within moments of onset, the seizure generalizes to involve both sides of the body, and the patient loses consciousness for the duration of the ictus.

EEG = electroencephalogram.

to give rise to a seizure as the patient becomes hyponatremic. In this case, management decisions need to be directed at maintaining appropriate fluid and electrolyte balance, as well as prescribing antitoxoplasmatic and anticonvulsant medications.

Etiologies of Seizures in the Patient with HIV

- CNS infections
  - Toxoplasmosis
  - Herpes encephalitis
  - Cryptococcal meningitis
- CNS neoplasms
  - Primary lymphoma
  - Metastatic neoplastic disease
- CNS vascular disease
  - Vasculitis
  - Bleeding
  - Ischemic stroke
- Metabolic/endocrinologic disorders
  - Hepatic failure
  - Renal failure
  - Hypoglycemia
  - Thyroid disease
  - Acidemia
- Electrolyte abnormalities
  - Hyponatremia
  - Hypernatremia
  - Hypocalcemia
  - Hypomagnesemia
- Drug withdrawal
  - Ethanol
  - Benzodiazepines
  - Anticonvulsants
- Drugs/toxins
  - Antidepressants
  - Antipsychotics
  - Analgesics
  - Anesthetics (local or general)

- Antimicrobials
- Antineoplastics
- Sympathomimetics
- Bronchodilators
- Hematologic disorders/anemias

Presentation and Assessment

Subjective

It is imperative to find a witness to characterize the seizure accurately. The patient cannot be considered a reliable historian for the event or the period following the event. If the clinician is a witness to the event, then the information is to be considered part of the objective assessment. The following data are collected regarding a history of seizures:

- Aura?
- Precipitating factors?
- Focal in onset?
- Motor manifestations?
- Behavioral manifestations?
- Characterize the postictal phase: Was there lingering focal neurologic deficits, such as weakness of a particular limb, or language difficulties that may help to localize an underlying focal brain abnormality that may have given rise to the seizure?
- What medications is the patient currently taking?
- Is there current or past alcohol or illicit drug use?
- Report past medical history of disorders that may be associated with seizures (e.g., diabetes mellitus and hypoglycemia) or history of head trauma.

Objective

The following physical examination is performed after a patient has experienced a seizure:

- Assess if there were any changes in the size of the pupils. Pupils during and immediately after a grand mal are usually dilated. Furthermore, pupil size and reactivity may be affected by possible toxins with sympathomimetic or anticholinergic (dilates pupils) vs. narcotic (constricts pupils) properties.

- Note the direction of the gaze during and after ictus. The frontal eye fields may have been affected. The patient looks away from the affected frontal eye field during ictus. Continued conjugate gaze laterally to one side following the apparent ictus has one of two implications: (1) the patient is looking toward a destructive lesion involving the frontal lobe or (2) the ictus is not over, but the process still involves neuronal discharge that causes the patient to look away from the lesion involving the frontal lobe.
- Assess if there was urinary or fecal incontinence that may have occurred in the ictal or postictal phase of a tonic-clonic seizure. The presence of urinary or fecal incontinence is also consistent with syncope.
- Assess the nature and duration of the aura, seizure, and postictal phase.
- Assess whether the patient was conscious or unconscious during the seizure, whether simple or complex.
- Determine the patient's behavior after the seizure. Was there lethargy, confusion, headache, muscle soreness, or language impairment? These observations can help in diagnosing the type of seizure and the areas of the brain involved.
- Assess whether there was any lateralizing weakness or paralysis of the extremities after the seizure. Lateralizing motor alterations (e.g., transient hemiplegia in Todd's paralysis) indicate asymmetric involvement of the motor cortex.

Related Medical Management

The medical management of seizures involves treatments directed at the underlying cause of the seizure disorder and the possible administration of the appropriate anticonvulsive medications. The goals of therapy in the seizure patient are centered around preventing the recurrence of seizures. The urgency of the medical intervention is dictated by the frequency and nature of the seizure, as well as the underlying process giving rise to the seizure. Several important but frequently neglected principles of therapy should be observed.

- Seizure patients have seizures. A single or infrequently recurrent seizure is usually not a malignant process in and of itself, and usually does not require acute medical intervention. Even generalized tonic-clonic seizures are generally a self-limited process, lasting only a few moments, and are then followed by a limited postictal phase of drowsiness and confusion.

- Benzodiazepines, such as diazepam (Valium), are not indicated for the single seizure. The patient who is suffering a seizure should most often be monitored and protected from injury during and after ictus. Indiscriminate use of benzodiazepines for a recurrent seizure will more often delay recovery needlessly from the postictal phase, as well as the subsequent clinical neurological examination.
- The occurrence of a seizure in the patient with AIDS in whom the underlying cause of the seizure is not well characterized should prompt the immediate investigation as to the nature and etiology of the underlying and possibly malignant disease process. Defining and administering directed therapy expeditiously to the underlying cause of the seizure most often affords the key to effective control of recurrent seizures.
- The purpose of antiepileptic medications is not to prevent the epileptic discharge, but to prevent the abnormal spread of the epileptic discharge over other areas of the cerebral cortex (Table 9.10). A patient who is prone to seizures but who is well-medicated with antiepileptic medications may continue to have an EEG that may manifest as an epileptic focus, although the spread of the focus and therefore the seizure is well controlled.
- Different antiepileptic medications have well-studied efficacy, or lack of efficacy, for controlling the recurrence of different types of seizures.

Table 9.10 Antiepileptic Medications

Seizure	Antiepileptic Medications
Generalized (primary)	
Tonic-clonic	Phenytoin (Dilantin), carbamazepine (Tegretol), valproate (Depakote)
Absence	Ethosuximide, valproate
Myoclonic	Valproate (Depakote), clonazepam
Atonic	Valproate (Depakote), clonazepam, ethosuximide
Partial (and secondarily generalized)	Phenytoin (Dilantin), carbamazepine (Tegretol), primidone, valproate (Depakote)

Therefore the type of seizure a patient is suffering must be well characterized before a rational antiepileptic medication regimen can be prescribed.
- Phenytoin and phenobarbital will decrease the plasma concentration levels of the protease inhibitor saquinavir.[27]
- Dilantin is a long-acting formulation of phenytoin administered once daily by mouth, and is available in 30-mg and 100-mg capsules that should not be crushed. Phenytoin is also available in IV and elixir forms, but must be administered more frequently, usually every 8 hours in the patient with normal liver function. Therefore, a patient taking dilantin 300 mg once daily may be switched to IV phenytoin 100 mg every 8 hours. Dilantin may cause sedation, so many patients choose to take it at bedtime.

Interventions

Prevention

Teaching the patient to recognize and control factors that can precipitate a seizure is important in preventing seizure activity. Prevention of seizures may involve the administration of anticonvulsants. Patient adherence to the anticonvulsant medication regimen is imperative to prevent seizures from occurring (see Chapter 21). The caregiver instructs the patient to take the exact dose of medication at the times prescribed. Missing doses, doubling doses, or taking extra doses can trigger a seizure. The patient or caregiver must be aware of possible adverse effects of the anticonvulsant medications. Bear in mind, the following:

- Adequate nutritional intake is important in the prevention of seizures. Instruct the patient to eat regular meals because skipping meals may lead to hypoglycemia. Hypoglycemia can cause unstable neurons to malfunction, thus triggering a seizure.[28,29]
- Alcohol consumption may trigger a seizure, so the patient needs to check with the physician to find out whether alcoholic beverages are permitted.[28,29]
- Excessive fatigue can precipitate a seizure, so adequate rest is important (see Chapter 16 and 17).
- Stress is another precipitating factor. Assist the patient in learning how to control stress through relaxation techniques.
- Treat a febrile episode early (see Chapter 20).

- Help the patient to identify and avoid other trigger factors such as flashing lights, hyperventilation, or loud noises.

Patient Information: Seizures

- Eat regular meals and eat snacks when you feel shaky, faint, or hungry to avoid hypoglycemic episodes.
- Alcohol and caffeine consumption can trigger a seizure.
- Take medications as ordered by the health care provider. It is important that the anticonvulsant medication be taken in the appropriate dose and at the appropriate time.
- If you miss a dose of the anticonvulsant, notify your health care provider.
- Do not take more or less of the anticonvulsant prescribed. Too much or too little of the anticonvulsant medication can cause a seizure.
- Make sure you do not take any over-the-counter medications without the health care provider's approval.
- Do not ever stop taking the anticonvulsant without your health care provider telling you it is okay to stop.
- Avoid fatigue by getting adequate rest and pacing activities.
- Illness and fever can trigger a seizure. If you do not feel well, notify your health care provider.
- It is important to wear a Medic-Alert bracelet or necklace in case a seizure occurs in public.
- If you feel a seizure coming on, lie down in the nearest safe place.

Caregiver Information: Seizures

If you know someone with a seizure disorder, it is important to know how to care for the person if a seizure occurs.

1. If the person loses consciousness, assist the person to the floor to prevent a fall.
2. Turn the person onto his side.
3. Loosen any tight clothing around the neck and waist. Remove the patient's glasses. Sharp and hard objects should be removed from around the person.
4. Do not put anything into the person's mouth. There is no danger that the person will swallow his tongue.

(continued)

5. When the seizure is over, the person will usually be confused. Tell the person what happened and where he is.
6. If the person is injured during the seizure or has another seizure right away, call the health care provider.
7. Stay with the person after the seizure until the person is no longer confused and can resume activities safely.

Seizure Management

ACUTE. Management of the patient who is experiencing a seizure focuses on safety. The health care provider assists the patient to a supine, side-lying position and protects the patient's head by placing a pillow or soft object under the head. The bed is placed in a low position and the side rails are raised. Restrictive clothing is loosened and glasses are removed. The area around the patient is cleared of hard and/or sharp objects. The caregiver does not try to force anything into the patient's mouth and does not attempt to restrain the person during the seizure.

After the seizure, the caregiver turns the patient to one side to allow saliva to drain from the mouth. Suctioning of the oropharynx should be available and used if the patient vomits. If the patient does vomit, the risk of aspiration is high and the patient's health care provider should be notified.

The patient may be confused and disoriented after the seizure. The caregiver reorients the patient after the seizure because the patient may have amnesia after the attack. The patient is not left unattended after the seizure. No food or liquids are offered to the patient until he is fully awake. Supplemental oxygen may be administered as needed.

CHRONIC. Unless the underlying cause of the seizure is treated, prevention of seizure activity is a lifelong process involving the administration of anticonvulsants. The patient needs to know about taking the medications in the correct dose, at the right time, and the common side effects to monitor (see Chapter 21).

Discharge planning and patient education is crucial. Patient teaching includes (1) precautions to take when ill, under stress, fatigued, or when workload increases; (2) diet and effects of alcohol; (3) driving restrictions, if any; (4) importance of follow-up visits with physicians; and (5) the need to wear a Medic-Alert bracelet or necklace.[28,29]

References

1. Levy R, Breseden D, Rosenblum M. Opportunistic CNS, pathology in patients with AIDS. *Ann Neurol.* 1988;23(suppl):S7–S12.
2. Adams RD, Victor M. *Principles of Neurology.* 4th ed. New York: McGraw-Hill Information Services; 1989.
3. Snyder M. *A Guide to Neurological and Neurosurgical Nursing.* 2nd ed. Albany, NY: Delmar Publishing; 1991.
4. Wells CE. *Dementia.* 2nd ed. Philadelphia: FA Davis; 1977.
5. Price RW, Brew BJ, Roke M. Central and peripheral nervous system complications of HIV-1 infection and AIDS. In: DeVita VT Jr, Hellman S, Rosenberg SA, eds. *AIDS: Etiology, Diagnosis, Treatment, and Prevention.* 3rd ed. Philadelphia: Lippincott; 1992:237–257.
6. American Psychiatric Association: Diagnostic and Statistical Manual of Mental Disorders, Fourth Edition. Washington, DC, American Psychiatric Association, 1994.
7. Hilton G. Neuroscience nursing and HIV. In: Barker E, ed. *Neuroscience Nursing.* St. Louis: Mosby-Year Book; 1994:143–159.
8. Maj M. Organic mental disorders in HIV-1 infection. *AIDS.* 1990;4:831–840.
9. Folstein MF, Folstein SE, McHugh PR. “Mini-mental state”: a practical method for grading cognitive state of patients for the clinician. *J Psychiatr Res.* 1975; 12:189–198.
10. Yarchoan R, Thomas RV, Grafman J, et al. Long-term administration of 3′-azido-2′,3′-dideoxythymidine to patients with AIDS-related neurological diseases. *Ann Neurol.* 1988;23(suppl):S82–S87.
11. Carlson DL, Fleming KC, Smith GE, Evans JM. Management of dementia-related behavioral disturbances: a nonpharmacologic approach. *Mayo Clin Proc.* 1995; 70:1108–1115.
12. Carmichael CG, Carmichael JK, Fischl MA. *HIV/AIDS: Primary Care Handbook.* Norwalk, CT: Appleton & Lange; 1995.
13. McArthur J. AIDS dementia—your assessment can make all the difference. *RN.* 1990;53:36–42.
14. Tackenberg J. Teaching caregivers about Alzheimer’s disease. *Nursing92.* 1992; 22:75–82.
15. Fleming KC, Evans JM. Pharmacologic therapies in dementia. *Mayo Clin Proc.* 1995;70:1116–1123.
16. Kirkpatrick C. Fungal infections in HIV patients. *Ann N Y Acad Sci.* 1990;616: 461–468.
17. Chuck S, Sande M. Infections with cryptococcal neoformans in acquired immunodeficiency virus: CT and MR imaging manifestations with clinical and pathologic correlations. *Radiology.* 1989;175:185–191.

18. Goldsmith SM, Whitley RJ. Herpes simplex encephalitis. In: Lambert HP, ed. *Infections of the Central Nervous System.* Philadelphia: BC Decker; 1991.
19. Boss BJ. Coma and cognitive deficits. In: Barker E, ed. *Neuroscience Nursing.* St. Louis: Mosby-Year Book; 1994:175–202.
20. Rubin M. The physiology of bedrest. *Am J Nurs.* 1988;88(1):50–56.
21. McLane AM, ed. *Classification of Nursing Diagnoses: Proceedings of the Seventh Conference.* St. Louis: CV Mosby; 1987.
22. Casey KM, Cohen F, Hughes A, eds. *ANAC's core curriculum for HIV/AIDS nursing.* Philadelphia: Nursecom; 1996.
23. Dalakas M, Pezeshkour G. Neuromuscular diseases associated with human immunodeficiency virus infection. *Ann Neurol.* 1988;23(suppl 1):S38–S48.
24. Newton HB. Common neurologic complications of HIV-1 infection and AIDS. *Am Fam Physician.* 1995;51:387–398.
25. Scherer P. How HIV attacks the peripheral nervous system. *Am J Nurs.* 1990; 90:66–70.
26. Tyor WR, Wesselingh SL, Griffin JW, McArthur JC, Griffin DE. Unifying hypothesis for the pathogenesis of HIV-associated dementia complex, vacuolar myelopathy, and sensory neuropathy. *J Acquir Immune Defic Syndr Hum Retrovirol.* 1995;9:379–388.
27. Heylen R, Miller R. Adverse effects of drug interactions of medications commonly used in the treatment of adult HIV positive patients. *Genitourin Med.* 1997;17:5–11.
28. Yanko JR. *Seizures. Teaching Patients with Acute Conditions.* Springhouse, PA: Springhouse Corporation; 1992.
29. O'Brein KO. Managing the seizure patient. *Nursing91.* 1991;21:63–65.

CHAPTER 10

Nutrition-Related Changes

Joyce Keithley, DNSc, FAAN

Chapter Preview

- Wasting
- Anorexia
- Oral/Esophageal Symptoms
- Nausea, Vomiting, and Retching
- Diarrhea

It is estimated that 80% or more of HIV-infected patients experience the adverse effects of malnutrition.[1,2] Similar to cancer cachexia, the mechanisms of HIV-related malnutrition are complex in nature. Wasting syndrome, anorexia, oral complications, nausea and vomiting, and diarrhea are major nutrition-related changes that are associated with malnutrition. These changes are subtle or subclinical in early HIV, become more prominent in middle-stage disease, and are severe and progressive in late-stage AIDS.

The end result of these changes is significant malnutrition, which influences immune function, disease progression, mortality, and quality of life. For example, it is well established that malnourished patients with HIV have decreased cell-mediated immunity, lower antibody response, and more OIs.[3] Because of the relationships among nutritional status, infectious disease, and the immune system, nutritional deficiencies are postulated to influence the natural history of this infection as well.[4,5] Timing of death also appears to be related to malnutrition. Kotler et al[6] found a close correlation between extent of wasting and mortality in patients with AIDS. Death occurred when body cell mass was 54% of normal and weight was 66% of normal. Similarly, Guenter et al[7] demonstrated a relationship between serum albumin and mortality. HIV-infected patients with a serum albumin <3.5 g/dl had a death rate that was 3.6 times greater than that for HIV-infected patients with normal serum albumin levels. Further, HIV-associated malnutrition is correlated with decreased quality of life, as a result of fatigue, weakness, and decreased ability to socialize and maintain employment.[8]

To prevent or minimize the adverse effects of malnutrition, the overall goals of nutrition intervention in HIV disease are

- Early assessment and treatment of nutritional deficiencies
- Prevention of body wasting
- Maintenance of quality of life and function

Specific interventions for meeting these goals include nutrition education regarding (1) eating a healthy diet, (2) preventing food-borne illness, (3) managing nutrition-related symptoms, (4) using nutritional supplements or nutrition support techniques, and (5) evaluating nutritional products and information. This chapter examines each of the major nutrition-related changes associated with HIV disease, as well as strategies for maintaining optimal nutritional status throughout the course of the disease.

Wasting

Wasting is a complex and severe complication of HIV infection. Extensive wasting is associated with decreased quality of life and more rapid disease progression.[6,7,9] Data from both prospective and retrospective studies indicate that 91 to 100% of people with AIDS experience wasting.[10,11]

Definition

Wasting is defined as a state of general ill health characterized by malnutrition, body composition changes and weight loss, weakness, and decreased quality of life.[12] The wasting syndrome associated with HIV infection, an AIDS-indicator condition, is defined by the CDC as a "profound involuntary weight loss greater than 10% of baseline body weight plus either chronic diarrhea (at least two loose stools per day for ≥30 days) or chronic weakness and documented fever (for ≥30 days, intermittent or constant) in the absence of concurrent illness or conditions other than HIV infection that could explain the findings (for example, cancer, TB, cryptosporidiosis, or other specific enteritis)."[13 (p 17)]

Biologic and Behavioral Basis/Etiologies Related to HIV Infection and Its Medical Treatment

HIV-related wasting is generally due to one or a combination of four mechanisms: (1) reduced intake, (2) excessive nutrient losses, (3) metabolic alterations, and (4) drug-nutrient interactions.

Mechanisms of Wasting in HIV Diseases

(1) Reduced nutrient intake
- GI symptoms (anorexia, nausea, oral lesions, taste changes)
- Psychosocial factors (depression, economic concerns, anxiety)
- CNS alterations (dementia, myoneuropathies)
- Pain

(2) Excessive nutrient loss
- Intestinal malabsorption (diarrhea, enteric pathogens, vomiting, malignancies)
- Functional alterations (decreased bile production, pancreatic insufficiency, decreased HCl production, villous atrophy)

(continued)

(3) Metabolic changes
- Hypermetabolism
- Cytokine mediators

(4) Drug-nutrient interactions
- Altered drug-nutrient absorption, metabolism, excretion, distribution (Table 10.1)

Table 10.1 Potential Adverse Nutritional Consequences of HIV/AIDS Medications[a]

Medication	Side Effects
A. ANTIVIRAL	
Acyclovir	Diarrhea Metallic taste Nausea/vomiting
Foscarnet	Hypocalcemia Hypermagnesemia Hyperphosphatemia
Ganciclovir	Anorexia Nausea/vomiting Diarrhea
B. ANTIRETROVIRAL	
ddI	Diarrhea Pancreatitis
ddC	Diarrhea Mouth/pharynx/esophageal ulcerations Nausea/vomiting Pancreatitis
Zidovudine	Abdominal pain Appetite/taste changes Nausea/vomiting Constipation Sweet intolerance
Indinavir	Nausea/vomiting
Ritonavir	Taste alterations, anorexia
Saquinavir	Nausea/vomiting

Table 10.1 *Continued*

Medication	Side Effects
C. ANTIFUNGAL	
Amphotericin B	Anorexia Diarrhea Fever/chills Hypokalemia Hypomagnesemia Nausea/vomiting
Fluconazole	Diarrhea Nausea/vomiting
Nystatin	Diarrhea, Nausea
D. ANTIMICOBACTERIAL	
Rifampin	Abdominal pain Diarrhea, Fever/chills Nausea/vomiting Pancreatitis
E. ANTIPARASITIC	
Dapsone	Anorexia Nausea/vomiting
Pentamidine	Hypoglycemia/hyperglycemia Nausea/vomiting Taste changes Pancreatitis
F. ANTIPROTOZOAL	
Clindamycin	Gastrointestinal toxicity Pseudomembranous colitis
G. ANTIBACTERIAL	
Trimethoprim-sulfamethoxazole	Diarrhea Glossitis/stomatitis Nausea/vomiting Pancreatitis

[a]Data culled from various sources.[14,15]

Food or energy intake can be compromised by anorexia, early satiety, nausea, pain, oral lesions, and taste changes. Depression, dementia, fatigue and weakness, myoneuropathies, and lack of economic resources may also reduce intake by limiting the patient's ability to purchase, prepare, and/or eat food.

Loss of nutrients through malabsorption occurs as a result of intestinal disease and alterations in GI function. Numerous enteric pathogens, most notably *Cryptosporidium parvum*, CMV, and *Mycobacterium avium intracellulare*, are associated with diarrhea, vomiting, and weight loss. In later stages of HIV infection, malignancies such as KS and NHL may invade the GI tract, causing decreased intake, nutrient losses, and wasting. Functional alterations that impair GI absorption include decreased bile production, pancreatic insufficiency, villous atrophy, altered oncotic pressure, bacterial overgrowth, and decreased hydrochloric acid production. Carbohydrates and fats are the two nutrients most commonly affected by these functional alterations, resulting in lactose intolerance and fat malabsorption respectively.[16]

A combination of hypermetabolism and cytokine mediators appears to be responsible for the metabolic alterations seen in HIV-related wasting. In early HIV infection, TNF, IL-1, IL-6, and IFNs may divert nutrients away from lean tissue and into fat stores via energy-wasting substrate cycles, producing changes in triglyceride, albumin, hemoglobin, and cholesterol levels.[11] Although hypermetabolism due to systemic infections and fever is widely reported in both asymptomatic HIV-infected patients and patients with AIDS, recent research indicates that reduced energy intake rather than elevated energy expenditure per se is the major reason for weight loss in HIV wasting.[17]

Drug-nutrient interactions are another cause of HIV-associated wasting. HIV pharmacologic therapies may alter nutrient intake, absorption, metabolism, or excretion, thereby resulting in adverse nutritional consequences. Medications such as acyclovir, IV pentamidine, zidovudine, and antibacterial agents are associated with appetite and taste changes, nausea and vomiting, diarrhea, and other nutrition-related side effects (see Table 10.1). Similarly, nutritional and GI status can alter drug absorption, metabolism, and distribution. For example, the presence of food in the stomach can either enhance or interfere with drug absorption. HIV medications that are better absorbed with food include atovaquone, invirase, and norvir. In contrast, HIV medications such as didanosine, zidovudine, and crixivan should be taken on an empty stomach. Decreased hydrochloric acid production from lack of food in the stomach or GI dysfunction reduces the absorption of other medications, such as dapsone and ketoconazole. Because most medications are transported bound to albumin, malnutrition causes greater levels of unbound drugs, enhancing their potentially toxic effects.[16]

Presentation and Assessment

HIV wasting usually presents with weight loss, loss of lean body and fat mass, anorexia, fatigue, fever, and diarrhea. Difficulty chewing or swallowing, altered taste, lactose intolerance, and steatorrhea may also be present. Patients at risk for or who already have wasting can be identified by performing a nutritional assessment. The nutritional assessment also provides baseline data for evaluating the effectiveness of nutritional interventions. A thorough nutritional assessment includes careful dietary and clinical histories, energy expenditure and body composition measures, physical examination, and biochemical parameters.

Subjective

Dietary and clinical histories identify risk factors for wasting. Estimates of dietary intake and patterns can be obtained by using 24-hour recalls, food diaries, or food frequency questionnaires. Particular attention should be paid to food likes and dislikes, food intolerances, special diets, use of dietary supplements, and use of nontraditional dietary therapies. The clinical history should focus on weight gain/loss patterns over the last 6 months; problems with anorexia or early satiety; drug side effects and drug-nutrient interactions; GI complications such as difficulty chewing and swallowing, nausea and vomiting, and diarrhea; fever and infections; pain; fatigue; functional, economic, and psychosocial status; and nutrition knowledge.

Objective

ENERGY EXPENDITURE AND BODY COMPOSITION MEASURES. Several methods can be used to estimate energy expenditure so that energy needs may be determined. Although indirect calorimetry is the preferred method, many clinical settings do not have the necessary equipment or it cannot be used reliably. The classic equations of Harris and Benedict[18] are, therefore, often used to estimate basal energy expenditure (BEE) based on weight, height, and age:

$$\text{BEE (men)} = 66.47 + 13.75\text{ W} + 5.0\text{ H} - 6.74\text{A}$$

$$\text{BEE (women)} = 655.10 + 9.56\text{ W} + 1.85\text{ H} - 4.68\text{A}$$

where W is weight in kilograms, H is height in centimeters, and A is age in years.

Activity and injury factors[19] are then multiplied by the BEE to estimate total energy expenditure:

$$\text{TEE} = \text{BEE} \times \text{activity factor} \times \text{injury factor}$$

where the activity factor may be confined to bed, 1.2; and ambulatory, 1.3; and the injury factor may be surgery, 1.1 to 1.2; infection, 1.2 to 1.8; trauma, 1.3 to 1.6; and burns, 1.5 to 2.0.

Body composition measures estimate body fluid and tissue mass status. For body weight, an unintentional weight loss of 5% over 1 month, 7.5% over 3 months, or 10% over 6 months is considered clinically significant.[20] Fat mass is usually estimated by measuring triceps skinfold thickness; and lean body mass is estimated by measuring mid arm muscle circumference. Body fat mass, lean body mass, and water can also be estimated accurately from bioelectrical impedance analysis (BIA) measures in clinically stable HIV- infected patients.[21] Body mass index (BMI), which is calculated by dividing weight (in kilograms) by height (in square meters), is another way to determine whether patients are at nutritional risk. Patients with a BMI of < 20 are considered underweight and are likely to need nutritional intervention. Body weight should be measured daily in at-risk inpatients; the other body composition parameters are measured every 2 to 4 weeks. For all of the body composition parameters except weight, measures of <90% of normal are indicative of malnutrition.[22]

PHYSICAL EXAM. The physical exam is used to evaluate patients for signs of nutritional deficiencies. In particular, assess for clinical signs of vitamin and mineral deficiency (most often detected in the skin and oral cavity), and fat and muscle wasting. Also assess for the presence of fever, hepatomegaly, splenomegaly, and edema.

BIOCHEMICAL PARAMETERS. Blood counts should be checked every 3 to 6 months for anemia, hypoalbuminemia, hypercholesterolemia, hypertriglyceridemia, and reduced total lymphocyte count. Fecal fat analyses and lactose intolerance tests are indicated in patients with malabsorption. In acutely ill inpatients, nitrogen balance and creatinine height index studies are sometimes used to estimate protein and lean body mass status.

Related Medical Management

Medical management is directed at early nutritional intervention, and treating OIs, fever, and malignancies. Ordering pharmacologic agents like Megace to stimulate appetite or to blunt metabolic alterations, and reviewing therapeutic and prophylactic drug regimens comprise other important components of effective medical management.

Interventions

Prevention

Early and ongoing nutritional assessment and counseling are essential if body wasting is to be prevented or minimized. A nutritional checklist (Figure 10.1) can be completed every 3 to 6 months by individuals with HIV infection to determine or monitor their nutritional risk. Persons at moderate nutritional risk (a score of 3 to 5) are referred to appropriate health care professionals and social agencies for preventive interventions (e.g., home meal delivery, assistance with shopping or cooking). High-risk persons (a score of 6 or more) require a thorough nutritional assessment.

Nutrition counseling should educate clients about the relationship between nutrition and HIV infection, the importance of maintaining adequate nutrient intake and reserve body weight (especially in clients who prefer to be thin), use of multivitamin and mineral preparations, food safety considerations, food misinformation, and available nutritional support options. Nutritional information is available from a variety of sources, including the American Dietetic Association (ADA), local health departments, the Food and Drug Administration (FDA), and nutritional or pharmaceutical companies. Selected examples of these resources are listed below.

The warning signs leading to poor nutritional health are often overlooked. Use this checklist to find out if you or someone you know is at nutritional risk.

Read the statements below. Circle the number in the column if the statement applies to you or someone you know. total your nutritional score.

• Without wanting to, I have lost 5 or more pounds over the last 2 months or 10 pounds or more over the last 6 months.	3
• I have 3 or more bowel movements per day that are significantly different from my usual bowel habits.	3
• I have had 2 or more unscheduled visits to my health care professional over the last 2 months due to HIV-related problems.	3
• I eat fewer than 2 meals per day.	3
• I take 3 or more different prescribed or over-the-counter medications a day.	1
• I have had a persistent fever and/or infection for 1 week or more.	3
• I am not always able to buy food, cook, or feed myself.	3
• I take 3 or more vitamin, mineral, and/or herb supplements a day.	1
• I have 3 or more drinks of beer, liquor, or wine almost every day.	2
• I eat very few fruits, vegetables, or milk products.	2
• I have limited food intake due to Nausea and/or vomiting Food aversions Chewing and/or swallowing difficulties	 2 1 2
Total	

Total your nutritional score.

If it's . . .

0-2 **Good!** Recheck your nutritional score in 3 months.

3-5 **You are at moderate risk.** Talk with your doctor, dietitian, or other health care professional to see what can be done to improve your eating habits.

6+ **You may be at high nutritional risk.** Show this checklist to your doctor, dietitian, or other qualified health professional. You may want to use a nutritionally complete supplement that is specifically designed to help provide effective nutritional management for people with HIV or AIDS.

Figure 10.1 HIV/AIDS Nutritional Checklist (From Cameron A. ed. Is nutrition important? *In Focus.* 1995;2(4):2. Reprinted with permission.)

Nutritional Information/Resources

- *Living Well with HIV and AIDS: A Guide to Healthy Eating*
  American Dietetic Association
  216 W. Jackson Boulevard
  Chicago, IL 60606-6995
  800-366-1655
- *Foodborne Illness in the Home: How and Why What You Eat Can Make You Sick*
  American Dietetic Association
  216 W. Jackson Boulevard
  Chicago, IL 60606-6995
  800-366-1655
- *Fight Back with Good Nutrition*
  Mead Johnson Nutritional Group
  2400 W. Lloyd Expressway
  Evansville, IN 47721
  800-247-7893
- *Nutrition and HIV: Practical Dietary Guidelines for People with HIV Infection or AIDS*
  Ross Products Division
  625 Cleveland Avenue
  Columbus, OH 43215-1724
  800-544-7495
- *HIV Disease Nutrition Guidelines: Practical Steps for a Healthier Life*
  Physicians' Association for AIDS Care
  101 W. Grant Avenue, Suite 200
  Chicago, IL 60610
  312-222-1326
- *Nutrition Guidebook for People Living with HIV/AIDS*
  Clintec Nutrition Company
  Three Parkway North, Suite 500
  PO Box 760
  Deerfield, IL 60015-0760
  847-317-2800

Management

ACUTE. Because short-term weight loss is related to reduced food intake, interventions during acute episodes should focus on providing adequate nutrients through oral, enteral, or parenteral routes. To maintain protein status, 1.0 to 1.4 g of protein per kilogram of body weight should be provided, while 1.5 to 2.0 g of protein per kilogram of body weight should be used for repletion of protein status. Acutely ill and febrile HIV patients generally have a total calorie need of 30 to 35 kcal/kg/day.[23] Meeting protein and calorie needs through oral intake is the preferred method for managing acute wasting. A daily multivitamin/mineral supplement that supplies 100% of the recommended daily allowance (RDA) is also recommended. When patients cannot consume enough protein and calories from food, oral high-calorie and high-protein supplements and snacks should be incorporated into the nutritional plan. Enteral nutrition should be considered when patients are unable to maintain adequate oral intake and the GI system is intact. Special formulas (e.g., contain peptides or medium chain triglycerides, or are low residue or low lactose) are available for patients with malabsorption, and special tubes (e.g., percutaneous endoscopic gastrostomy or jejunostomy) can be placed if esophageal lesions or aspiration are a problem. Indications for parenteral nutrition are intractable diarrhea and a nonfunctioning GI tract. If the duration of nutritional support is anticipated to be less than 7 to 10 days, the peripheral venous route should be used. Often, nutrition support involves a combination of the oral, enteral, and parenteral routes.[24-26]

CHRONIC. For chronic wasting, management focuses on early identification and treatment of factors that reduce energy intake or increase nutrient losses, especially anorexia, nausea and vomiting, and diarrhea. Strategies that can be used to offset reduced food intake and increased nutrient losses include small, frequent meals; nutrient-dense foods; convenience foods; calorie counts; and nutrition intake and symptom records. The following list gives the specific information for the patient.[24,25]

Patient Information: Wasting

- Eat a meal or snack every 1 or 2 hours.
- Make every bite count. Eat foods that are high in protein and calories, such as pizza, milkshakes, pudding, and peanut butter.

- Add protein and calories to foods by putting hard-boiled eggs, grated cheese, butter, cream, or chopped meat in vegetables, soups, casseroles, or salads.
- Make "double-strength milk" by adding 1 c powdered milk to 1 qt regular milk. Use double-strength milk in recipes or for making milk shakes. Add 4 to 6 tbls of powdered milk to hot cereals, soups, gravies, hamburger, casseroles, and cake and cookie recipes.
- Avoid eating foods that have few or no calories. Drink regular sodas, punch, or fruit juices instead of water, tea, coffee, and diet sodas. Use ice cubes made from juice or soda so that drinks are not watered down.
- Eat fruit canned in heavy syrup and munch on vegetables or fruit dipped in peanut butter, yogurt, or salad dressing.
- Check with your nurse, dietitian, or doctor about taking a vitamin and mineral supplement.
- Have family, friends, or volunteers help you with shopping and cooking.
- Order from take-out and delivery restaurants. Keep easy-to-prepare and convenience foods on hand.
- Try to walk or exercise a little before meals to improve appetite and muscle strength.
- Try drinking a nutritional supplement before going to sleep, or if you wake up during the night.
- Weigh yourself two times a week and keep a record of it.
- Tell your nurse or doctor if you are losing weight or if you are not able to eat enough.

Appetite stimulants, antiemetics, and antidiarrheal medications are recommended for patients in whom severe anorexia, nausea and vomiting, or diarrhea are the major underlying causes of wasting (see specific sections for details). Other pharmacologic agents such as anticytokines (e.g., fish oil, pentoxifylline), metabolic inhibitors (e.g., thalidomide), antioxidants (e.g., vitamins A and C), growth hormone (e.g., somatropin), and androgen therapy (e.g., testosterone, oxandrolone) may halt wasting for a period of weeks or months, but their long-term effects need to be clarified with further research.[27] Growth hormone and androgen therapy in particular are extremely expensive (several thousand dollars per month), limiting access for many HIV-infected patients. Another promising area of research indicates that exercise, in conjunction with nutrition and pharmacologic intervention, may promote weight gain and lean body mass retention.[28]

In end-stage AIDS, food and fluids should be provided as desired by the patient. Food and fluid administration can increase secretions, choking, aspiration, vomiting, and diarrhea, thus causing increased discomfort.[29]

Anorexia

Anorexia is often underestimated as an important cause of reduced food intake. It is considered to be a major factor in the involuntary weight loss associated with HIV infection.[17,30] Because of the many etiologies of anorexia, it is an especially challenging symptom for patients and caregivers to manage.

Definition

Anorexia is defined as a loss of desire to eat or a loss of appetite associated with a decrease in food intake.[31]

Biologic and Behavioral Basis

Normally, food intake is regulated by the interaction of two hypothalamic areas—the lateral "feeding center" and the medial "satiety center."[32] In HIV disease a constellation of biologic and behavioral factors can act singly or in concert to inhibit the feeding center or stimulate the satiety center. GI factors, endocrine disorders, nutrient deficiencies, cytokines, metabolic abnormalities, and medications are common biologic causes of anorexia. Behavioral cases include anxiety and depression. Fear of eating because of associated pain or diarrhea (sitophobia) and CNS disorders are other causes of anorexia and/or decreased intake.

Etiologies Related to HIV Infection and Its Medical Treatment

GI factors such as infections and malignancies can influence appetite and food intake significantly. A classic example is oral thrush, which causes pain, taste changes, and nausea and vomiting. Endocrine abnormalities are also thought to have an important influence on appetite. Documented endocrine abnormalities include adrenal insufficiency due to CMV adrenalitis; reduced secretion of GI hormones, testosterone, growth hormone, and insulinlike growth factors; and thyroid dysfunction.[33] These abnormalities may either affect the appetite directly or indirectly as a result of signs and symptoms of adrenocortical insufficiency, such as fatigue and nausea and vomiting. Specific nutrient deficiencies can have a major impact on anorexia as well.[4,34] Vitamin A and B6 deficiencies result in anorexia and decreased food intake; and a zinc deficiency decreases taste and smell, ultimately causing anorexia and reduced intake. Further, the levels of several intermediate metabolites such as peptides and lactic acid, and cytokines such as IL-1 and TNF are abnormal in HIV infection.[11,35] Their major impact is thought to be on appetite.

Most of the medications used to treat HIV and related OIs are anorexigenic.[14,15] For example, IV pentamidine prophylaxis for *Pneumocystis carinii* pneumonia can result in coughing, which in turn leads to gagging and a reduced desire to eat. In addition, HIV-related diseases, such as *P. carinii* pneumonia itself, can cause anorexia; and the oxygen therapy used to manage it heightens the anorexia by producing dry mouth and taste changes. Since it is not uncommon for patients in the later stages of HIV disease to be taking 20 to 40 pills per day, polypharmacy also can be a major cause of anorexia.

Appetite and food intake can be compromised by a number of other factors. Depression or anxiety related to HIV diagnosis or treatment can significantly reduce intake, as can a variety of socioeconomic factors, such as financial and employment concerns, social isolation, and substance abuse. Fear of eating (sitophobia) because of associated discomfort is another factor to be considered. With sitophobia, appetite may be normal, but food intake is curtailed to prevent unpleasant side effects, such as severe pain or diarrhea with eating. Similarly, CNS disorders such as ADC may limit intake despite a normal appetite.

Presentation and Assessment

Subjective and Objective

In evaluating anorexia it is important to assess for its various biologic and behavioral causes, as discussed. Subjective assessment should include a review of medications and nutritional, physiological, and psychosocial factors that may contribute to anorexia. Objective assessment should focus on clinical recording of weight loss, fat and muscle mass wasting, physical weakness, and psychological dysfunction, such as inappropriate effect or appearance.

Subjective Data
- Nutrition
  - When did anorexia start?
  - What causes the anorexia?
  - Is the anorexia associated with other symptoms such as pain, stomatitis, dysphagia, nausea and vomiting, taste changes, diarrhea?
  - What makes the anorexia worse? What helps?
  - Does anorexia interfere with eating?
  - How much?
  - Any associated weight loss?
  - Any food intolerances?
  - Able to force eating?
  - Fear of eating?
- Medications
  - Use of medications associated with anorexia?
  - Recent change in medication or new medications?
  - Use of multiple medications?
- General history
  - Depression? Anxiety?
  - Financial or employment concerns?
  - Social isolation?
  - Substance abuse?
  - Recent surgery, radiation, or chemotherapy?
  - Recent or current infections or malignancies?
  - Loss of functional ability? Fatigue?

Related Medical Management

Identifying and treating the causes of anorexia is the primary goal of medical management. When a biologic cause, such as infection, cannot be determined, referrals to a psychologist and/or social worker may help to pinpoint the underlying causes.

Interventions

Prevention

A record that tracks weight, food intake, and appetite is an important approach for preventing or minimizing anorexia. The form illustrated in Figure 10.2 is an example of an easy-to-use record that can be individualized

Date: ________________, _____ Weight: ________

TIME	MEAL	TYPE AND AMOUNT OF FOOD EATEN
	Breakfast	
	Snack	
	Lunch	
	Snack	
	Dinner	
	Snack	

APPETITE

1 2 3 4 5 6 7 8 9 10

Poor or Not Hungry at All — Good or Hungry — Excellent or Extremely Hungry

COMMENTS:

Figure 10.2 Food, Weight, and Appetite Record

by adding space for comments, medications, exercise, or other pertinent factors. It can be completed at each meal time or once a day at the end of the day. Patients should be encouraged to keep such a record even before weight loss occurs and to review it with their health care provider on a monthly basis to detect any changes. To reduce the anorexigenic effects of medications, changing the dose of medications, shifting medications, or prescribing short drug holidays is often beneficial.[14]

Management

ACUTE. A team approach consisting of a physician, pharmacist, nurse, dietitian, dentist, psychologist, and social worker can facilitate prompt detection and immediate treatment of acute episodes of anorexia. Infections, medications, oral problems, and socioeconomic concerns are the most frequent causes of short-term anorexia.

CHRONIC. Nutrition interventions, such as nutrition counseling and oral supplementation, are important ways to combat chronic anorexia. Counseling should include the importance of eating foods high in protein and calories, having a meal or snack every 1 to 2 hours, using nutrient-dense convenience foods, avoiding low-calorie and low-fat foods, eating in pleasant surroundings, taking appetite stimulants as prescribed, walking or exercising lightly before eating, and maintaining good dental health. When nutrient intake is inadequate, oral supplements can be used to supplement or replace dietary intake. The following provides instructions for the anorexic patient.[24,25]

Patient Information: Anorexia

- Eat small snacks and meals every 2 to 3 hours, rather than three large meals. Eat more food in the morning when appetite is best.
- Eat high-calorie, high-protein foods and snacks such as peanut butter, cheese, cottage cheese, whole milk, pudding, ice cream, candy bars, jelly, eggs, chips, nuts, and dried fruit. Avoid eating low-fat foods and using sugar substitutes.
- Drink high-calorie beverages—milk shakes, ice cream sodas or liquid supplements—rather than water, low-calorie soft drinks, tea, or coffee.
- Take your medicines with juices, chocolate milk, or instant breakfast drinks instead of water unless your doctor or nurse advises you otherwise.
- Eat cold or lukewarm foods if they have a better flavor than hot foods.
- Try drinking a small glass of wine or fruit juice before meals to improve your appetite. Do not drink liquids with meals if they fill you up. Drink liquids 1 hour before or after a meal.

- If fatigue or time is a problem, use prepared foods, frozen meals, or take-out or home-delivered foods. Keep a supply of ready-to-eat snacks on hand, such as trail mix, yogurt, or pudding cups.
- Take medicines for appetite or nausea 30 to 60 minutes before eating.
- Go for a walk or exercise lightly before eating to help stimulate appetite.
- Eat your favorite foods, and eat with other people in a pleasant, relaxed atmosphere to help improve your appetite.
- Tell your doctor or nurse if you notice any changes in your appetite or in the amount of food you eat that last more than 3 to 4 days.
- Let your doctor or nurse know if psychological or socioeconomic concerns are causing problems with eating. Examples are feeling depressed or not having enough money to buy food.

A variety of oral supplements specifically designed for HIV patients with added amounts of vitamins, minerals, and other nutrients known to be deficient in HIV are now available. They are produced not only in a variety of flavors, but also as soups and candy bars to prevent boredom or taste fatigue so common with liquid supplements. Selected examples of these products are listed in the Table 10.2. If oral supplementation is ineffective, tube feedings can be initiated if the GI tract is functional.

As an adjunct to nutrition interventions, appetite stimulants may be prescribed. Megestrol acetate (Megace) and dronabinol (Marinol) are two appetite stimulants currently approved for use in HIV. Megace is a synthetic progesterone derivative that was originally used to treat breast cancer. It has been shown to improve both appetite and weight gain, but the weight gain is mostly in the form of body fat rather than muscle mass.[30] Significant side effects include hypogonadism, muscle wasting, and lack of erection capability in men. These side effects are thought to be due to the inhibitory action of Megace on total testosterone secretion.[30,36] This might also explain why fat is gained and lean body mass is lost during Megace therapy. The use of exogenous testosterone, in the form of scrotal patches, is currently being trialed as a way to counter these effects.[37] Megace is available in 20-mg and 40-mg tablets and in liquid elixir form. Because up to 160 mg four times a day may be necessary, the liquid form (40 mg/ml) may be easier to take.

Dronabinol (Marinol), a synthetic derivative of marijuana, is also re-

Table 10.2 Selected Oral Nutritional Supplements for HIV/AIDS

Category			Polymeric Formulas		Elemental Formulas		Modular Nutrients		
Product	Advera	Impact	ImmunAid	Lipisorb	Peptamen	VIVONEX TEN	POLYCOSE Liquid	PROMOD	MICRO-LIPID
Calories/ml	1.28	1.0	1.0	1.35	1.0	1.0	2.0	42/10 g powder	4.5
Carbohydrate source (g/l)	Hydrolyzed cornstarch, sucrose, and soy polysaccharide (215.8)	Hydrolyzed cornstarch (130)	Maltodextrin (120)	Maltodextrin and sucrose (161)	Maltodextrin and starch (127)	Maltodextrin (206)	Hydrolyzed cornstarch (500)	1 g/10 g	0
Protein source (g/l)	Sodium caseinate, soy protein hydrolysate (60)	Sodium and calcium caseinates, L-arginine (56)	Intact lactalbumin and amino acids (80)	Sodium and calcium caseinate (57)	Partially hydrolyzed whey protein (40)	Free amino acids including glutamine and enriched with BCAAs (38.2)	—	Whey protein with lecithin (7.5 g/10 g)	0
Fat source (g/l)	MCT and oil (22.8)	Palm kernal and sunflower oil, menhad oil (28)	Canola and MCT oil (22)	MCT oil and sunflower oil (57)	MCT oil and sunflower oil (39)	Safflower oil (2.8)	—	1 g/10 g	Safflower oil; 50 g/100 ml
mOsm/kg	680	375	460	270	270	630	—	—	—
Sodium (mEq/l)	1,056	48	25.2	58.7	22	20	30	0.99	0
Potassium (mEq/l)	72.5	36	27.1	43.3	32	20	1.5	2.51	0

Vitamins (volume to meet 100% RDA; ml)	1,184	1,500	2,000	1,200	1,500	2,000	—	—	—
Caloric distribution (% CHO, PRO, FAT)	CHO: 65.5 PRO: 18.7 FAT: 15.8	CHO: 53 PRO: 22 FAT: 25	CHO: 48 PRO: 32 FAT: 20	CHO: 48 PRO: 17 FAT: 35	CHO: 51 PRO: 16 FAT: 33	CHO: 82.2 PRO: 15.3 FAT: 2.5	—	—	—
General characteristics	Lactose free, low fat, contains specialized peptides for easier absorption	Lactose free, provides arginine, fish oil, and RNA	Lactose free, powder that is reconstituted	Lactose free, available in powder and prepared forms	Contains small peptides and medium-chain triglycerides; requires minimal digestion	Low fat, elemental, used for impaired digestion or absorption	Carbohydrate source	Powdered protein source; add 100 cc water to 10 g powder when adding to concentrated formulas	Fat source

BCAA = branched chain amino acid; MCT = medium chain triglyceride; mOsm = milliosmoles; RDA = recommended dietary allowance; CHO = carbohydrate; PRO = protein; RNA = ribonucleic acid.

ported to increase appetite and weight gain in HIV infection.[38] Marinol is typically prescribed in 2.5-mg capsules taken twice a day, with the first dose taken 1 hour before lunch and the second dose taken 1 hour before dinner. In the absence of adverse effects and when further therapeutic effects are desired, the dinner dose can be increased to 5 mg. Patients should be taught that alcohol and drugs affecting the CNS (e.g., sedatives and hypnotics) can adversely interact with Marinol and are therefore contraindicated when Marinol is prescribed. Also, smoking marijuana while taking Marinol should be avoided because it can result in an overdose. Some of the side effects associated with Marinol are euphoria, hallucinations, tachycardia, palpitations, vasodilation, and exacerbation of depression and/or emotional instability. These side effects can be minimized by taking low doses (2.5–5 mg) of Marinol at bedtime, but then the positive effects on appetite are not as pronounced. Other medications used for appetite stimulation include prednisone, methylprednisolone, dexamethasone, cyproheptadine, and thalidomide.[39]

Oral/Esophageal Symptoms

The oral and esophageal portions of the GI tract are often sites of the initial symptoms of HIV infection. Common GI symptoms include dysphagia and odynophagia, mucositis (stomatitis, pharyngitis, and esophagitis), xerostomia, and taste changes. All of these symptoms can be significant sources of discomfort, anxiety, decreased quality of life, and reduced oral intake.

Definitions

Dysphagia is defined as difficulty swallowing and is often described as the sensation of "sticking" of food in the mouth, pharynx, or esophagus. *Odynophagia* refers to painful swallowing, which is usually characterized as having a burning or constricting quality. *Mucositis*, or inflammation of the mucous membranes, can affect the mouth (*stomatitis*), pharynx (*pharyngitis*), and esophagus (*esophagitis*) as well as other sites along the GI tract. *Xerostomia* denotes dryness of the mouth or a lack of saliva. Taste changes include *ageusia* (absence of sense of taste), *hypogeusia* (diminished taste sensitivity), and *dysgeusia* (disturbed sense of taste).[32]

Biologic and Behavioral Basis

A variety of neuromuscular and inflammatory conditions can alter normal oral, pharyngeal, and esophageal function, placing patients at significant nutritional risk. With difficult or painful swallowing, at least one of the four stages of swallowing is impaired: (1) *predeglutition,* in which food is broken down by chewing and saliva and is formed into a bolus on the anterior tongue; (2) *buccal pharyngeal,* in which the tongue pushes the bolus of food to the posterior pharynx; (3) *pharyngeal,* in which the soft palate closes off and seals the nasal passages, allowing the bolus to slide into the esophagus; and (4) *esophageal,* in which food passes through the esophageal sphincter and into the stomach as a result of peristalsis. Both voluntary and reflexive actions are involved in normal swallowing. The "swallowing center" is located in the brainstem and is made up of cranial nerves V, VII, IX, X, and XII. It can be triggered by either cortical influences or peripheral sensory stimuli.[32]

The oral mucosa keeps the mouth hydrated, aids in digestion, and provides a mechanical and chemical barrier to trauma and infectious organisms. The oral/esophageal mucosa is made up of multiple layers, namely the epithelial, lamina propria, and submucosal layers. The mucosal lining of the GI tract provides an important protective barrier against microorganisms. When any of these layers is damaged, pathogens can enter or exit the mucosa, causing regional or systemic infection and inflammation.[40]

In the oral cavity, the mucous membranes are protected and kept moist by saliva. Salivary secretion is under parasympathetic and sympathetic neural control. Most or about 70% of saliva is secreted by the submandibular and sublingual glands; the remaining 30% is secreted by the parotid glands. Saliva contains bactericidal, fungicidal, and viracidal agents (e.g., immunoglobulins, peroxidase); digestive enzymes (i.e., lipase, amylase); and mucins.[41] Saliva production is controlled by the salivatory nuclei located in the brainstem, which are regulated by certain tastes, odors, and tactile sensations. Excessive salivation may be associated with nausea since the salivatory nuclei and vomiting center are in close proximity in the brain.[32] Saliva limits microbial flora in the mouth and facilitates chewing and swallowing by moistening food. When saliva production is reduced by 50% or more,[42] these protective and functional properties are lost.

Similarly, taste can be affected by changes in oral integrity. The taste buds are located in the epithelial mucosa of the epiglottis, palate, pharynx, and fungiform and vallate papillae of the tongue. The round fungiform papillae are located near the tip of the tongue and contain as many as five taste buds per papilla, whereas the larger vallate papillae are arranged in a V shape on the back of the tongue and contain as many as 100 taste buds per papilla. The small conical filiform papillae that cover the dorsum of the tongue generally do not contain taste buds. The taste receptors, which are located in the taste buds, are activated and innervated by afferent nerve fibers in the lingual branch of the glossopharyngeal nerve. In all, there are about 10,000 taste buds. Sweet substances are tasted at the tip of the tongue, sour along the edges, bitter at the back, and salty just behind the tip of the tongue.[32] When taste buds are temporarily or permanently affected, significant taste changes can occur.

Etiologies Related to HIV Infection and Its Medical Treatment

Dysphagia is usually caused by *Candida* infection, while odynophagia is caused by CMV and HSV infections.[43] The initial site for these infections is the oral cavity.[44] Later, as the disease progresses and immunologic function declines, infections develop in or extend to the pharyngeal and esophageal areas. Up to 75% of patients with HIV develop candidiasis. Estimates of the prevalence of CMV infection in HIV range from 40 to 60%.[45] Chronic, persistent HSV is an AIDS-indicating condition.[13] *Candida*, CMV, and HSV infections cause ulcerations and inflammation, resulting in pain and luminal narrowing. In healthy adults, the esophageal lumen can distend to a diameter of 4 cm or more. When inflammatory conditions prevent the esophagus from dilating to more than 2.5 cm in diameter, dysphagia can occur. Dysphagia is always present when the esophageal diameter cannot distend beyond 1.3 cm.[46] Other potential causes of dysphagia and odynophagia include neuromuscular changes from CMV encephalitis or fatigue; medications, such as ddC; radiation-induced stomatitis and glossitis; other oral infections or malignancies such as KS, lymphoma, or HIV-associated aphthous lesions; xerostomia; dehydration; and gingivitis and periodontitis.[15]

In HIV/AIDS, stomatitis is most often due to secondary infections, such as candidiasis and HSV; side effects of medications, such as trimethoprim-sulfamethoxazole; or reaction to local radiation therapy.[47] These factors result in inflammation of the oral mucosa and, in severe cases, reduced ability of the oral mucosa to repair or replace damaged tissue. Pain, difficulty eating, and increased risk of local and systemic infection are among the adverse outcomes of stomatitis. Other causes of stomatitis are periodontal diseases and nutritional deficiencies, especially vitamins B and C, which cause alterations in lip (cheilosis) and oral mucosa (scurvy).[45]

Xerostomia may be temporary or permanent. Among the temporary causes are medication side effects, such as from the administration of atropine, antihistamines, tricyclic antidepressants, or phenothiazines; infection or destruction of the salivary glands by CMV, HSV, or oral malignancies; dehydration; and emotional factors such as fear. Local radiation to the head and neck area may produce a more permanent xerostomia due to destruction of the salivary glands.[43-45,47] Dryness of the mouth or lack of saliva alters taste; impairs swallowing; causes dental caries; reduces the immune properties of saliva; and increases the risk of bacterial, fungal, and viral invasion. Taste changes are usually the result of oral infections, medications, and radiation therapy. By coating the taste buds, oral infections such as candidiasis and oral hairy leukoplakia interfere with normal taste perception. Patients with oral candidiasis also often report that everything tastes salty.[48] Medications are linked to a variety of taste changes. Trimethoprim-sulfamethoxazole, acyclovir, and pentamidine are associated with bitter or metallic tastes, as well as lack of taste altogether.[49] Zidovudine is associated with an overly sweet taste to foods. Radiation therapy to the head and neck area may cause local destruction of the taste buds, altering taste receptivity. Frequent use of alcohol and tobacco products, xerostomia, gingivitis, periodontitis, and certain nutritional deficiencies such as zinc may also contribute to taste changes by interfering with normal taste receptor function.[15,16,23,43,45]

Presentation and Assessment

Patients with oral/esophageal symptoms present with general complaints of anorexia, inability to eat, and weight loss. Complaints specific to each symptom are also part of the presentation. Dysphagia and odynophagia are accompanied by difficulty swallowing and epigastric and substernal pain, and sometimes dry mouth or dehydration. Mouth pain and lesions, and difficulty chewing are the major symptoms associated with oral mucositis. Xerostomia is accompanied by dry mouth, difficulty chewing and swallowing, and taste changes. Patients with taste changes may have a dry or painful mouth, and may complain of food aversions and intolerances. The nursing assessment of oral symptoms is listed below.

Subjective Data

- Any changes in appetite, taste, smell, chewing, or swallowing ability? What is the change? When did you first notice the change? What types of foods are problematic? Is choking or regurgitation a problem?
- Any change in weight over the past 6 months? How much did you lose or gain? Over what period of time? Reason for weight change?
- Recent surgery or radiation treatments in the head and neck area? What type? When did this occur? Did this cause any changes in food intake?
- Any food allergies, intolerances, or unpleasant tastes? What are they? When did this occur?
- Presence of mouth, throat, epigastric, or substernal pain? How long? Severity of pain? What makes the pain better or worse?
- Any new medications? What types? How much? For how long?
- Use of alcohol or tobacco products? How much? How often?
- Dental caries, periodontal disease, oral lesions, or dry mouth? How long? How managed? Date of last dental exam?
- Recent activities or stress that caused oral trauma or infection? Which ones or what kind? Hard, hot, spicy, or acidic foods? Poorly fitting dentures? Oral sex? Other?
- Inadequate fluid intake or excessive losses? Reason for this? How long?

Objective Data

- Use a penlight and tongue blade to visualize all areas of the mouth, including the lips, teeth, tongue, mucous membranes, hard and soft palate, and oropharynx.
- Check for the presence of ulcerated lesions, white patches and plaques, nodules on the hard palate, loose teeth, inflammed gums, excessive or lack of saliva, and alterations in the appearance of taste buds and Stensen's (parotid gland opening) and Wharton's (submandibular gland opening) ducts. Palpate the parotid, sublingual, and submandibular glands for tenderness and enlargement.

The clinical manifestations of the most common HIV-related oral/esophageal infections and malignancies are presented in Table 10.3. Because the clinical features of oral infections, nutritional deficiencies, and poor oral hygiene may be similar or occur concurrently, definitive differential diagno-

Table 10.3 Common HIV-Related Infections and Malignancies of the Oral/Esophageal Area

Infection/Malignancy	Clinical Manifestation
Candidiasis	Creamy white curdlike patches on the mucous membranes that, if scraped, reveal a raw bleeding surface
Kaposi's sarcoma	Purplish pink, flat macular lesions that progress to purplish brown plaques or nodules; most often located on the palate
Oral hairy leukoplakia	White villiform or "hairy" areas on the lateral surfaces of the tongue; can occur concurrently with candidiasis, but cannot be rubbed off like candidiasis
Herpes simplex virus	Single or clustered vesicles that progress to ulcerated, crested lesions; usually painful and causes inflammation and bleeding
Cytomegalovirus	Large, shallow, superficial ulcers
HIV-associated aphthous ulcers	Painful, shallow pseudomembrane-covered ulcers surrounded by a ring of erythema; usually located on soft palate

sis is made by culture or biopsy and histologic examination. Keep in mind that oral/esophageal lesions may be indicative of other lesions lower in the GI tract.

Related Medical/Dental Management

Physicians and dentists work collaboratively to evaluate and treat oral/esophageal problems. Lesions are evaluated by oral and endoscopic cultures and biopsies, and are treated with topical or systemic medications. Oral/esophageal malignancies may require surgical or laser excision followed by radiation therapy and/or chemotherapy. Associated dental and periodontal problems are treated aggressively.

Interventions

Prevention

Good oral hygiene, regular dental care, preventive nutritional counseling, and other health maintenance strategies can help to prevent some of the problems associated with oral/esophageal symptoms. Oral hygiene should be performed after each meal and before bedtime. To avoid trauma to the mucous membranes, a soft toothbrush and toothpaste for sensitive gums and mucosa should be used, and teeth should be carefully flossed. WaterPiks and electric toothbrushes may be too abrasive and should be used cautiously. Normal saline or saline and bicarbonate mouthwashes are preferred because many commercial mouthwashes contain alcohol, glycerin, or phenol, which can be irritating or drying. Hydrogen peroxide solutions are also contraindicated since they can impair tissue healing. When salivary flow is decreased, the use of topical fluoride rinses or gel to prevent caries is advisable.[41,42,45] Patients should be taught to perform objective daily oral assessments (as listed earlier) and to keep dental and teeth-cleaning appointments at least every 6 months. Preventive nutritional counseling focuses on avoiding foods or products that can irritate or traumatize mucous membranes, such as pretzels, chips, tobacco, and alcohol; keeping the oral cavity moist by eating foods with a high moisture content or sipping beverages throughout the day; and maximizing taste bud function by eating highly seasoned foods and citrus fruits or juices.[25] Strategies to avoid or minimize trauma during oral sex should also be reviewed, including the use of soft protective barriers and not brushing or flossing teeth before oral sexual activity to reduce risk of infection through irritated tissue.[45]

Management

ACUTE. Because many acute episodes of oral/esophageal symptoms have an infectious origin, pharmacological therapy is the mainstay of management. Teaching patients how to maximize the therapeutic effects of prescribed medications and to minimize side effects will ensure optimum outcomes (Table 10.4). Certain medications and radiation therapy may cause acute flare-ups, but their adverse effects are usually managed on a more chronic basis.

When acute manifestations of oral symptoms make nutritional intake difficult or impossible, patients should be fed through an enteral tube. This approach reduces the risk of further trauma, bleeding, and pain, as well as aspiration.

CHRONIC. Nutritional recommendations for chronic oral/esophageal symptoms generally emphasize high-calorie, high-protein soft foods, liq-

Table 10.4 Pharmacological Management of Common Oral Infections[a]

Infection	Management	Comments
A. FUNGAL		
Oral candidiasis	Clotrimazole (Mycelex) troches dissolved in the mouth five times/day for 2 weeks or until plaques clear *or* nystatin oral suspension "swish and swallow," 4 to 6-ml swish retained in mouth for as long as possible, then swallowed, qid until 48 hours after symptoms have resolved	Teach patients to rinse their mouth of all foods before using lozenges or suspensions. For refractory cases, administer ketoconazole 200-mg tablets qid until infection clears (1–2 weeks). Instruct patients to take ketoconazole with orange juice or other acidic juices and not with food.
Esophageal candidiasis	Ketoconazole 200-mg tablets bid until symptoms resolve (7–10 days) *or* fluconazole 200-mg tablets qd until symptoms resolve	Fluconazole is more expensive than ketoconazole and should be used only when ketoconazole is ineffective. Intravenous (IV) amphotericin or IV fluconazole is used in patients unresponsive to oral therapy.
B. VIRAL		
Herpes simplex	Acyclovir 200-mg tablets five times a day until ulcers heal	For chronic therapy, acyclovir 200-mg tablets one to three times daily is used.
Cytomegalovirus	Ganciclovir 5 mg/kg IV q12h for 14 to 21 days	Foscarnet is used for breakthrough infection.

[a]Data culled from various sources.[48,50–52]

uids, shakes, or supplements. These foods are easier to swallow and less irritating to inflammed and painful oral lesions. Patients with taste changes usually find that highly seasoned or strongly flavored foods (e.g., chili, tacos) are better tolerated. Sometimes very sweet foods (e.g., ice cream, cookies) can combat unpleasant tastes.[49] Specific nutritional strategies for each oral/esophageal symptom are covered in the following lists.[24,25]

Patient Information: Difficulty Swallowing

- Eat soft foods such as stews, soups, canned fruits, or foods prepared in a blender. Cut or chop up foods into smaller pieces so they are easier to swallow.
- Add sauces or gravies to meats and vegetables to make them easier to swallow.
- Make hard foods softer by dipping them in liquids like coffee for bagels or milk for cookies.
- Thick liquids are usually easier to swallow than thin liquids. You can make liquids thicker by adding milk, cream, gravy, mashed potatoes, oatmeal, or Thickit.
- Eat foods that are cold or lukewarm. They are usually easier to swallow than hot or warm foods.
- Avoid sticky foods like peanut butter or carmels.
- Avoid milk if it makes you choke or gag.
- Try tilting your head back to make it easier to swallow.
- Let your doctor or nurse know which foods are hard to swallow or if you are having trouble swallowing pills.

Patient Information: Mouth Sores or Mouth Pain

- Eat soft foods, such as casseroles, noodle dishes, yogurt, soups, custards, and milk shakes.
- Use a straw to drink beverages and soups.
- Cold foods, such as popsicles, Italian ices, ice cream, and frozen commercial nutritional supplements can be comforting to your mouth.
- Avoid hot or spicy foods or beverages that can burn or hurt your mouth. Also avoid hard foods, such as hard bread and chips, which can hurt the inside of your mouth.
- Avoid acidic foods like oranges, lemons, tomatoes, and pineapples. Try apple juice or milk instead.

- Before you eat, use the medicines for pain that your doctor or nurse told you to use.
- Use a soft toothbrush to brush your teeth.
- Avoid over-the-counter mouthwashes that contain alcohol or glycerin. Use a mild salt or baking soda mouthwash instead (1 tsp salt or baking soda in a glass of water).
- Try putting Kaopectate, Maalox, Mylanta, or Mouth-Kote on the place that hurts in your mouth.
- Tell your doctor or nurse where your mouth hurts, what causes it to hurt, how much it hurts, and what makes it feel better or worse.

Patient Information: Dry Mouth

- Add gravies or sauces to foods or dip food in coffee, tea, milk, or cocoa.
- Choose juicy or soft foods such as oranges, melon, fish, casseroles, pot pies, and soups; or tuna, chicken, or ham salad sandwiches.
- Steam or microwave foods to make them easier to chew and swallow.
- Drink small amounts of beverages with meals to make it easier to swallow.
- Sip on nonalcoholic drinks during the day to keep your mouth wet or carry a squirt bottle of water or juice with you.
- Try eating citrus fruits and drinks and pickled foods; they may stimulate the taste buds.
- To avoid dental caries, suck on sugar-free hard candies or ice chips, or chew sugar-free gum to keep your mouth moist.
- Use a saliva substitute, such as Oralube or Salivart as directed. Put lip balm or petroleum jelly on your lips.
- Use a humidifier or vaporizer to add moisture to the air.
- Take care of your mouth and teeth before and after you eat and before you go to bed.
- Check with your dentist about using a mouthwash that has fluoride in it to prevent dental caries.

Patient Information: Taste Changes

- Eat foods that smell and taste good to you.
- Try rinsing your mouth with carbonated water before eating if you have a bad taste in your mouth.

(continued)

- If meat tastes bad, try eating meat substitutes such as eggs, cheese, peanut butter, and beans. Try marinating meats to make them taste better.
- Try eating spicy foods, such as chili, tacos, and barbecued ribs.
- Try eating citrus fruits and drinks, and or pickled foods.
- Try new seasonings or spices, or add onions and garlic to foods.
- Let hot foods cool and cold foods warm up before you eat them to bring out food flavors.
- Suck on hard candies or eat cookies, ice cream, and other sweet foods if you have a bad taste in your mouth.
- Avoid smoking before meals since smoking makes foods have a bland taste.
- Wait 10 or 15 minutes after brushing your teeth before you eat. Most toothpastes contain products that can make it harder to taste food.
- Let your doctor or nurse know which foods taste bad or have an "off" flavor.

To reduce pain associated with oral symptoms, several soothing mouthwashes are available, including Xylocaine 2% viscous, Orabase, Dyclonine, and Tylenol with codeine elixir. Other strategies to reduce mouth pain include using Cetacaine or Hurricane spray or Oratect Gel 30 minutes before meals. Systemic pain medications such as oral or subcutaneous morphine or transdermal Duragesic given at regular intervals are also useful.[41,48,52]

Saliva production can be stimulated with saliva substitutes such as Oralube, Salivart, or Polyox, which tend to be expensive[41]; by sipping liquids or spraying the mouth with water; or by chewing sugarless gum or sucking on hard sugarless candy or popsicles. Other strategies to maximize mouth comfort include regular oral hygiene and dental care, avoiding hot or hard foods, avoiding carbonated beverages, avoiding alcohol and tobacco use, applying lip lubricants, and using a room humidifier. As with other nutrition-related changes, symptom assessment tools are helpful in evaluating changes (Figure 10.3 and Table 10.5).

not at all unpleasant	0	1	2	3	4	5	6	7	8	9	10	extremely unpleasant

Figure 10.3 Subjective Taste Change Assessment[49].

Table 10.5 Stomatitis Grading Scale[71]

Grade	Description
Mild	Erythema observable and the patient experiences burning or pain in the oral cavity
Moderate	Isolated ulcerations and/or white patches present on examination; patient experiences intraoral pain but is generally able to eat or drink
Severe	Confluent ulcerations with white patches covering >25% of the oral mucosa on examination; the patient is often unable to eat or drink

Nausea, Vomiting, and Retching

Definition

Nausea, vomiting, and retching usually occur together, but are separate phenomena that can occur independent of one another. As immensely unpleasant GI symptoms, they can significantly impair nutritional, and fluid and electrolyte status. *Nausea* is the subjective feeling of an imminent desire to vomit, usually referred to the throat or epigastrium. *Vomiting* is the forceful expulsion of gastric contents, and *retching* is the labored rhythmic respiratory activity that commonly precedes vomiting.[53]

Biologic and Behavioral Basis

Nausea often antecedes or accompanies vomiting. It is usually associated with diminished stomach, duodenum, and small-intestine motility. Following severe nausea, altered autonomic (especially parasympathetic) activity may be present, exemplified by skin pallor, increased perspiration and salivation, and hypotension and bradycardia.

Vomiting is due to a series of involuntary visceral and somatic motor events under the control of two distinct medullary centers: the vomiting center and chemoreceptor trigger zone (CTZ; Figure 10.4). The vomiting center, located in the medulla, receives direct emetic impulses via afferent stimulation of the vagus nerve and sympathetic nervous system or by increased intracranial pressure. It may also be stimulated indirectly by visceral receptors in the GI tract, kidneys, heart, and uterus. The CTZ, which is located on the floor of the fourth ventricle, can be activated by

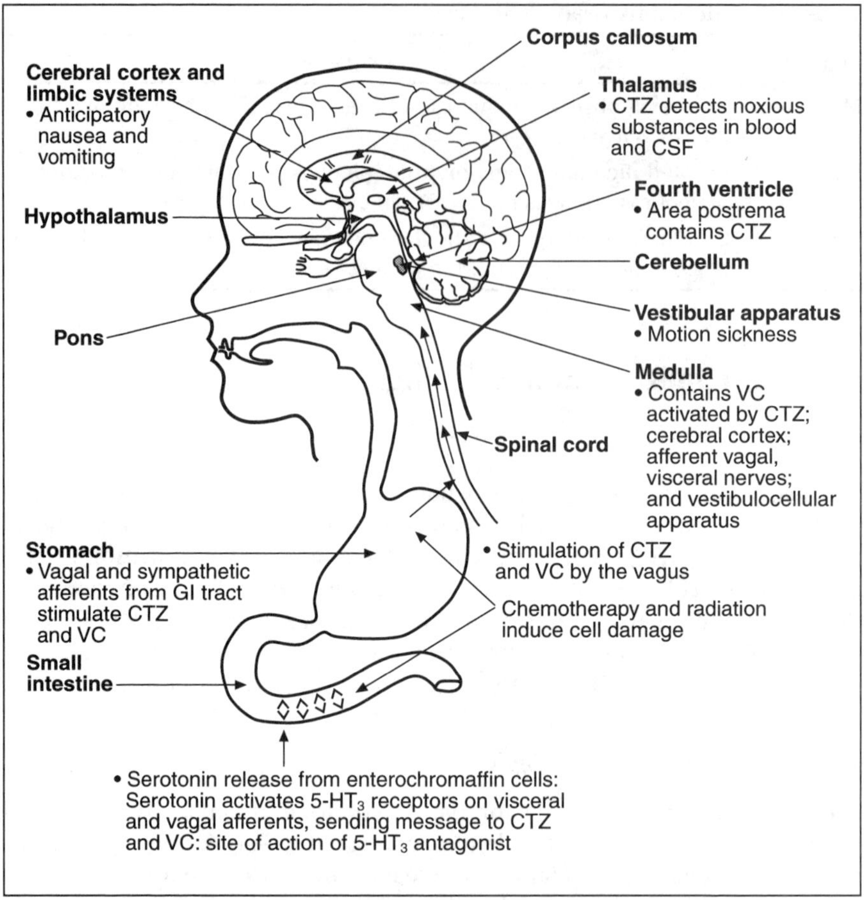

Figure 10.4 Nausea and Vomiting Pathways. CTZ = chemoreceptor trigger zone; VC = vomiting center; 5-HT_3 = 5-hydroxytryptaminek$_3$. (Groenwald, Frogge, Goodman, Yarboro: Cancer Nursing Principles and Practice, Third Edition © 1995 Boston: Jones and Bartlett Publishers. Reprinted with permission.)

vestibular stimuli associated with motion sickness, or by chemical stimuli associated with drugs or toxins. Most antiemetic drugs work in the CTZ by blocking receptors for neurochemicals, such as serotonin, acetylcholine, or dopamine. In addition, the cerebral cortex can cause nausea and vomiting by responding to emotions, stress, noxious odors, tastes, sights, and pain. Anticipatory nausea, vomiting, and retching are learned phenomena that can be triggered by association with unpleasant events or situations. Prolonged vomiting may lead to dehydration and loss of gastric secretions (especially hydrochloric acid), resulting in metabolic alkalosis with hypokalemia.[32]

Viral, bacterial, and parasitic infections of the intestinal tract may cause severe nausea and vomiting. Food intolerances such as fatty food can also provoke nausea and vomiting. The side effects of many drugs include nausea and vomiting. In some patients this is due to gastric irritation, which stimulates the medullary vomiting center.

Etiologies Related to HIV Infection and Its Medical Treatment

Nausea, vomiting, and retching in HIV disease are usually the result of medication side effects (especially amphotericin B, zidovudine, pentamidine, trimethoprim-sulfamethoxazole); OIs; GI neoplasms; radiation therapy; psychological factors (e.g., fear, anxiety); food intolerances; CNS disorders; pain; or noxious odors, sights, and tastes.[8,15,16,23]

Presentation and Assessment

The following list summarizes subjective and objective information that should be obtained from HIV-infected patients with nausea and vomiting.

Subjective

- Onset of nausea and vomiting?
- Intensity? Frequency? Duration?
- Precipitating factors such as medication, food intolerance, recent travel?
- Appearance and odor of vomitus?
- Amount of vomitus?

(continued)

- Any accompanying symptoms such as heartburn, abdominal pain, headache, diarrhea, constipation, or fever?
- Factors that aggravate or alleviate?
- What foods eaten in last 24 hours?
- Any partners, friends, family members with same symptoms in last 24 hours?
- Any projectile vomiting?
- Effect on functioning?

Objective
- Weight loss, including amount and time period?
- Changes in vital signs?
- Altered serum electrolytes (especially chloride and potassium)?
- Signs of dehydration (poor skin turgor or "tenting," dry mouth, decreased urine output)?
- Signs of generalized malnutrition (temporal wasting, fat and muscle mass loss)?
- Presence of projectile vomiting?
- Evidence of blood, bile, food, or feces in vomitus?

Related Medical Management

The goals of medical management are to identify and treat the underlying causes, provide symptomatic relief, and correct fluid and electrolyte imbalances.

Interventions

Prevention

Patient teaching to prevent nausea and vomiting should emphasize the importance of taking antiemetic medications as prescribed, avoiding problematic foods, and minimizing pain, stress, and other noxious stimuli.[24,25]

Patient Information: Nausea and Vomiting
- Take medicines for nausea and vomiting as directed by your nurse or doctor.
- Eat small meals or snacks every 2 to 3 hours rather than three big meals a day.

- Eat slowly and chew your food thoroughly for easier digestion.
- Eat food that is cold or lukewarm to avoid strong smells.
- Avoid sweet, spicy, fried, or greasy foods if they cause problems. Eat bland or salty foods (unless you have mouth sores) instead.
- Eat crackers, or dry toast or cereal first thing in the morning.
- Stay out of the kitchen while food is being cooked if food odors are a problem.
- Drink liquids 1 hour before or after a meal.
- Sip flat sodas, noncitrus juices, water, or weak tea through a straw, or suck on ice chips or popsicles.
- Rest in a chair and do not do any heavy work for 1 to 2 hours after eating.
- Breathe in and out deeply and slowly when feeling nauseated.
- Take medicines that may cause nausea at least 60 minutes after eating.
- Brush your teeth and rinse your mouth often throughout the day.

If nausea and vomiting occur, a self-report tool may be helpful in tracking the causes and severity of nausea and vomiting, evaluating the effectiveness of pharmacologic or nonpharmacologic therapies, and preventing future occurrences.[54] An example of such a tool and scale is illustrated in Figure 10.5.

Management

ACUTE. For nausea, vomiting, or retching that interferes with intake or occurs frequently throughout the day, pharmacologic therapy is indicated (Table 10.6). It is most effective when administered on a regular or around-

0	1	2	3
no nausea; no episodes of vomiting	slight nausea; 2 to 5 episodes of vomiting; maintains intake	moderate nausea; 6 to 10 episodes of vomiting; reduced intake	severe nausea; >10 episodes of vomiting; no intake

Figure 10.5 Nausea and Vomiting Assessment (Groenwald, Frogge, Goodman, Yarbro. *Cancer Nursing Principles and Practice.* 3rd ed. © 1995. Boston: Jones and Bartlett Publishers. Reprinted with permission.)

Table 10.6 Antiemetics for HIV-Associated Nausea and Vomiting[72]

Drug	Action	Clinical Uses	Dosage and Administration	Adverse Reactions/ Precautions
A. PHENOTHIAZINES				
Prochlorperazine (Compazine)	Depressant effect on CTZ; suppresses vomiting center	Management of severe nausea and vomiting	Oral: 5–10 mg every 6 to 8 hours; spansules: 10 mg every 12 hours; rectal: 25 mg every 12 hours; IM: 5–10 mg every 3–4 hours; IV: 2.5–10 mg (up to 40 mg/ day, dilute in saline)	Extrapyramidal symptoms, drowsiness, dizziness, blurred vision, hypotension, neutropenia, agitation
Thiethylperazine (Torecan)	Depressant effect on CTZ and vomiting center	Relief of nausea and vomiting	Oral, IM: 10 mg every 6 to 8 hours	Extrapyramidal symptoms, allergic-type reaction, dizziness, drowsiness; IV administration is contraindicated due to severe hypotension
B. ANTIHISTAMINES				
Trimethobenzamide (Tigan)	Depressant effect on CTZ	Control of nausea and vomiting	Oral: 100–250 mg every 6 to 8 hours; IM: 100–200 mg every 6 to 8 hours; rectal: 200 mg every 6 to 8 hours	Drowsiness; rare reports of parkinsonian symptoms

C. OTHERS				
Dronabinol (Marinol)	Affects the CNS	Treatment of anorexia with weight loss and nausea and vomiting that does not respond to conventional antiemetic therapy	Oral: 2.5–5 mg/m^2 every 6 hours (up to 15 mg/m^2 per dose)	May exacerbate psychiatric illnesses, CNS depression when used with alcohol or other CNS depressants
Metoclopramide (Reglan)	Increases GI motility; blocks dopamine receptors in CTZ	Short-term (4–12 weeks) therapy for symptomatic gastroesophageal reflux; prevention of nausea and vomiting	Oral, IM, IV: 10–20 mg 3–4 times per day	Sedation; rarely extrapyramidal symptoms
Cisapride (Propulsid)	Increases ACTH release from postganglionic nerves in myenteric plexus	Treatment of heart-burn due to gastroesophageal reflux	Oral: 10–20 mg four times per day before meals and at bedtime	Rare cases of serious cardiac arrhythmias; can effect absorption of other medications
Ondansetron (Zofran)	Blocks subclass of serotonin receptors ($5\text{-}HT_3$) in CTZ	Prevention of severe nausea and vomiting	Oral, IV: 0.15 mg/kg every 8 hours	Constipation, obstipation, transient blurred vision or dizziness with IV infusion
Granisetron (Kytril)	Blocks subclass of serotonin receptors ($5\text{-}HT_3$) in CTZ	Prevention of severe nausea and vomiting	IV: 10 $\mu g/kg$ (dilute in saline)	Headache, drowsiness, diarrhea, constipation, obstipation

CTZ = chemoreceptor trigger zone; ACTH = adrenocorticotropic hormone; $5\text{-}HT_3$ = 5-hydroxytryptamine 3.

the-clock, rather than prn, basis. The most commonly used antiemetics are the phenothiazine derivatives, such as thiethylperazine (Torecan) and prochlorperazine (Compazine). They function by blocking the stimuli that may trigger nausea and vomiting, and by having a sedative action on the CTZ.[55] In high doses or with long-term use, these medications can be associated with extrapyramidal symptoms and other adverse reactions, including drowsiness and dizziness. Trimethobenzamide (Tigan), which also acts on the CTZ, is another frequently used antiemetic.

Metoclopramide (Reglan) and cisapride (Propulsid) are prescribed when delayed gastric emptying, gastric reflux, or decreased GI motility are causing or contributing to nausea and vomiting. Two newer drugs, ondansetron (Zofran) and granisetron (Kytril), are also highly effective antiemetics.[23] Both are serotonin antagonists that work by selectively blocking the 5-hydroxytryptamine$_3$ (5-HT$_3$) receptors, a subclass of serotonin receptors located in the CTZ. Because of their considerable expense and propensity to cause severe constipation or obstipation, they should be used only to control severe nausea and vomiting.[55,56] Different combinations of antiemetics such as Reglan, Tigan, and Marinol are also useful.[14] Most of the antiemetics are available in oral, rectal suppository, IM, and IV forms. The IV and IM routes are used for patients with more severe nausea and vomiting, while oral and rectal antiemetics are used for milder cases of nausea and vomiting. With acute vomiting, fluid and electrolyte imbalances—especially hydrogen ($H+$) and chloride ($Cl-$) losses—can develop and result in alkalosis. IV fluids and electrolytes should be administered according to the amount and type of deficits. Other nursing interventions are accurate recording of intake and output, including frequency and amount of vomitus; monitoring vital signs; assessing for signs of dehydration; positioning weak or debilitated patients to prevent aspiration; administering antiemetics as prescribed; assessing antiemetic efficacy; weighing daily; and monitoring lab results for sodium, potassium, and chloride levels.

CHRONIC. Dronabinol (Marinol) is used to treat chronic nausea and vomiting in patients who fail to respond to conventional antiemetics.[14] It acts by depressing the CNS and is typically administered in 5-mg doses three or four times a day 30 minutes prior to meals. In addition to suppressing nausea and vomiting, Marinol has the additional advantage of stimulating appetite. Nonpharmacologic interventions such as visual imagery, acupressure wrist bands, and progressive muscle relaxation—either alone or in combination with pharmacologic agents—may also be useful in alleviating chronic nausea and vomiting.[56,57]

When liquids can be tolerated, fluids lost during vomiting can be replaced by sipping on room temperature, noncarbonated sodas, Gatorade or other sports drinks, noncitrus juices, weak tea, or broth, and by sucking on ice chips or popsicles. Commercially available oral rehydration solutions, such as Equalyte, also facilitate fluid and electrolyte replacement. Bland, easily digested foods (e.g., dry toast, crackers, baked potatoes, cereal with milk) are generally well tolerated. They should be eaten in small amounts to avoid stomach distention. Foods that are usually poorly tolerated include sweet, greasy, acidic, and spicy items.[23,25] Other useful strategies are maintaining an odor-free environment and sitting in an upright position for 1 to 2 hours after meals. Antiemetic drugs are most effective if administered 30 minutes before meals; nausea-promoting medications should be taken at least 60 minutes after eating. Lowering the dosage, changing the route of administration, or switching to another medication may lessen the emeticlike effects of pharmacological agents used to treat HIV and related OIs.[14]

Diarrhea

Diarrhea is perhaps the most distressing GI disturbance for people with HIV infection. Up to 50 to 90% of persons with AIDS will have diarrhea at some time.[43] In 1993 diarrhea became part of the CDC case definition of AIDS. Chronic diarrhea associated with wasting syndrome is an AIDS-indicator-condition, and diarrhea lasting longer than 1 month is a category B or symptomatic condition.[13] (See Appendix A.)

Definition

Diarrhea is defined as an increase in the frequency, fluidity, or volume of stools relative to usual patterns.

Biologic and Behavioral Basis

Diarrhea is an alteration in the normal fluid and electrolyte transport within the GI system. Approximately 9 l of fluid enter the duodenum each day. One to 1.5 l crosses the ileocecal valve and 0.2 l crosses the rectum. GI absorption of fluid and electrolytes involves a sodium chloride (NaCl) transport system. This system can be inhibited by second messengers such as cyclic adenosine monophosphate (cAMP), cyclic guanosine monophosphate (cGMP), diacylglycerol (DAG), and calcium (Ca^{++}). Absorption can occur both in the small intestine and the large intestine. Secretion in the GI tract is a Cl^{-}-dependent system. This secretion is potentiated by the same second messengers. Secretion can occur both in the small intestine and the large intestine.[58]

Diarrhea can be classified on the basis of duration (acute or chronic) or type (secretory, osmotic, or mixed). Acute diarrhea has an abrupt onset; lasts for less than a week; and may be associated with nausea, vomiting, and fever. Chronic diarrhea is diarrhea that lasts longer than 1 month and recurs over time.[59,60]

Osmotic diarrhea results from an unabsorbed, intraluminal solute that causes an osmotic load, drawing fluid into the GI tract. Secretory diarrhea results from actual fluid secretion from crypt cells into the GI tract. Mixed diarrhea is a combination of both osmotic and secretory diarrhea.[61]

Osmotic diarrheas occur when osmotically active substances such as fatty acids from fat malabsorption, hypertonic medications or formula, or sorbitol are present in the GI tract lumen. Other causes of osmotic diarrheas include mucosal disorders of the intestines, diabetes, GI bacterial overgrowth, GI motility disorders, or gastrinomas.[61]

Secretory diarrheas usually have infectious—viral, bacterial, or protozoal—etiologies. Most viral diarrheas tend to be self-limited, resolving in days to weeks. Bacterial secretory diarrheas are usually due to an endotoxin, such as seen with *Escherichia coli.* Antibiotic use may contribute to overgrowth of another bacteria, *Clostridium difficile*, resulting in secretory diarrhea. Secretory diarrheas may also be caused by endocrine tumors producing vasoactive intestinal peptide (VIP); and, occasionally, inflammatory bowel disease may have a secretory component.[62]

Etiologies Related to HIV Infection and Its Medical Treatment

An acute self-limiting diarrhea, often called *seroconversion diarrhea*, occurs early after infection with HIV. As the disease progresses, a more chronic, low-volume diarrhea due to *Salmonella*, *Campylobacter jejuni*, *Yersinia*, *Entamoeba histolytica*, and HSV commonly occurs. In later stage disease, *Cryptosporidium parvum*, *Microsporidia*, *Mycobacterium avium intracellulare*, *Isospora belli*, and CMV may cause chronic, high-volume diarrhea. When CD4 counts drop, below 50 cells/mm^3, CNS changes or CMV infection of the spinal cord can result in fecal incontinence that is sometimes mistaken for diarrhea.[43,47,63,64] (See Chapter 11.)

HIV-associated diarrhea is usually due to enteric pathogens or medications. Other less frequent causes include GI malignancies, hypoalbuminemia, and dietary intolerances. Some of the causes of diarrhea in HIV-infected patients are listed below, with the most frequent causes denoted by an asterisk.

Causes of Diarrhea in HIV-Infected Individuals

- **Bacterial**
  - *Campylobacter jejuni**
  - *Clostridium difficile*
  - *Mycobacterium avium intracellulare**
  - *Salmonella* species*
  - *Shigella flexneri**
- **Protozoal**
  - *Cryptosporidium parvum**
  - *Isospora belli**
  - *Microsporidia**
- **Neoplasmic**
  - KS
  - NHL
- **Viral**
  - Adenovirus
  - CMV*
  - HSV*
  - Other viruses (rotavirus, astrovirus, picornavirus, calcivirus, HIV)*
- **Medications**
  - Acyclovir
  - Ganciclovir
  - ddI
  - ddC
  - Antibiotics
- **Other**
  - Hypoalbuminemia
  - Enzyme deficiency
  - Hypochlorhydria
  - Emotional factors

Three protozoal agents—*C. parvum*, *I. belli*, and *Microsporidia*—are identified in approximately 15 to 20% of HIV-related diarrheas.[63] The proximal small bowel, generally the jejunum, is the usual site of protozoal infestation. In addition to voluminous diarrhea, patients complain of abdominal pain and fever. This form of secretory diarrhea is also accompanied by wasting and malnutrition.

Among the major bacterial organisms causing HIV-associated diarrheas are *M. avium intracellulare*, *Salmonella* species, *Shigella* species, and *C. jejuni*. Diarrhea from bacterial infection has a more acute clinical presentation, including fever, abdominal pain, and bacteremia. MAI more frequently involves the small intestine, and is therefore associated with higher volume diarrhea and weight loss. The other three bacterial pathogens (*Salmonella* species, *Shigella* species, and *C. jejuni*) often involve the colon and are associated with tenesmus and bloody diarrhea.[65] Contaminated food is an important vector for enteric pathogens such as *Salmonella* species and *Shigella* species.

The most common viral agents that cause diarrhea in the HIV-infected individual include CMV, HSV, and HIV.[43] CMV may present with either low- or high-volume diarrhea; CMV proctitis usually causes tenesmus. HSV symptoms include bloody or nonbloody rectal discharge, abdominal pain, and tenesmus. Perianal HSV infection may produce low-volume diarrhea, but is more likely to cause constipation.

When enteric pathogens are not identified, HIV infection of enterocytes may be the cause of diarrhea. In addition to its digestive and absorptive functions, the GI tract plays an important role in the body's immune system. It is the largest immune organ and serves as the first line of defense against foreign antigens. The gut-associated lymphoid tissue (GALT) contains Peyer's patches or lymphoid aggregates, specialized mucosal cells known as *M cells*, intraepithelial lymphocytes, and plasma cells that secrete IgA.[40] When HIV infects the GI tract, GALT immune responses are impaired, accounting for the frequent opportunistic intestinal infections and reinfections that occur, and the development of some malignancies. Alterations in the immune factor that contribute to HIV-associated diarrhea include a decline in CD4 numbers, decreased CD8 activity, decreased B- and T-cell activity, and a reduction in secretory IgA.[66] Although KS and NHL are occasionally cited as etiologies, they are uncommon causes of diarrhea in HIV disease.

Certain pharmacological agents routinely prescribed to treat HIV infection and its complications are responsible for medication-induced diarrhea. Antiviral and antiretroviral medications used to inhibit HIV infection, such as acyclovir and ddI, and medications used to treat enteric infections, such as rifampin and trimethoprim-sulfamethoxazole, are examples of diarrhea-causing agents. Additionally, it is estimated that 10 to 15% of HIV-related diarrhea is positive for *C. difficile*, which is due to antibiotic use.[66]

When infectious organisms and medications cannot be identified, the possibility of hypoalbuminemia, enzyme deficiencies, hypochlorhydria, and emotional factors such as stress and anxiety should be explored.[16]

Presentation and Assessment

When evaluating patients with diarrhea, it is important to consider the nature of the diarrhea and obtain their recent dietary, medication, travel, and emotional history. The physical exam should include an abdominal exam, a perianal exam, assessment of hydration status, and examination of a stool specimen.

Subjective data

- *Elimination:* Consistency, volume, frequency, color and odor of diarrhea? Duration? Severity? Aggravating and alleviating factors? Associated symptoms such as abdominal pain, bloating, fever, or pain or tenderness in the perianal area?
- *Nutrition:* Type of diet? Food intolerances such as lactose, caffeine, or spicy or greasy foods? Use of nutritional supplements with high osmolality? Vitamin C or magnesium megadosing? Ingestion of contaminated food?
- *Medications:* Changes in medications? Recent or current use of antibiotics or other medications associated with diarrhea?
- *General history:* Recent infection? Oral-anal contact or anal intercourse? Recent international travel or travel to a remote area? Emotional factors such as stress, anxiety, or fear?

Objective data

- *Abdominal exam:* Hyperactive bowel sounds in all four quadrants, abdominal tenderness, abdominal distention?
- *Perianal exam:* Lesions, discharge, tenderness, tissue breakdown?

(continued)

- *Hydration status:* Postural hypotension, tachycardia, poor skin turgor, dry mucous membranes, weakness, decreased urinary output, concentrated urine?
- *Stool:* Color, odor, and consistency of stool; presence of blood, pus, mucous, fat, or parasites in stool?

Diagnostic testing for diarrhea includes stool studies and endoscopy. Stool specimens are tested for ova and parasites, culture and sensitivity, *C. difficile* toxin, white blood cell count (WBC), fecal fat, and D-xylose. If a fever is present, blood cultures should be obtained. When these diagnostic studies are negative, sigmoidoscopy and rectal biopsy are indicated in patients who have low-volume diarrhea, tenesmus, or hematochezia. Patients with high-volume diarrhea should undergo upper endoscopy with small-bowel biopsy and duodenal aspiration for histology and culture.[65,66] An algorithm to evaluate diarrhea is shown in Figure 10.6.

Related Medical Management

The goal of medical management is to treat the underlying cause or causes of diarrhea. Although surgical resection or radiation therapy are sometimes

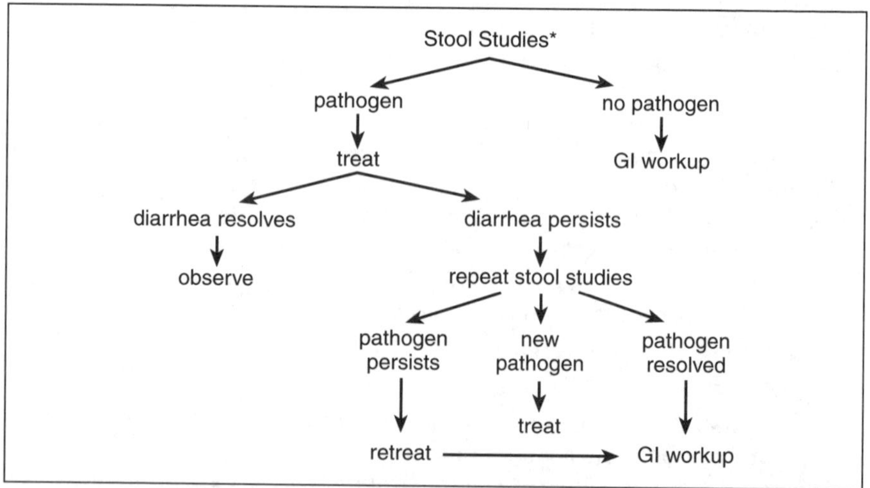

Figure 10.6 Evaluation of Diarrhea. (From Simon DM. AIDS-associated diarrhea. *Nutr HIV/AIDS.* 1992;1:34. Reprinted with permission.)
*Culture and sensitivity, ova and parasite exam, and *C. difficile* toxin.

employed for GI malignancies, pathogen-specific pharmacologic therapy is the key management modality for HIV-associated diarrhea. Pharmacologic agents that are effective in treating OIs that cause diarrhea are covered in Chapter 5.

Interventions

Prevention

Because some of the enteric pathogenic infections that cause HIV-related diarrhea are transmitted through contaminated food and water,[67] food safety counseling is an important aspect of diarrhea prevention (see Chapter 5). To decrease the risk of food- and water-borne infection, patients should be counseled on safe handling, storage, and preparation of food; careful cleaning of cooking utensils; and drinking safe water and milk.[68,69] The following list details these and other food safety guidelines.[68,69] In addition, patients should be instructed to avoid unprotected oral or anal sex because infection can occur through transmission of enteric cysts or pathogens.

Food Safety Recommendations

- Wash hands thoroughly with soap and hot water before handling or eating foods.
- When shopping, select perishable items last. Wrap meats in plastic bags and return home with perishables as soon as possible. Refrigerate or freeze perishable items as soon as possible.
- Store foods at safe temperatures. Keep foods refrigerated at or below 40°F or frozen at or below 0°F. Avoid letting food sit at room temperature for more than 2 hours.
- Thaw frozen food in a refrigerator or microwave oven to prevent prolonged exposure to unsafe temperatures. Marinate raw meat and poultry in the refrigerator.
- Protect opened foods with the use of airtight containers, plastic wrap, or foil. Discard leftover foods after 2 days.
- Never use foods that may be spoiled. Buy groceries in quantities that can be consumed before they spoil. Do not use foods after the recommended expiration date on the label.
- Never use cans with bulges, dents, or leaks.

(continued)

- Wash or scrub all fresh fruits and vegetables under running tap water before consumption.
- Use separate utensils and cutting boards for raw and cooked foods. Wash all utensils, dishes, and cutting boards in hot, soapy water or a dishwasher.
- Avoid using wooden cutting boards or cutting boards that are cracked. Never use dishes that are chipped or cracked.
- Avoid eating uncooked eggs, meat, poultry, fish, and seafood. Always use pasteurized milk and milk products. Discard cracked eggs.
- Cook meat and poultry until well done: all red meat (160°F) and poultry (180°F). Use a meat thermometer to judge internal temperatures.
- Stuff raw foods, such as turkey, right before cooking. Remove stuffing before refrigerating or freezing.
- Cook eggs thoroughly: boiled eggs for 7 minutes, fried eggs for 3 minutes *on each side*, poached eggs for 5 minutes, scrambled eggs for 1 minute.
- Thoroughly reheat dry leftovers at a temperature of 165°F. Bring wet leftover foods to a rolling boil. When using a microwave oven, rotate food during cooking and let it stand the recommended time before serving.
- Sponges, dishcloths, and dishtowels are breeding grounds for bacteria. Use clean ones daily or use paper towels.
- Avoid drinking untreated surface water or unsafe well water.
- Clean the inside of the refrigerator and microwave oven regularly according to manufacturer's instructions to control mold and pathogens.

Management

ACUTE. The goals of initial management of acute diarrhea are to provide symptomatic relief, minimize fluid and electrolyte imbalances, and prevent weight loss. (See Chapters 5 and 6.) For symptomatic relief, antidiarrheal agents—antimotility agents, luminal agents, or hormonal agents—should be used (Table 10.7). Most diarrhea can be controlled within 24 to 48 hours by giving Imodium and Lomotil in adequate amounts and at regular administration times. If adequate control is not achieved, stronger antimotility drugs such as deodorized tincture of opium, paregoric, or oral opiates should be prescribed, keeping in mind that they frequently cause constipation. Combining luminal agents with antimotility agents is also helpful in controlling diarrhea.[65] Luminal or bulk-forming agents such as Kaopectate or Metamucil can be taken every 4 to 6 hours to slow chronic, watery diarrhea, but they do not stop it.

Octreotide or Sandostatin, a relatively new hormonal antidiarrheal agent, may be useful for controlling secretory diarrhea. It acts by suppressing secretion of gastrin and the gastroenteropancreatic peptides. Sandostatin can be used alone or in combination with antimotility and luminal agents.[69] Antidiarrheal agents should not be given to treat diarrhea that is due to an infectious organism, since these agents slow the passage of stool through the GI tract, prolonging exposure of the gut mucosa to infectious toxins.

To minimize fluid and electrolyte imbalance, patients should drink at least 8 glasses of fluid or commercially available oral rehydration solutions, such as Equalyte, a day. In severe cases of diarrhea, IV fluid and electrolyte replacement is indicated.

For diarrhea related to small-bowel disease, the Task Force on Nutrition Support in AIDS[24] recommends small, frequent meals that are low fat, low lactose, low residue, and caffeine free. For diarrhea related to large-bowel disease, the Task Force recommends using either low-fat foods or adding commercially available medium-chain triglyceride (MCT) oil to foods and recipes, and following the small-bowel guidelines. For mixed diarrhea, the Task Force recommends adding a bulking agent, such as pectin, and eating low-lactose and low-fat foods.[24,25]

Patient Information: Diarrhea

- Try to eat small meals every 2 to 3 hours.
- If milk or milk products are a problem, buy lactose-free or lactose-reduced milk like Lactaid or Dairy Ease. You may be able to eat yogurt and aged hard cheeses like cheddar, swiss, and parmesan.
- Reduce or avoid carbonated and alcoholic beverages and beverages containing caffeine, such as coffee, tea, hot chocolate, and some soft drinks.
- Eat foods that are easy to digest, such as peeled, cooked fruits and vegetables; bananas; applesauce; cooked cereal; and rice.
- If fat is a problem, avoid foods that are high in fat, such as fried or greasy foods, sour cream, cheese, and butter. *(continued)*

Table 10.7 Antidiarrheal Agents[72]

Medication	Clinical Uses	Dosage and Administration	Comments/Side Effects/ Contraindications
A. ANTIMOTILITY AGENTS[72]			
Imodium (loperamide HCl)	Used for acute, nonspecific diarrhea; slows intestinal motility	Oral: 4 tsp or 2 caplets after first loose stool, then 2 tsp or 1 caplet after loose stools, not to exceed 8 tsp or 4 caplets in 24 hours	Constipation, nausea, and CNS depression are uncommon side effects
Lomotil (diphenoxylate/ atropine)	Adjunctive therapy in managing diarrhea	Oral: 2 tablets (5 mg) or 2 tsp (10 ml) every 6 hours	Inhibits peristalsis and may result in fluid retention in intestine, aggravating dehydration and electrolyte imbalance
Deodorized tincture of opium	Slows intestinal motility	Oral: 0.6 cc every 6 hours	See above
Paregoric	Slows intestinal motility	Oral: 5–10 cc every 6 hours	See above

B. Luminal-Acting Agents			
Metamucil (psyllium)	Used to slow chronic, watery diarrhea	Oral: 1 tbs (sucrose containing) or 1 tsp (sugar free) mixed with 8 oz liquid one to three times a day	Taking this product without adequate liquid may cause it to swell and block the throat or esophagus, causing choking
Kaopectate (kaolin plus pectin)	Used to slow chronic, watery diarrhea	Oral: 2 tbs after first loose bowel movement and each subsequent loose bowel movement, not to exceed 14 tbs in 24 hours	Teach patient to drink adequate liquids to prevent dehydration
C. Hormonal Agents			
Sandostatin (octreotide)	Treatment of profuse watery diarrhea associated with VIP-secreting tumors	IV: 50–100 µg every 8 hours (diluted in 50–200 ml saline or dextrose solutions and infused over 15–30 minutes)	Inhibits gallbladder contractility, decreases bile secretion, and may alter fat absorption

HCl = hydrochloric acid; VIP = vasoactive intestinal peptide.

- Avoid spicy foods like peppers and chili powder, and gassy foods like beans, cabbage, and onions if they cause problems.
- Drink at least eight glasses of liquid each day, preferably between meals rather than with meals. Water; tea; Gatorade or other sports drinks; apple, grape, peach, or pear juices; Italian ices; popsicles; broth; and jello are good choices.
- Replace lost minerals by eating bananas, fish, lean meat, potatoes, canned or processed foods, and adding salt to foods.
- Prevent infections by cooking meats, eggs, and fish until well done; not drinking raw milk or untreated water; and cleaning pots and pans and cutting boards with hot, soapy water.
- Try a medicine such as Metamucil to slow the diarrhea.
- If a medicine is prescribed to help with the diarrhea, take it about one-half hour before meals and on a regular schedule.
- Stay close to the bathroom or a bedside commode, or keep a bedpan handy.
- Wash and dry the anal areas thoroughly each time you have diarrhea. Put a skin paste or spray on your skin as instructed to prevent sores.
- Tell your nurse or doctor if you notice any of the following:
  - Urinating small amounts of dark urine
  - Very dry mouth or skin
  - Chills or fever of 100.8°F or higher
  - Dizziness or weakness
  - Diarrhea mixed with blood
  - Abdominal pain
  - Being unable to drink liquids
  - Painful sores in the anal area

Enzyme and hydrochloric acid supplements are sometimes beneficial in patients with fat and lactose malabsorption. Other management strategies include monitoring fluid and electrolyte status (blood pressure, pulse, urine output, urine specific gravity, skin turgor, sodium and potassium lab values); observing stool volume, frequency, and consistency using a stool assessment tool (Figure 10.7); and providing meticulous perianal skin care (thorough cleaning after each bowel movement, use of skin protectants, and perianal pouch).

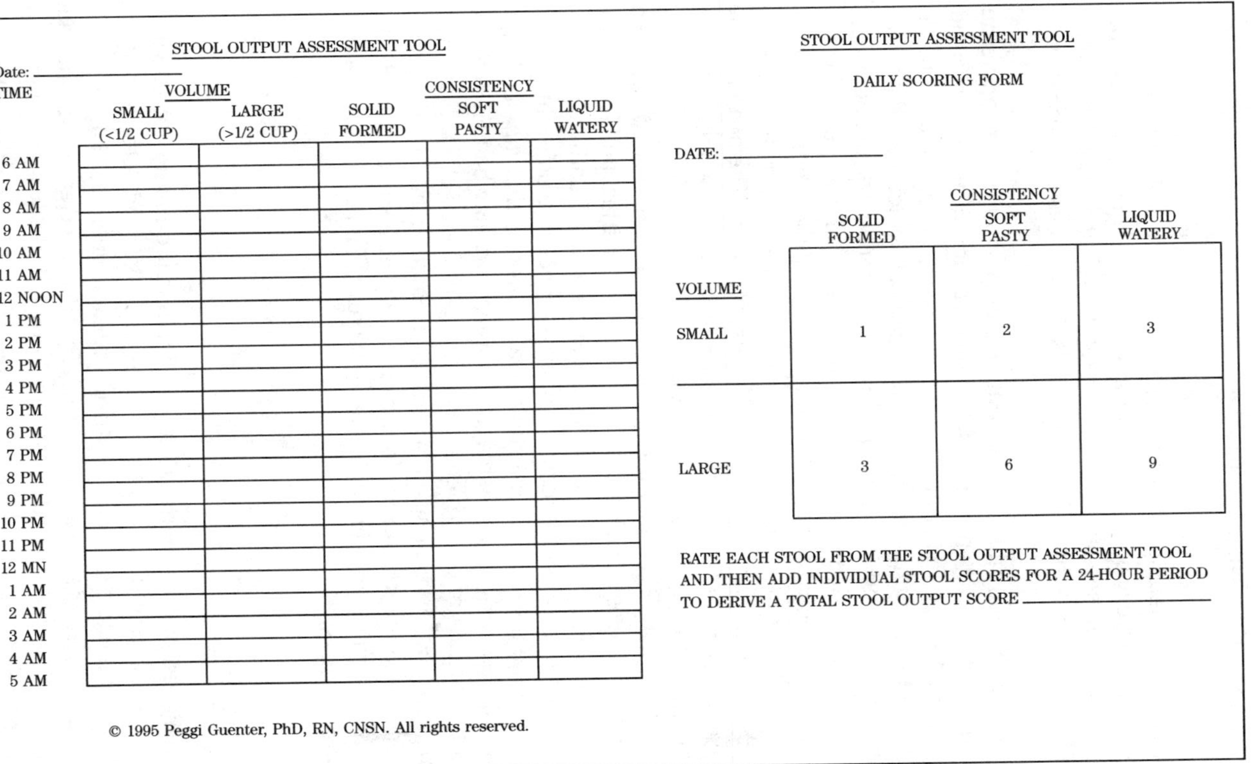

STOOL OUTPUT ASSESSMENT TOOL

Date: ____________

TIME	VOLUME SMALL (<1/2 CUP)	VOLUME LARGE (>1/2 CUP)	CONSISTENCY SOLID FORMED	CONSISTENCY SOFT PASTY	CONSISTENCY LIQUID WATERY
6 AM					
7 AM					
8 AM					
9 AM					
10 AM					
11 AM					
12 NOON					
1 PM					
2 PM					
3 PM					
4 PM					
5 PM					
6 PM					
7 PM					
8 PM					
9 PM					
10 PM					
11 PM					
12 MN					
1 AM					
2 AM					
3 AM					
4 AM					
5 AM					

STOOL OUTPUT ASSESSMENT TOOL

DAILY SCORING FORM

DATE: ____________

VOLUME	CONSISTENCY SOLID FORMED	CONSISTENCY SOFT PASTY	CONSISTENCY LIQUID WATERY
SMALL	1	2	3
LARGE	3	6	9

RATE EACH STOOL FROM THE STOOL OUTPUT ASSESSMENT TOOL AND THEN ADD INDIVIDUAL STOOL SCORES FOR A 24-HOUR PERIOD TO DERIVE A TOTAL STOOL OUTPUT SCORE ____________

Figure 10.7 Stool Output Assessment Tool

CHRONIC. Persistent diarrhea is also a serious problem because of its more insidious effect on weight, hydration, and psychological well-being. Small dietary changes, such as increasing intake of soluble fiber and decreasing intake of insoluble fiber and foods that increase intestinal motility, often help.

Fasting or the consumption of a BRAT diet (bananas, rice, applesauce, and tea or toast) during episodes of diarrhea is generally not recommended. Neither provides the nutritional intake necessary to prevent GI mucosal atrophy and hypoalbuminemia, both of which can exacerbate diarrhea.[16,25]

Oral and enteral nutrition are the preferred routes for maintaining the normal physical and immune barrier properties of the gut. When oral feedings are inadequate, enteral feedings may be given either alone or in conjunction with oral or parenteral nutrition. Isotonic, lactose-free polymeric or elemental formulas are usually tolerated best. The need for bowel rest, loss of adequate GI tract function, and inability to achieve GI access are indications for parenteral nutrition.

Psychological interventions are important because of related body image and lifestyle changes (e.g., need to stay close to a bathroom, need to wear a perianal pouch). Involving the individual and significant others in problem solving, providing opportunities to express concerns, using humor, and emphasizing the positive are psychological strategies that may be helpful.

Nontraditional or complementary therapies that may be beneficial, but for which evidence of effectiveness is lacking, include (1) *Saccharomyces boulardi*, an active yeast used widely to treat diarrhea in Europe; (2) vapreotide, a somatotropin analog under study in France; and (3) traditional Chinese medicine, including acupuncture, Chinese herbs, and hot-cold food theories.[70]

Summary

In summary, despite its many etiologies, malnutrition is not an inevitable consequence of HIV. Early nutritional assessment and intervention can prevent or minimize the major nutrition-related changes that contribute to malnutrition; namely, wasting, anorexia, oral/esophageal symptoms, nausea and vomiting, and diarrhea. As our knowledge advances, new nutritional guidelines and technology will further enhance our ability to provide individualized and effective nutritional care to patients with HIV infection.

References

1. Ysseldyke LL. Nutritional complications and incidence of malnutrition among AIDS patients. *JADA.* 1991;91:217–218.
2. Hellerstein MK. HIV-associated metabolic disturbances and body composition abnormalities: therapeutic implications. *AIDSFILE.* 1994;8:1–4.
3. Prasad C, Chandra RK. Nutrition and immunity. In: Kotler D, ed. *Gastrointestinal and Nutritional Manifestations of AIDS.* New York: Raven Press; 1991:35–49.
4. Beach RS, Mantero-Atienza E, Shor-Posner G, et al. Specific nutrient abnormalities in asymptomatic HIV-1 infection. *AIDS.* 1992;6:701–708.
5. Tang AM, Graham WMH, Kirby AJ, McCall LD, Willett WC, Saah AJ. Dietary micronutrient intake and risk of progression to acquired immunodeficiency syndrome (AIDS) in human immunodeficiency virus type 1 (HIV-1)-infected homosexual men. *Am J Epidemiol.* 1993;138:937–951.
6. Kotler DP, Tierney AR, Wang J, Pierson RN. Magnitude of body cell mass depletion and timing of death from wasting in AIDS. *Am J Clin Nutr.* 1989;50:444–447.
7. Guenter P, Muurahainen N, Simons G, et al. Relationships among nutritional status, disease progression, and survival in HIV infection. *J Acquir Immune Defic Syndr.* 1993;6:1130–1138.
8. Kotler DP. Nutritional effects and support in the patient with acquired immunodeficiency syndrome. *J Nutr.* 1992;122:723–727.
9. Timbo BB, Tollefson L. Nutrition: a cofactor in HIV disease. *J Am Diet Assoc.* 1994;94:1019–1022.
10. King AB. Malnutrition in HIV-infection: prevalence, etiology, and management. *PAAC Notes.* 1990;2:122–129.
11. Grunfeld C, Feingold KR. Metabolic disturbances and wasting in the acquired immunodeficiency syndrome. *N Engl J Med.* 1992;327:329–337.
12. Hellerstein MK. Pathophysiology of lean body wasting and nutrient unresponsiveness in HIV/AIDS: therapeutic implications. *Nutr HIV/AIDS.* 1992;1:17–25.
13. CDC. Revised classification system for HIV-infection and expanded surveillance case definition for AIDS among adolescents and adults. *MMWR.* 1992;41:1–19.
14. Cimoch PJ. Current agents for the management of wasting and malnutrition in HIV/AIDS. *Nutr HIV/AIDS.* 1992;1:27–32.
15. Raiten DJ. *Nutrition and HIV Infection: A Review and Evaluation of the Extant Knowledge of the Relationship between Nutrition and HIV Infection.* Washington, DC: Center for Food Safety and Applied Nutrition, US Food and Drug Administration, Department of Health and Human Services; 1990:1–99.
16. Fields-Gardner C. A review of mechanisms of wasting in HIV disease. *Nutr Clin Pract.* 1995;10:167–176.
17. Macallan DC, Noble C, Baldwin C, et al. Energy expenditure and wasting in human immunodeficiency virus infection. *N Engl J Med.* 1995;333:83–88.

18. Harris JA, Benedict FG. *A Biometric Study of Basal Metabolism in Man.* Washington, DC: Carnegie Institute; 1919:189–193.
19. Long CL. Energy and protein requirements in stress and trauma. *Crit Care Nurs Curr.* 1984;2:7–12.
20. Jeejeeboy KN. Assessment of nutritional status. In: Rombeau JL, Caldwell MD, eds. *Clinical Nutrition—Enteral and Tube Feeding.* Philadelphia: WB Saunders; 1990:118–126.
21. Suttman U, Ockenga J, Selberg O, Hoogestraat L, Deicher H, Muller MJ. Incidence and prognostic value of malnutrition and wasting in human immunodeficiency virus-infected outpatients. *J Acquir Immune Defic Syndr Hum Retrovirol.* 1995;8:239–246.
22. Blackburn GL, Bistrian BR, Maini BS, Schlamm HT, Smith MF. Nutritional and metabolic assessment of the hospitalized patient. *J Parenter Enter Nutr.* 1977; 1:11–22.
23. Beal JA, Martin BM. The clinical management of wasting and malnutrition in HIV/AIDS. *AIDS Patient Care.* 1995;4:66–74.
24. Task Force on Nutrition Support in AIDS. Guidelines for nutrition support in AIDS. *Nutrition.* 1989;5:28–36.
25. Newman CF. The role of nutritional assessment and nutritional plans in the management of HIV/AIDS: an overview of the PAAC initiative. *Nutr HIV/AIDS.* 1992;1:57–106.
26. ASPEN Board of Directors. Guidelines for the use of parenteral and enteral nutrition in adults and pediatric patients. *J Parenter Enter Nutr.* 1993;17: 7SA–11SA, 13SA–14SA.
27. Hellerstein M, Kohn J, Mudie H, Viteri F. Current approach to the treatment of human immunodeficiency virus-associated weight loss: pathophysiologic considerations and emerging management strategies. *Semin Oncol.* 1990;17:17–33.
28. Von Roenn J. Management of HIV-related bodyweight loss. *Pract Ther.* 1994; 47:774–783.
29. McCann RM, Hall WJ, Groth-Juncker A. Comfort care for terminally ill patients: the appropriate use of nutrition and hydration. *JAMA.* 1994;272:1263–1266.
30. Von Roenn JH. Randomized trials of megestrol acetate for AIDS-associated anorexia and cachexia. *Oncology.* 1994;51S:19–24.
31. Grant MM. Nutritional interventions: increasing oral intake. *Semin Oncol Nurs.* 1986;2:35–43.
32. Ganong WF. Review of medical physiology. 17th ed. Norwalk, CT: Lange; 1995: 171–173, 215, 448–450.
33. Coodley GO, Loveless MO, Nelson HD, Coodley MK. Endocrine function in the HIV wasting syndrome. *J Acquir Immune Defic Syndr.* 1994;7:46–51.
34. Baum M, Cassetti L, Bonvehi P, Shor-Posner G, Lu Y, Sauberlich H. Inadequate dietary intake and altered nutrition status in early HIV infection. *Nutrition.* 1994;10:16–20.

35. Lahdevirta J, Maury CPJ, Teppo A, Repo H. Elevated levels of circulating cachectic/TNF in patients with acquired immunodeficiency syndrome. *Am J Med.* 1988;85:289–291.
36. Oster MH, Enders SR, Samuels SJ, et al. Megestrol acetate in patients with AIDS and cachexia. *Ann Intern Med.* 1994;121:400–404.
37. Rabkin JG, Rabkin R, Wagner G. Testosterone replacement in HIV illness. *Gen Hosp Psych.* 1995;17:37–42.
38. Gorter R. Management of anorexia-cachexia associated with cancer and HIV infection. *Oncology.* 1991;5:13–17.
39. Grauer PA. Appetite stimulants in terminal care: treatment of anorexia. *Hospice J.* 1993;9:73–83.
40. Langkamp-Henken B, Glezer JA, Kudsk KA. Immunologic structure and function of the gastrointestinal tract. *Nutr Clin Pract.* 1992;7:100–108.
41. Ganley BJ. Effective mouth care for head and neck radiation therapy patients. *Med Surg Nurs.* 1995;4:133–141.
42. Goodman M, Ladd LA, Purl S. Integumentary and mucous membrane alterations. In: Groenwald SL, Frogge MH, Goodman M, Yabro CH, eds. *Cancer Nursing: Principles and Practice.* 3rd ed. Boston: Jones and Bartlett; 1993: 768–822.
43. Chui DW, Owen RL. AIDS and the gut. *J Gastroenterol Hepatol.* 1994;9:291–303.
44. Gallagher D. Gastrointestinal manifestations of HIV/AIDS. *Crit Care Nurs Clin North Am.* 1993;5:121–126.
45. Zakarian AJ. Oral complications of HIV infection. In: Kotler D, ed. *Gastrointestinal and Nutritional Manifestations of AIDS.* New York: Raven Press; 1991: 51–64.
46. Johnson LR, ed. *Physiology of the Gastrointestinal Tract.* 3rd ed. New York: Raven Press; 1994:903–928.
47. Dietrich DT, Poles MA, Lew EA. GI manifestations of HIV disease. In: Broder S, Marigan TL, Bolognesi D, eds. *Textbook of AIDS Medicine.* Baltimore: Williams & Wilkins; 1994:541–554.
48. Sulis C. Candidiasis. In: Libman H, Witzburg RA, eds. *Clinical Manual for the Care of the Adult Patient with HIV Infection.* Boston: Boston City Hospital; 1990:197–198.
49. Glover J, Dibble S, Miaskowski C, Giebert R. Changes in taste associated with intravenous administration of pentamidine. *J Assoc Nurses AIDS Care.* 1995; 6:43–48.
50. Friedman SL. Gastrointestinal symptoms in AIDS. *AIDS Clin Care.* 1989;3:19.
51. Berger T. Dermatologic manifestations of HIV infection. *AIDS Clin Care.* 1990; 2:57–64.
52. Craven DE. Cytomegalovirus infection. In: Libman H, Witzburg RA, eds. *Clinical Manual for Care of the Adult Patient with HIV Infection.* Boston: Boston City Hospital; 1990:177–183.

53. Guyton A. *Textbook of Medical Physiology.* 9th ed. Philadelphia: WB Saunders; 1995:849–850.
54. Camp-Sorrell D. Chemotherapy: toxicity management. In: Groenwald SL, Frogge MH, Goodman M, Yabro CH, eds. *Cancer Nursing: Principles and Practice.* 3rd ed. Boston: Jones and Bartlett; 1993:339–340.
55. Shlafer M. *The Nurse, Pharmacology, and Drug Therapy.* 2nd ed. Redwood City, CA: Addison-Wesley; 1993:837–847.
56. Cotanch PH. Relaxation training for control of nausea and vomiting in patients receiving chemotherapy. *Cancer Nurs.* 1983;6(4):277–283.
57. Wickham R. Managing chemotherapy-related nausea and vomiting: the state of the art. *Oncol Nurs Forum.* 1989;16:563–574.
58. Donowitz M, Welsh MJ. Regulation of mammalian small intestinal secretion. In: Johnson LR, ed. *Physiology of the Gastrointestinal Tract.* 2nd ed. New York: Raven Press; 1987:1351–1370.
59. Hecht F. Diarrhea and AIDS. *Ann Intern Med.* 1990;113:804–805.
60. Tanowitz H, Simon D, Wittner M. Gastrointestinal manifestations of AIDS. *Med Clin North Am.* 1991;76(suppl 1):45–62.
61. Greenberger N. Diagnostic approach to the patient with a chronic diarrheal disorder. *Disease-a-Month.* 1990;36(3):139–179.
62. Kane MG, O'Dorisio TM, Krejs GJ. Production of secretory diarrhea with intravenous infusion of vasoactive intestinal polypeptide. *N Engl J Med.* 1983;309:1482–1485.
63. Kotler D, Francisco A, Clayton F, Sholes JV, Orenstein JM. Small intestinal injury and parasitic diseases in AIDS. *Ann Intern Med.* 1990;113:444–449.
64. Wanke CA. Intestinal microsporidial infection in HIV patients. *AIDS Clin Care.* 1994;6:45–49.
65. Simon DM. AIDS-associated diarrhea. *Phys Assoc AIDS Care.* 1992;1:33–39.
66. DuPont HL, Marshall GD. HIV-associated diarrhea and wasting. *Lancet.* 1995;346:352–356.
67. Vakil NB, Schwartz SM, Buggy BP, et al. Biliary cryptosporidiosis in HIV-infected people after the waterborne outbreak of cryptosporidiosis in Milwaukee. *N Engl J Med.* 1995;334(1):19–23.
68. US Department of Health and Human Services. *Eating Defensively: Food Safety Advice for Persons with AIDS.* Washington, DC: Public Health Service/Food and Drug Administration/HFI-40, OHHS. 1994 Publication no. (FDA) 92-2232.
69. Romeu J, Miro J, Sirera G, et al. Efficacy of octreotide in the management of chronic diarrhea in AIDS. *AIDS.* 1991;5:1495–1499.
70. Flaskerud J. AIDS and traditional food therapies. In: Watson R, ed. *Nutrition and AIDS.* Boca Raton: CRC Press; 1994:235–247.
71. Goodman M, Stoner C. Mucous membrane integrity, impairment of: stomatitis. In: McNally J, Somerville E, Miaskowski C, Rostad C, eds. *Guidelines for Oncology Nursing Practice.* 2nd ed. Philadelphia: WB Saunders; 1991:241–247.
72. *Physician's Desk Reference.* 50th ed. Montvale, NJ: Medical Economics; 1996.

CHAPTER 11

Fecal Incontinence

Alice Basch, RN, MSN, ET

Chapter Preview

- Definition
- Biologic and Behavioral Basis
- Fecal Incontinence in HIV-Infected People
- Presentation and Assessment
- Related Medical Management
- Interventions

Definition

Fecal incontinence, the inability to control the elimination of stool or flatus, is one of the most emotionally difficult aspects of a progressive illness, often leading to embarrassment and a feeling of isolation. In addition, financial costs are associated with the use of diapers and containment devices, increased laundry, alteration in skin integrity, and an increased infection rate. Information is limited about the cause, extent, or solutions to fecal incontinence in either the general population or the HIV population.

Biologic and Behavioral Basis

The Defecation Process

A combination of factors in the GI tract maintain continence. Transit of digested food and liquid is accomplished by peristatic waves through the small and large intestines. Fluid, both ingested and secreted during digestion, is absorbed throughout the GI tract creating a bolus of waste material. Fluid content up to 100 cc remains in the descending colon and is stored in the rectum until a signal is sent through the neurologic pathways to the brain that the need to defecate is present. The internal anal sphincter, which normally maintains a slight contraction, relaxes as the external anal sphincter contracts to prevent leakage of solid, liquid, or gas. If the individual cannot or does not desire to complete the defecation process, the sensation of rectal fullness subsides in about 60 seconds, to begin again at a later time. If defecation is initiated, the individual strains, causing an increase in pressure in the abdomen. At the same time, the rectal-anal angle straightens to allow gravity to assist and the stool is eliminated. If any one factor in this process does not function properly, fecal incontinence can occur.

Causes of Fecal Incontinence

In the general population, fecal impaction due to medications, dietary factors, and aging are the primary cause of fecal incontinence. Intestinal transit time may be decreased due to medications or lack of activity, allowing for greater fluid absorption. A diet deficient in fluid or roughage can also lead to hard, difficult-to-pass stools. Hard, impacted stool can cause a weakening of the internal anal sphincter, allowing for poor resting tone and a leakage of stool or gas. Seepage of fluids may also occur around the impacted stool, resulting in a misdiagnosis of diarrhea. Intermittent or short-duration incontinence may occur during stressful situations or periods of increased stool volume when a weak muscle tone, due to disease or age, is unable to compensate. An increase in transit time from disease, infection, medication, or dietary causes will result in increased stress or pressure on the internal and external anal sphincters. If voluntary muscle control is diminished or absent, leakage occurs.

Neurological dysfunction is seen in people with diabetes, stroke, multiple sclerosis, paraplegia and quadraplegia, and women who have had difficult or lengthy childbirths. Innervation of the rectopubalis muscle, which controls voluntary constriction of the external anal sphincter, may be absent or weakened. Often, a lack of coordination or an inability to contract these muscles results and leakage occurs. Another factor in neurological deficits is the lack of sensation of rectal filling. Normal sensation of rectal filling is first felt at 10 to 15 cc. If sensation of fullness has not been identified by 60 cc, an overflow of stool can result.

Fecal Incontinence in HIV-Infected People

People with HIV infection may experience alterations in bowel function and an inability to store feces related to OIs, malignancies, neurological deficits, and dementia. Diarrhea is a common problem in HIV-infected people, occurring in about 60% of patients.[1] Leigh and Turnberg,[2] and Swash[3] have found in the general population that 50% of patients referred for diarrhea in reality had fecal incontinence. One can then extrapolate that upward of 30% of HIV-infected patients may have episodes of incontinence at some time. This may be as mild as a slight staining of undergarments or the more severe inability to store the feces until one reaches a bathroom or commode. The problem may be intermittent, chronic, or may occur during episodes of HIV-related infections or malignancies.

Causes of fecal incontinence include viral, bacterial, and fungal infections such as *Cryptosporidium* and *Mycobacterium avium*, which impair intestinal cell function and cause malabsorption and high-volume stools.[4,5] High-volume liquid stool places increased stress on the resting tone of the internal anal sphincter. If neurological deficits are also present, contraction of the external anal sphincter may also be compromised and leakage or spotting may occur. Neurological deficits from AIDS-related dementia or neuropathies may interfere with the signals relayed to the brain to initiate voluntary contraction or defecation. If undetected, fecal impactions can result and may lead to leakage or overflow incontinence. Confusion, disorientation, and memory loss may present barriers to the individual's ability to recognize the need to defecate, manipulate clothing, or find the appropriate toileting facilities. Peripheral neuropathies may make it difficult to manipulate buttons and zippers, interfering with the ability to maintain continence.

Presentation and Assessment

Subjective

Assessment of incontinence requires direct questions that elicit the extent of the problem.

Sample Questions for Fecal Incontinence History

- Describe a normal bowel movement (stool pattern). Are your stools hard? Loose? Watery?
- Describe your current bowel movements (stool pattern)? Are your stools hard? Loose? Watery?
- When did your normal pattern change? After a recent trip? Over the last few years? Yesterday? After the birth of your last child? After being diagnosed with . . . ?
- Do you leak solid stool? Liquid stool only? Gas only?
- Do you leak stool more than once a day? More than once a week but less than once a day? More than once a month?
- Do you use special panties or pads (paper towels, sanitary napkin, etc.)?
- How often each day do you change your panties or pads?
- Do you avoid going places because you are concerned about odor or leakage of stool?
- Do people complain of odor when they are near you?

In addition, drug and diet intake should be explored. A 3-day diet and stool history may detect patterns, and simple measures for eliminating offending substances can be taken if a relationship to diarrhea and incontinence is found. All food and additives should be listed, along with the time eaten. A parallel list of stool, incontinence episodes and amounts should be maintained (Figure 11.1). Common foods that frequently cause diarrhea include dairy products, caffeine, nonabsorbed carbohydrates (sorbitol),

Time	Food	Amount	Stool Consistency
7 A.M.	Coffee with artificial sweetener, eggs scrambled in margarine	2 cups, 1 tsp each 2 eggs 1 pat margarine	
8 A.M.			Loose stool
10:30 A.M.	Diet soda	12 oz	
11 A.M.			Loose stool
12:15 P.M.	Grilled cheese sandwich Apple Chocolate chip cookies Coffee with artificial sweetener	2 slices bread, 1 slice cheddar, 1 pat margarine, 1 apple, 2 cookies, 1 cup, 1 tsp	
1 P.M.			Loose stool
2:30 P.M.	Diet soda	12 oz	
3:30 P.M.			Loose stool
6:00 P.M.	White wine	4 oz	
7:00 P.M.	Grilled salmon Asparagus with lemon Biscuit with butter Green salad with dressing Rice Chocolate ice cream Decaf coffee with artificial sweetener	3 oz 6 spears 1, 1 tsp 2 tbsp ½ cup 1 scoop 1 cup, 1 tsp	
8:15 P.M.			Loose stool

Figure 11.1 Sample Diet and Stool History

alcohol, gluten, and raw fruits or vegetables. Herbal remedies and alternative diets should also be examined for effects on the GI tract. Additionally, attention should be paid to numerous prescription and over-the-counter medications that include lactose, which may lead to problems for lactose-intolerant individuals. Recreational drugs should also be reviewed. Narcotic use, along with poor dietary intake, may contribute to a decrease in parastaltic activity and may lead to constipation. The following medications alter stool consistency. Lactose-containing medications are indicated by an asterisk.

Prescription drugs (partial)

- Anthroquinone
- Floxuridine
- Ativan*
- Gemfibrozil
- Phenergen*
- Vasotec*
- Capoten*
- Guanethidine
- PenVee K Tab*
- Xanax*
- Catapres
- Levodopa
- Propranolol
- Zovirax*
- Colchicine
- Lopressor*
- Premarin*
- Amoxicillin
- Coumadin*
- Cephalexin
- Provera*
- Ampicillin
- Digoxin*
- Lovastatin
- Restoril*
- Sulfasalazine

- Dilantin*
- Macrodantin*
- Ritalin HCL*
- Cyclosporine
- Dyazide*
- Nitrostat*
- Seldane*
- Ciprofloxin
- Fiorinal*
- Nonsteroidal anti-inflammatory agents
- Synthroid*
- Clindamycin HCl
- Furosemide*
- Tavist-D*
- Dexamethasone
- 5-Fluorouracil
- Theophylline
- Erythromycin
- Mitomycin
- Miconazole
- Nechlorethamine penicillin
- Fluoxetine
- Quinine
- Tetracycline

Nonprescription drugs (partial)

- Anthraquinone
- Magnesium
- Actifed*
- Imodium A-D caps*
- Afrin*
- Lactulose
- Phenolphthalein
- Sleepinal*
- Bisacodyl
- Senna
- Bayer Enteric ASA*

(continued)

- Triaminic Cold Tabs*
- Benadryl 25*
- Ricinoleic acid
- Cascara
- Unicap Chewable Tabs*
- Centrum High Potency Multivitamin*
- Ascorbic acid
- Chlor-Trimaton*

Objective

During the physical assessment, the skin and anal structure may reveal fissures, abscesses, lesions, and skin denudement due to caustic stools, straining, disease, or injury. Lesions commonly found in the perineal area of an immunosuppressed patient are lesions of viral, fungal, pressure, or moisture origin. The most common skin problem seen associated with fecal incontinence is skin irritation related to the caustic chemicals found in liquid stool. Fungal infections are also seen in areas of moisture and stool. These appear as a rash; thick, reddened areas with satellite lesions around the edges; or as an open bleeding area. Fungal infections can also be found in fecally denuded skin and may be difficult to visualize. Satellite red lesions extending beyond the denuded skin are one marker.

A defect in the anus, similar in appearance to a keyhole, may indicate previous surgery, injury, or neurological deficit. Stool present at the anal opening suggests leakage of stool due to sphincter deficits. To rule out hygiene or cognitive factors, a simple test of the strength and contractability of the anus should be measured. A digital exam, if tolerated, measures angle and tone of the puborectalis muscle. On withdrawal of the finger, a closing reflex should be seen. A gentle stroke of a blunt pin along the side of the anus will elicit the "anal wink" if neurologically intact. A stool mass, if present, can also be examined. A hard stool may indicate impaction. Finally, an abdominal exam is performed to rule out masses due to impaction or disease.

Related Medical Management

On occasion, fecal incontinence and pain on defecation is so severe that bypass surgery is performed. Usually a temporary colostomy is constructed with reanastomosis in 3 to 6 months if resolution of the problem is achieved. Some reasons for surgical intervention may include rectal lymphoma, severe abscesses or fissures, and severe herpetic infection. If other disease processes are minimal, laparoscopic colostomy surgery may be performed to minimize hospitalization and side effects from anesthesia.

Interventions

Although fecal incontinence is a devastating problem, much can be done to provide comfort. Identification and recognition of the problem is the first step. Medication and dietary changes, manipulation of the environment, appropriate clothing and containment devices, and muscle strengthening can resolve many of the problems. Skin care and comfort measures are imperative if incontinence is present.

Foods are used to thicken and normalize stool consistency to allow for greater control when high-volume liquid stool is present. In addition to the familiar BRAT diet of bananas, rice, applesauce, and toast, other foods that thicken stool include strained tapioca, yogurt, marshmallows, and pasta. If a lactose intolerance is present, goat, rice, or soy milk can be substituted or live acidophalus culture may be added to regular milk.

To prevent or control diarrhea with enteral feedings, formulas should be isotonic and advanced slowly, starting at about 50 ml/hour. Use of formulas containing bulk agents can be used or bulk agents can be added to the formula. Antidiarrheal agents may also be necessary until nutritional status and bowel function improves. Witholding of feedings may cause worsening of the problem and should never be used as an intervention for diarrhea or incontinence.

Treatment of skin problems begins by eliminating the cause of the irritation. Comfort measures are utilized when appropriate. Gentle cleaning after each bowel movement and application of a moisture-barrier product should be performed as soon as diarrhea or incontinence presents. Tepid water, pH-balanced soaps, or commercial skin cleaners are used and the area is patted dry. A moisture barrier is applied immediately. Moisture barriers are usually zinc oxide or petrolatum based. Products come in cream and ointment form. The choice of a particular brand is based on product information obtained from manufacturers or other clinicians in the field regarding the effectiveness, convenience, availability, and cost of the product.

A more aggressive treatment is required when the skin has been denuded. A skin-barrier powder can be applied directly to the denuded area and covered with a moisture-barrier product. An alternative may be to mix the powder into the cream or ointment prior to application. Numerous products are now on the market that have been formulated to stick to moist, weeping tissue and can be used directly on irritated skin. Some practitioners have also had success with the use of hydrocolloid wafer dressings over the denuded areas. Caution should be taken if a viral or fungal lesion is suspected, because the use of occlusive dressings may cause worsening of the problem.

In some situations a prophylactic treatment for yeast such as a powder containing nystatin or miconazole is routinely used instead of the skin-barrier powder when antibiotics are being taken or immunosuppression is present. Moisture barriers containing miconazole are also available and can be obtained over the counter from some medical supply companies or pharmacies.

When abscesses, fissures, and herpetic lesions (which are usually quite painful on defecation) are present, comfort meaures can include local pain relievers such as topical xylocaine without alcohol, and oral medication if the pain is severe. Sitz baths and hemorrhoidal preparations can be helpful. Oral solutions developed for mouth ulcers containing 20% benzocaine have also been used successfully. Keeping stools soft or using glycerin suppositories for smoother passage are other recommendations. For cleansing sensitive skin, commercial cleansers are available that contain mild soaps and surfactants that loosen debris and minimize rubbing. Sitz baths and bidets have also been used for cleansing. Plastic bottles that can be squeezed to produce a gentle stream of water are another option for cleansing.

The use of diapers should be minimized because the plastic outer layer traps moisture against the skin, causing maceration. Patients should be placed on absorbent pads containing polymer fibers to absorb liquids. Pads should be changed when soiled, followed by skin cleansing and application of a moisture barrier. Diapers and absorbent pants can be used during ambulation. Some newer products use polymer fibers in disposable pads with mesh-type pants to hold the pad in place. These products allow for greater air circulation and wicking of fluid from the skin.

Fecal incontinence collectors are another option when frequent stooling is a problem. Successful application depends on a consistent caregiver, clean perianal skin, and removal of surrounding hair. Pouches remain in place 24 hours to 3 days depending on the product and skill in application. Stool is emptied from the bottom of the pouch or it can be attached to bedside drainage for high-volume liquid stool. Although these devices are most commonly used in the bed-bound patient, if a good seal is maintained, ambulatory patients may receive benefits as well.

If a cognitive deficit is present, interventions that manipulate the environment may be appropriate. Clothing that is easy to remove by using Velcro closures or elastic and draw-string pants may be beneficial. Well-marked bathrooms, easy-grip door handles, and support bars near the toilet can be used. Clean, easy-to-reach commodes and bedpans should be available.

A toileting program may work for individuals who "forget" to go to the bathroom or have decreased rectal sensation. A toileting program developed with the patient and caregiver can help in decreasing accidents. This may be a simple reminder to toilet at an established time each day. More formal bowel training would include use of rectal stimulation with a mild suppository or gloved finger, timed evacuation after a meal to take advantage of the gastrocolic reflex, and use of the left-sided lying or squat position for easier stool passage. Diet, fluid, and exercise should be discussed as appropriate.

If a neurological deficit or muscular weakness is present, sphincter exercises can be tried to improve sensation and tone in the internal and external sphincters. Kegel exercises are taught by instructing the individual to squeeze the perineal area. Methods of exercise vary among practitioners but commonly include a series of 5 to 10 squeezes, repeated several times throughout the day. Kegels may be difficult to teach unless a method of evaluation can be used. A finger in the rectum (or vagina in females) can provide feedback for identifying the proper muscles. If available, biofeedback equipment can utilize external sensors to identify muscles, muscle strength, and ongoing improvement.

References

1. Gee G. *AIDS: Concepts in Nursing Practice.* Baltimore: Williams & Wilkins; 1988.
2. Leigh RJ, Turnberg LA. Faecal incontinence: the unvoiced symptom. *Lancet.* 1982;1:1349–1351.

3. Swash M. New concepts in the prevention of incontinence. *Practitioner.* 1985; 229:1377–1398.
4. Friedman S, Sande MA, Volberding PA. Diarrhea. In: Cohen PT, ed. *The AIDS Knowledge Base.* 2nd ed. Boston: Little, Brown; 1994:5.19-1–5.19-13.
5. Rosenthal Y, Haneiwich S. Nursing management of adults in the hospital. *Nurs Clin North Am: AIDS.* 1988;23:707–718.

CHAPTER **12**

Respiratory Changes

Susan Janson, DNSc, RNc, ANP, FAAN
Virginia Carrieri-Kohlman, RN, DNSc, FAAN

Chapter Preview

- Dyspnea
- Cough

Dyspnea

Definition

Dyspnea is the subjective, unpleasant sensation of difficult breathing. It includes both the perception of labored breathing and the reaction to that sensation by the patient.[1] Thus, the experience of dyspnea includes the physical sensation or sensory component as well as an affective response. It is a subjective sensation that can only be described precisely by the individual experiencing it. Dyspnea is a cardinal symptom of pulmonary complications of HIV infection and often presents first as dyspnea on exertion.

Biologic and Behavioral Basis

Dyspnea is a sensation primarily of respiratory effort, but it is also related to increased respiratory drive.[2,3] The sensation is mediated through a variety of receptors in the diaphragm and intercostal muscles, the carotid bodies, receptors in the interstitium of the lung, and the respiratory center in the medulla. The exact mechanisms causing dyspnea in HIV-associated diseases are unknown. However, the combination of decreased lung compliance secondary to interstitial disease processes or the hypoxemia that results from decreased alveolar ventilation in pneumonia are probable causes. Hypoxemia usually occurs due to profound ventilation-perfusion mismatching and stimulates chemoreceptors in the carotid body that trigger central neuroreceptors and increase respiratory drive, resulting in an increased minute ventilation.[4] In addition, respiratory muscle fatigue or weakness and muscle wasting contribute to the inability of the thoracic muscular pump to meet ventilation requirements.

The perception of dyspnea can be increased in both acute and chronic anxiety states.[5] The anxious patient often complains of a "smothering" feeling or inability to take a deep breath, with associated symptoms of palpitations, dizziness, lightheadedness, and numbness of the hands and feet. Depression has also been associated with dyspnea. Depression and associated negative feelings are thought to produce an altered central perception of incoming afferent sensations. The relationship of depression and anxiety to dyspnea specific to HIV infection has not been studied.

Etiologies Related to HIV Infection and Its Medical Treatment

The most common pulmonary complications of HIV infection are PCP, bacterial pneumonia, cryptococcal pneumonia, pulmonary *Mycobacterium tuberculosis*, and pulmonary KS. The frequency of occurrence of most of these conditions, based on 79,674 adult and adolescent US cases reported to the CDC in 1994,[6] is shown in Table 12.1.

PCP

PCP is the most frequent AIDS-defining OI,[7] accounting for approximately 70% of respiratory presentations, whereas 30% are due to a variety of infections and neoplasms. The disease classically presents with fever, nonproductive cough, and dyspnea, frequently accompanied by constitutional complaints of fatigue, night sweats, and weight loss. The symptoms appear insidiously and gradually progress for weeks to months prior to diagnosis. Occasionally PCP presents with asthma-like symptoms of chest tightness and wheezing. A definitive diagnosis requires microscopic visualization of *Pneumocystis carinii* cysts or trophic forms. Physical examination of the lung is normal in approximately 50% of cases, with fine rales, rhonchi, or wheezes audible at times. The WBC count varies with immune status, use of bone marrow suppressive treatments, and presence of concurrent illness. LDH is elevated in most patients with PCP, but this test is nonspecific. The most common chest radiographic findings in PCP are diffuse, bilateral interstitial infiltrates, with occasional thin-walled cysts also visible. Pulmonary function testing reveals a decreased diffusion capacity in the majority of patients. A presumptive diagnosis of PCP requires (1) a history of dyspnea on exertion or nonproductive cough within the last 3 months, (2) either a chest radiograph or a gallium scan with evidence

Table 12.1 AIDS-Indicating Conditions in the United States, 1994[6]

Indicator Conditions	N	%
Pneumocystis carinii pneumonia	15,187	19.1
Bacterial pneumonia	2,252	2.8
Pulmonary *Mycobacterium tuberculosis*	3,392	4.3
Kaposi's sarcoma	3,467	4.4

of diffuse bilateral pulmonary disease, and (3) either an arterial blood gas of less than 70 mmHg or an increased alveolar-arterial oxygen tension gradient or diffusing capacity of less than 80% predicted. Severity of PCP is classified by degree of alveolar oxygen pressure (PaO_2) and A-a gradient abnormality. PCP severity is mild if PaO_2 is >70 mmHg or the A-a gradient is ≥35 mmHg; and moderate to severe if the PaO_2 is ≤70 mmHg or the A-a gradient is ≥35 mmHg. Degree of hypoxemia measured by PaO_2 may correlate roughly with the severity of dyspnea reported by the patient, especially dyspnea during exertion. (See Chapter 5 for PCP prevention and treatment.)

Bacterial Pneumonia

Recurrent bacterial pneumonia became an AIDS index diagnosis in 1993. It may have a higher incidence than PCP. A recent study reported that bacterial pneumonia accounted for 45.5% of admissions for HIV-infected persons hospitalized for a respiratory illness, while PCP accounted for 27% of admissions.[8] Bacterial pneumonia can occur and recur at any time during the course of HIV infection and at any CD4 count. The clinical presentation of community-acquired bacterial pneumonia in HIV-infected persons is similar to that seen in immunocompetent individuals. The most common symptoms are acute onset of fever, shaking chills, and cough productive of purulent sputum. Some patients also complain of pleuritic-type chest pain. Physical examination of the chest reveals the classic signs of focal lung consolidation, including decreased or absent breath sounds; flat percussion note; and egophony, bronchophony, and/or whispered pectoriloquy on auscultation. The WBC count is often elevated with a large increase in the number of immature white blood cells (polys). Arterial blood gas analysis reveals evidence of hypoxemia and respiratory alkalosis. The chest x-ray reveals focal disease with segmental, lobar, or multilobar consolidation. Diagnosis depends on clinical presentation, identification of organisms by sputum Gram stain, and blood cultures. Pneumonia produces a localized severe mismatch of ventilation to perfusion, resulting in hypoxemia, which causes dyspnea.

Cryptococcal Pneumonia

Cryptococcal pneumonia is the most common systemic fungal infection affecting the lungs in persons with HIV. Fever, cough, and dyspnea are the most common signs and symptoms of cryptococcal pneumonia, although pleuritic chest pain and productive cough occur occasionally. Symptoms are often subtle, nonspecific, and indistinguishable from those characteristic of other respiratory illnesses. Findings on physical examination are also nonspecific, with occasional fine rales. The most sensitive diagnostic laboratory test is serum cryptococcal antigen. Chest X-ray most often shows diffuse, bilateral interstitial infiltrates but this is also not specific to cryptococcal pneumonia. Definitive diagnosis is made by culture of *Cryptococcus neoformans* from sputum, bronchial alveolar lavage fluid, or transbronchial biopsy. Dyspnea associated with cryptococcal pneumonia results from hypoxemia and restriction of involved areas of the lung.

Pulmonary TB

Mycobacterial TB occurs frequently in HIV-infected persons but more often presents with fever and productive cough rather than dyspnea. Because cough is the presenting symptom, refer to the section entitled Cough later in this chapter.

Pulmonary KS

KS is the most common malignancy affecting HIV-infected homosexual or bisexual men. (See Chapter 6.) The most common visceral sites of KS involvement are the GI tract and lungs. Pulmonary KS most often presents with nonproductive cough, dyspnea, and fever. Signs of lung involvement noted on physical examination vary with the site of the KS lesions and the degree of airflow obstruction. The chest X-ray is abnormal with evidence of bronchial wall thickening, nodules, Kurley B lines, and/or pleural effusions. Pulmonary KS is diagnosed by bronchoscopy and biopsy. Visualization of multiple, cherry-red raised lesions in the trachea or at the bifurcations of airways is considered diagnostic of KS. These lesions can cause both intraluminal airflow obstruction and extrinsic compression and restriction of the lung due to tumor and lymph node enlargement. Dyspnea associated with KS results from increased metabolic demands, altered gas exchange, and decreased lung compliance.

Presentation and Assessment

The differential diagnosis of dyspnea can be approached by thinking of the three major physiologic categories of etiology:

1. Conditions that increase the work of breathing, such as airway narrowing, decreased lung compliance, and increased minute ventilation caused by hypoxemia
2. Reduced respiratory muscle function, such as weakness or fatigue of the inspiratory muscles
3. Abnormal central perception, such as occurs during anxiety, panic, and depression

Subjective

Like pain, dyspnea is a subjective symptom that can only be rated accurately by the person who is experiencing it. Direct measurement of dyspnea can only be self-report. Objective measures, such as pulmonary function tests, are indirect. They are used to detect the presence of physiological dysfunction as a cause of dyspnea. As with all symptoms, important characteristics to identify are onset (sudden or gradual), pattern (variable or constant), and duration; quality (what it feels like, intensity on a scale of 1–10); location (areas of the body affected); setting (what the patient was doing when the symptom occurred); associated manifestations (other symptoms or sensations that occurred at the same time); aggravating factors (what makes it worse); and alleviating factors (what makes it better).

INSTRUMENTS TO MEASURE DYSPNEA. The simplest yet least sensitive measurement of dyspnea is to ask that patient whether he or she is short of breath. This yes-no categorization is the method used most frequently, however it does not give information about the nature and extent of the symptom.

The instruments most frequently used and validated to measure dyspnea in conscious patients are the Visual Analogue Scale (VAS; Figure 12.1) and the Modified Borg Scale (MBS; Table 12.2).

The VAS is a vertical or horizontal 0- to 100-mm line anchored at either end by descriptive words such as "not at all breathless" to "worst imaginable breathlessness." The patient marks the line at the point representing

Not at all breathless	____________________	Worst imaginable breathlessness

Figure 12.1 The Visual Analogue Scale

Table 12.2 Modified Borg Scale for Measuring Dyspnea

Rating	Description
0	Nothing at all
0.5	Very, very slight (just noticeable)
1	Very slight
2	Slight
3	Moderate
4	Somewhat severe
5	Severe
6	Severe
7	Very severe
8	Very severe
9	Very, very severe (almost maximal)
10	Maximal

Used with permission. Burdon, JGW, Juniper, EF, Killian, KJ, et al. The perception of Breathlessness is Asthma. *Am Rev Resp* Dis 1982; 126:835–828 Figure 1.

the degree of dyspnea felt.[9] It is important to specify the time frame you wish the patient to rate, such as "rate how short of breath you are right now" or "rate how short of breath you have been over the last 24 hours." The MBS is a categorical scale in which numbers from 0 on the top to 10 on the bottom are labeled with words describing degrees of shortness of breath.[10] The VAS and MBS correlate (r = .90)[11] and have similar attributes and reproducibility.[12] When taking the patient's history, dyspnea can be measured indirectly by the minimum level of activity that is associated with the subjective report of shortness of breath. This approach is especially useful for people with chronic dyspnea. Severity of breathlessness can be assessed by asking patients what level of activity brings on their shortness of breath (SOB). (Table 12.3).[13] One other measures of dyspnea based on assessment of functional impairment is the Baseline Dyspnea Index (BDI) and the Transition Dyspnea Index (TDI), which has been developed and tested extensively.[13] The BDI includes five grades that reflect increasing severity of dyspnea for each of three categories: functional impairment, magnitude of task, and magnitude of effort. Ratings for each

Table 12.3 American Thoracic Society Grade of Breathlessness Scale

Grade	Degree	Activity Causing Dyspnea
0	None	Not troubled with breathlessness except with strenuous exercise
1	Slight	Troubled by shortness of breath when hurrying on the level or walking up a slight hill
2	Moderate	Walks slower than people of the same age on the level because of breathlessness or has to stop for breath when walking at own pace on the level
3	Severe	Stops for breath after walking about 100 yards or after a few minutes on the level
4	Very severe	Too breathless to leave the house or breathless when dressing or undressing

From Brooks, S.M. Task group on surveillance for respiratory hazards in the occupational setting. *ATS News* 1982; 8:12–16. Reprinted with permission.

category, ranging from 0 to 4, are determined by an interviewer following specific criteria. The TDI is used to evaluate breathlessness ratings from the baseline condition (BDI) of each category. Ratings for each category of the BDI on the TDI range from +3 (major improvement) to −3 (major deterioration). This instrument has been tested for reliability and related to physiological lung function, oxygen consumption, exercise capacity, and the efficacy of medical therapies.

Dyspnea with changing activities and emotional situations can be monitored by the patient at home. A daily log to monitor shortness of breath has been used successfully to evaluate changes in the therapeutic regimen, to target breathing strategies, and to prescribe energy conversation depending on the intensity of dyspnea and its triggers. At the initial visit, a baseline dyspnea measurement can be obtained with a VAS or MBS. The worst and usual dyspnea level with and without activity should be measured at each clinic visit to determine patterns over time, seasonal variation, with varying activities, and in different environments. Scales to measure dyspnea with activities are reviewed in depth elsewhere.[14]

Recently, a clinical score based on respiratory rate, degree of fever, cough, dyspnea, chest tightness, and chest radiographic findings was reported that predicts early death from *P. carinii* pneumonia in HIV-infected patients.[15] The clinical score is based on respiratory rate, cough frequency, degree of chest tightness, degree of dyspnea, need for supplemental oxygen, body temperature, and chest radiographic findings, and is shown in Table 12.4. The score is a sum of each item and ranges from 0 to 53. This clinical score was found to differentiate between survivors and nonsurvivors at 45 days of treatment and is thought to be useful in predicting PCP treatment failure.

Objective

Observable signs or pulmonary function measures can be used as additional indirect measures of dyspnea to compare with the subjective rating or to estimate shortness of breath if the patient is unable to communicate.

OBSERVABLE MANIFESTATIONS. Signs or manifestations that are observable to others and indicative of increased work of breathing or changes in breathing pattern are often associated with shortness of breath. Healthy subjects and patients with chronic obstructive pulmonary disease (COPD) who use accessory neck and rib cage muscles for ventilation are more likely to report an increase in the sensation of dyspnea.[16] An increase in minute ventilation and respiratory rate alone has been associated with an increase in dyspnea in normal subjects and in hospitalized patients.[17,18]

Behaviors or observable signs associated with dyspnea include increased respiratory rate; restlessness; diaphoresis; use of accessory respiratory muscles; labored breathing; rapid and open mouth breathing; audible wheezing; gasping breaths; coughing; pallor; interrupted or "staccato" speech; tremulousness; large, staring eyes; a frozen immobile position; and appearing withdrawn and uncommunicative. Use of learned strategies, such as pursed lip breathing, may also be objective manifestations of increasing dyspnea. Physiological correlates that can be used in the indirect measurement of dyspnea include lung volumes and flows, and arterial blood gas changes.

PULMONARY FUNCTION TESTS. Diagnostic and periodic lung function testing can provide important data on lung capabilities over time, and indicates progression of disease and/or response to treatment. Lung diffusion studies are useful to assess progression of interstitial lung diseases, such as PCP. Spirometric measures of airflow, such as the forced vital capacity and forced expiratory volume in 1 second, are useful to detect

Table 12.4 PCP Prognostic Score

Parameter	Score
Respiratory rate	0 = ≤16/min 2 = 17–22/min 4 = 23–28/min 6 = 29–39/min 8 = ≥40/min
Cough	0 = None 1 = Mild: coughing less than 1/15 min 2 = Moderate: between 1/15 min and 1/5 min, and cough interfering with sleep 3 = Severe: 1 or more/5 min and cough interfering with both conversation and sleep
Chest tightness	0 = None 1 = Mild 2 = Moderate: present but does not interfere with daily activities 3 = Severe: constant, noticeable with every breath or conversion limiting
Dyspnea	0 = None 2 = Forced to slow walking pace 4 = Forced to interrupt walking 6 = Forced to stop every few minutes or after about 9 meters 8 = Breathlessness with dressing or undressing 10 = Breathlessness at rest
Supplemental oxygen	0 = No supplemental oxygen required for comfort 2 = FI_{O2} of 22–30% (1–2 l O_2/min nasal cannula) 4 = FI_{O2} of 31–40% (3–4 l O_2/min nasal cannula) 6 = FI_{O2} of 41–50% (5–6 l O_2/min nasal cannula) 8 = FI_{O2} of 50–100% or in need of mechanical ventilation
Fever	0 = <37.6°C 2 = >37.6 but <38.5°C 4 = >38.6 but <39.5°C 6 = >39.6°C
Chest radiograph	Entry: 0 = Normal, 6 = Abnormal Follow-up: 0 = Changes resolved, 3 = Improvement since entry, 9 = Worsening since entry

O_2 = oxygen; FI_{O2} = fraction of inspired oxygen concentration.

Adapted from Vanhems P, Tome E. Evaluation of a Prognostic Score for *Pneumocystis carinii* Pneumonia in HIV-infected Patients. *Chest* 1995; 107: 97–112.

bronchial obstruction to airflow, such as that caused by endobronchial lesions or airway inflammation.

In summary, many parameters that have been observed clinically when patients are experiencing dyspnea now have been validated in the laboratory or clinical setting. The following objective physiological measures can be used to measure indirectly and thus estimate shortness of breath: (1) increased respiratory rate and tidal volume, (2) use of accessory muscle, (3) paradoxical and dysynchronous breathing, (4) hypoxia, (5) hypercapnia, (6) decreased forced expiratory volume (FEV1), and (7) fatigue.[19] If the patient is unable to rate shortness of breath, these indirect objective manifestations can be used to estimate the dyspnea felt by the patient. Any of these may be important but the severity of aberration in any one of them should alert the clinician to trouble.

Related Medical Management

The medical management of HIV-associated dyspnea depends on making the correct diagnosis of the infectious cause and beginning appropriately selected treatment early. Dyspnea often diminishes soon after beginning appropriate treatment for the underlying cause. Recurrence or exacerbation of dyspnea usually indicates recurrent or new OI. Treatment of pulmonary opportunistic infections is described in detail in the section on treatment of opportunistic infections (See Chapter 5.)

Oxygen therapy decreases respiratory drive and ventilation during rest and exercise, and some investigators have found that individuals with COPD can walk farther and are less breathless when breathing higher than room air oxygen concentrations.[20] Clinically, hypoxemic patients with COPD have been shown to experience a significant reduction in dyspnea and an increase in their quality of life when on a regimen of low-flow oxygen.[21] However, not all hypoxemic patients experience reduced dyspnea with oxygen therapy. Although the value of oxygen therapy is accepted in chronically hypoxemic patients, the value of oxygen for the relief of dyspnea when the PaO_2 is above 55 to 60 mmHg is less apparent. In a British study,[20] however, supplemental oxygen was shown to increase walking distance and improve exercise-induced dyspnea in patients with chronic lung disease and near normal resting PaO_2 values.

Opiates, especially morphine, decrease the perception and increase tolerance of breathlessness in many patients with chronic persistent dyspnea due to chronic lung conditions.[22] Morphine can be given by several routes. Doses are usually started low and increased until relief is obtained. Potential benefits such as decreased respiratory drive, improved efficiency of exercise, and decreased dyspnea may be offset clinically by the risk of respiratory depression and side effects, although the actual incidence of respiratory depression has been low in most studies.[22] Therefore, the risks of using morphine to control dyspnea are minimal and the potential benefit is large. If morphine is prescribed for severe dyspnea, the patient should start slowly with a low dose of approximately 4 mg/ml under constant supervision until there is a measured decrease in dyspnea.[23] Morphine sulfate has long been a standard treatment for pain in end-stage lung cancer patients. The efficacy of this medication in relieving severe dyspnea in lung cancer or end-stage pulmonary disease is being studied and is often used to relieve intractable dyspnea as death nears. Both oxygen and opiate therapy may be appropriate interventions for treatment of unrelenting severe dyspnea in end-stage HIV, although neither have been specifically studied in people with AIDS. In addition, these therapies may be appropriate earlier in the disease for those patients who are bothered so much by dyspnea that their quality of life has deteriorated. The decision of when to use opiate therapy depends on clinical judgment and the agreement of the individual patient.

Interventions

Prevention

The best way to prevent or minimize severe dyspnea is to teach and encourage patients to use strategies to conserve energy by simplifying work, to relax during periods of difficult breathing, and to pace themselves and control the rate and depth of breathing. This approach is very important if dyspnea interferes significantly with ADLs.

Breathing Strategies

PURSED LIPS BREATHING (PLB). PLB decreases dyspnea in some patients, probably because it makes them breathe in more slowly and exhale more completely, thereby decreasing the respiratory rate and increasing the tidal volume.[24,25] If patients are to benefit from PLB they should be instructed to perform the following steps:

1. Breathe in normally through the nose while counting to two.
2. Purse lips as if about to whistle.
3. Breathe out slowly through pursed lips, while counting to four or take at least twice as long to exhale as inhale.

If patients can successfully perform PLB, they should be instructed to use it during exertion and coordinate movement with exhalation. If patients are unable to purse their lips, they can be instructed to exhale through a fist held up to their mouths. Patients should be warned not to breathe too deeply, which can cause dizziness and not to exhale too vigorously because forced exhalations increase airway collapse and may trigger bronchospasm. Most patients with chronic lung disease adopt a PLB pattern naturally, indicating that it is a physiologically adaptive response. However, PLB is not helpful for all dyspneic patients. Individuals with HIV who have restrictive processes in the lung, such as pneumonia, may not be helped by PLB.

PACED BREATHING. Paced breathing is the coordination of inspiration and PLB during expiration with activities such as walking, stair climbing, and bending. Activities are paced to match ventilatory capacity. The patient is instructed to (1) breathe in while at rest before performing a strenuous activity, such as lifting an object, and (2) exhale slowly and gently through pursed lips while doing the work. The patient should be encouraged to focus on the prolonged exhalation and should be warned not to hold his breath, because breath holding during exertion constitutes a Valsalva-like maneuver. This increases intrathoracic pressure and impairs cardiac return, contributing to a subsequent drop in cardiac output that can actually increase dyspnea and perceived effort.

Position Changes

Position changes decrease the intensity of dyspnea for some individuals. Patients should be allowed to choose the most comfortable position for activities and to sit whenever possible, avoiding bending or stooping. Standing still, finding a "breathing station," having some place to sit or lean, or just being "motionless," "keeping still," or "staying quiet" are behaviors that other people have described to help them decrease their shortness of breath. Patients will usually discover for themselves their "best" position for physiological benefit and should be encouraged to assume this position whenever dyspnea occurs or increases. The "leaning forward" position with the arms supported on a table often helps relieve dyspnea. This position permits the abdominal organs to drop away from the diaphragm, promoting better diaphragmatic excursion, increasing accessory muscle use, and stabilizing the upper chest while still allowing freedom of movement of the lower chest.[26]

Relaxation Techniques

Relaxation can take many forms depending on patient choice. Most relaxation methods include a quiet environment, comfortable position, loose clothing, some type of word or imagery repeated in a systematic fashion, slow abdominal breathing with deep breaths and slow expirations, and systematic tensing or relaxing of muscles while concentrating on the muscles. Individualized tape recordings by a therapist can be used to coach patients through a session in the home.[27]

PANIC CONTROL MEASURES. The panic that may accompany the sensation of dyspnea often exacerbates the sensation. It may be possible to help the patient control panic by initial rapid, panting respirations, then gradually coaching the patient, breath by breath, to slow the respiratory rate by extending the expiratory time. This kind of breath-by-breath coaching should continue until the patient relaxes.[28]

DISTRACTION. Active distraction can increase tolerance and decrease psychological distress from dyspnea. During acute dyspnea, distraction is often effective because it is difficult to focus on two activities at once. Listening to music can distract people from their breathing and thus help them to relax.

GUIDED IMAGERY. Guided imagery is a form of distraction that is used for the management of many chronic symptoms, including pain and nausea. Patients are instructed to close their eyes, assume a comfortable position, and allow their minds to visualize a pleasant scene as a standard guided imagery script is read.[29] Although the effectiveness of this strategy remains unproved, it may be clinically helpful for some patients.

Additional Strategies for Chronic Dyspnea

Adjunct strategies may help the patient live with the symptom and possibly decrease symptom intensity when dyspnea becomes a chronic problem.

EXERCISE. Patients with shortness of breath are often reluctant to exercise or to perform daily activities. A cycle of decreasing activity and increasing dyspnea results in deconditioning of skeletal muscles. Muscles that are "deconditioned" use more oxygen so that deconditioning may make patients feel increasingly short of breath with activity. Exercise helps "condition" muscles so that oxygen is used efficiently, and exercise has been shown to decrease dyspnea in chronic lung disease.[30,31] If exercise conditioning is undertaken, it is important to spend time doing "quality exercise" that conditions and tones skeletal muscles.

In persons with chronic lung disease, increasing the amount and duration of exercise has been found to decrease the anxiety and panic that sometimes occurs with increasing shortness of breath.[32] Walking with a supportive, trusted friend may decrease the fear of dyspnea while building confidence in the ability to control it. The friend or relative can act as a "coach" by reinforcing the learned breathing strategies and providing encouragement.[33] Distractions of any kind such as music, TV, or reading have been found to help people to continue to exercise.

Information for the Patient

Education

Although the effect of education on dyspnea is unknown, knowledge about what causes the symptom and what is "appropriate" may decrease anxiety, fear, and pain. When patients are given information about their illness or dyspnea management, anxiety decreases while feelings of well-being and confidence increase.[34] Knowledge may decrease dyspnea by increasing the patients' belief that they can control the symptom with the techniques they have learned. Clinically, it has been observed that the perception of personal self-efficacy or control does help buffer pain, and presumably this is also true of dyspnea.[35] When patients believe they have behavioral strategies to cope with a distressing symptom, the distress associated with that symptom is diminished.[36]

An organized problem-solving approach should be used with patients to help them develop strategies to cope with dyspnea. The nurse and patient should build on what the patient already does to decrease shortness of breath, extending and expanding these skills with strategies known by the clinician. Describing the sensations related to dyspnea helps patients believe they have control by clarifying what they should expect, showing them how important their role is in decreasing the symptom, finding meaning in the symptom for them, and acknowledging the importance of techniques they have learned on their own.

Patients should be taught about the nature of the symptom itself and the pathophysiologic processes that may be the reason for the onset of their dyspnea. As with all coping strategies, knowledge about each medication and its role in decreasing dyspnea is important because patients often manipulate multiple medications daily. Education during subsequent visits should cover all strategies previously described, such as PLB, breathing exercises, energy conservation, graduated exercise regimens, relaxation, and panic control. It is most important to listen to the patient and family to (1) tailor information to their concerns, (2) answer questions they may have about what they can do and how short of breath they can be, and (3) support any strategies they have developed on their own.

Social Support

It is generally accepted that social support is positively associated with desirable health outcomes and buffers stress in chronic diseases and stressful situations. It is frequently recommended as an intervention to improve psychological and physical health. Chronic lung symptoms often decrease social interaction and may produce isolation. In a recent meta-analysis of several research studies on social support and health, the availability and adequacy of social support were the most important factors in determining overall perception of health.[37] Many people develop extensive networks and resources that provide a high level of social support.[38] However, it is important to remember that each individual will have a personal interpretation of what is helpful and supportive.

Some patients find help in structured support groups that give people the opportunity to see that they are not alone and to learn strategies from others who have been coping with chronic dyspnea. Family and significant others also find great benefits in attending support groups and hearing from others. Being with others who have the same problems and who have tested successful ways to decrease the symptom can be a powerful confidence-building experience.[39]

Other patients with dyspnea isolate themselves. They begin to limit their interactions with friends and family either because social interaction is fatiguing or their shortness of breath prevents them from participating in recreational activities that provided the basis for their network of friends and social resources. People may sometimes benefit from isolating themselves from others in certain situations. Permission to withdraw and isolate oneself in periods of severe dyspnea can be helpful both physically and psychologically.

Activity Modification and Energy Conservation

For people with chronic, severe shortness of breath, learning to pace activities, slow down, and conserve energy are difficult tasks. Patients may have made or need to make major lifestyle changes as shortness of breath begins to affect their tolerance of activities. Activities can be substituted that are pleasurable but require less effort. For example, a walking regimen can replace more strenuous exercise.

Crucial balance is required between pacing or resting and appropriate exercise. A "daily outline," can be used to divide the day into morning, afternoon, late afternoon, and early evening. After deciding what daily tasks must be done, they can be divided across the day, leaving time for scheduled rests and pleasurable activities. Rest periods are a high priority. Frequent, short rest periods are of more benefit than fewer long rests because they prevent undue fatigue and allow more energy for other activities. HIV-infected patients with dyspnea should be counseled to stop working and to rest before exhaustion.

Graduated exercise to stay physically conditioned can continue even though patients may need to move at a slower pace. It is important to teach patients to save energy for small tasks while delegating those that can be done by others. Rushing through activities only increases dyspnea and should be avoided. Selection of strategies for simplifying work and conserving energy should be individualized for patient needs, severity of dyspnea, and living situation.

Potential self-care strategies for minimizing shortness of breath include:

- Sit during as many activities as possible, such as when you brush your teeth or apply makeup.

- Shower rather than bathing, using a chair in the shower.
- Intersperse activities with frequent rest periods.
- Sit on the edge of the bed or chair to dress, dressing the lower body first, and use slip-on shoes.
- Organize tasks and break them down into small steps.
- Avoid rushing through tasks, which may increase dyspnea.
- To change the bed, change one side at a time. Start with the bottom sheet, top sheet, blanket, and spread on one side and continue to the other side.
- For meal preparation, gather all necessary food and utensils from cupboards and the refrigerator. Use PLB for reaching and moving supplies. Break activities into several steps. Put a stool in the kitchen so meal preparation can be done sitting down, and allow plenty of time to avoid rushing.

Cough

Definition

Cough is the forceful expulsion of air from the lungs. Stimulation of the cough reflex results in inspiration, glottic closure, and tightening of abdominal and intercostal muscles. As a result, positive pleural pressures reach as high as 100 to 200 mmHg, producing the forceful exhalation.

Biologic and Behavioral Basis

Cough is initiated by stimulation of irritant receptors at any of a number of locations. The irritant receptors are found primarily in the upper airway (nose, sinuses, and pharynx) and lower airway (larynx, trachea, and major bronchi at points of bifurcation). Cough receptors are particularly dense in the central airways. Afferent cough signals reach the brain via the trigeminal, glossopharyngeal, superior laryngeal, or vagus nerves.

Etiologies Related to HIV Infection and Its Medical Treatment

The major causes of cough in HIV-infected individuals are inflammatory processes in the airways caused by infection, endobronchial lesions, and parenchymal disease. In addition, some treatments cause cough. The most notable is the cough caused by inhaled pentamidine for prophylaxis of PCP.

Mycobacterium tuberculosis is an important and virulent respiratory pathogen in patients with AIDS. The organism may not require the same degree of immunosuppression to produce disease as other OIs.[40] Pulmonary TB tends to occur in groups of persons with a high background prevalence of TB, such as IV drug users, indigent and immigrant populations, and those living in crowded conditions. HIV infection increases the risk of developing both primary and reactivated TB. HIV-infected persons exposed to *M. tuberculosis* can develop TB rapidly.[41] The clinical presentation is similar to that seen in patients without HIV infection and develops insidiously rather than acutely. Although most patients with HIV infection manifest either systemic symptoms or pulmonary symptoms, TB can present with no symptoms and merely an abnormal chest x-ray. Systemic symptoms include fever, night sweats, weight loss, anorexia, and fatigue. Pulmonary symptoms consist of cough, sputum production, hemoptysis, and occasionally chest pain. Physical examination sometimes reveals crackles or rales over the affected areas of the lung. Sometimes evidence of pleural effusion is present. Diagnosis is made by sputum smear and culture. HIV-infected patients with TB tend to die sooner and progress to AIDS faster than HIV-infected patients without TB.[42]

Presentation and Assessment

Subjective

History is the key to diagnosis of cough. It is important to elicit information about precipitating causes, time of onset, association with sputum production, frequency, current pharmacologic and nonpharmacologic treatments, and past history of respiratory illnesses. Cough is described as dry or wet; productive or nonproductive; and hacking, coarse, or barking. Cough is a common presenting complaint in HIV-associated pulmonary conditions. A brief questionnaire has been described recently that allows rapid assessment for the presence of 12 common symptoms of HIV-related infection, including cough and dyspnea.[43]

Objective

The physical examination must be an active exam to diagnose cough, which means you need to listen to the patient cough while you are examining the chest. It is important to listen to the cough and note its frequency and quality. Note whether respiratory maneuvers, such as deep breathing, precipitate coughing. If they do, it suggests interstitial lung disease. The upper airway should be carefully inspected, including the nose, for drainage, throat for visible mucus, and sinuses for tenderness. Drainage from the nose and sinuses into the back of the throat is a frequent cause of cough and, if identified, directs treatment. Decreased breath sounds and the presence of rales, rhonchi, and wheezes are of obvious importance in detecting lung disease, and suggest the etiology of cough is parenchymal lung processes. Beyond the physical exam, sputum analysis and chest X-ray are the most useful tests to search for an infectious cause of cough. Gross examination of sputum is preferable to reliance on the patient's descriptions. Microscopic examination of sputum will show the presence of white cells and bacteria. Sputum culture is necessary to diagnose bacterial, mycobacterial, or fungal infections.

Differential Diagnosis

Cough is usually due to increased or abnormal mucus, stimulation of cough receptors by secretions or organisms, aspiration of mucus or gastric contents, or psychological factors, such as anxiety. Any of these causes are relevant to HIV infection and the diagnosis of OI. A new cough or a change in cough may be associated with an acute infectious process, such as bronchitis or pneumonia.[44] Chronic cough is usually a symptom of a chronic disease process, such as chronic airway inflammation or chronic bronchitis.[44] Coughing may also be caused by non-HIV problems, such as exposure to allergens or irritants, postnasal drip, aspiration, pulmonary lesions, pneumonia, or TB. Timing of the cough may suggest further diagnostic possibilities that complicate the clinical picture of HIV. A nocturnal cough suggests asthma, heart failure, or esophageal reflux. Cough with deep breathing or laughing is common in patients with interstitial lung processes or airway inflammation. Worsening of cough in certain specific environments may be due to exposure to allergens or airway irritants. Some medications cause cough through a variety of mechanisms. Cough in association with fever and night sweats suggests TB or bacterial pneumonia. Sputum production and hemoptysis may occur with pulmonary infection and pneumonia. Dark-yellow or green sputum suggest ongoing lower respiratory bacterial infection. Hemoptysis occurs with pneumonia but can also be caused by erosion of small capillaries of endobronchial lesions.

Sinusitis is a very important cause of postnasal drip and cough in HIV-infected individuals. Purulent nasal discharge and pain or fullness over the sinuses are helpful signs of sinusitis.

Related Medical Management

Treatment of cough is most effective when it is directed at its underlying cause. The treatment of PCP, bacterial pneumonia, and TB will often greatly improve if not eradicate coughing. Persistent cough due to lung disease that cannot be eradicated requires nonspecific therapy, such as expectorants, cough suppressants, airway rest, and reassurance. Expectorants and humidification are popular, but there is no convincing proof of their efficacy. Cough suppression can be attempted with dextromethorphan 15 to 60 mg three to four times daily, codeine 15 to 30 mg every 6 hours, or local anesthetics such as nebulized lidocaine. Airway rest is accomplished with a period of bed rest and sedation, and many patients report decreased cough when this is accomplished. Opiates such as codeine and morphine are used widely for the palliative treatment of symptoms in end-stage HIV infection, including both dyspnea and cough.[45]

Interventions

Prevention

In patients subject to persistent, recurrent coughing, sudden respiratory maneuvers should be avoided or minimized. Patients are the best judge of what triggers prolonged coughing episodes and they will develop their own strategies for avoiding stimulation of cough. In patients receiving aerosolized pentamidine, pretreatment with a beta agonist bronchodilator can relieve cough and enhance uniform pentamidine distribution.[46]

Acute

Acute, severe coughing suggests a change in disease status and the need for prompt reevaluation. New infectious processes can trigger cough and will respond better to treatment if intervention occurs early.[47] Acute onset of cough may be alarming, triggering fear and panic about the possible cause. Reassurance and encouragement to seek treatment are important first-line nursing interventions.

If abnormal secretions are present, interventions to promote airway clearance may be needed, including (1) therapeutic coughing, (2) forced exhalation techniques, (3) abdominal push maneuver, and (4) postural drainage. Therapeutic coughing is accomplished by having the patient sit upright, inhale deeply and slowly, and lean forward while producing two or three short coughs on the same exhalation. Forced exhalation or *huffing* enhances secretion clearance in patients who have large quantities of sputum. This technique consists of a series of short, quick exhalations (huffs) following a slow, deep inhalation and a short breath hold. In patients who are very weak, an assistant can perform an abdominal push to assist airway clearance by pushing on the abdomen during forced exhalation following a deep inspiration. Postural drainage consists of positioning the patient so that gravity enhances the drainage of lung segments. This may be difficult to accomplish if the patient is very dyspneic, but postural drainage is still practiced as an effective measure for draining peripheral portions of the lung.

Chronic

When there is not a therapeutic purpose to coughing, such as clearing mucus from the airways, chronic, persistent coughing can be debilitating. Reassurance and support are helpful, but every effort must be made to find an effective method of cough suppression. Concerns about potential respiratory depression from narcotics are misplaced when the goal is to provide comfort and palliation to a suffering patient. The combination of cough suppression with bed rest and sedation may interrupt the cycle of chronic coughing and allow a period of rest and relief. In some patients who have spirometric and bronchoscopic evidence of airway inflammation, cough will improve with steroid therapy.[48] Corticosteroid therapy is recommended as adjuvant therapy for PCP when PaO_2 is <70 mmHg or the alveolar-arterial oxygen tension gradient is >35 mmHg (i.e., moderate to severe PCP). It reduces the occurrence of respiratory failure and may improve survival when given over 2 to 3 weeks as a burst with a tapering dose (i.e., 40 mg PO bid for 5 days, 20 mg PO bid for 5 days, then 20 mg PO qd to the end of therapy).[49,50]

In summary, dyspnea and cough are common, frequent manifestations of HIV infection. The symptoms are reduced with early etiologic diagnosis and intervention. When they become chronic, debilitating symptoms that cause severe distress, every attempt should be made to provide amelioration through a combination of pharmacological and nonpharmacological interventions. Many of these strategies can be taught and encouraged in the home care and community setting by nurses who are skilled in the management of chronic illness.

References

1. Comroe JH. Some theories of the mechanisms of dyspnea. In: Howell JB, Campbell EJM, eds. *Breathlessness*. Boston: Blackwell Scientific; 1965:1–7.
2. Killian KJ, Campbell EJM. Mechanisms of dyspnea. In: Mahler DA, ed. *Dyspnea*. Mt. Kisco, NY: Futura Publishing; 1990:55–73
3. Cherniack NS, Altose MD. Mechanisms of dyspnea. *Clin Chest Med*. 1987;9: 237–248.
4. Chronos N, Adams I, Guz A. Effect of hyperoxia and hypoxia on exercise-induced breathlessness in normal subjects. *Clin Sci*. 1988;74:531–537.
5. Bess C, Gardner W. Emotional influences on breathing and breathlessness. *J Psychosom Res*. 1985;29:599–609.
6. CDC. *HIV/AIDS* Surveillance report. Atlanta: US Department of Health and Human Services, Public Health Service, CDC, 1995:3–4, 30–4 (Vol 7, no. 1).
7. CDC. 1993 revised classification system for HIV infection and expanded surveillance case definition for AIDS among adolescents and adults. *MMWR*. 1992; 41(RR-17):1–19.
8. Magnenat JL, Nicod LP, Auckenthaler R, Junod AF. Mode of presentation and diagnosis of bacterial pneumonia in human immunodeficiency virus-infected patients. *Am Rev Respir Dis*. 1991;144:917–922.
9. Cockcroft A, Adams L, Guz A. Assessment of breathlessness. *QJM*. 1989;72: 669–676.
10. Burdon J, Juniper E, Killian K, Hargreave F, Campbell E. The perception of breathlessness in asthma. *Am Rev Respir Dis*. 1982;126:825–828.
11. Lush M, Janson-Bjerklie S, Carrieri V, Lovejoy N. Dyspnea in the ventilator-assisted patient. *Heart Lung*. 1988;17:528–535.
12. Wilson RC, Jones PW. A comparison of the Visual Analogue Scale and Modified Borg Scale for the measurement of dyspnea during exercise. *Clin Sci*. 1989; 76:277–282.
13. Mayler DA, Guyatt GH, Jones PW. Clinical measurement of dyspnea. In: DA Mahler, ed. *Dyspnea*. New York: Marcel Dekker, 1998:149–181.
14. ACCP/ACVPR Pulmonary Rehabilitation Guidelines Panel. Pulmonary Rehabilitation. *Chest* 112(5):1363–96.
15. Vanhems P, Toma E. Evaluation of a prognostic score for *Pneumocystis carinii* pneumonia in HIV-infected patients. *Chest*. 1995;107:107–112.

16. Breslin EH, Garoutte BC, Carrieri VK, Celli BR. Correlations between dyspnea, diaphragm, and sternomastoid recruitment during respiratory resistive breathing in normal subjects. *Chest.* 1990;98:298–302.
17. LeBlanc P, Bowie DM, Summer E, Jones N, Killian K. Breathlessness and exercise in patients with cardiorespiratory disease. *Am Rev Respir Dis.* 1986; 133:21–25.
18. Mahler DA, Faryniarz K, Lentine T, Ward J, Olmstead EM, O'Connor GT. Measurement of breathlessness during exercise in asthmatics. *Am Rev Respir Dis.* 1991;144:39–44.
19. Carrieri-Kohlman V. Dyspnea in the weaning patient: assessment and intervention. *AACN Clin Issues Crit Care Nurs.* 1991;2:462–473.
20. Woodcock AA, Gross ER, Geddes DM. Oxygen relieves breathlessness in "pink puffers." *Lancet.* 1981;i:907–909.
21. Dean NC, Brown JK, Himelman RB, Doherty JJ, Gold WM, Stulbarg MS. Oxygen may improve dyspnea and endurance in patients with chronic obstructive pulmonary disease and only mild hypoxemia. *Am Rev Respir Dis.* 1992;146: 941–945.
22. Light RW, Muro JR, Sato RI, Stansbury DW, Fisher CE, Brown SE. Effects of oral morphine on breathlessness and exercise tolerance in patients with chronic obstructive pulmonary disease. *Am Rev Respir Dis.* 1986;139: 126–133.
23. Stulbarg MS, Belman MJ, Ries AC. Treatment of dyspnea: physical modalities, oxygen, and pharmacology. In DA Mahler, ed. *Dyspnea.* New York: Marcel Dekker, 1998:321–354.
24. Mueller RE, Petty TL, Filley GF. Ventilation and arterial blood gas changes induced by pursed lips breathing. *J Appl Physiol.* 1970;28:784–789.
25. Thoman RL, Stoker GL, Ross JC. The efficacy of pursed-lips breathing in patients with chronic obstructive pulmonary disease. *Am Rev Respir Dis.* 1966; 93:100–106.
26. Sharp JT, Drutz WS, Moisoan T, Foster J, Machnach W. Postural relief of dyspnea in severe chronic obstructive pulmonary disease. *Am Rev Respir Dis.* 1980;122:201–213.
27. Horsman J. Using tape recordings to overcome panic during dyspnea. *Respir Care.* 1978;23:767–768.
28. Weiser PC, Mailer DA, Ryan KP, Hill KL, Greenspon LW. Dyspnea: symptom assessment and management. In: Hodgkin JE, Connors GL, Bell CW, eds. *Pulmonary Rehabilitation.* Philadelphia: Lippincott; 1993:478–511.
29. Moody LE, Fraser M, Yarandi H. Effects of guided imagery in patients with chronic bronchitis and emphysema. *Clin Nurs Res.* 1993;2:478–486.
30. Ries AL, Kaplan RM, Limberg TM, Prewitt LM. Effects of pulmonary rehabilita-

tion on physiologic and psychosocial outcomes in patients with chronic obstructive pulmonary disease. *Ann Intern Med.* 1995;122:823–832.
31. Reardon J, Awad E, Normandin E, Vale F, Clark B, ZuWallack RL. The effect of comprehensive outpatient pulmonary rehabilitation on dyspnea. *Chest.* 1994; 105:1046–1052.
32. Carrieri-Kohlman V, Douglas MK, Gormley J, Stulbarg MS. Exercise training decreases dyspnea and the distress and anxiety associated with it. *Chest* 1996; 110:1526–35.
33. Carrieri-Kohlman V, Gormley JM, Stulbarg MS. Monitored exercise and coached exercise decrease dyspnea intensity, dyspnea anxiety, and increase walking self-efficacy. *Ann Behav Med.* 1993;15:S168.
34. Hudson LD, Tyler ML, Petty TL. Hospitalization needs during an outpatient rehabilitation program for severe chronic airway obstruction. *Chest.* 1976;70: 606–610.
35. Goldstein RS, Girt EH, Avendano MAA, Guyatt GH. Randomized controlled trial of respiratory rehabilitation. *Lancet.* 1993;344–397.
36. Thompson SC. Will it hurt less if I can control it? A complex answer to a simple question. *Psychol Bull.* 1981;90:89–101.
37. Smith CE, Fernengel K, Holcroft C, Gerald K, Marien L. Meta-analysis of the associations between social support and health outcomes. *Ann Behav Med.* 1994;16:352–353.
38. Janson-Bjerklie S, Carrieri VK, Hudes M. The sensations of pulmonary dyspnea. *Nurs Res.* 1986;35:154–159.
39. Burkhardt CS. Coping strategies of the chronically ill. *Nurs Clin North Am.* 1987;22:543–550.
40. Barnes PF, Bloch AB, Davidson PT, Snider DE Jr. Tuberculosis in patients with human immunodeficiency virus infection. *N Engl J Med.* 1991;324:1644–1650.
41. Daley CL, Small PM, Schecter GF, et al. An outbreak of tuberculosis with accelerated progression among persons infected with the human immunodeficiency virus. *N Engl J Med.* 1992;326:231–235.
42. Lane HC. Recent advances in the management of AIDS-related opportunistic infections. *Ann Intern Med.* 1994;120(11):945–955.
43. Whalen CC, Antani M, Carey J, Landefeld CS. An index of symptoms for infection with human immunodeficiency virus: reliability and validity. *J Clin Epidemiol.* 1994;47:537–546.
44. Wallace JM, Rao AV, Glassroth J, et al. Respiratory illness in persons with human immunodeficiency virus infection. The Pulmonary Complications of HIV Infection Study Group. *Am Rev Respir Dis.* 1993;148(6, pt 1):1523–1529.
45. George RJ, Robinson VH, Edwards D, Jennings AL. Opiates and symptom

control in end stage HIV disease. Proceedings of Int Conf Aids Jun 6–11;9(1): 518. Abstract PO-B33-2296.
46. Harrison KS, Laube BL. Bronchodilator pretreatment improves aerosol deposition uniformity in HIV-positive patients who cough while inhaling aerosolized pentamidine. *Chest.* 1994;106:421–426.
47. Smith GH. Treatment of infections in the patient with acquired immunodeficiency syndrome. *Arch Intern Med.* 1994;154:949–953.
48. Hammett RJ, Pigott P. Chronic cough in HIV—a retrospective review. Proceedings of Ann Conf Austral Soc HIV Med 1994 Nov 3–6;6:118, 1994.
49. Bozzette SA, Sattler FR, Chiu J, et al. A controlled trial of early adjunctive treatment with corticosteroids for *Pneumocystis carinii* pneumonia in the acquired immunodeficiency syndrome. *N Engl J Med.* 1990;323:1451–1457.
50. Gagnon S, Boota AM, Fischl MA, Baier H, Kirksy OW, LaVoie L. Corticosteroids as adjunctive therapy for severe *Pneumocystis carinii* pneumonia in the acquired immunodeficiency syndrome: a double-blind, placebo-controlled trial. *N Engl J Med.* 1990;323:1444–1450.

CHAPTER 13

Hematologic Abnormalities

Carole S. Viele, RN, MS

Chapter Preview

- Neutropenia
- Thrombocytopenia
- Anemia

Among the hematologic changes experienced by the patient with HIV infection are neutropenia, thrombocytopenia, and anemia. These alterations may be the result of HIV itself, the OIs and malignancies associated with HIV infection, or their treatment.

Neutropenia

Neutropenia is a decrease in the number of circulating neutrophils, which are a subset of leukocytes or WBCs. Leukocytes are responsible for fighting infection, and a normal WBC count ranges from 5,000 to 10,000 cells/mm^3. Neutrophils comprise 50 to 60% of the WBC population.

Etiologies Related to HIV Infection and Its Medical Treatment

Neutropenia is a common complication of HIV infection, often associated with progressive immune suppression.[1] The exact mechanism of this phenomenon is varied and may even be idiopathic. An autoimmune mechanism involving antigranulocytic antibodies and/or impaired granulopoiesis may play a role in the development of neutropenia, however this is not yet proved.[2] In addition, many of the pharmacological therapies for HIV infection are myelosuppressive. Zidovudine in particular is associated with neutropenia, especially in association with other antiviral agents such as ganciclovir. Agents that may induce neutropenia are listed below.

- Zidovudine
- Ganciclovir
- Foscarnet
- Amphotericin
- Flucytosine
- Trimethoprim-sulfamethoxazole
- Pentamidine
- Most antineoplastic agents
- IFN
- Sulfonamides
- Dihydrofolate reductase inhibitors

Presentation and Assessment

Assessment of neutropenia includes regular evaluation of the neutropenic potential of all medications the patient is receiving. Neutropenia is most often asymptomatic, and assessment consists of regular laboratory monitoring. The formula used to calculate the absolute neutrophil count (ANC) to determine if a patient is neutropenic is

$$\text{ANC} = \text{total WBC count} \times \text{percent (neutrophils + bands)}$$

Related Medical Management

The World Health Organization criteria for management of neutropenia are summarized in Table 13.1. The first step in the management of drug-induced neutropenia is lowering the dose or discontinuing potentially myelosuppressive medications. When patients require additional intervention, colony stimulating factors (growth factors) are frequently employed. Both G-CSF and granulocyte/macrophage colony stimulating factor (GM-CSF) have been used in HIV-infected neutropenic patients. However, there is concern that GM-CSF will encourage HIV replication through stimulation of the macrophage line. Infected monocytes and macrophages stimulated with GM-CSF express increased amounts of HIV in vitro.[1] Therefore, G-CSF, a growth factor that stimulates only the granulocyte line and has not been shown to stimulate HIV-infected monocytes or macrophages in vitro,[2] is more commonly used.

Side effects associated with these growth factors range from mild bone pain to fever, myalgias, and pain at the injection site. Occasionally the patient may complain of severe bone pain, requiring the use of nonsteroidal anti-inflammatory agents to ameliorate symptoms. Generally, patients receiving GM-CSF experience more symptoms than those receiving G-CSF.

Nursing Interventions

Nursing management of the neutropenic patient begins with a careful review of all of the patient's medications for potential neutropenic effects and assurance that the patient understands the potential side effects. If a colony stimulating factor is prescribed, the patient needs additional instructions regarding the rationale for therapy, possible side effects, self-injection techniques, storage information, and the importance of site rota-

Table 13.1 World Health Organization Criteria for Neutropenia

Grade	Absolute Neutrophil Count (cells/mm^3)	Risk of Infection	Intervention
I	1,500–2,000	Minimal	None
II	1,000–1,500	Increased	Watchful waiting
III	500–1,000	Increased	Careful monitoring
IV	<500	Significant	Prophylactic antibacterials, growth factors, neutropenic precautions

tion. Patient education should begin before therapy and should include the list below.

- Instructions for self-administration
  - The importance of clean technique and what that entails
  - How to pick an injection site
  - How to clean the site
  - How to evaluate for signs and symptoms of infection
  - Where to document injection sites (calendar, diary, etc.)
  - Noting the date of injection, because all colony stimulating factors are not given daily
- How to draw up medication
- Storage instructions
  - Do not shake
  - Do not freeze
- Safe needle, syringe, and vial disposal (Make sure patient has a needle box at home and knows where to return the box when it is full.)

Although neutropenia is common in the HIV-infected patient, serious bacterial infections as a result of the neutropenia are not. However, extrapolating from other profoundly neutropenic populations, the implementation of strategies to decrease the risk of bacterial infections is prudent. It is imperative that patients, family members, and significant others understand the rationale for these precautions to encourage adherence. The following lists some neutropenic precautions.

- Restrict your diet.
  - No fresh fruits or vegetables
  - All fruits and vegetables should be cleaned and washed prior to cooking
  - No fresh-squeezed juices
  - No unpasteurized milk
  - No raw fish, shellfish, or meat
  - All foods need to be cooked thoroughly
  - If using dried herbs, all products should be cooked or heated to boiling to destroy bacteria
- Avoid crowds and individuals with colds or the flu.
- Avoid fresh flowers, as the water may be contaminated with *Pseudomonas*.

(continued)

- Do not clean litter boxes or handle pet excreta during the period of neutropenia.
- Do not handle soil or plants during periods of neutropenia.
- When working outside, wear a mask to avoid inhaling any organisms, and wear gloves to prevent entry of organisms through cuts or scratches.
- Do not submit to rectal exams or use suppositories.
- Use a good hand-washing technique; that is, wash hands with soap and water for at least 15 seconds (or the time it takes to sing the first verse to "Yankee Doodle Dandy").
- Monitor your body temperature twice a day.

Thrombocytopenia

Thrombocytopenia is a decrease in the number of circulating platelets. Platelets are a key element in the process of clotting, hemostasis, and thrombus formation. A normal platelet count is 150,000 to 350,000 cells/mm^3. The risk of bleeding increases as the platelets fall to <50,000 cells/mm^3, with the risk of life-threatening bleeding occurring when platelets are <10,000 cells/mm^3.

Etiologies Related to HIV Infection and Its Medical Treatment

Thrombocytopenia is a common manifestation of HIV disease. It appears that HIV diminishes the capacity of megakaryocytes to produce platelets during times of increased demand.[1] Whether this is due to viral infection of the marrow or some other mechanism is unknown. A number of other possible etiologies have been described, including immune-mediated destructive, thrombotic thrombocytopenic purpura and impaired hematopoiesis. Impaired hematopoiesis may be the result of any infectious or neoplastic condition involving the bone marrow or may reflect myelosuppression caused by medications. In addition, thrombocytopenia may develop from causes such as alcohol use, splenomegaly, liver disease, recreational drug use, or from the heparin used in vascular access devices.

In the presence of HIV, thrombocytopenia is frequently the result of platelet-associated Ig, which coats platelets, inducing the spleen and the reticuloendothelial system to remove them from circulation, believing them to be foreign agents or "nonself." Typically this is a relatively early phenomenon, and as the immune system deteriorates, an increase in circulating immune complexes and gamma globulin occurs. These circulating proteins flood the spleen and the reticuloendothelial system, resulting in the sparing of platelets, and a spontaneous reversal of the thrombocytopenia may be observed.

Presentation and Assessment

Patients with thrombocytopenia are assessed according to the National Cancer Institute's (NCI) common toxicity criteria.[3] A normal platelet count ranges from 150,000 to 350,000 cells/mm^3. Patients are noted to be thrombocytopenic when platelets drop to $\leq$100,000 cells/mm^3 and exhibit clinically significant symptoms such as recurrent or severe epistaxis, gingival or subconjunctival hemorrhage, or GI hemorrhage. Table 13.2 summarizes the grading scale for thrombocytopenia.

Medical evaluation of thrombocytopenia requires a bone marrow biopsy to identify cytotoxic or alcohol-related marrow effects. Examination of the marrow includes both cultures and pathological evaluation to identify lymphoma or OIs such as fungus or mycobacteria, which would result in decreased platelet production. Other causes of peripheral platelet destruction such as splenic sequestration, liver disease resulting from portal hypertension, drug-induced thrombocytopenia, or the presence of disseminated intravascular coagulation are also considered.

Related Medical Management

The choice of therapy for thrombocytopenia depends on the underlying etiology. Lower grade thrombocytopenia may simply be observed. Medical

Table 13.2 National Cancer Institute's Grading of Thrombocytopenia

Grade	Platelet Count (cells/mm^3)	Clinical Risk
I	>75,000	None
II	50,000–74,999	Low
III	25,000–49,999	Moderate
IV	<25,000	Marked increase risk of bleeding from nose, gastrointestinal tract, and any invasive procedure

From Division of Cancer Treatment. Common toxicity criteria. *National Cancer Institute Investigator's Handbook*, Washington, DC: NIH, 1977.

interventions include plasma pheresis; the administration of fresh, frozen plasma or IV Ig, corticosteroids, or dextran, or a splenectomy. The combination of zidovudine (AZT) and IFN-α is sometimes effective. The mechanism of action of corticosteriods is unknown, although it is thought to help differentiate marrow cell lines. Administering IV Ig floods the spleen with Ig, forcing it to remove the Ig and ignore the coated platelet preferentially. Removal of the spleen removes the organ sequestering the platelets and results in increased platelet counts.[4] Dextran is used to ameliorate the autoimmune process that may play a role in platelet destruction.

Nursing Interventions

Acute

In the event that platelet transfusions are required, the risk/benefit ratio, specifics regarding the type of platelets required (i.e., leuko-poor, random pheresis, HLA or platelet cross-match), and after care need to be explained to the patient. Instruct the patient on the need for premedication, as well as the symptoms to expect and report during the transfusions. Observe the patient for fever, chills, rigors, SOB, rash, hives, or other allergic phenomena during transfusion.

Chronic

Evaluate all medications for thrombocytopenic potential. Check for use of aspirin, nonsteroidals, anticoagulants, codeine, indomethacin, or sulfa drugs. These agents may not necessarily reduce the total number of platelets but they do interfere with platelet function. Patients should be instructed to discontinue all of these medications when the platelet count drops below 50,000 cells/mm^3, unless otherwise instructed by their health care provider. The skin should be inspected regularly for petechiae and ecchymosis. The nurse's role also involves reducing the patient's anxiety about a significant bleed, allowing the patient to verbalize her concerns, answering all her questions, and instructing her on risk reduction techniques.

Information for the Patient

The following bleeding precautions are strategies (1) to minimize the risk of inducing a bleed and (2) to evaluate the mucous membranes for bleeding (gums, nose, and rectum).

- Inspect skin for petechiae and ecchymosis daily.
- Report changes in respiratory pattern, SOB, dyspnea on exertion, or hemoptysis.
- Instruct patients to blow nose gently and try not to Valsalva or strain at stool.
- Initiate stool softeners.
- Use only electric razors, not safety razors.
- Women should keep track of the number of pads or tampons used during menstruation. If the number doubles, the health care provider should be notified.
- Avoid aspirin, nonsteroidal anti-inflammatory medication, anticoagulants, indomethacin, and sulfa-containing compounds.
- Avoid IM injections.
- Avoid rectal exams or suppositories.
- Avoid flossing teeth.
- In the case of severe thrombocytopenia (platelet count < 10,000 cells/mm^3), avoid eating foods that may induce oral trauma, for example, crusty breads, potato chips, and pretzels.

Anemia

Anemia, which is defined as a decrease in the number of circulating erythrocytes, is the most common hematologic abnormality associated with HIV infection. The degree of anemia increases as the immune system declines. The prevalence of anemia is between 66 and 85% of patients diagnosed with AIDS.

Etiologies Related to HIV Infection and Its Medical Treatment

Etiologies of anemia in the context of HIV infection include deleterious effects on the bone marrow of infections, medications, and neoplastic processes. Organisms infecting the bone marrow and reported to induce anemia are B19 parvovirus, MAC, *Mycobacterium tuberculosis*, histoplasmosis, *Cryptococcus neoformans*, *Coccidioides immitis*, CMV, and rarely *Pneumocystis carinii*.[2,5] The anemia seen in these patients closely resembles the anemia of chronic disease and is characterized by abnormal mobilization of iron, inhibition of erythropoietin production, failure to respond to endogenous erythropoietin production, and humoral inhibition of erythropoiesis. Typically, the anemia is described as normocytic and normochromic.[6] HIV-infected patients frequently have both low reticulocyte counts and low erythropoietin levels, suggesting that a basic mechanism for the stimulation and production of red blood cells is malfunctioning.[1,5] Adequate iron stores are often present, but an inability to incorporate the stored iron into the erythroid precursors results in normocytic, normochromic anemia. Ineffective erythropoiesis may be a consequence of HIV infection or result from inappropriate release of cytokines, particularly TNF, which inhibits red blood cell production in vitro.[5] Other infectious agents may induce anemia through the direct invasion of the bone marrow with organisms. Once in the marrow, they replicate, inhabiting space normally occupied by stem cells and the colony-forming units. The cells of the marrow are unable to replicate when this space is not available, and anemia (neutropenia or thrombocytopenia) may result.

Drug-induced anemia is associated with many of the treatments for HIV infection. The drug most commonly implicated is zidovudine (AZT). Manifestations of AZT-induced anemia are marrow erythroid hypoplasia, aplasia, and megaloblastic maturation.[6] This phenomenon was reported more frequently when the dose of AZT was 1,000 to 1,200 mg/day. Since the recommended dosages have been reduced by half (500–600 mg/day), less anemia has been observed.[2,6] Other drugs often implicated are the sulfa drugs (sulfamethoxazole), dapsone, pentamidine, foscarnet, and ganciclovir.

The malignant complications of HIV infection are sometimes associated with anemia. Chronic blood loss from GI invasion of both KS or lymphoma may lead to anemia. In addition, the therapeutic options for any malignancy in the HIV patient most likely include multiple myelosuppressive agents. These agents have significant ability to induce anemia, ranging from mild to profound.

Presentation and Assessment

Subjective

Signs and symptoms of anemia are listed below.

- Fatigue
- Muscle weakness

- Shortness of breath
- Headache
- Lightheadedness
- Feeling faint
- Tachypnea
- Tachycardia
- Hypotension

The nurse should also be alert to more subtle or unusual signs of anemia. For example, patients may complain of being able to hear their heart pounding in their ears, or family members may note a mental status change, which may indicate anemia. Performance status should be evaluated with each visit to the hospital or clinic.

Objective

The degree of anemia is measured by the size of the decrease in hemoglobin, hematocrit, and red cell laboratory values. The NCI grades toxicity by hemoglobin level (Table 13.3). A normal hemoglobin is 12 to 15 g/dl.

Related Medical Management

Medical management of the anemia of HIV is etiology dependent. Treating the underlying infection, discontinuing medications, and using erythropoietin are options for medical management of anemia associated with AIDS. However, most of these methods do not produce immediate results, and in fact can take days to months to have an effect, if one is obtained at all.

Table 13.3 National Cancer Institute's Grading of Anemia

Grade	Hemoglobin Level (g/dl)
I	10.0–normal
II	8.0–9.9
III	6.5–7.9
IV	<6.5

From Division of Cancer Treatment. Common toxicity criteria. *National Cancer Institute Investigator's Handbook*, Washington, DC: NIH, 1977.

Therefore, the cornerstone of therapy for profound anemia (hemoglobin < 8 g/dl), when immediate results are required, remains the transfusion of red blood cells. Many patients continue to need transfusions during the course of their illness, despite other interventions. For patients with overt or covert bleeding, arresting the bleeding is the primary concern, but in many patients the bleeding is more of a continual oozing with no "lesion" to repair. In these patients transfusions are the treatment of choice to maintain an adequate level of hemoglobin.

Nursing Interventions

The nurse's role in transfusion administration encompasses instructing the patient about the risks and benefits of blood transfusion, and assessing the patient prior, during, and after the transfusion. It is important to note that 20% of all transfusions result in some type of reaction. Patients need to be instructed to report fever, chills, pruritus, urticaria, rash, or SOB experienced during the actual transfusion or within a week after the transfusion. Any change in the color of urine or stool could also be an indication of a transfusion reaction and should be reported. To help patients understand the need for transfusions, it is incumbent on the nurse to know the suspected etiology of the anemia and the plan of care.

For patients receiving erythropoietin, instructions on self-administration, including drawing up the product, storage, disposal, and special handling issues, should be provided. Instructions for patients who are self-injecting should include how to pick an injection site, how to evaluate injection sites for signs or symptoms of infection, self-injection technique, and the importance of keeping track of injection sites and the date of injection (see Table 13.1).

References

1. Doweiko J. Management of the hematologic manifestations of HIV disease. *Blood Rev.* 1993;7:121–126.
2. Northfelt D. Hematologic aspects of HIV infection. In: Cohen P, Sande M, Volberding P, eds. *The AIDS Knowledge Base.* Boston: Little, Brown; 1994:5.16–5.17.
3. Division of Cancer Treatment. Common toxicity criteria. *National Cancer Institute Investigator's Handbook*, Washington, DC: NIH, 1997.

4. Aster R. Thrombocytopenia in the HIV-infected patient. *Hosp Pract.* 1994;29: 81–86.
5. Northfelt D, Mitsuyasu R. Hematologic complications of HIV infection. In: DeVita V, Hellman S, Rosenberg S, eds. *AIDS Etiology Diagnosis, Treatment and Prevention.* Philadelphia: JB Lippincott; 1992:337–346.
6. Hambleton J. Hematologic complications of HIV infection. *Oncology.* 1996;10: 671–680.

CHAPTER **14**

Skin Problems

Cecily Cosby, PhD(c), FNP

Chapter Preview

- Immunologic Function of the Skin
- General Assessment of the Skin
- Definitions and General Changes
- Itching (Pruritus)
- Skin Lesions and Rashes

The clinical and psychological significance of dermatologic problems related to HIV infection cannot be overstated. Since cutaneous manifestations increase as T-helper (CD4+) cells decline, skin findings act as early indicators of HIV infection as well as signal HIV disease progression. Skin problems in HIV may be atypical in appearance, symptomatically more severe than in the normal host, frequently refractory to usual treatments, and associated with significant emotional distress. Patients should be counseled that as a target organ of HIV, skin symptoms may flare unpredictably with changes in the immune system. Many acute and chronic conditions may elude definitive diagnosis, with symptom management often the primary strategy.

Immunologic Function of the Skin

The dermis contains a major T-cell population (Figure 14.1) and is an integral part of the immune system.[1] Animal models have shown anatomic, molecular, and functional similarities between the epithelial cells of the skin and thymus. Langerhans' cells (dendritic cells with an immunologic function) are derived from bone marrow. They comprise about 5% of the cells of the epidermis and are identical to tissue macrophages. They present antigens to lymphocytes and have cell-membrane receptors for certain immunologic molecules. As the first line of immunologic defense in the skin, they are responsible for the immunizing capacity of topically applied antigen. Changes in the immune system, including CD4+ cell function, antigen response, shifting cytokine expression, as well as a propensity for autoimmune reactions underlie the skin immunodysfunction that occurs with HIV infection.[2]

General Assessment of the Skin

Because dermatology is a visual science, it is important for clinicians to evaluate skin complaints in good lighting with the patient adequately disrobed. Becoming familiar with the morphological (structural) characteristics of skin lesions is important for purposes of description and documentation. The HIV disease stage of the patient, CD4+ count, history of OIs, allergies, and current oral and topical medications are important informa-

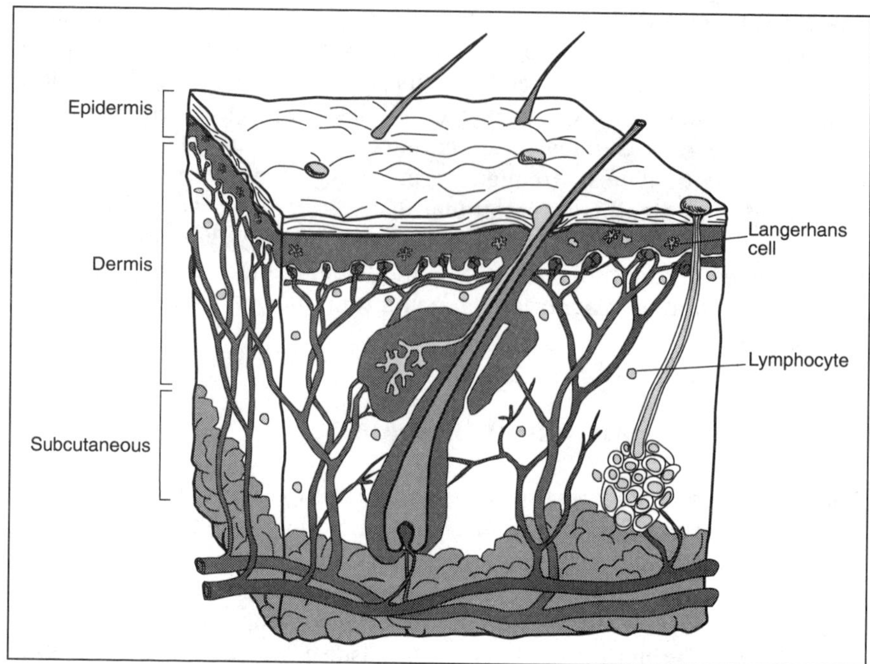

Figure 14.1 Anatomy of the Human Skin

tion when assessing skin complaints. Dietary habits, environmental exposures, sexual preferences and exposures, travel history, pets, skin care habits, and social and family history are additional factors to consider.

Definitions and General Changes

Changes of the Skin

Common skin changes associated with HIV infection, even in the absence of secondary conditions, include hyperkeratosis (horny layer hypertrophy), hyperpigmentation, and xerosis (dry skin).

- **Skin**
  - Xerosis
  - Hyperkeratosis
  - Hyperpigmentation
- **Hair**
  - Thinning
  - Patchy alopecia
  - Lash elongation
- **Nails**
  - Pigmentation
  - Fungal infections

Hyperkeratosis

Hyperkeratosis refers to any horny superficial growth and appears as thickening of the skin, especially of the palms and soles. There may be areas of pustulation within keratotic plaques. Hyperkeratosis may be an isolated finding or may be a feature of Reiter's syndrome, psoriasis, cutaneous fungal infection, or KS. It may be unsightly and uncomfortable. The use of keratolytic agents (salicylic acid and propylene glycol [e.g., Keralyt gel]) can be helpful, but must be used with caution to avoid skin irritation and worsening dryness (Table 14.1).

Hyperpigmentation

Hyperpigmentation results from enhanced melanin production and may follow any skin inflammation. It is most commonly seen in dark-skinned individuals and may involve the skin, oral mucosa, or nails. It may be associated with sun exposure or certain medications, especially zidovudine (Retrovir, AZT). Frequently with HIV infection there is an increase in the number of nevi and freckles, and preexisting ones may become darker. No treatment is indicated. Suspicious nevi should be evaluated for biopsy.

Dry Skin (Xerosis)

Dry skin is the most common cause of itching with no visible rash and the most common HIV-associated scaling dermatosis. *Asteatotic eczema*, *xerotic eczema*, and *winter itch* are other names given to this pruritic condition. It may resemble acquired ichthyosis, a defect of the horny layer

Table 14.1 Nursing Interventions for Skin Conditions Associated with HIV Infection

Problem/Symptom	Patient Education/Nursing Observations and Care
General care	Counsel regarding nature of skin as a target organ of HIV; prevention strategies: moisturize and wear sun protection; maintenance strategies: develop new skin care habits; avoid length exposure to hot water, avoid vigorous towel drying, pat skin dry, use emollients and bath oils on damp skin (caution slippery!), limit daily bathing and soap use except to axilla and genitalia, avoid overuse of soap and deoderants, and maintain supply of skin care products
Alopecia (general change)	Nature of hair growth cycle; evaluate for infectious processes and medication side effects; if progressive or severe, request dermatologic assessment and treatment
Drug rash (inflammatory/hypersensitivity)	Counsel regarding nature of HIV skin hypersensitivity; monitor closely for systemic complaints of Stevens-Johnson syndrome (e.g., fever, stomatitis, headache, malaise); symptom management: see "Itching"; early identification of suspicious medications
Dry skin (xerosis; general change)	Counsel regarding worsening symptoms in winter; see "General care"; symptom relief: manage itching, administer oral antihistamines; avoid scratching, keep nails short; limit water exposure and use of soap; avoid daily bathing; use cool water for bathing and showers; keep skin moisturized
Eosinophilic folliculitis (inflammatory/ hypersensitivity)	Counsel regarding chronic nature; encourage maintance therapy with topical and oral therapies as prescribed, due to chronicity; provide reassurance and emotional support due to high visibility; symptom management: see "Itching"; prevent secondary infection
Folliculitis (infectious)	Counsel regarding skin hygiene, association with shaving and staph on skin, nature of nasal carriage; encourage intermittent use of antibacterial soaps, moisturizers; follow instructions when using prescribed oral antibiotics and applying mupirocin to nares; evaluate for development of cellulitis, abscess formation

Fungal infections, nails (general changes/infectious)	Dry feet and hands well; use cool blow dryer to toes, web spaces; change socks frequently; wear open-toe shoes; reassure as to benign nature; counsel regarding chronicity, slow response, need for daily use of topical therapies
Herpes (infectious)	Counsel as to nature of sexual and/or other transmission, hand washing, use of gloves and hygiene; review suppressive adherence strategies, regular dosing; consider any ulceration herpes until proved otherwise and don't cover with occlusive dressings; provide adequate pain control
Hyperkeratosis (general change)	Check palms and soles, consider Reiter's syndrome; consider cautious removal of plaques; prevent secondary infection
Hyperpigmentation (general change)	Counsel as to skin response to trauma, sun exposure; reassure as to benign nature, may fade over time; avoid sun exposure, especially to areas of recent injury or infection, and use sun screen; evaluate suspicious nevi, other for biopsy
Insect bites (inflammatory/hypersensitivity)	Assess distribution on lower extremities; see "Itching"; treat animal and environment
Itching (pruritus) (general change)	See "General care" and "Dry skin"; assist in identifying and treating underlying cause (localized vs. generalized, new medication?); symptom management: topical anti-inflammatory creams/ointments, antifungals as indicated, antihistamines; consider scabies; use gloves, other protective measures
Kaposi's sarcoma (neoplastic)	Counsel as to nature of hyperpigmentation, lymphedema; not universally progressive; treatment options: cryotherapy, radiation, and intralesional, systemic chemotherapy
Molluscum contagiosum (infectious)	Avoid picking, shaving, as bacterium spreads easily; requires aggressive, frequent treatment and might still persist

(continued)

Table 14.1 *Continued*

Problem/Symptom	Patient Education/Nursing Observations and Care
Photosensitivity (inflammatory/ hypersensitivity)	Avoid sun exposure, especially 10 A.M. to 2 P.M.; use sun protection (≥SPF 15); wear hats, protective clothing; counsel regarding increased risks associated with certain medications (sulfa, tetracycline, dapsone, NSAIDs)
Pigmentation, nails (general change)	Counsel regarding association to medications (zidovudine); provide reassurance
Psoriasis (inflammatory/papulosquamous)	Counsel regarding medications that may increase symptoms (beta blockers, lithium, NSAIDs); assess for associated arthritis, nail pitting, and secondary infection; nature of condition as chronic, recurrent; symptom management: topical steroids; regular maintenance may control severity of flares
Rash/lesions (inflammatory, infectious, neoplastic)	Counsel regarding nature of increased dermatoses, often chronic nature, refractory to treatments, atypical; consider systemic etiologies, disseminated disease (syphilis, *Cryptococcus*); transmission precautions, hand washing, gloves; symptom management
Scabies (inflammatory/hypersensitivity)	Have high index of suspicion for any rash/itching; use gloves, hand washing; counsel regarding risks and exposures, contagion; reinforce instructions for treatment: wash all linens, underclothing, etc., in hot-cycle machine; use medication as prescribed and don't wash hands after applying; treat household and sexual contacts; counsel that symptoms may persist even after successful treatment; symptom relief for itching, don't use Kwell on open skin
Seborrheic dermatitis (inflammatory/ papulosquamous)	Counsel regarding daily use of topical therapies to prevent acute flares; treat scalp as well as face; use combination topical anti-inflammatory and antifungal ointments; may have associated blepharitis; distinctive distribution: face, scalp, body folds

Thinning hair (general change)	See “Alopecia”; suggest over-the-counter products for fullness and body; provide reassurance
Tinea (infectious)	Counsel regarding association with heat, moisture; symptom management: topical, occasionally systemic antifungals
Varicella zoster (infectious)	Counsel as to risk of primary infection to children, other susceptible hosts; use of VZIG for exposures; assess for disseminated disease; complications such as headache and fever suggestive of meningitis; initiate therapy at first sign of vesicles
Warts, anogenital (infectious)	Counsel regarding nature of sexual transmission, association with carcinoma, and need for Paps smears and regular follow-ups
Warts, skin (infectious)	Counsel regarding transmission; typically worsen and increase with advancing HIV; may require multiple treatments

NSAIDs = nonsteroidal anti-inflammatory drugs; VZIG = varicella zoster immune globulin.

of the epidermis, with diminished sweat and sebaceous secretion causing dry and thickened skin. Those with a history of asthma, hay fever, or atopic dermatitis are predisposed to dry skin, which is more symptomatic in winter months. It often presents as itching and dryness with areas of erythematous papules and fine scales on the posterior arms and lower legs.[3] The differential diagnosis includes scabies, fungal infections, eczema, and contact dermatitis.

Dry air and exposure to soap and water contribute to the loss of moisture and cause the skin to chap and crack. Unfortunately, improvement in the level of systemic hydration does not diminish the signs or symptoms of this cutaneous condition. Nursing management approaches are listed in Table 14.1.

Changes of the Nails

Common conditions affecting the nails include fungal infections and pigmentation.

Fungal Infections (Dermatophytosis)

Fungal infections from *Candida* and *Tinea* can affect the cuticle (paronychia) or nail bed (onychomycosis) respectively. The fungi produce proteases that digest keratin, which enables fungal invasion of the nail. The nails often appear brittle and lusterless, and may be thickened (hypertrophic) and friable. Chronic water exposure can predispose to these infections. The diagnosis is most often made by appearance. Infections of the toenails are difficult to cure, the fingernails respond better. Oral and topical antifungal agents are employed. Nursing management is summarized in Table 14.1.

Pigmentation

Pigmented nail bands and/or blue lunae (pigmented proximal nails) are commonly seen with HIV infection. They are likely due to increased melanin deposits and are commonly associated with zidovudine therapy. Typically it appears within 4 to 8 weeks after the initiation of therapy with zidovudine. When due to zidovudine, this phenomenon is usually reversible after dosing is suspended. No treatment is indicated.

Changes of the Hair

Hair changes associated with HIV may include premature graying, premature frontal recession of the hairline, diffuse thinning, elongation of the eyelashes, and alopecia areata.

Diffuse Thinning

Patients may complain that their "hair is falling out." This is most often not noticeable to others, but of great concern to the patient. This condition may be secondary to medications or as a result of chronic disease and the HIV infection itself. The normal hair growth cycle may include periods of noticeable hair loss. It is often self-limiting and there is no treatment other than identifying potential contributory medications.

Elongation of the Eyelashes

This condition may be associated with any severe illness and results from the prolongation of the hair growth phase.

Alopecia Areata

This is patchy hair loss with discrete bald areas. It is thought to be an autoimmune condition and possibly related to an abnormality in T lymphocytes. The area should be evaluated for fungal or bacterial conditions. After those have been ruled out, the involved area can be evaluated for treatment with steroid injections by a dermatologist.

Itching (Pruritus)

Pruritus, a sensation exclusive to the skin, produces the desire to scratch. Itch, touch, temperature, and pain sensations are all mediated by the same receptors. Chemical, mechanical, thermal, and electric stimuli may elicit itching. Psychic trauma, stress, absence of distractions, anxiety, and fear may all enhance itching. It is commonly most severe at bedtime. Itching is the most common symptom of skin diseases. For people with HIV, it may be the major complaint and is often severely disruptive.

Assessment

It is important to determine if the itching is caused by a skin or systemic disorder. Two important distinctions should be made during the assessment of itching. First, is the itching generalized or localized? Secondly, is it associated with a rash, and if so, is the rash from scratching or did it precede, accompany, or follow the itching? Patients with generalized itching require a complete medical history and physical examination. Screening tests for systemic etiologies might include a CBC, differential count, liver and renal function tests, thyroid profile, and chest radiograph.

Etiology

Considerations for itching without a rash include dry skin (xerosis), neurodermatitis, fungal infections, and systemic disease (endocrine, renal, hepatic, or hematologic). Scabies, contact dermatitis, or drug reactions may be itchy prior to a rash. Typical lesions or rashes that may itch include scabies, contact dermatitis, drug reactions, folliculitis, seborrheic dermatitis, and insect bites.

Nursing Interventions

Management and preventive measures are directed at the specific cause of itching once determined. Since the likelihood of mixed processes is high, combination therapies are often indicated. As a symptom associated with a number of conditions, attempts to provide symptom relief from itching should begin prior to establishing a definitive diagnosis (see Table 14.1).

Skin Lesions and Rashes

Skin lesions and rashes are generally the result of inflammatory, infectious, or neoplastic causes. They can be solitary, grouped, or disseminated lesions, or involve discrete, diffuse, or confluent areas.

Inflammatory

Inflammatory causes of skin disorders include hypersensitivity reactions and papulosquamous conditions.

- **Papulosquamous conditions**
  - Seborrheic dermatitis
  - Psoriasis
- **Hypertensivity reactions**
  - Drug reaction
  - Photosensitivity
  - Eosinophilic folliculitis
  - Papular pruritic eruptions
  - Scabies
  - Insect bites
  - Atopic and contact dermatitis

Hypersensitivity

Hypersensitivity reactions occur frequently in HIV-infected persons, suggesting that normal numbers of T cells are not necessary for many hypersensitivity reactions.[3] Hypersensitive conditions include eosinophilic folliculitis, papular pruritic eruptions, scabies, insect bites, photosensitivity, and drug reactions. Other hypersensitive conditions not discussed here include irritant and allergic contact dermatitis, and atopic dermatitis.

EOSINOPHILIC FOLLICULITIS. Eosinophilic folliculitis is a unique manifestation of HIV disease that occurs in persons with CD4+ counts usually <200 cells/mm³.[3] It is a pruritic folliculitis with distinctive clinical and laboratory features. Primary lesions consist of discrete, erythematous, urticarial follicular papules measuring 3 to 5 mm.[4] Frequently there is excoriation and crusting. Lesions are generally scattered on the trunk, the head and neck, and the proximal aspect of the extremities. Ninety percent of the lesions are above the nipple line and occur in a chronic, waxing-and-waning course. Positive histological diagnosis is made by skin biopsy, and is essential to rule out other conditions such as bacterial folliculitis.

This is a particularly difficult condition for patients due to its high visibility and chronic nature. Ultraviolet phototherapy can be beneficial and itraconazole (Sporanox) 200 to 400 mg daily for 3 weeks has been successful. After signs and symptoms have responded, therapy can be tapered to the lowest effective dose.[5]

PAPULAR PRURITIC ERUPTIONS. Most patients with pruritic papular eruptions have folliculitis. Causes may include *Staphylococcus aureus* folliculitis, eosinophilic folliculitis, demodex mites, insect bite reactions, and granulomas with no identifiable infectious agent.[3] Empiric treatment for *Staphylococcus* can be initiated with a semisynthetic penicillin (dicloxacillin) or a first-generation cephalosporin (Keflex) while awaiting results of skin biopsy.[3] With the increasing use of testosterone therapy there are reports of associated follicular outbreaks. These conditions resolve with the decrease or suspension of dosing with testosterone.

SCABIES. Scabies is a highly contagious mite infestation characterized by severe itching. With HIV disease progression, the infestation may exaggerate, spare the characteristic areas, and become refractory to treatment.[3] Areas of the body most commonly involved are the interdigital web spaces, the flexor areas of the wrists, the axillae, buttocks, lower back, penis, scrotum, and breasts. The pathognomonic lesion is the burrow—a short, wavy line that often follows skin lines. Typical erythematous, firm, 5- to 8-mm papules will be seen. As few as eight organisms can cause generalized pruritus.

A KOH preparation or mineral oil to identify the mite, its eggs, or fecal material can establish the diagnosis. However, failure to make the diagnosis on microscopic examination should not delay empiric treatment if clinical suspicion is high. Scabies should be considered in any patient with an unexplained pruritic eruption or dermatitis. All family members and sexual contacts should be treated. A typical treatment program for scabies instructs the patient to apply the antiscabietic cream over the entire body once a week for 4 weeks. Avoid washing the hands after the application and take a cool shower the next morning. It may take several weeks following therapy for symptoms to resolve. A nonpruritic form, true crusted (Norwegian) scabies, which requires more aggressive treatment, may occur in patients with advanced HIV disease.[6]

INSECT BITES. Insect bites from fleas or mosquitoes can cause a papular urticaria. Lesions may be vesicular or may include large, tense bullae. They are frequently found on the lower extremities in the case of fleabites, and on exposed skin areas with mosquitoes. A skin biopsy is usually not necessary but can confirm the diagnosis. Insect protection combined with oral antihistamines and topical antipruritic agents will offer some relief.

Treating the flea-carrying animal and the infested environment is also necessary.

DRUG REACTION. The most common manifestation of a drug eruption is a maculopapular rash. Other types of reactions include urticaria (hives), exfoliative erythroderma, fixed drug eruption, erythema multiforme (severe, acute eruption of macules, papules, or vesicles in a multiform appearance), and toxic epidermal necrolysis. These reactions are most often due to antibiotics, especially trimethoprim-sulfamethoxazole (Septra) and the penicillins. Stevens-Johnson syndrome is a severe, at times fatal, variety of erythema multiforme. There is typically an abrupt onset manifested by fever, headache, malaise, and soreness of the throat and mouth. Constitutional symptoms become more severe, and stomatitis is an early and conspicuous symptom. These patients require hospitalization and aggressive, rapid treatment.

PHOTOSENSITIVITY. Photodermatitis is a phototoxic or photoallergic response and can be either acute or chronic. The severity of this reaction is a result of the concentration of the photosensitizing substance and intensity of light. It may occur with topical or ingested substances. Patients at any stage of HIV are at risk. Medications typically implicated include trimethoprim-sulfamethoxazole, tetracycline, and NSAIDS. Other medications frequently used in HIV infection that may cause photosensitive reactions include some antihistamines, antipsychotics, antidepressants, and ciprofloxacin (Cipro).

The reaction appears as a papular or scaly pruritic eruption that may become exudative and may appear similar to contact dermatitis. It is largely resitricted to sun-exposed areas and may resemble seborrheic dermatitis when it appears on the face. The dorsa of the hands, extensor forearms, and sides of the neck and face are most often involved. The diagnosis is made by history and distribution. Topical steroids, plus patient education regarding sun avoidance and protection and sunscreens, are the primary treatment and preventative measures.

Papulosquamous Conditions

Papulosquamous conditions are cutaneous eruptions with both papules and scales. These conditions most often occur when the CD4+ count is <100 cells/mm^3.

SEBORRHEIC DERMATITIS. Seborrheic dermatitis occurs in as many as 83% of people with HIV and is a frequent cause of blepharitis (eyelid inflammation) and otitis externa. Seborrheic dermatitis is located in areas of the skin where the sebaceous glands are most active, such as the face, scalp, and body folds and may involve the trunk, groin, and extremities. Typically it appears red and scaly, and sticky crusts and fissures are common. Pruritus is variable. The differential diagnoses include psoriasis, *Tinea*, and contact dermatitis.

Because seborrheic dermatitis is a chronic condition, maintenance therapy is often required. Mild symptoms are treated with mild topical steroids, tar shampoos, and topical imidazoles applied twice daily. Scalp treatments with selenium sulfide shampoo can improve facial symptoms. Patients should be instructed to leave shampoo lather on their scalp for 5 to 10 minutes. Extensive involvement can be treated carefully with more potent topical steroids and tar applications.

PSORIASIS. Psoriasis is a common, chronic, recurrent inflammatory disease of the skin characterized by round, circumscribed, erythematous, dry, scaling patches of various sizes covered by grayish white or silvery white overlapping scales.

The clinical appearance of psoriasis is similar in HIV-infected and noninfected persons. The lesions are commonly found on the scalp, nails, extensor surfaces of the limbs, the elbows, the knees, and the sacral region. The lesions are usually symmetrical and may vary from a solitary macule to countless plaques. The frequency of psoriasis in those with HIV infection is similar to that of the general population—as many as 3%. Nail pitting and dystrophy, arthritis, pruritus, and secondary infection may be other features. The severity varies greatly from one patient to another, and for each patient over time.

Although HIV infection may be associated with exacerbations of longstanding stable psoriasis, many patients may have stable psoriasis even as immunodeficiency progresses.[3] The disease may be affected by systemic medications, some of which may cause flaring (beta blockers, lithium, some nonsteroidal anti-inflammatory agents) and others such as zidovudine, which have been shown to improve symptoms.[7] Stress has been implicated as an aggravating factor.

Infectious

Typical infectious causes of skin lesions include bacterial, viral, and fungal conditions.

- **Bacterial**
  - *Staphylococcus*
  - *Bartonella*
  - *Mycobacterium avium*
  - Syphilis
- **Fungal**
  - *Candida*
  - *Tinea*
  - *Cryptococcus*
  - *Histoplasma*
  - Sporotrichosis
- **Viral**
  - Herpes simplex (types 1 and 2)
  - Varicella Zoster virus
  - Cytomegalo virus
  - *Molluscum contagiosum*
  - Human papilloma virus
  - HIV

Definitive care involves identifying and treating the underlying infection. Gloves and good hand-washing techniques for both patient and care providers are essential. Any persistent ulcer in an HIV-infected individual should be considered infectious. Any genital lesion should be evaluated to rule out primary syphilis. Even sacral lesions in a bed-bound patient should not be assumed to be decubital. Avoid occlusive dressings, which can make herpetic lesions worse. Secondary bacterial infections of these lesions are common. Patients should be instructed to use gloves and good hand-washing techniques when cleansing or touching lesions.

Nursing Interventions

Patient complaints associated with skin conditions are common and distressing. By nature dermatology is baffling to many patients and clinicians. As with many HIV-related conditions, having the "right diagnosis" initially may be less important than identifying the acuity of the problem and initiating strategies for symptom control. Nurses make a significant contribution through patient and family education, assisting in the care and management of distressing conditions, providing comfort and reassurance, and by advocating on behalf of the patient. Expedient and appropriate management of chronic and acute skin conditions can contribute to enhanced quality of life for people with HIV infection. As many skin conditions are infectious, nurses must use and teach good hand-washing techniques, and inform the patient when the use of gloves and other precautions are appropriate. See Table 14.1 for detailed nursing interventions associated with each condition.

References

1. Edelson RL, Fink JM. The immunologic function of the skin. *Sci Am.* 1985;252: 46–53.
2. Duvic M. Human immunodeficiency virus and the skin: selected controversies. *J Invest Dermatol.* 1995;105:1179–1219.
3. Berger T. Dermatologic manifestations of HIV infection. In: Cohen PT, Sande MA, Volberding PA, eds. *The HIV Knowledge Base.* 2nd ed. Boston: Little, Brown; 1994:5.3.1 1–31.
4. Rosenthal D, Leboit PE, Klumpp L, Berger T. Human immunodeficiency virus-associated eosinophilic folliculitis. *Arch Dermatol.* 1991;127:206–209.
5. Blanchet KD. Cutaneous manifestations of HIV disease. *AIDS Patient Care.* 1995;60–66.
6. Drabick JJ, Lupton GP, Tompkins K. Crusted scabies in human immunodeficiency virus infection. *J Am Acad Dermatol.* 1987;17:142. Letter.
7. Duvic M, Rios A, Brewton GW. Remission of AIDS-associated psoriasis with zidovudine. *Lancet.* 1987;ii:627. Letter.

CHAPTER 15

Psychosocial Responses

Barbara Munjas, PhD, RN, FAAN
Catherine A. Oliver, MS, RN
Brenda J. Luna, MS, RN, CS, FNP

Chapter Preview

- Definition and Relationship of Psychosocial Responses: Anxiety, Grief, Depression, Mania, Psychosis, and Suicide
- Presentation and Assessment
- Interventions

The psychological impact on the person with HIV infection is as pervasive and profound as the physiological effects of this chronic and terminal illness. After HIV diagnosis, the individual has to cope not only with the illness itself, but with increased stress arising from family, friends, and society. Psychosocial responses that the person with HIV infection experiences include fear, anxiety, grief, loss, depression, mania, psychosis, and suicide. Anxiety, grief, and depression are the most frequent responses.

Health care professionals must be able to identify stressors and negative life events encountered by persons with HIV. They must also recognize their clinical significance in the development of psychiatric illness and disorders. Because nurses are present and actively involved at every stage of the HIV illness continuum, they are in a position to assess continually and to identify emotional and psychosocial distress. Early assessment, planning, intervention, and evaluation can reduce distress, decrease the impact and suffering associated with these common psychosocial responses, and decrease the risk of clinically significant psychiatric complications, of which suicide is the most serious.[1]

Persons diagnosed with HIV infection succumb to a multitude of physiological and psychosocial sequela. The advancement of prophylactic intervention and medical management of HIV has received greater attention, often overlooking its tremendous psychosocial impact. However, the growing recognition that the psychosocial and emotional sequela associated with a diagnosis of HIV significantly affects the person's quality of life, social support systems and relationships, health status, and ability to follow medical protocols, supports the need for increased scientific inquiry in this area.[1–3]

Persons who are asymptomatic or experiencing new onset of HIV symptoms have greater levels of psychological distress and psychiatric complications than those with an AIDS diagnosis.[1–4] This is also true for those contemplating HIV testing as a result of their perceived risk of infection.[5] Interestingly, HIV-infected individuals with a preexisting psychiatric diagnosis, IV drug abusers, substance abusers, and those with alternative lifestyles tend to experience greater psychological distress than other HIV-infected individuals.[1,6–8]

Persons with HIV infection follow a psychosocial trajectory, along which *junctures* in the trajectory represent the psychosocial transitions they experience similar to and simultaneously with the disease trajectory.[9] Duffy[3] proposed 14 *crisis points* from identified stressors experienced by those testing HIV positive and persons with AIDS that may precipitate a psychological crisis along the HIV illness continuum:

1. Testing procedure results—fear of the waiting period/results
2. Others' illness/death—own mortality becomes evident; feelings of anxiety, depression, guilt
3. Family/friend notification—feelings of fear, pain, guilt, concern for impact on family/friends
4. Lifestyle changes—loss of independence, employment/income, social, support, home, leisure
5. Physical illness—increased body awareness, fear of physical changes, loss of control
6. Decision to self-test—anonymous vs. confidential resting, decision of testing site
7. Medication treatment—reminder of illness, acknowledgment of immune system deterioration
8. Symptoms of HIV infection—illness progression, uncertainty
9. Terminal care decisions—advance directives, arrangements for care of family
10. Friends/acquaintances HIV positive—disease becomes more personal, breaks through own denial
11. Obtaining medical care—deciding when and where to obtain care, fear and embarrassment
12. Risk behavior awareness—first conscious awareness of own risk behaviors and threat to self
13. First hospitalization—prospective suffering and death, helplessness, depression
14. Diagnostic change—diagnosis of AIDS, threat of death, own demise

While the factors listed here represent identified precipitators of increased psychological distress in HIV persons, this list is not all inclusive nor will every person experience these stressors and their negative sequela.[3,10]

Patterns of fear, anxiety, grief, and loss have been reported in persons with HIV infection.[3,11] Progression of a person's HIV infection, as demonstrated by the increased presence of symptoms, is associated with the presence of psychological distress manifested by such symptoms as depressed mood, increased anxiety, insomnia, anorexia, inability to concentrate, and anhedonia. Similarly, the presence of pain presents the same relationship in HIV-infected persons demonstrated previously in cancer patients. The presence of pain may intensify depression and sleep disturbances, act as a reminder of one's illness, and significantly increase suicidal risk.[4,12] Present factors that contribute to the increased prevalence of emotional and psychological distress experienced in HIV-infected persons, in addition to those identified earlier are listed below.[1,6–8,10,12,14]

- **Psychosocial factors**
  - Real/perceived lack of social support
  - Sexual, physical, and/or emotional abuse
  - External locus of control
  - Social isolation, withdrawal
  - Low socioeconomic status
  - IV drug abusers, substance abusers
  - Marital/family problems
  - Sexual dysfunction
  - Inability to meet ADLs, functional decline
  - Perception of self as "victim"
  - Difficulty communicating with health care providers
  - Negative response of caregivers to diagnosis/person's lifestyle
  - Poor coping/problem-solving skills, poor sense of self-worth
  - Same-sex orientation
  - Inability to meet responsibilities/needs: financial, family, home, medical
- **Demographic factors**
  - Female
  - Homeles
  - Age 22 to 44 years
  - Low socioeconomic status
- **Medical factors**
  - Preexisting psychiatric diagnosis and hospitalization
  - IV drug abusers, substance abusers
  - Dual psychiatric diagnosis
  - Comorbid medical illness, acute or chronic
  - Medication, adverse side effects
  - Genetic predisposition/family history of psychiatric disorders
  - Pain
  - Vitamin B12 deficiency

Effective use of clinical judgment and expertise in the appraisal of the crisis points and contributing factors will enable nurses and other primary care professionals to provide anticipatory guidance for successful coping and problem-solving skills. Along with providing anticipatory guidance, referrals to community resources and other members of the multidisciplinary team should be made. Primary care providers have a responsibility to provide overall management of the person's health care, including assessment of support systems and quality of life issues; provision of psychosocial support; appropriate psychological assessment, evaluation, treatment and referral; and integration into the health care system.[15]

Current trends in the health care industry to decrease hospital time, streamline health care services, and move toward managed care make it inevitable that increased numbers of persons with early HIV infection will be seen in the primary care setting. Mental health professionals are unprepared to care for their HIV-related physical care. At the same time, primary care providers are equally unprepared to address their growing mental health needs.[16] Mental health issues constitute an integral part of their health care because psychological factors influence functioning of the immune system.

Definition and Relationship of Psychosocial Responses

The psychosocial responses of fear, anxiety, grief and loss, depression, mania, psychosis, and suicide, will be defined, contrasted, and compared. An understanding of the concepts of fear, anxiety, and grief and loss, and the application of appropriate interventions may aid in the successful resolution of the grief process and reduce the risk of the HIV-infected person's progression to a diagnosis of clinical depression or the act of suicide. Early intervention can promote a more positive clinical outcome for the person by reducing the severity and frequency of symptom exacerbations. It can also help to determine whether the symptoms are induced by psychosocial factors related to the HIV infection or are the result of neurological deterioration.[1,3,6,7,10,17]

Fear

Fear is a response to a real or perceived danger that the individual validates.[18] The identification of the stressor makes it possible to deal with the fear by fighting it or fleeing. This is known as the *fight-or-flight re-*

sponse. This response acts as a direct outlet for the physiological and psychological tension resulting from fear. The following list summarizes many of the sources of fear response associated with the thought of HIV infection or an actual HIV diagnosis.[19,20]

- Rejection by loved ones
- Stigma
- Social isolation
- Loss of financial security
- Dependency on others
- Pain and suffering
- Early death
- Loss of control over destiny
- Acceptance of AIDS as a terminal illness
- Loss of function
- Medical treatment

Anxiety

Anxiety is a vague, unpleasant feeling with a source that is nonspecific or unknown. Components of anxiety may be uncertainty, agitation, dread, brooding, fear, doubt, powerlessness, and tension.[21] When a person experiences anxiety, he cannot distinguish it from fear, so the psychological response of "fight or flight" is the same. Anxiety warns a person that something is wrong, however an identifiable source is not present. Levels of anxiety are categorized as mild, moderate, severe, and panic (Table 15.1). The ability to differentiate and to identify the levels of anxiety enable the practitioner to initiate the appropriate interventions accurately.[22]

Different psychosocial issues creating anxiety emerge over the course of the HIV illness. The experience of anxiety in the earlier stages of the disease occurs as a result of uncertainty about the disease process, clinical course, treatment, and outcomes. It is also experienced as a result of rejection and social isolation.[23] New onset of symptoms that herald disease progression acts as a constant reminder of the person's illness and its ultimate outcome. Person's with AIDS eventually have to deal with issues of death, dying, and resolution of unfinished business.[3,24]

Table 15.1 Response: Anxiety

Levels of Anxiety	Description
Mild	Causes person to be alert and increase perceptual field
	Motivates learning, problem solving, growth, productivity
Moderate	Allows person to focus on immediate concerns
	Perceptual field narrows and failure to notice certain aspects of the experience may occur
Severe	Focus is on one specific detail; fails to think about anything else
	Perceptual field greatly reduced
	All behavior directed at obtaining relief
Panic	Feeling of terror, loss of rational thought, disorganization of the personality, and inability to relate to others
	Level incompatible with life if behavior continues for extended periods
	Results in exhaustion/death without immediate intervention

Grief and Loss

Grief is a process that consists of the emotional reaction focused on or surrounding the longing for someone or something that is no longer there. It is not simply a reaction to a real or perceived loss, but may be triggered in anticipation of a loss.[11]

Grief and loss associated with HIV infection extend from the moment an individual contemplates testing until death. The central issue confronting the person with HIV infection is that death is an eventual certainty. Little by little, the person loses pieces of himself through decreases in psychological and physical well-being. Unlike many chronic illnesses, HIV infection strikes primarily young to middle-age adults who are at the prime of life and thus have great difficulty coping with terminal illness and premature death. The person is forced to confront such issues as the search for the meaning of life, purpose of the illness, and his place in the world.[19] Religious and social condemnation associated with HIV infection further complicate the grief process and can lead to a very intense grief reaction with increased risk of prolonged or pathological grief outcomes.[20] The stages of the grief continuum are emotional responsiveness, uncomplicated grief reaction, suppression of emotions, and delayed grief reaction (Table 15.2). Grief may progress to maladaptive depression or mania, which are abnormal extensions, or overelaborations of sadness and grief.[25] In *Grief and AIDS*, Sheer[11] discusses how a diagnosis of HIV may result in dramatic grief, and the variety of losses that may be experienced (Table 15.3).

Depression

The term *depression* has been used to describe feelings (sad, blue, depressed), symptoms (medication side effects, medical condition), and mood disorders (major depressive disorder, bipolar disorder). Depression is a disturbance in mood that is an elaboration of grief and a reaction to an actual, threatened, or perceived loss. It is a common and often

Table 15.2 Response: Grief

Class	Description
Emotional responsiveness	Awareness of feelings
	Active participant of internal and external world
Uncomplicated grief reaction	Emotions focused on or surrounding the longing for someone or something that is no longer there
	May be triggered in anticipation of a loss
	Faces the reality of the loss, immersed in the work of grieving
Suppression of emotions	Able to use coping strategies and mechanisms of defense to reduce the effect of strong emotion, enabling maintenance of normal performance
Delayed grief reaction	Persistent absence of emotional response to a loss, reaction may continue for months to years
	Pathological
	Further loss and less significant experiences of sadness act as triggers to grief onset

Table 15.3 Losses Associated with an HIV Diagnosis

Type of loss	Description
Health	Good health can no longer be taken for granted; individual may face sudden and unexpected periods of illness
Relationships	HIV infection may dramatically affect relationships; the relationship may be enhanced or there may be a negative effect in the presence of HIV infection
Sex	There may be curtailment of previously enjoyed behavior at a time when expression of love and intimacy may be especially desired
Future	The individual's future is cut short
Certainty	Much human endeavor is founded on some degree of certainty; HIV diagnosis questions such certainty
Life	HIV infection challenges individual's meaning of life and the goals they have set for themselves
Job	Dramatic effects on employment; the loss of a job may cause economic deprivation, social limitation, curtailed career, and loss of sense of purpose and ambition
Family/loved ones	HIV diagnosis may cause rejection and condemnation by family and friends; with the increase in the number of HIV infections and death, the individual may be faced with a concentration of losses with her families, friendship networks, and communities

incapacitating condition seen in both the hospital environment and in primary care settings.[26] Depression is the most frequently diagnosed psychiatric disorder in persons with HIV infection.[2,27] It goes beyond grief in duration and intensity, and is increasingly incapacitating in all aspects of the person's life.[28] Depression impairs a person's coping skills, judgment, physical and mental capacity, and ability. Grothe[13] describes depression as a physical illness caused by an imbalance of neurotransmitters in the brain. An abnormal receptor-neurotransmitter relationship is affected by various factors, resulting in an abnormality in the storage, release, and uptake primarily of serotonin and norepinephrine.

Risk factors for depression listed below apply universally to all people.

- Prior episodes of depression
- Family history of depressive disorder
- Prior suicide attempt
- Female gender
- Age of onset <40 years
- Postpartum period
- Medical comorbidity
- Lack of social support
- Stressful life events
- Substance abuse

Additional factors that result in psychological distress, such as those listed earlier, increase the risk of clinical depression. Pain is also a risk factor for depression and is most often associated with a chronic illness. Control or alleviation of the pain frequently results in resolution of the depressive symptoms.

Symptoms indicative of depression are also associated with HIV infection and may be signs of early neurological involvement[2,27,29]: Symptoms of depression include:

- Appetite or weight change
- Decreased interest or pleasure
- Sad or depressed mood
- Fatigue, loss of energy
- Sleep disturbance
- Trouble concentrating, indecisiveness
- Delusions or hallucinations
- Feelings of worthlessness or excessive guilt
- Physical agitation or retardation
- Thoughts of death or suicide

Differentiation of depression induced as a result of neurological impairment in ADC is discussed in Chapter 9. The 1993 Agency for Health Care Policy Research (AHCPR) Clinical Practice Guidelines[30] on depression provide a comprehensive review and stepwise guide for the identification, diagnosis, and management of depression, as well as other mood disorders closely resembling or associated with clinical depression (available from http://www.ahcpr.gov). Depression in HIV-infected persons may occur as a result of psychological reactions, side effects of medications, substance abuse, concomitant medical conditions, or organic damage to the brain.[2,31] It is imperative to identify the correct cause of the depression to ensure proper treatment and effective interventions.

Mania

Persons with HIV infection may at some point along the illness continuum exhibit behaviors associated with mania. While only approximately 8% of the HIV-infected population have been reported to suffer from mania,[32] it is important to understand and recognize mania as a possible sign of neurological involvement, substance abuse, reaction to medication, or preexisting psychiatric disorder.

Mania is described as a syndrome characterized by periods of elation or irritability, psychomotor agitation, and ideas of self-importance.[31–33] Mania by itself is an illness episode, but more often it is associated with *bipolar disorder*, which was previously known as *manic-depressive disorder.*[30] The manic person presents with feeling generally happy, cheerful, and optimistic. Other symptoms associated with mania are decreased need for sleep, thoughts of grandiosity or persecution, increased distractibility, decreased inhibition, and rapid pressured speech. Along with increased psychomotor agitation, appetite is increased, requiring the person to eat often, quickly, and greedily. Persons suffering from mania are apt to be impulsive, displaying poor judgment and a distorted sense of the world around them. Some patients present as irritable rather than euphoric, and others vacillate between the two extremes.[29]

Medications such as antivirals, used in the treatment of HIV infection, may precipitate depression or mania. Substance abuse, psychosocial stressors, antidepressant therapy, electroconvulsive therapy, and childbirth can all influence the progression of mania. Due to strong evidence supporting the hereditary aspect of bipolar disease,[34] persons who exhibit signs of mania need to be assessed for prior episodes of mania and depression indicating a psychiatric disorder not related to HIV infection. Episodes of mania may also indicate disease progression, representing organic affective disorder resulting from neurological involvement. Because it is uncommon to see purely manic states without any associated depressive manifestations, manic behaviors should alert the care provider to possible psychiatric history or neurological deficits.[34] It is essential that anyone presenting with signs or symptoms of an acute manic episode be referred for evaluation and inpatient treatment.

Psychosis

Psychosis is a mental disorder that impairs the person's ability to meet the ordinary demands of life. It is characterized by an impairment in the person's reality orientation. Behaviors indicative of the many forms of psychosis are cognitive impairment, delusions, hallucinations, agitated behavior, and incoherent or pressured speech. While a number of reports have cited the presence of psychoses exclusive of organic signs such as schizophreniform and paranoid psychosis, these are rare within the HIV population.[2] However, Leavitt and Sullivan[35] point out that individuals diagnosed with disorders presenting with psychotic symptoms, such as bipolar disorder and schizophrenia, are at increased risk for HIV infection as a result of disorder-related behaviors (impaired judgment, poor impulse control, decreased inhibition), socioeconomic status, educational level, and minimal access to HIV education and community services.

An individual diagnosed with HIV experiences various levels of depression and anxiety, often as a component of an adjustment disorder. Some experience a psychotic reaction that may occur prior to diagnosis, with HIV diagnosis, or later during the course of the illness as a result of life stressors or CNS involvement. The person most often is unaware of the inappropriateness of his behavior and is not cognizant of the change. A portion of persons with HIV infection have previous psychiatric diagnoses. Those with a prior diagnosis of major depression or personality disorder are more likely to experience recurrent depressive symptoms and disorders, and lifetime anxiety disorders.[2,5,7,27,35] According to the National Institute of Mental Health, 5 to 20% of persons admitted to mental health facilities with chronic and severe mental illness tested positive for the HIV antibody.[36] This compounds the difficulty in differentiating an exacerbation of a previous condition vs. a new onset of mental impairment. Accurate assessment of a person's current mental health status, prior mental health history, and its impact on the person's life and physical health is needed to ensure appropriate diagnosis, treatment, and referral. An acute exacerbation of a psychiatric illness with a psychotic presentation can be mistaken easily as an organic dementia resulting from HIV.

One form of psychosis that may occur in a person with HIV is *alcoholic psychosis*, which is associated with excessive alcohol use. Delirium tremors, Korsakoff's syndrome, alcohol hallucinosis, and alcoholic paranoia may be evident. Another form of psychosis is known as *brief reactive psychosis*, or more commonly, *situational psychosis*. This form occurs as a result of a reaction to a recognizable and distressing life event. It is of sudden onset and lasts for less than a month. Presenting symptoms may include incoherence, loose associations, delusions, hallucinations, and disorganized or catatonic behavior. *Depressive psychosis* occurs as a result of major depression, with or without an adjustment disorder component, and includes psychotic symptoms. Alcoholic, brief reactive, and depressive psychosis may all be considered under the heading of functional psychosis in which no apparent organic disease or dysfunction is found. Alcoholic psychosis may have an organic basis related to alcoholic encephalopathy and other disease states. Psychosis resulting from CNS involvement is pathological and is known as ADC (see Chapter 9).

Suicide

Suicide is the greatest psychiatric complication of depression, with depression being the greatest precipitant of suicide. *Suicide* is the intentional performance of lethal acts that result in self-inflicted death. *Attempted suicide* is the performance of potentially lethal acts in an effort to kill oneself. It can also be a nonlethal gesture for attention-seeking purposes, such as mild overdoses and wrist cutting. "Life threatening illnesses increase the incidence of depression and suicide."[1(p 134)]

Persons diagnosed with HIV have a suicide rate 40 to 66 times greater than that of the general population.[37,38] Deaths previously attributed to HIV infection were later found to have resulted from suicide, with a higher prevalence occurring in person's who were asymptomatic.[39] Other research suggests that the risk of suicide increases with disease progression, most notably from the asymptomatic to symptomatic stages.[38] A person's risk of suicide is based on whether she has a plan, and the lethality of the plan. Risk factors associated with suicide should be assessed as part of the psychological profile for all HIV-infected individuals, including:

- **Psychosocial factors**
  - Hopeless, helpless, depression
  - Caucasian race

(continued)

  - Male gender
  - Advanced age
  - Living alone, social isolation
  - Single
- **History**
  - Prior suicide attempts
  - Family history of suicide attempts
  - Family history of substance abuse
  - Physical or sexual abuse
- **Diagnostic**
  - General medical illness
  - Psychosis (schizophrenia)
  - Substance abuse
  - Depression

Behaviors associated with potential suicide, listed below, are highly correlated to depression.

- Hopelessness about the future
- Suicide note or verbalization
- Writing, art, conversation with death themes
- Giving away possessions
- Quitting a job or volunteer work
- Symptoms of major depression
- Psychosis

Suicides in the HIV population are preventable and can be managed with appropriate interventions. Factors that contribute to suicide include:

- Combination of psychiatric illness and psychosocial factors
- Major depression and bipolar disorder
- Substance abuse
- Psychotic disorders
- Terminal medical disorder

Most suicidal persons do not desire to die, but rather desire to relieve the feelings associated with depression, alleviate clinical symptoms and pain, and regain some sense of control.[1] Pain has been shown repeatedly to be the most common factor associated with suicide in persons suffering from a terminal illness.[38,40] Studies have shown that the risk of suicide increases immediately before or after inpatient admission and with changes in medication, treatment program, and counselors and physicians.[38,40] Increased risk of suicide is also associated with the number and quality of frequent losses.[38,40] Identification of events that potentiate the risk of suicide enables the health care provider to be aware of periods when increased support and preventive interventions may need to be implemented.

Often a person who either attempts or succeeds at suicide has seen their primary care provider or therapist within 2 weeks.[37,40] A large number of these persons evaluated by their primary care provider were seen for the chief complaints of physical symptoms without evidence of suicidal ideation. This suggests that the persons focused on their physical symptoms, such as pain, and did not identify their depression or suicidal ideation as a problem.[37] These findings support the need for all levels of health care providers to be aware of and assess the signs, symptoms, and risk factors of depression and suicide, as well as the psychosocial stressors associated with this chronic and terminal illness. These responses are all interrelated and, left undetected and untreated, may result in not only a decrease in the quality of life that may be achieved, but also premature loss of life.

Presentation and Assessment

Health care providers must be knowledgeable and skilled in the assessment, planning, and management of emotional or psychiatric stressors in all health care settings. Pharmacological and non-pharmacological interventions are often employed simultaneously. Assessment data provide the foundation on which the clinician builds the framework of interventions that promote and enhance the person's physical and emotional well-being, development, and problem-solving and coping capacities. The caregiver must be alert to verbal and nonverbal messages throughout any interaction. Although assessment is an ongoing process, the initial assessment can facilitate the identification of current problems and provide a baseline for the clinician to identify subtle changes over time.

Assessment of a person encountering psychosocial crisis as a result of HIV infection requires a biopsychosocial approach.[41,42] Often, health care providers use what is known as the Mini Mental State Examination (see Figure 9.1, pp. 250–251) to get an overview of the patient's emotional and mental functioning. The more comprehensive Mental Status Exam (MSE) assesses the patient's appearance, behavior, speech, thought, perceptions, mood and affect, and intellectual functioning.[43] These areas are assessed to evaluate abnormalities in a patient's level of consciousness, thinking, feeling, perception, memory, and behavior.[9,43] Each area of assessment on the MSE is listed below.

Appearance
- Manner of dress
- Grooming/general self-care
- State of health
- Physical features such as scars, obesity, emaciation, deformities

Behavior
- Activity level
- Cooperativeness, eye contact
- Gestures and mannerisms
- Motor behavior
- General attitude
- Signs of extrapyramidal symptoms (EPS) if on psychotropic, medication

Speech
- Rate of speech/tone
- Word choice and sequences
- Lack of speech
- Degree of spontaneity
- Presence of abnormalities
- Pressured speech or rhyming

Thought content
- Magical, bizarre, unusual thoughts
- Paranoia/obsessions
- Preoccupation
- Delusional ideas of reference

Processes
- Clarity of thought
- Logical or illogical
- Organized
- Circumstantial
- Associations

Perceptions
- Sensory awareness
- Interpretation of the environment
- Illusions, hallucinations
- Depersonalization

Mood and affect
- How client states he feels; observed mood
- Observed emotional response and feelings
- Demeanor
- Tone of voice
- Body movement
- Affect flat, labile, blunt, constricted
- Whether affect and mood are appropriate and congruent
- Intellectual functioning
- Orientation: Person, place, time, events

Registration and recall: Able to state name of physician,

nurse, health care, provider; can name three to five unrelated objects immediately and after 5 minutes
Concentration: Is client able to follow and carry out instructions; can client subtract by threes or sevens from 100
Language: Does client state details of life that are verifiable; can client provide historical data such as medical history, previous addresses, life events
Thought processes: Can client nurse, health care provider; can name correctly interpret a proverb; is the thinking concrete, bizarre, or nonsensical; is the thinking logical and coherent or difficult to understand
Insight: Able to assess current situation
Judgment: Chooses appropriate actions; able to make decisions and follow through; sees alternatives

A variety of formalized questionnaires and standardized tests are available as additional methods of assessing the presence and severity of emotional, psychological, and cognitive dysfunction and disorders. Rating scales most commonly encountered are either observer ratings or self-report. The Brief Psychiatric Rating Scale (BPRS) is an assessment tool that has been used extensively and can assist the practitioner in integrating outcome assessment into clinical practice. It is a clinician-based rating scale that provides an efficient means of evaluating psychiatric symptoms seen in both outpatient and inpatient settings.[44] The BPRS consists of 18 items measured on a 7-point continuum, ranging from not present to extremely severe.

Scales commonly in use are the Beck Depression Inventory, Center for Epidemiologic Studies-Depression Scale (CES-D), Beck Anxiety Inventory, Anxiety Disorders Interview Schedule-Revised, Anxiety Sensitivity Index, Social Interaction Anxiety Scale, and the Hamilton Anxiety Scale.[42,43] Based on the client interview and outcome of the psychosocial/health history, physical exam, provider observations, and psychological testing, medical and nursing diagnoses are developed. Interventions are based on these diagnoses and the person's individual needs.

Medical diagnosis of the presenting problem requires an understanding of the difference between a medical disorder and a mental disorder. The *Diagnostic and Statistical Manual of Mental Disorders (DSMIV-R)*,[45] provides guidance in understanding the boundaries, concepts, criteria, and differential diagnoses currently accepted and in use. A *medical disorder* is formed based on abstractions that include pathology, symptoms, physiological deviation, and etiology. Mental disorders are formed based on concepts of significant behavioral or psychological patterns and syndromes associated with distress, disability, or loss of freedom, in which the cause is a manifestation of either behavioral, psychological, or biologic dysfunction. It should be understood that a medical disorder may present with components of a mental disorder and a mental disorder may present with components of a medical disorder.[45]

The more common medical diagnoses that may be incurred in persons with HIV infection as a result of psychosocial stressors are adjustment disorder, acute stress disorder, generalized anxiety disorder, bereavement, major depressive disorder/episode, and psychological factor affecting medical condition. Many diagnoses closely resemble each other. The use of professional resources that provide clear diagnostic criteria should be employed to ensure proper diagnosis and intervention. In the HIV-infected person, it should be kept in mind that the presenting symptoms and resulting psychiatric diagnosis may be induced by medication, a comorbid medical condition, or a preexisting psychiatric condition.

Interventions

Medical management includes further testing, pharmacotherapy, psychotherapy, specialized medical care, referral to community and other resources, and close follow-up and professional collaboration. Hospitalization may be indicated in persons suffering from a severe response or if safety is an issue. Patient teaching is provided by all health care providers and ancillary services based on assessment of individual needs. These medical interventions are applicable to each of the psychiatric diagnoses presented. Variances in medical treatment occur in the pharmacotherapy, type of counseling or psychotherapy, referrals made, and frequency of follow-up. These variances are based on the client's perception of his health status, diagnosis, severity of symptoms, and overall psychosocial assessment with an emphasis on his social support system.

Medications commonly used to treat psychiatric disorders are antidepressants, anxiolytics, sedatives and hypnotics, and antipsychotics. The prescribing and administering of these medications to persons diagnosed with HIV requires the clinician to be cognizant of the interaction and sensitivity that may be experienced. Often, decreased doses must be given. The individual's physiological status must be considered because medications such as hypnotics and anxiolytics can depress an already depressed respiratory system in a person suffering from *Pneumocystis carinii* pneumonia. Antidepressants have been shown to have potentially adverse effects on sexual functioning by altering the libido, inducing priapism and ejaculatory difficulties, and interfering with achieving orgasm. For the person with HIV infection, the loss of sexual function can result in decreased self-esteem, anxiety, anger, fear of abandonment, and fear of loss of their sexual partner and loss of control over her life. Drugs frequently used in the treatment of symptoms, disorders, and diseases associated with HIV that have the potential to induce psychiatric side effects are listed in Table 15.4.

Nursing interventions reflect the actions taken or performed to assist the client achieve a desired outcome. They are planned steps taken to facilitate the altering of etiologic factors associated with psychosocial responses to a diagnosis to improve the person's overall health status or address an identified deficit. In instances when the etiology of a specific behavior or symptom is unknown, the interventions should be directed toward symptomology. Interventions require establishing goals, prioritizing those goals, and a means of measuring the effectiveness of the intervention. Intervention is based on the clinician's professional evaluation of the individual's response to his health problems and treatment, life processes, emotional and social well-being, and care needs.

Evaluation of interventions is a continual process that often results in modification of the goals and interventions planned. Methods to evaluate the effectiveness of an intervention should be presented in a measurable format and should be realistic. The planned goals and desired outcomes are not presented in the diagnostic and treatment overviews. However, in the planning of interventions to alter the etiology or symptomology of a diagnosis, the process of setting and prioritizing goals and specifying outcomes is conducted.

The diagnostic and treatment overviews presented in Tables 15.5 through 15.7 review the diagnostic criteria, symptom/response, interventions, and evaluation applicable to some of the diagnoses as a result of the individual's psychosocial response.[45–48] There are many other identifiable

Table 15.4 Common Medications with Psychiatric Side Effects Used in the Treatment of HIV[49]

Drug	Reaction	Comment
Acyclovir	Paranoia, delusions, depression, insomnia, fearfulness	High doses; especially chronic renal failure
Albuterol	Hallucination, paranoia	—
Amphetaminelike drugs	Paranoia, delusion, manic symptoms, anxiety, depression	With overdose, abuse, inhaler use
Amphotericin B	Delirium	—
Anticholinergics, atrophine	Paranoia, delirium, confusion, memory loss, depression, fear, agitation, bizarre behavior	—
Anticonvulsants	Hallucinations, paranoia, delusions, agitation, depression, delirium, mania	—
Antidepressants, tricyclic	Paranoia, delusions, delirium, hypomania, mania	In 10% of patients; also in withdrawal
Bactrim	Delusions, psychosis, depression, disorientation	—
Barbiturates	Hyperactivity, depression, excitability, delirium, tremorlike syndrome	—
Benzodiazepines	Paranoia, mania, rage, hostility, delirium, depression, nightmares	During treatment or withdrawal

Beta adrenergic blockers	Paranoia, delusion, depression, confusion, mania	With usual doses including ophthalmic use
Bromocriptine	Paranoia, delusion, mania, aggressive behavior, depression, anxiety	Not dose related; symptoms persist for weeks after stopping the drug
Cephalosporins	Paranoia, confusion, disorientation	—
Ciprofloxacin	Delirium, psychosis	—
Corticosteroids	Hallucinations, paranoia, mania, depression, confusion	Withdrawal occurs with inhalation
Histamine H_2 receptor antagonist	Hallucinations, paranoia, mania, bizarre behavior, delirium, depression, disorientation	—
INH	Hallucinations, paranoia, depression, agitation	—
Ketaconazole	Hallucinations	—
Narcotics	Paranoia, dysphoria, nightmares, agitation, euphoria, depression, anxiety	—
NSAIDS	Paranoia, delusions, depression, anxiety	Not all drugs in this class
Zidovudine	Hallucinations, paranoia, mania	—

INH = isoniazid; NSAIDS = nonsteroidal anti-inflammatory drugs.

Table 15.5 Major Depressive Disorder

Definition: Mood disorder characterized by one or more Major Depressive Episodes, often following a severe psychosocial stressor (see MDE).

Presentation & Assessment: Sadness, apathy, feelings of worthlessness, hopelessness and helplessness, weight loss or gain, anorexia, anhedonia, sleep disturbance, suicidal thoughts. Adolescents may exhibit behaviors associated with social isolation, acting out, negative attitude.

Differential Diagnosis:
Mood Disorder Due to a General Medial Condition
Depressive Disorder Not Otherwise Specified
Adjustment Disorder with Depressed Mood Attention-Deficit/Hyperactivity Disorder
Substance Induced Mood Disorder
Manic Episode with Irritable Mood
Bereavement
Dementia

Diagnostic Criteria	Psychosocial Response	Interventions	Evaluation
I. **Major depressive disorder (MDD), single episode** A. Presence of a single major depressive episode (MDE) B. MDE not accounted for by schizoaffective disorder and not superimposed on schizophrenia, schizophreniform disorder, delusional disorder, or psychotic disorder; not otherwise specified	I. **Violence self-directed, resulting from feelings of hopelessness:** The presence of risk factors for suicide resulting from a perceived lack of alternatives or personal choices	I. A. Initiate appropriate safety protocols B. Assess intent/plan; contract for safety C. Assist in identifying sources of depression and hopelessness utilizing warm, caring, nonjudgmental manner D. Help identify positive qualities in self E. Administer appropriate medications	I. A. Does not harm self B Contracts for safety; states will not harm self; contacts someone when anxious or experiencing suicidal thoughts C. Expresses feelings of depression and anxiety, identifying their source D. Identifies positive qualities of self E. Expresses need for ongoing treatment and support; adheres to medication regime

C. No history of manic episode, mixed episode, or hypomanic episode unless episodes are substance or treatment induced, or due to direct physiological effects of a general medical condition		F. Provide phone numbers/resources for crisis centers, counselors, hot lines	F. Identifies support resources
II. Major depressive disorder, recurrent A. Presence of two or more MDEs B. Same criteria as B above C. Same criteria as C above	**II. Grieving, dysfunctional:** An individual's exaggerated, delayed, prolonged, or absent response to a loss of a significant person, ideal, status, object, or body part	**II.** A. Observe for lack of grieving B. Assist in working through excessive, distorted, and delayed emotional reactions C. Provide support; explain that grieving is normal and painful D. Discourage rumination about guilty feelings; encourage expression of feelings such as sadness, anger, and helplessness	**II.** A. Discusses loss and associated feelings B. States acceptance and understanding that feelings of sadness, anger, denial, and guilt are part of the normal grieving process

Table 15.5 Major Depressive Disorder *Continued*

Diagnostic Criteria	Psychosocial Response	Interventions	Evaluation
	III. Coping, ineffective individual: A lack of effective adaptive behaviors to cope with difficult life situation	**III.** A. Provide information about cause, diagnosis, and treatment of MDD B. Help analyze current situation and evaluate effectiveness of coping strategies C. Teach and discuss alternatives to ineffective behaviors	**III.** A. Verbalizes causes, symptoms, and appropriate treatment of MDD B. Discusses emotions triggered by illness and usual coping behaviors C. Describes at least one situation solved by identifying the problem and choosing an appropriate alternative coping method
	IV. Social isolation: The unwanted social isolation resulting from a combination of physical, psychological, social, and environmental factors	**IV.** A. Provide time for expression of concern over effect of illness on social life B. Assist in identifying factors contributing to social isolation C. Involve in the planning of care D. Help identify social activities that can be initiated independently E. Encourage to express feelings associated with increased dependence	**IV.** A. Discusses concern and effects of illness on social aspects of life including feelings of dependency B. Describes factors contributing to social isolation C. Actively participates in planning care D. Seeks and accepts assistance in increasing social contacts and participates in support groups/volunteer activities associated with HIV/AIDS

Table 15.6 Bereavement (Grief)

Definition: The psychological response to a perceived or actual loss. It should be noted that bereavement varies considerably among different cultural groups.
Presentation & Assessment: Sadness, restlessness, insomnia, decreased appetite, social withdrawal, guilt or blame of others.
Differential Diagnosis:
Major Depressive Disorder
Adjustment Disorder

Diagnostic Criteria	Psychosocial Response	Interventions[a]	Evaluation[b]
A. Symptoms are present for ≥1 to 2 months B. Absence of symptoms characteristic of a major depressive disorder C. Emotional symptoms are interspersed with normal feelings	I. **Grieving, anticipatory:** State in which the individual experiences feelings in response to an expected loss II. **Grieving:** The state in which the individual experiences feelings to a loss III. **Grieving, dysfunctional:** An individual's exaggerated, delayed, prolonged, or absent response to the loss of a significant person, idea, status, object, or body part incurred due to the HIV illness continuum	A. Discuss the normal course of grieving and provide an opportunity for the client to talk about loss and express feelings of sadness and anger B. Encourage involvement in daily activities C. Assist in creating meaningful rituals D. Encourage participation in support groups E. Encourage active participation in health care, AIDS organizations, and research F. Instruct in ways to divert emotions by using activity and relaxation	A. Verbalizes the normal grief reaction and discusses his losses, expressing feelings of sadness and anger B. Verbalizes continued involvement in interests and activities C. Able to identify meaningful rituals and verbalizes participation in AIDS marches, attending funerals, and support activities D. Attends and actively participates in AIDS support groups E. Performs health-promoting behaviors and is a member of a research study group

Table 15.6 Bereavement (Grief) *Continued*

Diagnostic Criteria	Psychosocial Response	Interventions[a]	Evaluation[b]
		G. Evaluate readiness to discuss death and initiate discussions as soon as ready	F. Performs guided imagery and progressive relaxation, and is working out three times a week
		H. Educate regarding prescribed medication, side effects, drug interactions and precautions, as well as any other treatment modality that may potentially alter the clients lifestyle, feelings of well-being, and/or the normal grief process	G. Is able to discuss the death and dying process H. Verbalizes the expected side effects, interactions, and precautions, and the impact treatment has on his activities of daily living (ADLs), and the effect these have on his grieving process

[a]Interventions provided are appropriate for each listed response.
[b]Evaluation based on interventions implemented for each response.

Table 15.7 Generalized Anxiety Disorder

Definition: Excessive anxiety and worry for a period of at least 6 months which is evidenced by both psychological and physical symptons (see MDE).

Presentation & Assessment:

Psychological: Fearful anticipation, irritability, insomnia, night terrors, restlessness, poor concentration, repetitive worrying thoughts, depression

Physical: Headache, dizziness, tinnitus, dry mouth, dysphagia, epigastric discomfort, chest tightness/discomfort, dyspnea, palpitations, polyuria, frequent/loose bowels

Differential Diagnosis:

Anxiety Disorder Due to a General Medical Condition
Adjustment Disorder
Obsessive-Compulsive Disorder
Substance Induced Anxiety Disorder
Post Traumatic Stress Disorder
Panic Disorder
Mood Disorder

Diagnostic Criteria	Psychosocial Response	Interventions	Evaluation
A. Excessive anxiety and worry occurring more days than not for at least 6 months, about a number of events or activities B. The person finds it difficult to control the worry C. The anxiety and worry are associated with three or more of the following six symptoms (with at least some symptoms present for more days than not for the past 6 months):	I. **Fear:** The response to a real or perceived danger associated with HIV infection	I. **Fear:** A. Discuss fears and anxiety known to be associated with HIV/AIDS and help identify those currently being experienced B. Help anticipate and respond to symptoms C. Counsel regarding aspects of illness that can be affected	I. **Fear:** A. Is able to identify own fears and sources of anxiety, and verbalizes feelings B. Describes course of illness, symptoms, and aspects of life that may be affected C. Utilizes alternative methods to overcome physical and psychological limitations

Table 15.7 General Anxiety Disorder *Continued*

Diagnostic Criteria	Psychosocial Response	Interventions	Evaluation
restlessness or feeling keyed up, on edge; being easily fatigued; difficulty concentrating, mind going blank; irritability; muscle tension; sleep disturbance (difficulty falling or staying asleep; restless, unsatisfying sleep) D. Focus of anxiety and worry are not confined to features of another axis I disorder E. The anxiety, worry, or physical symptoms cause clinically significant distress or impairment in social, occupational, or other important areas of functioning F. The disturbance is not due to the direct physiological effects of a substance or general medical condition and does not occur exclusively during a mood, psychotic, or pervasive developmental disorder		D. Assist in understanding and accepting limitations, identifying alternative methods to live life to its fullest E. Develop clinical services that mobilize social support systems F. Assist in understanding relationship between psychological distress and physical symptom	D. Verbalizes relationship between physical and psychological symptoms related to HIV infection
	II. **Decision-related conflicts:** A state of uncertainty about health-related courses of action when choice involves risk, loss, or challenges to personal life	II. **Decision-related conflicts:** A. Encourage and assist to make decisions regarding own health care B. Provide clear and concise explanations, in terms the patient can understand, of treatment regimen; avoid information overload that may impair cognitive abilities	II. **Decision-related conflicts:** A. Makes appropriate care-related decisions B. Verbalizes understanding of treatment plan, potential side effects, and outcomes, and demonstrates ability to adhere to treatment regimen C. Verbalizes acceptance of limitations imposed by HIV infection

	C. Assist patient in recognizing physical and psychological limitations, encourage acceptance of limitations, and identify strengths that can be mobilized to overcome limitations	
III. Anxiety: A vague, unpleasant feeling in response to multiple psychological and physiological stressors experienced as a result of HIV infection	**III. Anxiety:** A. Assist in recognizing anxious behaviors and identify their source B. Listen attentively and encourage verbalization of feelings C. Assist to accept that the patient is no less worthy as a result of an HIV diagnosis D. Assist in identifying and utilizing community support systems and resources E. Encourage involvement of family, friends, and significant others in assisting with planning and decision processes	**III. Anxiety:** A. Reports feelings of anxiety and describes anxiety-inducing situations B. States positive aspects of self C. Engages in conversation and activities with significant others, caregivers, and other support systems

problems, interventions, and methods of evaluation that are appropriate to these diagnoses and these should be determined individually. Those presented represent examples of those that may be applied to any of the diagnoses presented based on an individual's response. Medication management, psychotherapy, and other intervention and treatment modalities previously presented could be applied to any of the overviews presented.

References

1. Servellen G, Aguirre MG. Symptoms, symptom management, and psychological morbidity among persons with HIV disease. *AIDS Patient Care.* 1995;9(3): 134–139.
2. Miller D, Riccio M. Non-organic psychiatric and psychosocial syndromes associated with HIV-1 infection and disease. *AIDS.* 1990;4(5):381–388.
3. Duffy VJ. Crisis points in HIV disease. *AIDS Patient Care.* 1994;2:28–32.
4. Gil F, Arranz P, Lianes P, et al. Physical symptoms and psychological distress among patients with HIV infection. *AIDS Patient Care.* 1995;9(1):28–31.
5. Jadresic D, Riccio M, Hawkins DA, et al. Long-term impact of HIV diagnosis on mood and substance use—St. Stephen's cohort study. *Int J STD AIDS.* 1994; 5:248–252.
6. McGurk D, Miller TW, Eggerth DE. HIV status, substance dependency, and psychiatric diagnosis. *AIDS Patient Care.* 1994;8(6):328–330.
7. Johnson JG, Williams JBW, Rabkin JG, et al. Axis I psychiatric symptoms associated with HIV infection and personality disorder. *Am J Psychiatry.* 1995; 152(4):551–554.
8. Davis RF, Metzger DS, Meyers K, et al. *AIDS.* 1995;9(1):73–79.
9. Luis S, Grained RD, McDonnell WA, et al. *Manual of Psychosocial Nursing Interventions: Promoting Mental Health in Medical-Surgical Settings.* Philadelphia: WB Saunders; 1989.
10. Kyle RD, Sachs LG. Perceptions of control and social support in relation to psychosocial adjustment to HIV/AIDS. *AIDS Patient Care.* 1994;December: 322–327.
11. Sheer L, ed. *Grief and AIDS.* West Sussex, England: John Wiley & Sons; 1995.
12. Brady MJ, Cella DF. Helping patients live with their cancer. *Patient Care.* 1995; 29(10):41–51.
13. Grothe D. Barriers to effective treatment of depression. *Drug Topics.* 1994; May:51–64.
14. Perkins DO, Stern RA, Golden RN, et al. Mood disorders in HIV infection:

prevalence and risk factors in a nonepicenter of the AIDS epidemic. *Am J Psychiatry.* 1994;151(2):233–236.

15. Sande MA, Carpenter CC, Cobbs CG, et al. Antiretroviral therapy for adult HIV-infected patients: recommendations from a state-of-the-art conference. *JAMA.* 1993;270(21):2583–2589.
16. Knox MD, Davis M, Friedrich MA. The HIV mental health spectrum. *AIDS Patient Care.* 1995;9(1):20–27.
17. Roberts SJ. Somatization in primary care: the common presentation of psychosocial problems through physical complaints. *Nurse Pract.* 1994;19(5): 47–55.
18. Carpenito L. *Handbook of Nursing Diagnosis.* 5th ed. Philadelphia: Lippincott; 1993.
19. Vader B, Wrubel B, Vader M. Death, dying, and the patient with acquired immunodeficiency syndrome. *Clin Pediatr Med Surg.* 1992;9(4):993–996.
20. Carson V, Soeken K, Shanty J, et al. Hope and spiritual well-being essentials for living with AIDS. *Perspect Psychiatr Care.* 1990;26(2):28–34.
21. Whitley G. Concept analysis of anxiety. *Nurs Diagn.* 1992;3(3):107–116.
22. Ziegler SM. *Theory-Directed Practice.* New York: Springer; 1993.
23. Holland J, Tross S. The psychosocial and neuropsychiatric sequelae of the acquired immunodeficiency syndrome and related disorders. *Ann Intern Med.* 1985;103:760–764.
24. Chuang H, Devins G, Hunsley J, et al. Psychological distress and well-being among gay and bisexual men with human immunodeficiency virus infection. *Am J Psychiatry.* 1989;146(7):886–890.
25. Stuart G, Sundeen S. *Principles and Practice of Psychiatric Nursing.* 5th ed. St Louis: Mosby; 1995.
26. Simon GE, VonKorff M. Recognition, management, and outcomes of depression in primary care. *Arch Fam Med.* 1995;4:99–105.
27. Rabkin JG, Ramien RH. Depressive disorder and HIV disease: an uncommon association. *FOCUS: A Guide to AIDS Research and Counseling.* 1995;10(9): 1–5.
28. Peternelj-Taylor CA, Hartley VL. Living with mental illness: professional/family collaboration. *J Psychosoc Nurs.* 1993;31(3):23–28, 40–41.
29. Wilson SE. AIDS dementia complex: a comprehensive approach to care. *AIDS Patient Care.* 1989;3(5):20–22.
30. ACHPR. *Depression in Primary Care.* Vols. 1 and 2. Rockville, MD: US Department of Health and Human Services; 1993.
31. Baker J. Treatment of mood disorders. *FOCUS: A Guide to AIDS Research and Counseling.* 1993;8(8):1–5.
32. Lyketosos CG, Hanson AL, Fishman M, et al. Manic syndrome: early and late in the course of HIV. *Am J Psychiatry.* 1993;150:326–327.

33. Gelder M, Gath D, Mayou R. *Concise Oxford Textbook of Psychiatry.* New York: Oxford University Press; 1994.
34. Goodwin FK, Jamison KR. *Manic-Depressive Illness.* New York: Oxford University Press; 1990.
35. Leavitt E, Sullivan P. HIV and chronic mental illness. *FOCUS: A Guide to AIDS Research and Counseling.* 1993;8(4):1–5.
36. Sacks M, Dermatis H, Looser-Ott S, Burton W, Perry S. Undetected HIV infection among acutely ill psychiatric inpatients. *Am J Psychiatry.* 1992;149(4):544–545.
37. Valente SM. Evaluating suicide risk in the medically ill patient. *Nurse Pract.* 1993;18(9):41–50.
38. Pugh K. Suicide in patients with HIV infection and AIDS. In: Sherr L, ed. *Grief and AIDS.* West Sussex, England: John Wiley & Sons; 1995.
39. Motto JA. Rational suicide: then and now, when and how. *FOCUS: A Guide to AIDS Research and Counseling.* 1994;9(5):1–4.
40. Earle KA, Forquer SL, Volo AM, et al. The relationship between acute psychiatric symptoms, diagnosis, and short-term risk of violence. *Hosp Commun Psychiatry.* 1994;45(2):133–137.
41. Adinolfi A. The role of the nurse in the care of patients with HIV infection. In: Bartlett JA, ed. *Care and Management of Patients With HIV Infection.* Research Triangle Park, NC: Glaxco; 1993.
42. Barlow DH. *Clinical Handbook of Psychological Disorders: A Step-by-Step Treatment Manual.* 2nd ed. New York: Guilford Press; 1993.
43. Maxmen JS, Ward NG. *Essential Psychopathology and Its Treatment.* 2nd ed. New York: WW Norton; 1995.
44. Sederer L, Dickey B. *Outcomes Assessment in Clinical Practice.* Baltimore: Williams & Wilkins; 1995.
45. *Diagnostic and Statistical Manual of Mental Disorders.* 4th ed. Washington, DC: American Psychiatric Association; 1994.
46. Bulechek GM, McClossky JC. *Nursing Interventions: Essential Nursing Treatments.* 2nd ed. Philadelphia: WB Saunders; 1992.
47. Dyer JG, Sparks SM, Taylor CM. *Psychiatric Nursing Diagnoses: A Comprehensive Manual of Mental Health Care.* Springhouse, PA: Springhouse; 1995.
48. Moller MD, Knudsvig LG. Successfully living with mania: helpful hints to families and professionals. *Innov Res.* 1993;2(2):61–68.
49. *Med Lett.* 1993;35:65–70.

CHAPTER 16

Fatigue

Barbara F. Piper, DNSc, RN, AOCN, FAAN

Chapter Preview

- Definition
- Biologic and Behavioral Basis
- Presentation and Assessment
- Related Medical Management
- Interventions
- Information for Patients about HIV-Associated Fatigue

Despite the fact that fatigue is one of the most commonly experienced and bothersome symptoms in people infected with HIV,[1] it has not been well studied.[2,3] Fatigue may even precede the diagnosis of HIV infection, CNS involvement,[4] OIs,[1] and AIDS.[1] A fatigue prevalence rate of 17 to 60% has been documented in HIV-infected adults prior to the diagnosis of AIDS.[5–10] For people with AIDS, the prevalence rate is reported to be between 43 to 70%.[3,8,11] Although fatigue may occur across all stages of HIV,[8,11–13] its prevalence may actually increase as the disease progresses and CD4 counts decline.[11,14]

Fatigue is a prevalent and significant problem[11] for HIV-infected individuals.[15–18] It can affect negatively overall health,[3,19] functional status,[20–22] ADLs,[11,19–21] disability,[19] employment and wage-earning abilities,[11,23] and quality of life.[19,24]

Definition

Fatigue is the perception of unusual or abnormal whole-body tiredness disproportionate to or unrelated to activity or exertion.[25] It may not be relieved by a good night's sleep or by rest. It is termed *acute*, when it is experienced for less than 1 month, or *chronic* when it lasts 1 month or longer.[25]

Biologic and Behavioral Basis

Although few studies have determined the specific etiologies of fatigue in HIV infection,[3] HIV-related fatigue (HRF) is most likely multifactorial, as with fatigue experienced in other clinical conditions.[3,25] Various theories and models have been proposed to explain how fatigue occurs in clinical populations.[25–29] Figure 16.1 depicts one such framework—the Integrated Fatigue Model (IFM).[26–28] Because it is the most frequently cited framework used to guide assessment and theory development in cancer-related fatigue,[28] it is thought to have comparable utility in HRF.[17]

In the center of the IFM are the manifestations or dimensions of fatigue: temporal, sensory, cognitive/mental, affective/emotional, behavioral, and physiological.[26] See Presentation and Assessment for further discussion of these dimensions. Surrounding the center of the IFM are the proposed

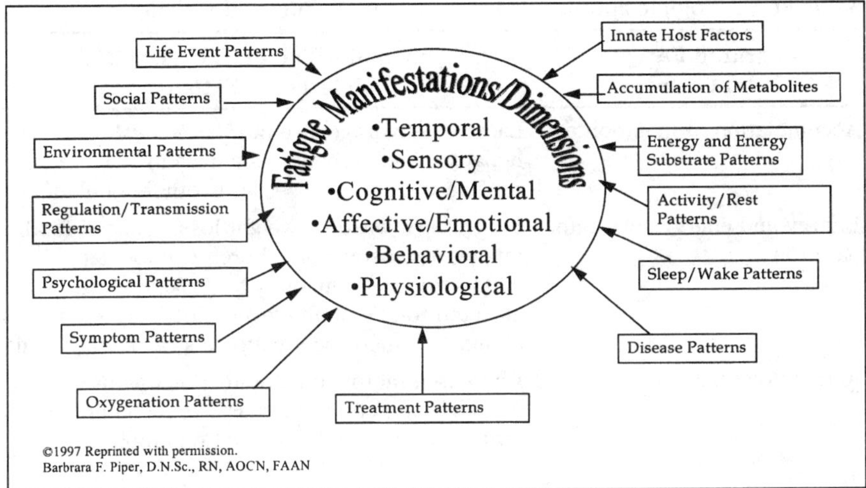

Figure 16.1 Integrated Fatigue Model

factors that may be associated positively and negatively with fatigue in clinical populations. As HIV can affect every organ system, HRF can occur because of the virus' effects on these systems.[30]

The IFM can be used to guide the health care provider's clinical assessment of HRF. The term *patterns* is used to indicate what may be usual or recurring characteristics over time for a specific individual. Changes in these characteristic patterns over time can suggest underlying etiologies and treatments for HRF. Table 16.1 describes the IFM patterns and the factors that have been associated with HRF.

Presentation and Assessment

Subjective

Subjective manifestations of fatigue may include feeling tired, weary, listless, weak, or worn out. Common complaints include lack of energy, stamina, or endurance. Emotionally the person with fatigue may become more irritable or impatient and may lack motivation. Behaviorally the person

Table 16.1 Biologic and Behavioral Basis for HIV-Related Fatigue

Integrated Fatigue Model Patterns	Variables/Factors Potentially Related to Fatigue
Accumulation of metabolites	Lactate dehydrogenase in *Pneumocystis carinii*, hepatitis, and hemolytic anemias in HIV[11] and in cardiac and muscle diseases in other populations[31]
Energy and energy substrate patterns	Progressive wasting, weight loss, reduced food intake, malabsorption, altered metabolism, malnutrition[3,22,32]; inability to cook/shop for food[17]; elevated total globulin levels (total protein minus albumin)[11]; Increased resting energy metabolism[33]
Activity/rest patterns	Decreased motor functioning[4]; myopathies[23]; decreased functional status[20,21,34]; deconditioning;[28] fatigue has a negative impact on employment status[3]
Sleep/wake patterns	Insomnia is common[4,15,35] and also is associated with AZT[36]; fatigue increases total hours of sleep needed[11]
Disease patterns	Lower CD4 counts are associated with a higher prevalence of fatigue[11,14]; site of HIV involvement, such as the lungs[37] and heart[38]; presence of HIV-associated endocrinopathies[39] and comorbidities, such as fibromyalgia[3]
Treatment patterns	Zidovudine (AZT) causes anemia in 12–40%[40,41] and mitochondrial toxicity in approximately 17%[42,43]; reduced muscle carnitine occurs[44]; depletion of phosphocreatine suggests mitochondrial impairment of oxidative metabolism[42,43,45,46]; fatigue may or may not be dose limiting[47–49] or intensified when AZT is combined with other agents[48,50]; fatigue can occur as a side effect of medications[8] such as foscarnet,[51] from a low white blood cell count,[22] and from radiation[28] and biotherapies[52]
Oxygenation patterns	Anemia is experienced by 70–90%[19]; HIV-related lung disease[37]; HIV-related cardiomyopathy[39]
Symptom patterns	Pain, diarrhea, night sweats[8]; increased number and distress of symptoms[14,22,53,54]

Table 16.1 *Continued*

Integrated Fatigue Model Patterns	Variables/Factors Potentially Related to Fatigue
Psychological patterns	Anxiety, depression, lack of motivation[25]; mental health problems[3,4,22]
Regulation/transmission patterns	Adrenal insufficiency[55]; humoral mediators such as interferon, tumor necrosis factor, interleukins, neurotransmitters, neurohormones,[25] and electrolyte imbalances[56]
Environmental patterns	Noise, heat, allergens, altitude[25]
Social patterns	Social,[3,25] economic, cultural, and ethnic[25]; sexual preferences and drug abuse patterns[53]
Life event patterns	Job changes or losses, moving, illness, or death of friends[25]
Innate host factors	Age, gender[57,58]; race[3,25,53]; genetic makeup[25]

may say that it takes longer to do things, more effort is required, or certain activities are no longer undertaken because of the fatigue.[25]

All HIV-infected individuals should be considered at risk for fatigue. Patients should be screened and rescreened periodically over time at their routine follow-up appointments for HRF to identify quickly those who may be experiencing moderate to severe levels of fatigue (i.e., 5 or greater), or for whom fatigue is a problem. Simple numeric intensity rating scales (0, not at all, to 10, a great deal), visual analog scales (0 mm, no fatigue, to 100 mm, overwhelming fatigue), or verbal descriptor scales (0, none; 1, mild; 2, moderate; 3, severe; 4, overwhelming) can be used. Asking the following questions often can give the health care provider an immediate assessment of fatigue: Are you experiencing any unusual fatigue? How intense is your fatigue on a scale of 0 to 10? Does your fatigue affect your daily activities and if so, how?

In those individuals for whom fatigue is a problem, responses to the intensity scale and the three previously mentioned questions can be followed by a more in-depth assessment of fatigue.[29] While no consensus exists about which subjective or objective dimensions constitute fatigue, fatigue is considered to be multidimensional, and questions designed to evaluate the following dimensions are recommended[26,29]: (1) *temporal*, refers to the timing/circadian pattern, onset/duration, and pattern over time; (2) *sensory*, refers to intensity and local or systemic symptoms of fatigue; (3) *cognitive/mental*, refers to changes in concentration, ability to remember/think clearly/direct attention, and degree of alertness; (4) *affective/emotional*, refers to irritability, impatience, lack of motivation, depression, and emotional meaning ascribed to fatigue; (5) *behavioral*, refers to fatigue's impact on ADLs; and (6) *physiologic*, refers to laboratory, radiographic, and physical examination findings. Table 16.2 describes specific questions that can be used to assess subjectively these multiple dimensions.[26,27,30]

Objective

Table 16.3 describes the tests that have been used clinically to assess the physiological dimension.

Differential Diagnoses

Anemia

Because anemia can cause HRF and is one of the variables that can predict the development of AIDS in HIV-infected patients,[61] it is important to detect and treat anemia when it occurs (see Chapter 13).

Depression

In the differential diagnosis of depression vs. HRF, it is important to recall that many of the somatic symptoms of depression such as fatigue and lack of motivation often overlap with similar HIV-related somatic symptoms. Because depression inventories, such as the CES-D, contain both somatic and cognitive-affective items to diagnose depression, false-positives can occur when these inventories are used in HIV[62] (see Chapter 15).

For this reason, Kalichman et al[62] believe that it is appropriate to use depression inventories to screen and diagnose depression during the early stages of HIV infection when patients are asymptomatic from their HIV. In HIV-symptomatic patients, it is appropriate initially to use the depression inventory's cognitive-affective items or subscale alone for screening purposes. A negative result would rule out depression, while a positive result

Table 16.2 Subjective Assessment–Examples of Questions to Assess Subjective Fatigue Multidimensionally[a]

Dimension	Questions
Temporal dimension	A. Timing/circadian pattern
	1. Are you experiencing fatigue now?
	2. When during the day does fatigue usually occur?
	3. Is it better/worse in the mornings/afternoons/evenings?
	B. Onset/duration
	1. When did you first notice the fatigue?
	2. How long has it lasted (i.e., seconds, minutes, hours, days, weeks, months)?
	C. Pattern
	1. Brief, momentary, acute, transient, intermittent?
	2. Seldom, infrequent, often, frequent?
	3. Constant, continuous, chronic?
	4. Changes in this pattern over time?
	5. How does the fatigue you are experiencing now compare with the fatigue you have experienced in the past/before your illness/with previous forms of HIV treatment?
Sensory dimension	A. What are the problems that you experience that let you know that you are fatigued?
	1. Tired eyes, legs, arms (i.e., localized)?
	2. Whole-body fatigue, lack of energy/endurance/stamina, perceptions about exertion/weakness/loss of strength (i.e., generalized)?
	B. What makes your fatigue worse?
	C. What do you do to make your fatigue better? What works?

(continued)

Table 16.2 *Continued*

Dimension	Questions
Sensory dimension *(cont.)*	
	D. Overall, how severe is your fatigue?
	1. Use 0 to 10 scale *or*
	2. Mild, moderate, severe, overwhelming?
	E. What other symptoms are you experiencing at this time? How severe are these symptoms? (Use 0 to 10 scale)
Cognitive/mental dimension	A. How has fatigue affected your mental processes?
	1. Your ability to concentrate?
	2. Your ability to focus attention on something/your attention span?
	3. Your ability to remember?
	4. Your ability to think clearly?
	5. Your alertness (i.e., alert, drowsy, or sleepy)?
Affective/emotional dimension	A. How has your mood been affected by your fatigue?
	1. Have you become more irritable or impatient?
	2. Have you become more depressed?
	3. Are you less motivated to do things?
	4. Are you less interested or become easily bored with things?
	B. How distressing is this fatigue to you?

	C. Does this fatigue have any particular meaning or significance to you? Is your fatigue 1. Normal vs. abnormal? 2. Usual vs. unusual? 3. Protective vs. destructive? 4. Other meanings?
Behavioral dimension	A. How has fatigue affected your ability to carry out your usual activities of daily living or to do the things that you most like to do? 1. Bathing/dressing/shopping/cooking 2. Social activities (i.e., social relationships/activities/sexual patterns) 3. Employment/work activities 4. Physical activity/exercise activities 5. Sleep/rest/nap activities 6. Nutritional/eating activities 7. Hobbies/interests
	B. Have you noticed that it takes longer for you to do certain activities because of the fatigue?
	C. Are there activities that you no longer can do because of your fatigue?

[a]Data culled from various sources.[26,27,29]

Table 16.3 Objective Assessment of HIV-Related Fatigue

Physiologic Dimension	Parameter Studied
Physical assessment	Significant findings from physical examination General appearance, vital signs, weight for height, lymph nodes, HEENT, musculoskeletal, nervous system, neck, thorax and lungs, heart and circulation, abdomen
Laboratory tests	CD4+ and T lymphocytes,[11] electrolytes (K+, Na+, Mg++, Ca++)[56] hemoglobin and hematocrit,[11,59] lactate dehydrogenase,[11] serum carnitine,[44,60] serum creatine kinase,[42] serum erythropoietin,[59] thyroid hormone levels,[25] total globulin (total protein minus albumin,[11] WBC count[11]

HEENT = head, eyes, ears, nose, throat.
WBC = white blood cell.

would suggest depression. These findings should be followed by administering the inventory's somatic items/subscale. A positive result on the somatic items or subscale alone, however, is insufficient to make the depression diagnosis.[62]

Related Medical Management

Medical management of fatigue is directed toward the diagnosis and treatment of the underlying disease, and its complications such as anemia and depression.

Pharmacologic Therapy

A variety of medications may be used to treat the underlying mechanisms of HRF. For example, recombinant human erythropoietin (rHuEPO) 4,000 to 8,000 units given subcutaneously 6 days/week in anemic AIDS patients who have serum erythropoietin levels of <500 can improve perceptions of energy and health in those who respond to treatment.[59] Oral carnitine supplements (L-carnitine) may improve HRF symptoms in patients with AZT-induced myopathy by facilitating the transport of long-chain fatty acids into the remaining healthy mitochondria, thereby increasing energy production within the muscle fibers.[44,60]

Other medications used to treat fatigue regardless of medical diagnosis include methylphenidate (Ritalin)[2] and amantadine.[3] IV porcine-derived hyperimmune immunoglobin is reported to have significantly ameliorated HRF in one phase I study.[63] Antidepressants may be helpful when depression is contributing to fatigue and decreased physical functioning[22] (see Chapter 15). Appetite stimulants may be helpful in malnutritional states (see Chapter 10).

Interventions

Prevention

When possible, fatigue and weakness should be prevented by maintaining adequate nutrition and by encouraging physical activity and light resistive exercise[23] to prevent the secondary fatigue associated with deconditioning. Patient teaching is directed toward earlier recognition and reporting of HRF to prevent normal tiredness from progressing to the more acute and chronic forms of HRF. Patients can be given preparatory sensory information regarding the commonly experienced symptoms associated with fatigue and information regarding when the onset of these symptoms may be anticipated, based on anecdotal reports of other patients.[25]

Management

Interventions should be tailored to the underlying causes of the fatigue and to the patient's condition.[25] The majority of interventions recommended for the treatment of HRF are unproven. No randomized clinical trials have been conducted that evaluate the efficacy of these proposed interventions on HRF-related outcomes.

Accumulation of Metabolites

Encouraging a minimum daily fluid intake of 8 to 10 glasses daily is recommended to promote the active excretion of cell destruction end products that may be causing HRF.[25]

Energy and Energy Substrate Patterns

Although no studies have examined nutritional status and nutritionally related therapies and fatigue, it seems reasonable to recommend a high-protein, high-calorie diet in HIV/AIDS individuals.[64] Megestrol acetate and dronabinol may be useful as appetite stimulants[64–67] to treat HRF indirectly (see Chapter 10).

Activity/Rest Patterns

ENERGY CONSERVATION. It is important to document fatigue patterns over the course of the day to establish diurnal patterns of fatigue. A fatigue diary maintained for a week is helpful to establish factors that may be causing, aggravating, or relieving fatigue. Energy-conserving activities include pacing and presheduling activities, and delegating and organizing the home or workplace to do activities more efficiently and with less effort.[25] Teaching patients to think about their "energy stores" as a "bank" where they have to make periodic deposits via nutrition, exercise, and reduction of stressors; conduct periodic energy audits; and make withdrawals can assist individuals in setting priorities and cultivating the "fine art of delegation."[18,25] Referral to occupational therapy for teaching and reinforcement of principles of energy conservation, setting priorities, and simplifying tasks also may be helpful.[2,23] Assistive devices such as adaptive equipment for bathrooms, gait aids for ambulation,[30] and wheelchairs[2,23] may be helpful in maintaining a level of mobility and may decrease the associated energy expenditure with mobility that can exacerbate fatigue.[2,23]

REST. No studies exist that formally define, describe, or test different forms of "rest" on fatigue.[25] Although rest is frequently viewed as an energy-conserving or energy-enhancing activity, too much rest is considered detrimental, particularly if it leads to a cycle of decreased energy and increased inactivity.[25]

EXERCISE. Gentle conditioning programs to maintain muscle strength and endurance should be encouraged,[2] although what exactly constitutes these programs has not been defined or tested. Light resistive exercise may be helpful in treating weakness.[68] Physical therapy may be helpful to decrease the lack of ". . . endurance secondary to general deconditioning, decreased pulmonary capacity, and . . . neurologic deficits."[2(p 94)]

Sleep/Wake Patterns

Patients report that napping and sleeping are among the most frequently tried and beneficial self-initiated interventions for fatigue.[25] Studies are limited that examine the relationship between fatigue and sleep disorders in HIV or that test and evaluate sleep-related interventions and/or medications for their effect on fatigue outcomes (see Chapter 17).

Symptom Patterns

HIV patients experience a multitude of different symptoms and side effects during the course of their disease and treatment. Interventions that are designed to control and/or alleviate these clinical problems can have a positive effect on HRF (see Chapters 9 through 20).

Oxygenation Patterns

In addition to the administration of rHuEPO mentioned earlier, hyperbaric oxygen therapy[69,70] and oral L-carnitine supplements to improve oxidative muscle metabolism[44] may be helpful in the treatment of HRF.

Psychological Patterns

Interventions designed to dissipate stressors and promote the expression of emotional reactions[18] through counseling or support groups may be helpful for some patients in treating the emotional exhaustion that frequently accompanies fatigue. Diversional activities such as reading, listening to music, doing crossword puzzles, and thinking about pleasant things have been consistently identified by patients as being effective in relieving fatigue in other populations.[25] These diversional or distracting activities are thought to produce an inflow of nerve impulses from the nonfatigued parts of the body to the facilitory part of the reticular formation, thus shifting the balance between inhibition of voluntary effort and facilitation to one of facilitation. Decreased mental fatigue symptoms may result.[25]

Information for Patients About HIV-Associated Fatigue

Everyone experiences tiredness. It is a universal sensation that is expected to occur normally at certain times of the day or after certain types of activity or exertion. It usually has an identifiable cause, is short lived, and is dissipated by a good night's sleep or by rest. In contrast to tiredness, the fatigue experienced by people who are infected with HIV or who have AIDS often is described as unusual or excessive whole-body tiredness, disproportionate to or unrelated to activity or exertion, and is not easily dispelled by sleep or by rest. Fatigue may be short term (acute), lasting less than 1 month; or may be more long term (chronic), lasting from 1 to 6 months or longer.

Fatigue, acute or chronic, can have a profound negative impact on the person's quality of life by interfering in the ability to perform the kinds of activities and roles that give meaning and value to life. As a consequence, fewer activities are undertaken, and those that are performed may take longer to complete and may require more effort. As fatigue begins to alter what individuals can do for themselves, family members and caregivers begin to assume many of the roles previously held by these individuals. These increased role demands can lead to fatigue in family members and the caregiver, and social isolation for family members, the caregiver, and the HIV-infected individual.

Causes of Fatigue

While no one knows exactly why people with HIV and other chronic illnesses experience this unusual fatigue, many factors may contribute. Lack of appetite, malabsorption of nutrients, an increased basal metabolism, and weight loss are frequent complications of HIV and may affect fatigue. Lack of energy may limit the ability to cook and shop for food. Disease complications and/or the side effects of treatment such as anemia, infection, and fever can create additional energy demands that usual food intake alone cannot supply, and nutritional supplements and therapy may be required. Diagnostic tests, HIV-related medications, radiation therapy, chemotherapy, biotherapy, and drug therapies used to control symptoms/side effects of treatment, such as pain and insomnia, can be associated with fatigue. For example, zidovudine (AZT) can cause anemia and changes in muscle metabolism that can lead to symptoms of fatigue, weakness, reduced endurance, and exercise intolerance. A common side effect of treatment—a low WBC count—is associated with fatigue. Fatigue has been associated with foscarnet as well. Specific drugs such as ddI may cause fatigue as a result of neurotoxicity and/or peripheral neuropathies.

As cells die in response to therapy, intracellular substances are released that may contribute to fatigue. Increased attention and research have been given recently to the possible role that cytokines play in the development of fatigue. Cytokines are natural cell products or proteins, such as the interferons and the interleukins, that are normally released by white blood cells, lymphocytes, and macrophages in response to infection and inflammation. These cytokines carry messages that regulate other elements of the immune and neuroendocrine systems. In high amounts, these cytokines can be toxic and may lead to persistent fatigue.

Changes in activity/rest patterns can play significant roles in the prevention, cause, and alleviation of fatigue. Unnecessary sedentariness, prolonged bed rest, and immobility contribute to loss of muscle strength and endurance. Muscle that is not exercised loses its ability to metabolize oxygen, thus more effort and oxygen is required to perform the same amount of work that can be performed by conditioned muscle. This is one of the reasons why aerobic, endurance exercise, such as walking three to four times per week for 20 to 30 minutes, is often recommended or prescribed.

Lack of restful or adequate sleep at night also can lead to fatigue, and increased sleepiness and napping during the day. Sleep disturbances are common in HIV and may be due to treatment and/or disease side effects such as night sweats. Insomnia, defined as difficulty falling asleep, staying asleep, and/or early morning awakenings, is a common symptom of depression. Other factors implicated in the cause of fatigue include age, gender, genetic, socioeconomic, and environmental factors.

What to Do About Fatigue

The best way to combat fatigue is to treat the underlying cause of the fatigue. Unfortunately it is not always easy to know the exact cause of the fatigue. More commonly, multiple factors may be involved that require *multimodal therapies*, particularly if the fatigue has become chronic. All possible causes must be assessed. For example, if fatigue is related to anemia, then medications or growth factors designed to increase red blood cell production, supplemental oxygen, and/or blood transfusions may be prescribed. Other causes may be managed on an individual basis and may include physical therapy and strength training, nutritional assessment and support, and psychological intervention. Specific actions for the patient are described in the following paragraphs.

Assessment

Conduct periodic fatigue/energy audits. Think about your personal energy stores as a "bank." Deposits and withdrawals need to be made over the course of a day and the week to ensure that a balance is achieved between energy conservation, restoration, and expenditure. Keep a diary for 1 week to identify the time of day when you are most fatigued or have the most energy and determine the contributing factors. Be alert to warning signs of impending fatigue such as tired eyes, legs, whole-body tiredness, stiff shoulders, boredom or lack of motivation, sleepiness, increased irritability, nervousness, anxiety, and impatience.

Activity/Exercise Patterns

Identify which activities or situations make your fatigue worse or better. Develop a plan to pace yourself, scheduling activities according to your fatigue/energy patterns. Try scheduling activities ahead of time during the day and throughout the week to avoid becoming unusually tired. Pace yourself and plan adequate rest and sleep periods to allow full energy recovery before undertaking additional activities.

Deliberately select the activities that are most important for you to do or that give you the most pleasure. Do these activities first, and let the others go or delegate them to others. Try to feel less "guilty" about restructuring your life as to what is really most important, and do what gives you the most pleasure! Reduce unnecessary energy expenditure by using assistive equipment or by placing equipment and supplies within easy reach. Physical therapy can help with bed and strengthening exercises, overhead trapezes, walkers, canes, and stair-climbing instruction. Occupational therapy can help with assistive equipment and energy-conserving activities. Begin to cultivate the "fine art of delegation."

Adhere to some form of individually tailored exercise program approved by your physician, nurse, or physical therapist. Walking is an activity most individuals may be able to do at certain times during their illness and treatment. Avoid exercising 24 hours before your lab tests and 24 hours after any IV therapy if possible. Avoid exercising if you are running a fever or have a low white blood cell count. Under these circumstances, consult your doctor or nurse.

Symptom Patterns

Monitor the effectiveness of medications and other strategies that you are using to control your other symptoms such as nausea, vomiting, pain, and lack of sleep. Are these symptoms and their treatments influencing your fatigue patterns?

Nutritional Patterns

Drink at least 8 to 10 glasses of water a day to maintain hydration and to excrete cell destruction end products or toxins that may be associated with fatigue. Try to eat a balanced diet that emphasizes complex carbohydrates (grains, legumes, vegetables), which provide a more sustained source of energy over time. Pursue dietary counseling, help with food preparation or shopping, or take advantage of Meals on Wheels to maximize and conserve your energy further and to prevent your fatigue from becoming unusual, excessive, or chronic.

Distraction

Use distraction techniques to focus on positive things other than your fatigue, illness, or treatments. These include listening to music, visiting with friends, watching television, or going for walks. Focus on those activities that may restore attention-depleting activities. These usually involve a change in activity or daily routine to vary the stimuli and avoid boredom. Pursue activities that catch your interest easily and that are enjoyable or at least pleasurable (i.e., appreciating nature; doing something creative such as drawing or writing; working on a hobby; or doing something socially with others with whom you enjoy). Contract with yourself to do these types of activities three times each week for at least 30 minutes at a time. Your mind, heart, and spirit need exercising too!

Psychological Patterns

Use methods to dissipate the negative effects of stressors. These include, exercise, progressive relaxation, visual imagery, meditation, prayer, talking with others, and therapeutic counseling. Social services can help with referrals to support groups for yourself and family members.

Sleep Patterns

Begin to advocate for yourself. Set limits on visitors if necessary, or have someone else "run interference" for you when you need to rest and do not wish to be disturbed. Sit or lie down often. Short rest periods are better than longer ones. Take naps as needed, as long as they do not interfere with your normal sleep patterns. Adhere to or reestablish bedtime "rituals" that help you to fall asleep, stay asleep, and enjoy a good quality of sleep. Sleep-enhacing aids and sleep medications may be helpful at certain times during your illness and treatment.

References

1. Whalen CC, Antani M, Carey J, et al. An index of symptoms for infection with human immunodeficiency virus: reliability and validity. *J Clin Epidemiol.* 1994; 47(5):537–546.
2. O'Dell MW. Rehabilitation medicine consultation in persons hospitalized with AIDS; an analysis of 30 cases. *Am J Phys Med Rehabil.* 1993;72(2):90–96.
3. O'Dell MW, Meighen M, Riggs RV. Correlates of fatigue in HIV infection prior to AIDS: a pilot study. *Disabil Rehabil.* 1996;18(5):249–254.
4. Perkins DO, Leserman J, Stern RA, et al. Somatic symptoms and HIV infection: relationship to depressive symptoms and indicators of HIV disease. *Am J Psychiatry.* 1995;152(12):1776–1781.
5. Hoover DR, Saah AJ, Bacellar H, et al. Signs and symptoms of 'asymptomatic' HIV-1 infection in homosexual men. *J Acquir Immune Defic Syndr.* 1993;6:66–71.
6. Kaslow RA, Phair JP, Friedman HB, et al. Infection with the human immunodeficiency virus: clinical manifestations and their relationship to immune deficiency. *Ann Intern Med.* 1987;107:474–480.
7. Lang W, Anderson RE, Perkins H, et al. Clinical, immunologic, and serologic findings in men at risk for acquired immunodeficiency syndrome. *J Am Med Assoc.* 1987;257:326–330.
8. Lubeck DP, Fries JF. Health status among persons infected with human immunodeficiency virus: a community-based study. *Med Care.* 1993;31:269–276.
9. Mather-Wagh U, Spigland I, Sacks HS, et al. Longitudinal study of persistent

generalized lymphadenopathy in homosexual men: relation to acquired immunodeficiency syndrome. *Lancet.* 1984;ii:1033–1038.
10. Metroka CE, Cunningham-Rundles S, Pollock MS, et al. Generalized lymphadenopathy in homosexual men. *Ann Intern Med.* 1983;99(5):585–591.
11. Darko DF, McCutchan JA, Kripke DF, et al. Fatigue, sleep disturbances, disability and indices of progression of HIV infection. *Am J Psychiatry.* 1992;149:514–520.
12. Perdices M, Dunbar N, Grunseit A, et al. Anxiety, depression, and HIV-related symptomatology across the spectrum of HIV disease. *Aust N Z J Psychiatry.* 1992;2:560–566.
13. Riley TA. Fatigue. In: Casey KM, Cohen F, Hughes AM, eds. *ANAC's Core Curriculum for HIV/AIDs Nursing.* Philadelphia: Nursecom; 1996:209–211.
14. Neidig JL, Nickel J, Smith B, et al. Self-reported symptoms in HIV infection. *Proceedings of the International Conference on AIDS (Vancouver).* 1996:231. Abstract TuB176.
15. de Boer J, van Dam FSAM, Sprangers MAG, et al. Longitudinal study on the quality of life of symptomatic HIV-infected patients in a trial of zidovudine versus zidovudine and interferon-α. *AIDS.* 1993;7:947–953.
16. Hurley P, Ungvarski P. Home healthcare needs of adults living with HIV/disease AIDS in New York City. *JANAC.* 1994;5(2):33–40.
17. Longo M, Spross J, Locke A. Identifying major concerns of persons with acquired immunodeficiency syndrome. *Clin Nurse Spec.* 1990;4:21–26.
18. O'Brien M, Pheifer W. Physical and psychosocial nursing care for patients with HIV infection. *Nurs Clin North Am.* 1993;28:303–316.
19. Cleary PD, Fowler Jr FJ, Weissman J, et al. Health-related quality of life in persons with acquired immune deficiency syndrome. *Med Care.* 1993;31(7):569–580.
20. O'Dell MW, Hubert H, Lubeck DP, et al. Disability in persons prior to AIDS. *Arch Phys Med Rehabil.* 1994;75:720. Abstract.
21. O'Dell MW, Hubert H, Lubeck DP, et al. Disability in persons with AIDS. In: *Proceedings of the International Rehabilitation Medicine Association Meetings.* Washington, DC: 1994: Abstract F-24.
22. Wilson IB, Cleary PD. Clinical predictors of functioning in persons with acquired immunodeficiency syndrome. *Med Care.* 1996;34(6):610–623.
23. Levinson SF, O'Connell P. Rehabilitation dimensions of AIDS: a review. *Arch Phys Med Rehabil.* 1991;72:690–696.
24. Tsevat J. Methods for assessing health-related quality of life in HIV-infected patients. *Psychol Health.* 1994;9:19–30.
25. Piper BF. Fatigue. In: Carrieri-Kohlman V, Lindsey AM, West CM, eds. *Pathophysiological Phenomena in Nursing: Human Responses to Illness.* Saunders, Philadelphia, PA. 2nd ed. 1993:279–302.

26. Fatigue in patients with cancer. In: *Oncology Nursing Focus: Distance Learning Video Series #4: Lesson Guide.* Pittsburgh: Oncology Nursing Society; 1996.
27. Piper BF, Lindsey AM, Dodd MJ. Fatigue mechanisms in cancer patients: developing nursing theory. *Oncol Nurs Forum.* 1987;14(6):17–23.
28. Winningham ML, Nail LM, Burke MB, et al. Fatigue and the cancer experience: the state of the knowledge. *Oncol Nurs Forum.* 1994;21(1):23–36.
29. Piper BF. Measuring fatigue. In: Frank-Stromborg M, Olsen SJ, eds. *Instruments for Clinical Health-Care Research.* Boston: Jones & Bartlett; 1997:482–496.
30. O'Connell PG. A medical rehabilitation perspective. *Occup Ther Health Care.* 1990;7(2–4):19–43.
31. Fischbach FT. *A Manual of Laboratory & Diagnostic Tests.* 5th ed. Philadelphia: Lippincott; 1996.
32. Parisien C, Gelinas MD, Cossette M. Comparison of anthropometric measures of men with HIV: asymptomatic, symptomatic, and AIDS. *J Am Diet Assoc.* 1993;93(12):1404–1408.
33. Schambelan M, Grunfeld C. Endocrinologic manifestations of HIV infection. In: Sande M, Volberding P, eds. *The Medical Management of AIDS.* 4th ed. Philadelphia: WB Saunders; 1995:343–357.
34. O'Dell MW, Lubeck DP, O'Driscoll P, et al. Validity of the Karnofsky performance status in an HIV-infected sample. *J Acquir Immune Defic Syndr Hum Retrovirol.* 1995;10:350–357.
35. Nokes KM, Kendrew J. Sleep quality in people with HIV disease. *J Am Nurs AIDS Care.* 1996;7(3):43–50.
36. Creagh-Kirk T, Doi P, Andrews E, et al. Survival experience among patients with AIDS receiving zidovudine. *JAMA.* 1988;260:3009–3015.
37. Murry JF, Mills J. State of the art: pulmonary complications of HIV infection. *Am Rev Resp Dis.* 1991;141:1356–1372.
38. Kaul S, Fishbein MC, Siegel RJ. Cardiac manifestations of acquired immunodeficiency syndrome: 1991 update. *Am Heart J.* 1991;122:535–544.
39. Grinspoon SK, Bilezikian JP. HIV disease and the endocrine system. *N Engl J Med.* 1992;327:1360–1365.
40. Fischl MA, Richman DD, Grieco MH, et al. The efficacy of azidothymidine (AZT) in the treatment of patients with AIDS and AIDS-related complex: a double-blind, placebo-controlled trial. *N Engl J Med.* 1987;317:192–197.
41. Fischel M, Galpin JE, Levine JD, et al. Recombinant human erythropoietin for patients with AIDS treated with zidovudine. *N Engl J Med.* 1990;322: 1488–1492.
42. Cupler EJ, Danon MJ, Jay C, et al. Early features of zidovudine-associated myopathy: histopathological findings and clinical correlations. *Acta Neuropathol.* 1995;90:1–6.

43. Sinnwell TM, Sivakumar K, Soueidan S, et al. Metabolic abnormalities in skeletal muscle of patients receiving zidovudine therapy observed by ^{31}P in vivo magnetic resonance spectroscopy. *J Clin Invest.* 1995;96:126–131.
44. Dalakas MC, Leon-Monzon ME, Bernardini I, et al. Zidovudine-induced mitochondrial myopathy is associated with muscle carnitine deficiency and lipid storage. *Ann Neurol.* 1994;35(4):482–487.
45. Soueidan S, Sinnwell T, Jay C, et al. Impaired muscle energy metabolism in patients with AZT-myopathy: a blinded comparative study of exercise ^{31}P magnetic resonance spectroscopy (MRS) with muscle biopsy. *Neurology.* 1992;42 suppl 3:146. Abstract.
46. Weissman JD, Constantinitis I, Hudgins P, et al. ^{31}P magnetic resonance spectroscopy suggests impaired mitochondrial function in AZT-treated HIV-infected patients. *Neurology.* 1992;42:619–623.
47. Gill PS, Bernstein-Singer M, Espina BM. Adriamycin, bleomycin and vincristine chemotherapy with recombinant granulocyte-macrophage colony-stimulating factor in the treatment of AIDS-related Kaposi's sarcoma. *AIDS.* 1992;6: 1477–1481.
48. Kovacs JA, Deyton L, Davey R, et al. Combined zidovudine and interferon-α therapy in patients with Kaposi sarcoma and the acquired immunodeficiency syndrome (AIDS). *Ann Intern Med.* 1989;111(4):280–287.
49. Kovacs JA, Vogel BS, Albert JM, et al. Controlled trial of interleukin-2 infusions in patients infected with the human immunodeficiency virus. *N Engl J Med.* 1996;335(18):1350–1356.
50. Fischl MA, Finkelstein DM, He W, et al. A phase II study of recombinant human Interferon-α_{2a} and zidovudine in patients with AIDS-related Kaposi's sarcoma. *J Acquir Immune Defic Syndr Hum Retrovirol.* 1996;11:379–384.
51. Sjövall J, Bergdahl S, Movin G, et al. Pharmacokinetics of foscarnet and distribution to cerebrospinal fluid after intravenous infusion in patients with human immunodeficiency virus infection. *Antimicrob Agents Chemother.* 1989;33(7): 1023–1031.
52. Piper BF, Rieger P, Brophy L, et al. Recent advances in the management of biotherapy-related side effects: fatigue. *Oncol Nurs Forum.* 1989;16(suppl 6): 27–34.
53. Palencik J, Nelson KE, Vlahov D, et al. Comparison of clinical symptoms of human immunodeficiency virus disease between intravenous drug users and homosexual men. *Arch Intern Med.* 1993;153:1806–1812.
54. Wu AW, Rubin HR, Mathews WC, et al. A health status questionnaire using 30 items from the Medical Outcomes Study. *Med Care.* 1991;29(8):786–798.
55. Kaplan LD, Wolfe PR, Volberding PA, et al. Lack of response to suramin in patients with AIDS and AIDS-related complex. *Am J Med.* 1987;82:615–620.

56. Yu-Yahiro JA. Electrolytes and their relationship to normal and abnormal muscle function. *Orthop Nurs.* 1994;13:38–40.
57. Semple SJ, Patterson TL, Temoshok LR, et al. Identification of psychobiological stressors among HIV-positive women. *Women Health.* 1993;20(4):15–36.
58. Vlahov D, Muñoz A, Solomon L, et al. Comparison of clinical manifestations of HIV infection between male and female injecting drug users. *AIDS.* 1994;8:819–823.
59. Revicki DA, Brown RE, Henry DH, et al. Recombinant human erythropoietin and health-related quality of life of AIDS patients with anemia. *J Acquir Immune Defic Syndr.* 1994;7:474–484.
60. DeSimone C, Tzantzoglou S, Famularo G, et al. High dose L-carnitine improves immunologic and metabolic parameters in AIDS patients. *Immunopharmacol Immunotoxicol.* 1993;15(1):1–12.
61. Saah AJ, Munoz A, Kuo V, et al. Predictors of the risk of development of acquired immunodeficiency syndrome within 24 months among gay men seropositive for human immunodeficiency virus type 1: a report from the Multicenter AIDS Cohort Study. *Am J Epidemiol.* 1992;135(10):1147–1155.
62. Kalichman SC, Sikkema KJ, Somlai A. Assessing persons with human immunodeficiency virus (HIV) infection using the Beck Depression Inventory: disease processes and other potential confounds. *J Pers Assess.* 1995;64(1):86–100.
63. Osther K, Wiik A, Black F, et al. PASSHIV-1 treatment of patients with HIV-1 infection: a preliminary report of a phase I trial of hyperimmune porcine immunoglobulin to HIV-1. *AIDS.* 1992;6:1457–1464.
64. Ungarvarski PJ, Hurley PM. Nursing research in HIV/AIDS home care: part 2. *Home Healthcare Nurse.* 1995;13(4):9–13.
65. Gorbach SL, Knox TA, Roubenoff R. Nutrition grand rounds: interactions between nutrition and infection with human immunodeficiency virus. *Nutr Rev.* 1993;51(8):226–234.
66. Oster MH, Enders SR, Samuels SJ, et al. Megestrol acetate in patients with AIDS and cachexia. *Ann Intern Med.* 1994;121:400–408.
67. Von Roenn JH, Armstrong D, Kotler DP, et al. Megestrol acetate in patients with AIDS-related cachexia. *Ann Intern Med.* 1994;121:393–399.
68. Spence DW, Galantino MLA, Mossberg KA, et al. Progressive resistance exercise: effect on muscle function and anthropometry of a select AIDS population. *Arch Phys Med Rehabil.* 1990;71:644–648.
69. Reillo M. Hyperbaric oxygen therapy for the treatment of debilitating fatigue associated with HIV/AIDS. *J Assoc Nurs AIDS Care.* 1993;4:33–38.
70. Reillo M, Altieri R, Neubauer R. Hyperbaric oxygen therapy. *AIDS Patient Care.* 1994;8(3):106–107. Letter.

CHAPTER 17

Sleep Alterations

Felissa Rose Lashley, RN, PhD, ACRN, FAAN

Chapter Preview

- Definition
- Biologic and Behavioral Basis
- Etiologies Related to HIV Infection and Its Medical Treatment
- Presentation and Assessment
- Related Medical Management
- Interventions

Definition

Sleep has been defined in various ways, many of which have been overly simplistic. *Sleep* is part of a normal, cyclic alteration of sleep and wakefulness. The sleep-wake rhythm is regulated and influenced by a variety of systems including a neural pacemaker, neurochemical systems, and conditions of light and darkness.[1,2] Sleep patterns have a characteristic association with age, as discussed later.

Sleep Disorders

Disorders of sleep and arousal have recently been reclassified[3] and are outlined in Table 17.1. Sleep disorders affect persons in all age groups. The National Commission on Sleep Disorders Research[1] has estimated that in the United States, 40 million people suffer from chronic sleep disorders and an additional 20 to 30 million have intermittent sleep problems. Among adults, population surveys[4–8] at various times consistently show that the most common sleep complaint is insomnia. In addition, medical and/or psychiatric illnesses may further affect sleep, and sleep disruptions may precipitate or exacerbate other illnesses and problems. Indeed, the effects of disturbed sleep and sleep disorders affect all aspects of life and can result in decreased alertness and daytime fatigue.[9]

Insomnia

Insomnia is a symptom rather than a disease and encompasses a wide range of parameters. It may include difficulty in falling asleep and/or difficulty in staying asleep, and results in subjective feelings of not feeling rested on awakening in the morning. Insomnia often results in excessive daytime sleepiness and impaired functioning. Insomnia has been classified as (1) transient, lasting 7 days or less; (2) short term, lasting more than 7 days to about 3 weeks; or (3) long term, lasting more than 3 weeks.[10] It is important to note that multiple factors can contribute to insomnia.[11] A final classification may not be possible when the person is first seen.

Biologic and Behavioral Basis

Sleep is a necessary process that is active rather than passive, with various stages occurring during the sleep period or night. Much of what is known

Table 17.1 Classification of Sleep Disorders

Classification	Example
A. DYSSOMNIAS	
Intrinsic sleep disorders	Idiopathic insomnia, narcolepsy, obstructive sleep apnea syndrome
Extrinsic sleep disorders	Inadequate sleep hygiene, hypnotic-dependent sleep disorder
Circadian rhythm disorders	Time zone change syndrome
B. PARASOMNIAS	
Arousal disorders	Sleepwalking
Sleep-wake transition disorders	Rhythmic movement disorder
Parasomnias usually associated with REM sleep	Nightmares
Other parasomnias	Sleep bruxism
C. SLEEP DISORDERS ASSOCIATED WITH MEDICAL/PSYCHIATRIC DISORDERS	
Associated with mental disorders	Psychoses
Associated with neurological disorders	Parkinsonism
Associated with other medical disorders	Sleeping pickiness
D. PROPOSED SLEEP DISORDERS	

REM = rapid eye movement.
Source: Diagnostic Classification Steering Committee. International Classification of Sleep Disorders: Diagnostic and Coding Manual. Rochester, MN: American Sleep Disorders Association; 1990.

about sleep stages comes from polysomnography, often called *a sleep study*. This technique is usually done overnight in a sleep laboratory.[12] The basic measurement in polysomnography is an EEG. Other standard assessment measures are (1) an electro-oculogram to measure eye movement, (2) an EKG, (3) muscle monitoring (usually the mentalis/submentalis muscles) by electromyography, and (4) respiratory parameters. Other parameters such as blood pressure, penile tumescence, esophageal pH, and core temperature determinations may also be done, as may more in-depth measurements of the standard parameters depending on the reason for the sleep study. Standardized guidelines and scoring are used to interpret these measurements, which must be recorded and interpreted by certified experts.[13]

Two major states comprise sleep: rapid eye movement (REM) sleep and nonrapid eye movement (NREM) sleep. NREM sleep is divided into stages whereas REM sleep usually is not. NREM and REM sleep states have distinctive characteristics on polysomnography, as does each stage of NREM sleep. REM sleep is associated with high brain activity, metabolism, spontaneous REMs, and dreams. NREM sleep stages are listed in Table 17.2.

The length of sleep per night and patterns within a sleep period vary with age. For young adults, "normal" sleep is considered to range from 6 to 10 hours/night with 7 to 9 hours being usual. Newborns are thought to spend about half of their sleep in the REM stage. Slow-wave sleep (stages 3 and 4) is at a maximum in children and is thought to be associated with growth. Slow-wave sleep decreases with age, and in older persons NREM stage 4 sleep may be absent. Older persons have been observed to have shorter sleep times, although this is not universal. Their total sleep time actually may not be much shorter, but may be distributed across 24 hours. Sleep fragmentation and more awakening during the night are more common in elders than in younger adults. Early-morning awakenings are also more common in elders.[14,15]

Etiologies Related to HIV Infection and Its Medical Treatment

The frequency of reported sleep disturbances is not related to the immune status of the patient as represented by the CD4+ count. The most commonly

Table 17.2 NREM Sleep Stages

NREM Stage	Sleep Description	% of Normal Adult Sleep
1	Drowsiness	5–10
2	Light sleep	45–55
3	Slow-wave, delta, or deep sleep	4–6
4	Slow-wave, delta, or deep sleep	12–15

NREM = nonrapid eye movement.

described sleep-related problems in persons with HIV infection include insomnia and excessive daytime sleepiness. Insomnia may result from a variety of causes that may interact and have a multiple impact. For example, the person with HIV infection might have insomnia due to side effects of medication; pain, such as headache; anxiety or worry; arising at night because of unrelieved diarrhea; and noise disturbances in the environment. Each cause may require a different approach to achieve a solution.

Pharmacologic management of HIV infection may also affect sleep. Some of the early major drugs used against HIV infection, such as zidovudine and zalcitabine, may result in insomnia as a side effect[16] and feelings of fatigue during the day. Excessive sleep has also been described as a result of HIV infection. HIV-related sleep disturbances can also result from infections or fever, neurological invasion of HIV, immune function disruption, cancers or infection accompanying HIV infection, or secondary to such psychiatric sequelae as depression or anxiety.[17–19] A large number of non-HIV-specific medications can result in sleep disorders in persons who are not HIV infected, and depending on the regimen of the HIV-infected person, any of them might play a part in the presenting sleep complaint. These medications include adrenergic and dopaminergic agonists, steroids, thyroid hormones, antihypertensives, anticonvulsants, narcotics, cancer chemotherapeutic agents, antidepressants, theophylline derivatives, antipsychotics, CNS depressants and stimulants, as well as the use of alcohol, tobacco, or caffeine.[11,20] Some medications used to induce sleep, such as secobarbital, can cause rebound insomnia after long-term use.

Presentation and Assessment

The majority of available HIV studies examined sleep disturbance as a reflection of objective parameters such as the EEG or as brief subjective reporting when ascertaining a multitude of symptoms. Darko et al[21] compared HIV-infected subjects and found that those with HIV infection slept more, napped more, had more early morning awakenings, and were less alert in the morning than those who were HIV negative. Ferini-Strambi et al[22] found decreased slow-wave sleep in their sample of 9 HIV-infected men when compared with age-matched controls. Darko et al[23] also described increased slow-wave sleep with early HIV infection and decreases with sleep fragmentation in advanced HIV infection. In a study by Epstein et al,[24] excessive daytime sleepiness resulted from obstructive sleep apnea due to adenotonsillar hypertrophy. Nokes and Kendrew[25] examined sleep in 56 HIV-infected persons (mostly male) and found that 96% reported at least some sleep disturbance. Thirty percent rated their subjective sleep quality as fairly or very bad, and 25% reported daytime dysfunction as somewhat of a problem. In the study of 50 HIV-infected persons by Cohen et al,[18] about two-thirds reported difficulty in falling asleep. Only 26% reported no restlessness; 50% rated their sleep as less than satisfactory, whereas 56% reported feeling tired in the morning.

The first step in regard to potential sleep problems is the assessment. While with some patients it is desirable and/or necessary to do a complete workup that includes polysomnography coupled with observation by video recording, sleep problems can often be elicited and explored using noninvasive methods. These include (1) self-report questionnaires, (2) sleep diaries, (3) interviews, (4) sleep logs, and (5) charts. (Cohen[26] reviews related instruments.) Sleep assessments may be obtained from the HIV-infected person and/or from the sleeping and/or living partner. These measures and others such as visual analogue scales or rating scales, are also used to evaluate the effectiveness of therapeutic approaches to the sleep problem. Day-to-day reports of sleep and wake activities can be cumbersome to maintain but can give a 24-hour picture of sleep and wake activities that form a pattern over a longer period of time. Diaries also have clinical relevance and provide some insight into patterns affecting sleep and the impact that is experienced by the patient. Diaries can be used to record activities or behaviors that affect sleep such as alcohol or drug use, medication use, smoking, caffeine intake, meals, snacks, exercise, and recreation. They may also record feelings such as tension, mood, mental activity, and energy level.

As part of the sleep history, health care providers should ascertain the information listed below.

- Usual bedtime
- Usual "lights out" time
- Time the patient falls asleep or how long it takes to fall asleep
- Is the patient tired when he goes to bed?
- Usual bedtime routine
- How often does he have difficulty in falling asleep?
- Does he take medications to help him sleep and taken how often?

- If he wakes up at night, why?
- How often does he wake up at night?
- Does the patient associate any event or reason for awakening?
- How long does it take to fall back to sleep?
- What helps to fall back to sleep?
- Does the patient get out of bed when he wakes up during the night? If so, what does he do?
- Does he dream during the night? If so, are the dreams disturbing?
- Quality of sleep
- What time the patient awakens in the morning
- What awakens the patient
- How well rested is he when he gets up in the morning?
- Does the patient take any daytime naps? If so, how many and for how long?
- Current daily activities
- Caffeine, alcohol, and tobacco intake daily
- Emotional factors, such as anxiety, depression, and stress

An environmental assessment of how the patient sleeps and sleeping preferences should be obtained as well.

- What is the usual sleep environment?
- Lighting: Is the bedroom dark? Is there a nightlight?
- Bedding: How many and what type of pillow is preferred? Any special bedding, such as covers, pad, or mattress?
- Temperature: What is the preferred temperature of the bedroom?
- Noise: Is the bedroom usually quiet? Does the person require quiet to facilitate sleep?
- Ventilation: Does the person like to sleep with the window or door open?
- Positioning: What is the person's usual sleep position?
- Behavioral: Does the person usually sleep alone?

These items should be modified slightly and assessed as they apply in the inpatient setting if that is where the patient is having sleep difficulties. In cases when the sleep difficulties do not exist outside the hospital environment, the problem is probably a transitory one. Therefore, the solution might lie in the short-term use of medications or in the removal of any identifiable impediments to sleep that can be accomplished readily within the framework of the anticipated stay.

In addition to the assessments just listed, a family history, history of current and past medication use, history of use of alcohol or drugs, and an evaluation for disorders such as depression should be obtained. HIV-related approaches include ascertaining (1) the presence of symptoms that can directly or indirectly affect sleep, (2) therapeutic regimens that may affect sleep, and (3) HIV-related concerns such as fear, worry, and anxiety. In the study by Cohen et al,[18] persons with HIV infection reported waking up at night because of diarrhea or the need to urinate, pain, night sweats, and worrying about some aspect of their disease.

Parameters such as mood, anxiety, hopelessness, fatigue, and depression assessed both at bedtime and on awakening add more specific information. Activities such as exercise, recreational activities, type of food eaten, and medications used and when should also be assessed as part of understanding the sleep problem and determining an approach.

Related Medical Management

The initial approach to sleep problems in the person with HIV infection is twofold: (1) addressing the disease state and its symptoms and treatment, and (2) applying basic sleep hygiene parameters. Sleep hygiene parameters are a group of actions that can be applied to persons with sleep problems regardless of the reason for the problem and independent of the disease.

Medical management of HIV-related sleep disorders may be direct or indirect. Indirect ways of managing problems are to institute adequate controls for symptoms that may disrupt sleep. For example, diarrhea resulting from cryptosporidiosis may be brought under better control by its medical treatment (see Chapter 5). Control of diarrhea and associated cramping may result in a lack of symptoms that usually awaken the patient during the night, thus disrupting sleep. Likewise, bringing pain under control will allow the patient to relax at bedtime and not be awakened by pain (see Chapter 19). Direct medical management of insomnia in HIV infection may take the form of drug prescription, depending on the length of time that the insomnia has been present, condition of the patient, and other factors. The usual agents prescribed for pharmacologic management of insomnia fall into the classes of the benzodiazepines and cyclopyrolone derivatives.[27] The main actions of benzodiazepines are hypnotic, anxiolytic, anticonvulsive, muscle relaxing, and amnesic. The extent of each of these actions depends on the specific agent being used, as does their rate of elimination. They also have different properties, such as onset of action and duration. Sometimes these agents may be used in combination with other agents such as antidepressants. Most of the disadvantages are related to long-term use, but rebound insomnia, hangover effects, and respiratory depression can occur short term. Examples of benzodiazepines in common use are flurazepam, lorazepam, temazepam, quazepam, and estazolam.[11,27–29] The decision to use these drugs requires careful consideration in light of their abuse potential and side effects. Zolpidem, an imidazopyridine, also is effective in treating insomnia.[11]

Medical management of insomnia caused by antiretroviral agents such as zidovudine may not be resolved easily because of the necessity of the primary treatment of the HIV infection. Newer classes of antiviral agents used to treat HIV may have less direct effects on sleep, but little definitive information is currently available. Approaches include dosage adjustments, combinations of agents, use of agents with fewer known sleep effects, and treatment of the insomnia with other drugs or with nonmedical approaches. The same problem exists for antineoplastic drugs such as IFN-α.[11] Other medical treatments may include psychotherapy or treatment of unprescribed drug or alcohol use, or other appropriate techniques.

Interventions

One of the first and most important parts of intervention in sleep disorders related to HIV infection is the assessment of the disorder. A systematic and thorough history not only of the sleep problem, but of the usual and present sleep rituals and environment should be obtained as described earlier. Alternative reasons for the sleep problem should be explored. For example, psychiatric disorders such as depression may complicate the picture and interfere with sleep. These can respond to appropriate treatment. Control of symptoms that interfere with sleep such as pain, cramping and diarrhea, headache, itching, burning, night sweats, anxiety, fever, cough, and dyspnea should be addressed before proceeding to other sleep-related therapies. Other strategies such as stress management, relaxation techniques, exercise, or sleep restriction may also be useful. Sleep hygiene techniques, listed below that apply generally can be instituted.[18]

- Get as much sleep as needed to feel refreshed during the next day, but not more than that
- Adhere to a regular time to wake up to strengthen circadian cycling; get up even if you did not have a good night's sleep
- Do not stay in bed for more than 15 minutes if you cannot fall asleep; move to another room until sleepy and then go back to bed
- Try not to worry about getting to sleep
- Establish a regular bedtime
- Avoid eating heavy meals near bedtime
- Avoid being hungry near bedtime; hunger may disturb sleep
- Avoid stimulating activities before bed
- Clear your mind and relax
- Restrict caffeine from late afternoon on
- Restrict medications with stimulating effects far enough before bedtime to minimize interference with sleep
- Restrict tobacco a few hours before bedtime
- Get regular daily exercise but stop 4 to 7 hours before bedtime; sporadic exercise does not necessarily improve sleep
- Develop and follow a bedtime routine; for example, read in bed
- Take a warm bath before bed
- Drink a warm beverage before bed; drinks containing milk may promote sleepiness
- Create an environment conducive to sleep
    - Clean, dry linens and bed clothes
    - Dark room
    - Quiet
    - Comfortable bed
    - Comfortable temperature
    - Comfortable pillow arrangement
- Use bed for sleeping only
    - Do not work in bed

  - Do not eat in bed
- Do relaxation exercises
- Do not nap during the day

In summary, sleep problems in the HIV-infected person may arise from a variety of causes. These include those directly related to HIV infection; due to symptoms resulting from HIV and its manifestations, such as headaches and diarrhea; associated with drug or alcohol abuse; from psychological causes such as anxiety; and from drug therapy of HIV infection or its side effects. It is important to conduct a comprehensive assessment of sleep history, habits, and environment before deciding on a treatment plan. The most common sleep-related problems reported in HIV infection are insomnia and excessive daytime sleepiness. Disturbed nighttime sleep may result in daytime symptoms such as fatigue and decreased alertness, and result in diminished quality of life. Pharmacological approaches should consider the cause or causes of the sleep problem. Nonpharmacological approaches such as sleep hygiene techniques are useful as sole therapy or adjunctive therapy depending on the cause of the sleep problem.

References

1. *National Commission on Sleep Disorders Research Report. Vol. 1. Executive Summary and Executive Report.* Bethesda, MD: National Institutes of Health; 1993.
2. Carskadon MA, Dement WC. Normal human sleep: an overview. In: Kryger MH, Roth T, Dement WC, eds. *Principles and Practice of Sleep Medicine.* 2nd ed. Philadelphia: WB Saunders; 1994:16–25.
3. Diagnostic Classification Steering Committee. *International Classification of Sleep Disorders: Diagnostic and Coding Manual.* Rochester, MN: American Sleep Disorders Association; 1990.
4. Bixler E, Kales A, Soldatos CR, Kales JD, Healey S. Prevalence of sleep disorders in the Los Angeles metropolitan area. *Am J Psychiatry.* 1979;136(10): 1257–1262.
5. Karacan I, Thornby JI, Anch M, et al. Prevalence of sleep disturbance in a primarily urban Florida county. *Soc Sci Med.* 1976;10(5):239–244.
6. Lavie P, Adam N, Nave N, Kremerman S. Prevalence of sleep complaints in Israel. *Sleep Res.* 1979;8:198.

7. McGhie A, Russell SM. The subjective assessment of normal sleep patterns. *J Mental Sci.* 1962;108(456):642–654.
8. Toufexis A. Drowsy America. *Time.* 1990;136(26):78–85.
9. Cohen FL. Narcolepsy: review of a common life-long sleep disorder. *J Adv Nurs.* 1988;13(50):546–556.
10. National Institutes of Health (NIH). Consensus Development Conference. Drugs and insomnia: the use of medication to promote sleep. *J Am Med Assoc.* 1984; 25:2410–2414.
11. Kupfer DJ, Reynolds CF III. Management of insomnia. *N Engl J Med.* 1997; 336(5):341–346.
12. Rechtschaffeu, Kales. 1968.
13. *American Encephalographic Society Guidelines.* 1992.
14. Kripke DF, Simons RN, Garfinkel L, Hammond EC. Short and long sleep and sleeping pills. Is increased mortality associated? *Arch Gen Psychiatry.* 1979; 36(1):103–116.
15. Webb WB, Swinburne H. An observational study of sleep of the aged. *Percept Mot Skills.* 1971;32(3):895–898.
16. *Physicians Desk Reference.* 51st ed. Montvale, NJ: Medical Economics Co.; 1997.
17. Casey KM, Cohen FL, Hughes A, eds. *ANAC's Core Curriculum for HIV Nursing.* Philadelphia: Nursecom; 1996.
18. Cohen FL, Ferrans CE, Vizgirda V, Kunkle V, Cloninger L. Sleep in men and women infected with human immunodeficiency virus. *Holistic Nurs Pract.* 1996;10(4):33–43.
19. Moeller AA, Oechsner M, Backmind HC, Popeseu M, Emminger C, Holsboer F. Self-reported sleep quality in HIV infection: correlation to the stage of infection and zidovudine therapy. *J Acquir Immune Defic Syndr.* 1991;4:1000–1003.
20. Cohen FL, Merritt S. Sleep promotion. In: Bulechek GM, McCloskey JC, eds. *Nursing Interventions.* 2nd ed. Philadelphia: WB Saunders; 1992:109–119.
21. Darko DF, McCutchan JA, Kripke DF, Gillin JC, Golshan S. Fatigue, sleep disturbances, disability, and indices of progression of HIV infection. *Am J Psychiatry.* 1992;149:514–520.
22. Ferini-Strambi L, Oldani A, Tirloni G, et al. Slow wave sleep and cyclic alternating pattern (CAP) in HIV-infected asymptomatic men. *Sleep.* 1995;18(6):446–450.
23. Darko DF, Muller JC, Gallen C, et al. Sleep electroencephalogram delta-frequency amplitude, night plasma levels of tumor necrosis factor alpha, and human immunodeficiency virus infection. *Proc Natl Acad Sci U S A.* 1995;19: 12080–12084.
24. Epstein LJ, Strollo PJ Jr, Donegan RB, Delmar J, Hendrix C, Westbrook PR. Objective sleep apnea in patients with human immunodeficiency virus (HIV) disease. *Sleep.* 1995;18(5):368–376.

25. Nokes KM, Kendrew J. Sleep quality in people with HIV disease. *J Assoc Nurs AIDS Care.* 1996;7:43–50.
26. Cohen FL. Measuring sleep. In: Frank-Stromborg M, Olsen S, eds. *Instruments for Clinical Health Care Research.* 2nd ed. Sudbury, MA: Jones and Bartlett; 1997:264–285.
27. Maczaj M. Pharmacological treatment of insomnia. *Drugs.* 1993;45(1):44–55.
28. Ashton H. Guidelines for the rational use of benzodiazepines. *Drugs.* 1994; 48(1):25–40.
29. Clark JBF, Queener SF, Karb VB. *Pharmacologic Basis of Nursing Practice.* 5th ed. St. Louis: Mosby; 1997.

CHAPTER 18

Visual Changes

Teri Dew, RN, MSN • Tracy A. Riley, MSN, RN, CS

Chapter Preview

Definition

A *visual sensory* or *perceptual alteration* is defined as a state in which an individual experiences a change in the amount or patterning of oncoming stimuli accompanied by a diminished, exaggerated, distorted, or impaired response to such stimuli.[1] As newer chemotherapeutic regimens delay progression of HIV to AIDS and delay or prevent the onset of some OIs, the threat of moderate to severe visual impairment for persons with advanced disease increases. Minimizing the consequences of visual loss is the challenge for the treatment team.

Etiologies Related to HIV Infection and Its Medical Treatment

The following lists the etiologies of visual changes in persons with HIV infection (also see Chapter 4).

- Viral
  - Cytomegalo virus (CMV)
  - Herpes Simplex Virus (HSV)
  - Varicella Zoster virus (VZV)
- HIV-associated "cotton wool" spots
- Syphilis
- Neurological
  - *Toxoplasma gondii*
  - PML
  - Lymphoma
- Other
  - *Cryptococcus neoformans*
  - Atypical mycobacteria

These changes cause a significant impact on lifestyle, autonomy, and self-esteem. Treatment is most often life long, expensive, and cumbersome. There is always a threat of relapse or of the development of resistance to therapy, and blindness if the underlying cause is left untreated.

The primary cause of disability related to visual impairment is CMV retinitis.[2] For HIV-infected persons, the lifetime risk has increased from 25 to 40%. Risk is greatest for those with CD4 counts of <50 cells/mm³. Infection is usually asymptomatic until it is quite advanced, and if untreated, it is progressive, permanent, and irreversible.

Other viral sources of visual impairment include HSV and VZV.[3] VZV may not be associated with cutaneous zoster and can lead to acute retinal necrosis (ARN) syndrome, which is a rapidly progressive necrosis of the peripheral retina. Marked vitreous and anterior chamber inflammation, optic neuritis, and scleritis can occur, with complete visual loss in the involved eye. Both eyes are involved in one half of patients.

Presentation and Assessment

Subjective

Patients may report floaters, light flashes, blurred vision, or scotomas (blind spots). Symptoms may be noted only when the unaffected eye is covered or when bilateral disease is present. Some patients are first aware of a new visual dysfunction when they notice distortion in newsprint such as blurring, blank spots, or a darker color.

Self-screening instruments include the Amsler grid[4] (Figures 18.1 and 18.2) and the Teich Target[5] (Figure 18.3). The Amsler grid, which detects only central (macular) involvement, indicates advanced disease. A positive test is one in which the lines of the grid are wavy, distorted, and broken, or missing lines are noted (see Figure 18.2).

The Teich Target (see Figure 18.3) is composed of concentric circles of varying colors and shades surrounding a black fixation point and intersected by radial lines. The central circle is red and incorporates a grid. When an appropriately sized chart is used at the correct viewing distance, the Teich Target detects deficiencies in up to 45 degrees of the central visual field (zone 1, vision threatening). For the home or office, use a 46-cm-diameter target viewed at 60 cm. For hospitalized patients, use a 23-cm-diameter target viewed at the bedside from a distance of 30 cm. The test is positive when the red circle appears faded to the involved eye.

Psychosocial assessment of the patient with a visual deficiency is important because there are a wide range of emotional responses to visual changes including denial, grief, anger, depression, guilt, and anxiety. Patients may fear the progression of visual loss and its impact on their ability

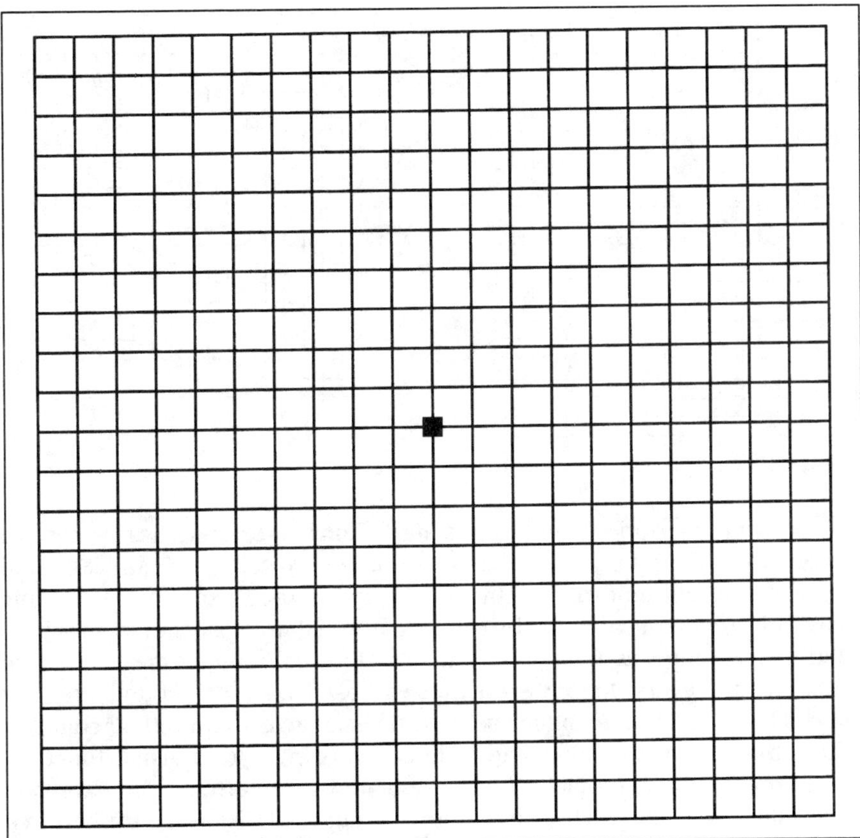

Figure 18.1 Normal Amsler Grid

to perform ADLs, to remain independent, to continue to work, or to drive a car. In addition, significant visual loss may emphasize the reality of living in an advanced stage of AIDS. Finally, assessment of the availability of supportive services, family, and friends is important for planning care.

Objective

Objective assessment variables include the date of the patient's last normal funduscopic/ophthalmic exam and her visual acuity after accounting for

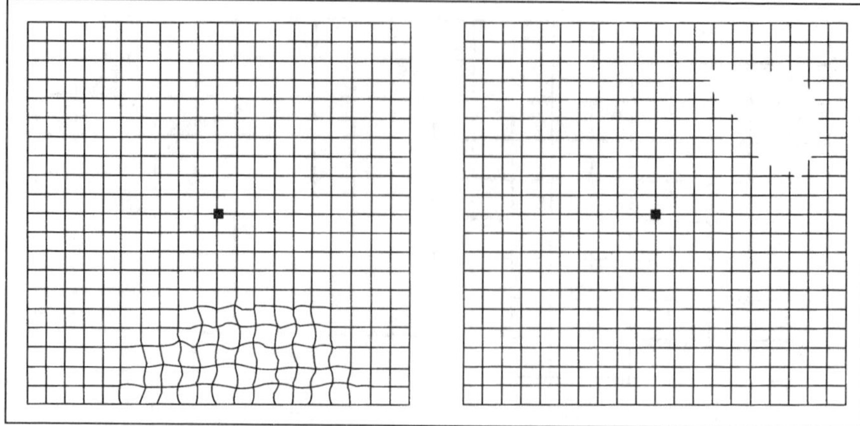

Figure 18.2 Abnormal Amsler Grids

corrective prescriptions and age-related changes. Routine assessment of vision is key, especially if the CD4+ count is <100 cells/mm^3, and it should *not* wait for self-reported problems. A funduscopic exam at each clinic visit and a regular evaluation by a skilled ophthalmologist should be scheduled every 6 months for patients with CD4+ cell counts between 50 to 100/mm^3, and every 3 months for those whose CD4+ cell counts are <50/mm^3. This evaluation should assess both visual acuity and retinal changes. When the patient or the provider detects any change in visual function, an urgent ophthalmologic exam is indicated to determine the extent of potential pathology, such as unilateral vs. bilateral disease, peripheral vs. central disease, and whether or not retinal detachment has occurred.

Financial and psychosocial barriers to prescribed care, including a mental status examination, should also be assessed to guide the development of a care plan (see Chapter 9).

Related Medical Management

The goals of medical management[2] of CMV retinitis are to preserve vision and prolong survival while maximizing convenience (see Chapter 5). When choosing one of the following current therapies, it is important to consider both ease of administration and toxicity:

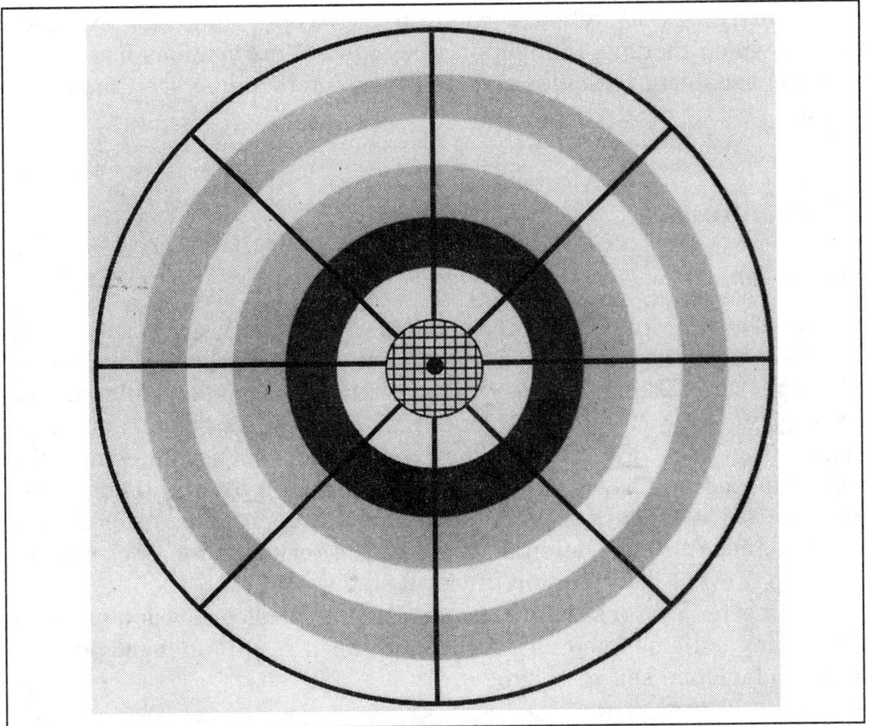

Figure 18.3 Black-and-white photograph of the Teich Target (© 1993, Steven A. Teich, pat. no. 370259). The concentric circles are of varying shades and colors; however, the central circle is red.
(Used with permission from SA Teich and originally published in Teich SA, Saltzman BR. Evaluation of a new self-screening chart for cytomegalovirus retinitis in patients with AIDS. *Journal of Acquired Immune Deficiency Syndrome and Human Retrovirology* 1996;13:336–342.)

- Ganciclovir IV bid for the induction phase, followed by a daily maintenance regimen; an oral formulation is available but is less effective; ganciclovir also may be administered via an intraocular insert, which must be replaced approximately every 8 months
- Foscarnet IV bid for the induction phase, followed by daily maintenance
- Cidofovir IV once a week for 2 weeks then every 2 weeks

Patients with CMV retinitis require frequent ophthalmologic examinations to guide therapy. In addition, the antiviral medications listed here all have significant toxicities and drug-drug interactions (see Chapters 3 and 5).

Interventions

Prevention

The small number of HIV-positive patients who are CMV seronegative may benefit by avoiding unprotected sexual contact (especially anal receptive) with CMV-seropositive persons, contact with CMV-shedding children, and transfusion with CMV-positive blood. CMV-seropositive persons may also benefit from these precautions if they are able to avoid new infection with superimposed strains of CMV. Adherence to antiretroviral therapy can prevent CMV if it delays progression of immunosuppression. After diagnosis, adherence to medication and monitoring regimens for CMV therapy can help prevent deterioration of visual status.

HIV-infected persons should be asked about changes in vision on every visit. Many patients keep an Amsler grid taped in a prominent place at home to facilitate self-screening.

Acute

Visual changes in an HIV-infected person are an emergency, and such patients should be referred for urgent ophthalmologic examination. Prompt diagnosis and initiation of therapy may be vision saving.

Chronic

Long-term management of CMV retinitis falls into two categories: nursing interventions related to the safe administration of IV medications and nursing interventions to assist patients with visual limitations in successful adaptation to their condition.

Patients and caregivers need detailed instructions regarding the administration of prescribed medications as scheduled and monitoring the side effects and drug interactions (see Chapters 3 and 5). They also require instruction about the care of venous access devices including flushing, site observation, dressing changes, and prevention of infection.

Patients who are visually impaired will benefit from environmental engineering to promote adaptation, safety, and optimal self-care. The following suggestions will help both nurses and family caregivers work with patients to provide a safe, supportive environment[6,7]:

- Ask the patient what she can or cannot do; ask whether assistance is needed.
- Arrange living space/hospital room with input from the patient.
- Speak in a normal voice (the patient is not deaf), speak directly to the patient, especially if she is with a sighted person; introduce yourself by name; inform her when you enter or leave the room; *speak before touching the patient.*
- It is not necessary to avoid such words as *see* or *look at*—they are commonly used in conversation.
- Approach the patient on the side of her better eye.
- Give directions, as specific as possible, using the words *right* or *left* from the direction the patient is facing.
- Encourage the use of optical assistive devices (such as a magnifying glass), and adaptive devices like talking clocks and books, special kitchen equipment, and check-writing guides.
- Write with large letters and use bold black pen on white paper.
- Suggest that the patient or family remove obstacles in the home such as throw rugs and sharp objects. Keep things in the same place. Use a bath bar, shower chair, and commode as indicated.
- Suggest that the patient avoid smoking when alone.
- Do not do for the patient what she can do for herself.
- Describe the location of food on the plate using clock positions.
- Develop a plan for self-administration of oral medications (e.g., Braille box, color coded).
- Encourage short, easy-care hairstyles and use of an electric shaver.
- Adjust lighting, contrast, and color to facilitate comfort and independence.
- Discuss side effects of medication, especially narcotic analgesics that could alter mental acuity.

- Encourage verbalization of feelings regarding visual impairment/loss (from patient, caregiver, or significant others).
- Utilize innovation and creativity to solve unique and individual problems.

Information for Patients

In addition to the education for prevention of CMV retinitis discussed in this chapter, many patients with visual impairment can benefit from community resources. In many communities there is a sight center for adaptive training and assistance as well as support groups, individual therapy, and Meals on Wheels programs. These may be useful in addition to services provided by the local community-based AIDS organization case management and buddy programs.

References

1. McCloskey JC, Bulachek GM. *Nursing Interventions Classification (NIC)*. 2nd ed. St. Louis: Mosby; 1996.
2. Masur H, Whitcup SM, Cartright C, et al. Advances in the management of AIDS-related cytomegalovirus retinitis. *Ann Intern Med.* 1996;125:126–136.
3. Sanford JP, Sande MA, Gilbert DN. *Guide to HIV/AIDS Therapy.* 5th ed. Antimicrobial Therapy, Inc: Dallas, Texas. 1996;5:30–32.
4. Amsler M. *Amsler charts manual.* London: Hamblin (Instruments) Limited, 1949.
5. Teich SA, Saltzman BR. Evaluation of a new self-screening chart for cytomegalovirus retinitis in patients with AIDS. *J Acquir Immune Defic Syndr Hum Retrovirol.* 1996;13:336–342.
6. Flaskerud JH, Ungvarski PJ. *HIV/AIDS, A Guide to Nursing Care.* 3rd ed. Philadelphia: WB Saunders; 1995.
7. The Lighthouse Inc. *Guidelines for Interacting with People Who Are Visually Impaired.* New York: The Lighthouse Inc.

Chapter 19

Pain

Patrick Coyne, MSN, CS, CRNH
Mary Ropka, PhD, RN, FAAN

Chapter Preview

- Definition
- Biologic and Behavioral Basis
- Etiologies Related to HIV Infection and Its Medical Treatment
- Presentation and Assessment
- Related Medical Management
- Interventions

Pain in individuals with HIV infection occurs across the spectrum of disease and varies widely in its occurrence, etiology, and impact.[1] Reports of the prevalence of pain in individuals with HIV infection are different depending on stage of disease, ranging from early-stage HIV infection to AIDS; care setting, including ambulatory, inpatient, or palliative; and study approach, involving retrospective vs. prospective data collection and diverse methods of pain assessment. Estimates of pain prevalence increase with disease progression.[2–7] Individuals with HIV infection often experience more than one type of pain concurrently.[3,8] In spite of evidence of its adverse impact on function and life quality,[3,9,10] HIV-associated pain is frequently undertreated.[10,11]

Definition

Pain is unique for each person. Although different for each individual, the experience of pain is similar in that it is multidimensional, comprised of physiological, sensory, affective, cognitive, behavioral, and sociocultural dimensions[12] (Figure 19.1). Awareness of the multidimensional nature of pain is essential for proper assessment and treatment. According to the International Association for the Study of Pain, pain is ". . . an unpleasant sensory and emotional experience associated with actual or potential tissue damage, or described in terms of such damage."[13,p. 250] In addition, the American Pain Society notes that pain is "always subjective. Objective observations of grimacing, limping, and tachycardia may be useful in assessing the patient, but these signs are often absent in patients with chronic pain known to be caused by structural lesions. There is no neurophysiological or chemical test that can measure pain. The clinician must accept the patient's report of pain."[14,p. 2] Margo McCaffery put the definition of pain most explicitly: "Pain is whatever the experiencing person says it is, existing whenever the experiencing person says it does."[15,p.]

Cancer pain provides a good model for understanding HIV-associated pain and its treatment. A French study describing pain in hospice practice found that patients with AIDS had frequency and intensity ratings similar to or greater than cancer patients.[16] Although certain aspects of the pain associated with HIV are unique, Jacox et al[17] noted that ". . . principles of pain assessment and treatment in the patient with HIV/AIDS are not fundamentally different from those in the patient with cancer and should

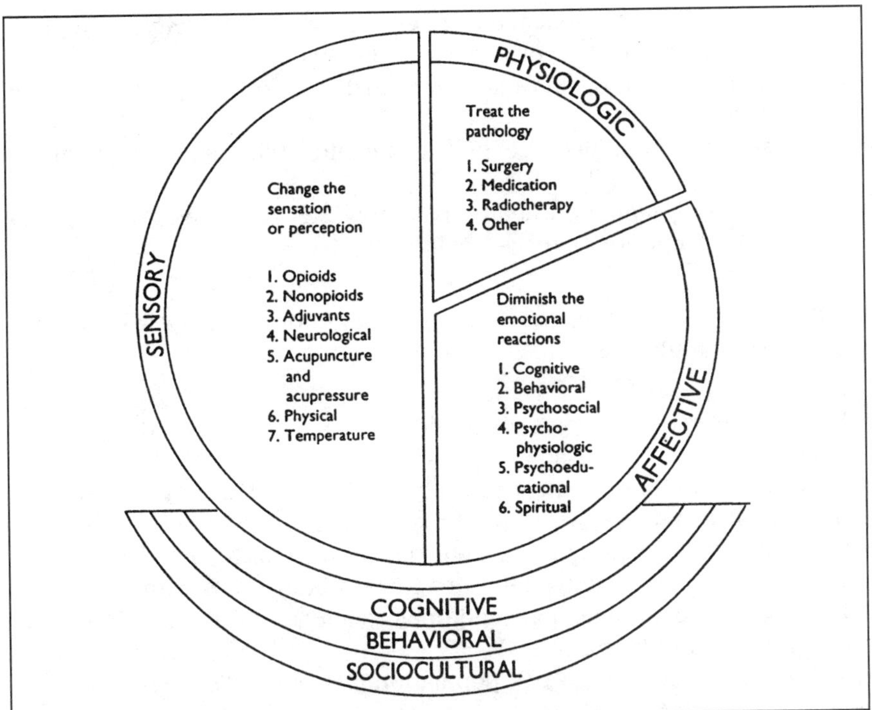

Figure 19.1 Treatment of Pain: A Multidimensional Approach (Reprinted with permission from McGuire DB, Yarbro CH, Ferrell BR. *Cancer Pain Management.* Boston: Jones & Bartlett, 1995:12.)

be followed for patients with HIV/AIDS."[17,p. 139] For the individual with HIV, pain management focuses primarily on aggressively treating infections rather than tumor. Unlike cancer, no controlled clinical trials have been conducted to examine the optimal management of HIV-associated pain. However, experience with the cancer population has demonstrated that utilizing the World Health Organization (WHO) analgesic ladder is effective in relieving 85 to 90% of all cancer pain.[18] Factors that affect cancer pain management have many important similarities with pain of HIV infection:

- Potential to enter a phase in which palliation becomes the treatment goal rather than cure of the disease

- Phases in which different pain patterns may predominate (acute; episodic; procedure-related; or chronic, stable pain)
- Comorbidity or altered pharmacokinetics due to concurrent disease and/or medications
- Increased suffering because of the meaning that pain holds for an individual
- Economic and human burden on patients, their family and friends, and society due to poorly managed pain

Other factors affecting pain management are different between cancer and HIV populations:

- HIV usually involves a younger individual who is less prepared psychologically for illness and disability.
- Compared with many cancer patients, individuals with HIV now live for more than 10 years.
- Cognitive impairment is more frequent in individuals with HIV.
- Society has more negative attitudes toward individuals with HIV.
- HIV may have preexisting conditions, such as substance abuse and chronic mental illness.
- A high proportion of the HIV population is socially disenfranchised.[19]

Biologic and Behavioral Basis

Pain is a complex process initiated by a noxious chemical (including damage to nerve tissue by medications), mechanical, or thermal stimulus. It is theorized that this stimulus initiates the release or production of numerous substances. These substances, which may include potassium, histamines, serotonins, acetylcholine, prostaglandins, bradykinin, and substance P, activate peripheral nerve afferent sensory fibers, initiating the ascending nerve pathway impulse. Pain is transmitted via the A delta and C fibers to the dorsal horn of the spinal cord. Here, it is theorized, a gate mechanism either stops or allows pain transmission to continue upward to the cortex of the brain, where perception of pain occurs.[20,21] The Gate Control Theory of Pain, originally introduced in 1965, provides a basic understanding of pain transmission.[22] An understanding of pain mechanisms is important because analgesic regimes work at various sites (Figure 19.2). With this knowledge, health care professionals can better plan a multimodal approach for maximal relief of pain and suffering with minimal side effects.

Etiologies Related to HIV Infection and Its Medical Treatment

Pain in the individual with HIV infection occurs as a result of HIV itself due to viral burden or immunosuppression, HIV treatment, or other coexisting

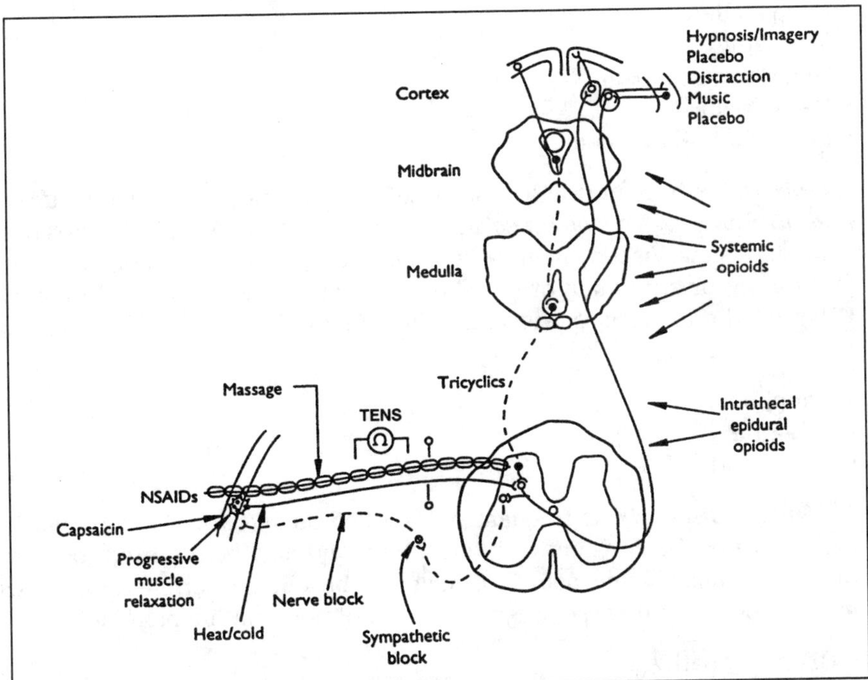

Figure 19.2 Schematic Diagram Showing Sites of Action of Commonly Used Pharmacologic and Behavioral Pain Therapies (From Fields HL, Levine JD. Pain-mechanisms and management. *West J Med* 141:350, 1984. Adapted by permission of the Western Journal of Medicine.)

conditions unrelated to HIV. HIV treatment-related pain and discomfort occur with diagnostic procedures such as endoscopy or lumbar puncture; chest tubes; radiation therapy or chemotherapy-associated mucositis; surgery; and some antiretrovirals.

Although HIV pain has the same basic etiologies, altered immune capability of the host, or the treatment of this altered immunity, it can be categorized as described in the following paragraphs.[8,23]

Somatic pain is typically well localized and constant. Adjectives used frequently by patients are *aching* or *gnawing*. Somatic pain originates from activation of peripheral nerve receptors in deep and cutaneous tissues. HIV-related etiologies common for somatic pain include

- Meningitis
- Encephalitis
- Myopathy
- Ulcerative esophagitis
- Rectal pain
- Procedure-related pain

Visceral pain is poorly localized and is frequently described as *deep*, *pressure*, *crampy*, or *squeezing* and may appear to "travel" or be referred to cutaneous sites. Visceral pain is usually caused by distension, compression, infiltration, or stretching of the abdominal or thoracic viscera. Common HIV-related etiologies for visceral pain include

- KS
- Lymphoma
- Infection
- Pancreatitis

Neuropathic pain is frequently described as *shocklike* or *burning* in nature. It may be constant or intermittent, and may be reported to move or travel. Neuropathic pain is thought to be due to peripheral or CNS injury. Common HIV-associated etiologies of neuropathic pain include

- HIV neuropathy
- Postchemotherapy with vincristine
- Postradiation therapy damage to nerves or nerve plexuses
- Postherpetic neuropathy
- HIV therapy with ddI, ddC, d4T, rifampin, and pentamidine

Headache is another common type of HIV-associated pain. Headache etiologies may derive from HIV infection itself or its treatment, including

- Encephalitis
- Tumor
- Meningitis
- Sinusitis
- ART with zidovudine
- Postlumbar puncture

Presentation and Assessment

Presentation

Although estimates of the incidence and prevalence of pain vary with stage of disease, setting, and demographic characteristics, the more common pain syndromes in HIV include

- Headache due to HIV or zidovudine
- Sensory peripheral neuropathy
- Pain due to KS
- Upper GI tract pain, including oral cavity, pharynx, and esophagus
- Abdominal pain
- Arthralgias and myalgias
- Dermatologic conditions
- Herpes zoster[4,7–9,19,24,25]

Assessment

Effective assessment of pain must depend on patient report. Pain assessment requires an ongoing process, similar to that of adjusting insulin for the diabetic, because the condition of HIV patients is likely to change. Pain assessment requires thorough and continuous investigation of the patient's complaint through a history that includes evaluation of pain intensity and character, careful physical assessment including a neurological examination, appropriate diagnostic tests, and a psychosocial assessment. Several algorithms have been published that outline the steps for workup of specific pain problems (headache, peripheral neuropathies, muscular pain, and abdominal pain) and can be found in *Pain in HIV/AIDS: La Douleur du SIDA/HIV.*[19] Additional information is available from the Roxane Pain Institute at 1-300-335-9100 or at *http://www.roxanne.com/Roxanne/RPI/AIDSPain/PainBook/index.html.* Pain assessment needs to be ongoing to determine the effect of pain management interventions and the need for changes in approach, because "the adequacy of pain management is directly related to the frequency of pain assessment."[26] The role of pain assessment cannot be overemphasized. It is important to remember that many patients will not volunteer information about pain, and it is not uncommon for an individual with HIV to have multiple HIV-associated pains at any given time.[9,11] Overall effectiveness in improving quality of life and decreasing suffering relies on good pain assessment skills and empathy with the patient's experience.

Subjective

Patient self-report of pain should be the primary source of pain assessment. The following provides an initial assessment plan.

Initial Pain Assessment

A. Assessment of pain intensity and character

1. **Onset and temporal pattern**—When did your pain start? How often does it occur? Has its intensity changed?
2. **Location**—Where is your pain? Is there more than one site?
3. **Description**—What does your pain feel like? What words would you use to describe your pain?
4. **Intensity**—On a scale of 0 to 10, with 0 being no pain and 10 being the worst pain you can imagine, how much does it hurt *right now*? How much does it hurt *at its worst*? How much does it hurt at its best?
5. **Aggravating and relieving factors**—What makes your pain better? What makes your pain worse?
6. **Previous treatment**—What types of treatments have you tried to relieve your pain? Were they effective in the past? Are they effective now?
7. **Effect**—How does the pain affect physical and social function?

B. Psychosocial assessment
Psychosocial assessment should include the following:

1. Effect and understanding of the HIV diagnosis and HIV treatment on the patient and the caregiver
2. The meaning of the pain to the patient and the family
3. Significant past instances of pain and their effect on the patient
4. The patient's typical coping responses to stress or pain
5. The patient's knowledge of, curiosity about, preferences for, and expectations about pain management methods
6. The patient's concerns about using controlled substances such as opioids, anxiolytics, or stimulants
7. The economic effect of the pain and its treatment
8. Changes in mood that have occurred as a result of the pain (e.g., depression, anxiety)

C. Physical and neurological examination

1. Examine site of pain and evaluate common referral patterns.
2. Perform pertinent neurological evaluation.
   - Head and neck pain—cranial nerve and funduscopic evaluation
   - Back and neck pain—motor and sensory function in limbs; rectal and urinary sphincter function

D. Diagnostic evaluation

1. Evaluate progression of HIV or tissue injury related to HIV treatment.
   - Laboratory test
   - Radiological studies
   - Neurophysiological (e.g., electromyography) testing
2. Perform appropriate radiological studies and correlate normal and abnormal findings with physical and neurological examination.
3. Recognize limitations of diagnostic studies.
   - Bone scan—false-negatives in myeloma, lymphoma, previous radiotherapy sites

(continued)

- CT scan—good definition of bone and soft tissue but difficult to image entire spine
- MRI scan—bone definition not as good as CT; better images of spine and brain

Adapted from Jacox A, Carr DB, Payne R, et al. *Management of Cancer Pain. Clinical Practice Guideline Number 9*. Rockville, MD: Agency for Health Care Policy and Research, US Department of Health and Human Services, Public Health Service, 1994. AHCPR publication no. 94-5-0592.

Establishing a routine approach to pain assessment and management can be facilitated by remembering the ABCDE mnemonic presented in *Management of Cancer Pain.*[17] This mnemonic emphasizes the importance of assessment:

A	**Ask** about pain regularly. **Assess** pain systematically.
B	**Believe** patient and family report of pain and what relieves it.
C	**Choose** pain management options that are appropriate for and acceptable to patient, family, setting, and culture.
D	**Deliver** pain management in a timely, logical, coordinated, and cost-effective, manner.
E	**Empower** patients and their families. **Enable** patients to control their care as much as possible.[17,p. 24]

Some patients are unable to verbalize their discomfort. People at increased risk of poor pain assessment—and subsequent inadequate management—include:

- Patients with end-stage disease
- Patients with impaired cognitive states
- Children
- Women
- Those who are not fluent in the caregiver's language
- Those unable or unwilling to utilize pain scales
- Elderly patients

In addition to those identified above, others who typically have their pain managed inadequately are minorities, individuals with active past history of substance abuse, and the poor.[27]

Use of an established pain assessment tool is recommended. Pain tools need to be understandable, easy to utilize, and used consistently. Three commonly used self-report measures for quantifying *intensity* of pain are 1) a numeric rating scale, 2) visual analogue scale (VAS), or 3) verbal descriptor scale (Figure 19.3). The easiest approach consists of asking the patient to rate their current level of pain from 0 to 10, where 0 represents the absence of pain and 10 represents the worst pain imaginable. Another category of pain assessment instrument is more complex because it evaluates the multidimensional nature of pain rather than just pain intensity. Examples include the McGill Pain Questionnaire, the Brief Pain Inventory (BPI), and the Memorial Pain Assessment Card. The BPI (Figure 19.4) is easily used.

Objective

One of the initial goals of pain management is to discover pain etiologies, such as infection, that can be treated to manage the pain. Findings from

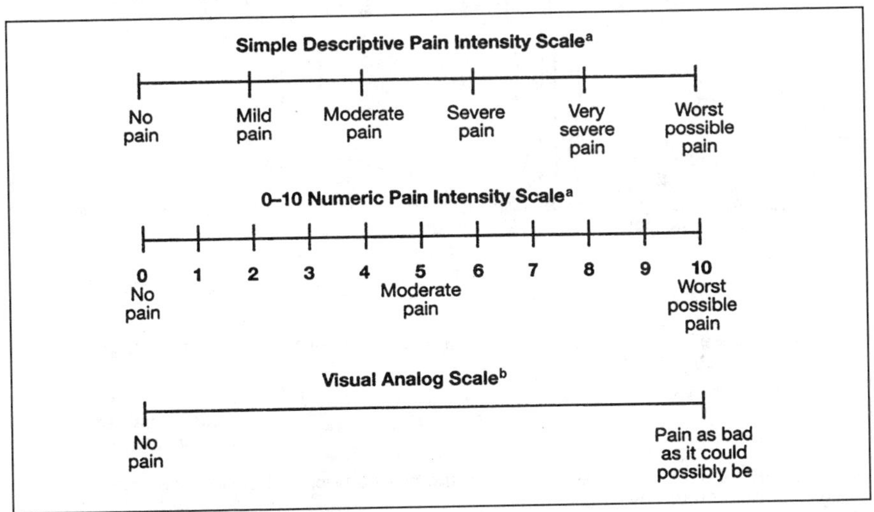

Figure 19.3 Pain Intensity Scales
[a]If used as a graphic rating scale, a 10-cm baseline is recommended.
[b]A 10-cm baseline is essential for VAS scales.
(Reprinted from Jacox A, Carr DB, Payne R, et al. *Management of Cancer Pain. Clinical Practice Guideline Number 9.* Rockville, MD: Agency for Health Care Policy and Research, US Department of Health and Human Services, Public Health Service; 1994:26. AHCPR publication no. 94-0593.)

Study ID#__________ Hospital#__________

Do not write above this line

Date: ____/____/____

Time:__________

Name:______________________ ______________________ ______
Last First Middle Initial

1) Throughout our lives, most of us have had pain from time to time (such as minor headaches, sprains, and toothaches). Have you had pain other than these everyday kinds of pain today? 1. Yes 2. No

2) On the diagram, shade in the areas where you feel pain. Put an X on the area that hurts the most.

Right Left Left Right

3) Please rate your pain by circling the one number that best describes your pain at its **worst** in the past 24 hours.

0 1 2 3 4 5 6 7 8 9 10
No pain — Pain as bad as you can imagine

4) Please rate your pain by circling the one number that best describes your pain at its **least** in the past 24 hours.

0 1 2 3 4 5 6 7 8 9 10
No pain — Pain as bad as you can imagine

5) Please rate your pain by circling the one number that best describes your pain on the **average.**

0 1 2 3 4 5 6 7 8 9 10
No pain — Pain as bad as you can imagine

Figure 19.4 Brief Pain Inventory (Short Form) (Reprinted from Jacox A, Carr DB, Payne R, et al. *Management of Cancer Pain. Clinical Practice Guideline Number 9.* Rockville, MD: Agency for Health Care Policy and Research, US Department of Health and Human Services, Public Health Service; 1994:228–229. AHCPR publication no. 94-0593.)

6) Please rate your pain by circling the one number that tells how much pain you have **right now.**

0 No pain	1	2	3	4	5	6	7	8	9	10 Pain as bad as you can imagine

7) What treatments or medications are you receiving for your pain?

____

8) In the past 24 hours, how much **relief** have pain treatments or medications provided? Please circle the one percentage that most shows how much relief you have received.

0% No relief	10%	20%	30%	40%	50%	60%	70%	80%	90%	100% Complete relief

9) Circle the one number that describes how, during the past 24 hours, **pain has interfered** with your:

A. General activity

0 Does not interfere	1	2	3	4	5	6	7	8	9	10 Completely interferes

B. Mood

0 Does not interfere	1	2	3	4	5	6	7	8	9	10 Completely interferes

C. Walking ability

0 Does not interfere	1	2	3	4	5	6	7	8	9	10 Completely interferes

D. Normal work (includes both work outside the home and housework)

0 Does not interfere	1	2	3	4	5	6	7	8	9	10 Completely interferes

E. Relations with other people

0 Does not interfere	1	2	3	4	5	6	7	8	9	10 Completely interferes

F. Sleep

0 Does not interfere	1	2	3	4	5	6	7	8	9	10 Completely interferes

G. Enjoyment of life

0 Does not interfere	1	2	3	4	5	6	7	8	9	10 Completely interferes

Figure 19.4 Continued

physical examination and diagnostic tests from the laboratory or radiology can be helpful in this regard. The area of pain should be examined through inspection, palpation, and manipulation. Dermatomal distribution, motor or sensory loss, and reflexes should be evaluated. Vital signs are not valid indicators of pain nor are behavioral changes, especially with chronic pain. Diagnostic tests can help investigate other problems related to the pain or pain treatment, such as confusion or altered consciousness.

Related Medical Management

Pain associated with HIV infection has many etiologies. Medical treatment of underlying causes of pain will often be the most effective method of relieving discomfort and should be the first step. Medical management techniques can be aimed at treating infections and tumors or decreasing inflammation with surgery, radiation therapy, chemotherapy, immunotherapy, antibiotics, antivirals, antifungals, or steroids. HIV treatments and procedures may be the etiology of the patient's pain, including antiretrovirals, antivirals, antimicrobacterials, PCP prophylaxis, chemotherapy, radiation therapy, surgery, and procedures. Table 19.1 displays information regarding conditions associated with HIV pain that benefit from primary medical treatment delivered concurrently with specific pain relief measures. The health care provider should strive to maximize patient comfort while awaiting the benefits of their medical treatment regime.

Interventions

Pain in HIV is often undertreated and requires frequent comprehensive assessment, evaluation, and intervention. Potential barriers to adequate HIV pain management are similar to those identified for cancer pain:

Barriers to HIV Pain Management

Barriers related to health care professionals

- Inadequate health care provider knowledge of pain management
- Poor assessment of pain

- Failure to believe the patient's report of pain
- Concern about controlled substance regulation of the HCP
- Fear of patient addiction, especially those with a history of substance abuse
- Concern about analgesic side effects
- Misperceptions regarding tolerance to analgesics
- Failure to elicit or believe the patient's pain report
- Phobia or fears of treating HIV-infected patients

Barriers related to patients

- Reluctance to report pain: concern about distracting health care provider from treatment of underlying HIV infection, fear that pain means HIV is worse, concern about not being a "good" patient
- Reluctance to take pain medications: fear of addiction or of being labeled an addict, worries about side effects, concern about developing tolerance to pain medications
- Past history of or current substance abuse
- Inability to pay for analgesics

Barriers related to the health care system

- Low priority given to pain treatment
- Inadequate reimbursement for pain management
- Restrictive regulation of controlled substances
- Problems with pain treatment availability or access
- Negative attitudes of society toward individuals with HIV

Adapted from Jacox A, Carr DB, Payne R, et al. *Management of Cancer Pain. Clinical Practice Guideline Number 9.* Rockville, MD: Agency for Health Care Policy and Research, US Department of Health and Human Services, Public Health Service, 1994:17. AHCPR publication no. 94-0593.

Although pain is as distinct as the individual, a standardized pain management approach can be helpful and improve overall results. Table 19.2 provides an example of a standard of care for the patient in pain. The goals of pain management are to relieve or diminish pain, minimize side effects, maximize comfort and function for improved life quality, and minimize cost. Effective pain management includes both pharmacological and nonpharmacological approaches.

Table 19.1 HIV-Associated Pain That Requires Initial Medical Management

Pain Location	Pain Cause
Chest	Pneumothorax, pulmonary tuberculosis, fungal infection of lungs, CMV, esophageal candidiasis, esophageal ulcers, postherpetic neuropathy (zoster)
Headache	Aseptic meningitis, CNS lymphoma, KS, toxoplasmosis, zidovudine, sinusitis
Oral cavity and esophagus	Candidiasis, KS, aphthous ulcers, herpes simplex
Peripheral neuropathy	HIV infection, ddI or ddC
Abdomen	Cholecystitis, ascending cholangitis, KS, perforation, *Mycobacterium avium cellulare* complex, pancreatitis, organomegaly, anorectal lesions
Musculoskeletal	Septic arthritis, metastatic disease related to lymphoma, Reiter's syndrome

CMV = cytomegalovirus; KS = Kaposi's sarcoma.

Table 19.2 Pain Management Standard of Care

Expected Outcome	Action
The patient/SO will understand the current or proposed pain relief plan and assessment technique. The patient/SO will readily discuss concerns, questions, or problems related to pain management.	Instruct patient/SO in the current pain control regimen. Instruct patient/SO to notify health care provider of unrelieved pain or unacceptable side effects. Involve patient/SO in discussions related to pain relief options such as IV PCA, oral, epidural analgesia, imagery, relaxation and making treatment decisions. Answer questions honestly. Supply educational materials to the patient/SO regarding pain relief. Believe the patient's complaint of pain. Accept the patient's complaint of pain as valid.

Table 19.2 *Continued*

Expected Outcome	Action
	Assess for presence of pain in a consistent manner using a standardized measurement tool (0 to 10 scale or slide algometer). Various other assessment tools may be utilized if the patient is unable to master the standard tools. Assess the nature of the pain, including quality, quantity, and location.
Patient will obtain/maintain an optimal level of comfort as noted by pain scores and the patient's verbalizations related to pain.	Notify the patient's health care provider if pain relief techniques fail to maintain a pain level below an agreed, tolerable level (0 to 10 scale or slide algometer). Change pain treatments as appropriate. Administer analgesic medications as needed or make sure the patient can. Monitor and evaluate the effectiveness of analgesics and/or interventions. Ensure that the patient receives pain medication in advance of painful procedures. Assume the patient is in pain if a physiological etiology exists and the patient is unable to communicate his complaint. Ask for SOs' input regarding their assessment as to whether patient is in pain. Incorporate adjunct pain relief techniques into the patient's plan of care as applicable: distraction, imagery, heat or cold, relaxation, positioning for comfort, TENS unit. Consult appropriate resources as required—dietitian, physical therapist, chaplain, advanced practice nurse.

(continued)

Table 19.2 *Continued*

Expected Outcome	Action
Patient's pain tolerance will be maintained and/or improved as demonstrated by pain scores.	Ensure adequate periods of rest. Maintain nutritional status. Promote safe, relaxing environment. Instruct and encourage the patient to initiate and maintain a pain log or diary if pain is anticipated to persist for an extended duration.
Patient will perform daily activities at optimal level.	Increase patient activity to ensure adequate pain relief with the optimal activity.
Patient will experience minimal side effects of analgesic therapy.	Monitor for side effects of analgesic therapy such as increased level of sedation, constipation, nausea, vomiting, pruritus, and respiratory depression. Initiate appropriate interventions to prevent, decrease, or eliminate side effects. Notify patient's health care provider of unacceptable side effects of analgesic therapy and obtain required interventions.

SO = significant other; PCA = patient-controlled analgesia; TENS = transcutaneous electrical nerve stimulation.

(Adapted from Coyne P. Standard of care for pain management interventions. *Oncol Nurs Forum.* 1995;22(9):1437–1438.)

Pharmacologic Approaches

The World Health Organizations (WHO) in 1986 introduced the three-step analgesic ladder. The WHO approach has five essential concepts that should be adhered to when possible:

1. *For the individual*: Individualize the approach. The right dose is the one that relieves the pain for that person at that time.

2. *By the clock*: Incorporate an around-the-clock regular administration schedule rather than PRN. Also provide for rescue doses for breakthrough pain.
3. *By the mouth*: The oral administration route is preferred because it creates a steady state, providing longer lasting pain relief.
4. *By the ladder*: Use the WHO analgesic ladder (Figure 19.5).
5. *Pay attention to detail.*

Three major classes of drugs are used alone or in combination to treat pain: (1) *nonopioids*, which include NSAIDs and acetaminophen; (2) *opioids*, which include agonists (such as codeine, morphine, hydromorphone, methadone, and fentanyl), partial agonists (such as buprenorphine), and mixed agonist-antagonists; and (3) *adjuvant drugs*, such as antidepressants, anticonvulsants, corticosteroids, local anesthetics, methotrimeprazine, baclofen, and capsaicin.

NSAIDs and Acetaminophen

The WHO ladder (see Figure 19-5), as its first step or rung, starts with NSAIDs or acetaminophen for mild pain, defined as less than 4 on a scale of 0 to 10. Acetaminophen has minimal anti-inflammatory effects and produces analgesia primarily by a central mechanism. NSAIDs have been shown to be opioid sparing in moderate to severe pain while effectively relieving mild discomfort.[17] No NSAID has been shown to be any more effective than another, although they do have different side effect profiles. The initial choice of an NSAID should be based on its efficacy,[17] safety, and relative expense. Generally, the least expensive NSAID should be utilized. If one NSAID is not effective, one from another class—proprionic acid derivatives (Ibuprofen, naproxen, fenoprofen, ketoprofen), indole derivatives (indomethacin, sulindac), or fenol acenic acid (diclofenac sodium)—sometimes is effective and is appropriate to try. Information regarding NSAIDs is summarized in Table 19.3. Contraindications include low platelet count, elevated creatinine, or GI bleed or gastritis. The patient should be monitored carefully for adverse effects of NSAIDs, including renal failure, hepatic dysfunction, prolonged bleeding, and GI effects. Low albumin makes patients more prone to NSAID side effects.

Opioid Therapy

The second step of the WHO ladder (see Figure 19.5) recommends a weak opioid that is usually a combination opioid. Its dose is restricted by

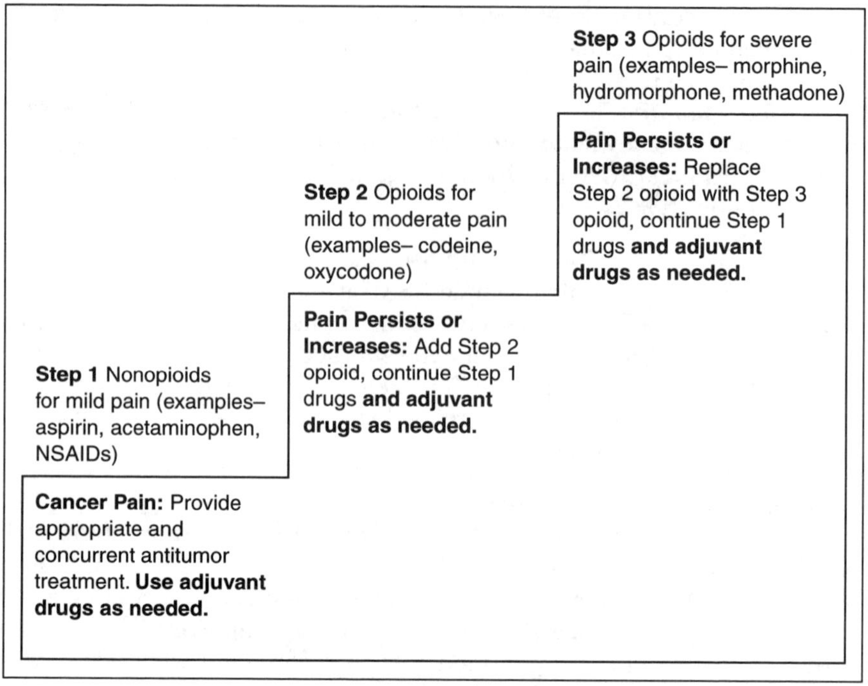

Step 3 Opioids for severe pain (examples– morphine, hydromorphone, methadone)

Pain Persists or Increases: Replace Step 2 opioid with Step 3 opioid, continue Step 1 drugs **and adjuvant drugs as needed.**

Step 2 Opioids for mild to moderate pain (examples– codeine, oxycodone)

Pain Persists or Increases: Add Step 2 opioid, continue Step 1 drugs **and adjuvant drugs as needed.**

Step 1 Nonopioids for mild pain (examples– aspirin, acetaminophen, NSAIDs)

Cancer Pain: Provide appropriate and concurrent antitumor treatment. **Use adjuvant drugs as needed.**

Figure 19.5 WHO Three-Step Analgesic Ladder (Reprinted from Jacox A, Carr DB, Payne R, et al. *Management of Cancer Pain. Clinical Practice Guideline Number 9.* Rockville, MD: Agency for Health Care Policy and Research, US Department of Health and Human Services, Public Health Service; 1994:14. AHCPR publication no. 94-0593.)

Table 19.3 Nonsteroidal Anti-inflammatory Drugs

Chemical Class	Generic Name (Trade Name)	Half-life (hours)	Dosing Schedule[a]	Recommended Starting Dose[b] (mg)	Maximum Dose Recommended (mg/day)	Comments
p-aminophenol derivatives	Acetaminophen (Tylenol®)	3–4	q4–6h	650	6000	Overdosage produces hepatic toxicity. No GI or platelet toxicity.
Salicylates	Aspirin	3–12	q4–6h	650	6000	Standard for comparison. May not be as well tolerated as some of the newer NSAIDs.
	Diflunisal (Dolobid®)	8–12	q12h	500	1500	Less GI toxicity than aspirin.
	Choline Magnesium Trisalicylate (Trilisate®)	8–12	q12h	500–1000	4000	Minimal GI toxicity. No effect on platelet aggregation.
	Salsalate (Disalcid®)	8–12	q12h	500–1000	4000	
Proprionic acids	Ibuprofen (Advil®, Motrin®, Nuprin®)	3–4	q6h	400	4200	Avaliable as a suspension.
	Naproxen (Naprosyn®)	1–3	q12h	250	1500	
	Fenoprofen (Nalfon®)	2–3	q6h	200	3200	
	Ketoprofen (Orudis®)	2–3	q6h	25	300	
	Flurbiprofen	5–6	q12h	100	300	
	Oxaprozin	40	q24h	600	1800	

(continued)

Table 19.3 *Continued*

Chemical Class	Generic Name (Trade Name)	Half-life (hours)	Dosing Schedule[a]	Recommended Starting Dose[b] (mg)	Maximum Dose Recommended (mg/day)	Comments
Acetic acids	Indomethacin (Indocine®)	4–5	q8h	25	200	Higher incidence of GI and CNS side effects than proprionic acid. Available in slow-release preparations.
	Tolmetin (Tolectrin®)	1	q8h	200	2000	
	Sulindac (Clinoril®)	14	q12h	150	400	
	Diclofenac sodium (Voltaren®)	2	q8h	25	200	
	Ketorolac (Toradol®)	4–7	q6h	30–60 load, then 15–30 q6h (parenteral), 10 q6h (oral)	150 Day 1, 120 Day 2 and after (parenteral) 40 (oral)	Experience limited to acute pain. Efficacy and safety with chronic use to be determined. Long-term use not recommended.
Oxicams	Piroxicam (Feldene®)	45	q24h	20	40	
Fenamates	Mefenamic acid	2	q6h	250	1000	
Pyranocarboxylic acids	Etodolac	7	q8h	200	1200	

[a]Dosing interval in hours.
[b]Starting dose should be one-half to two-thirds recommended dose in the elderly, those on multiple drugs, or those with renal insufficiency.
NSAID = nonsteroidal anti-inflammatory drug.
(Adapted with permission from McGuire DB, Yarbro CH, Ferrell BR. *Cancer Pain Management.* 2nd ed. Boston: Jones & Bartlett; 1995:91–92.)

the amount of NSAID or acetaminophen in the preparation. The same NSAID and acetaminophen risks mentioned previously should be considered. These classes of drugs serve as a small step, argued by some as not truly required, and are frequently skipped.

The use of opioids is recommended for relieving moderate (4 to 7 on a 10-point scale) to severe (8 or more on a 10-point scale) pain and may be used with or without adjunct medication. Opioids work directly in the dorsal horn to limit pain transmission and consequent perception of discomfort. Opioids are found to be most effective in visceral and somatic pain. Their effect on neuropathic pain is often disappointing. The correct dose of opioids is the one that manages the pain while producing minimal side effects. Morphine is typically the drug of choice, as it is relatively inexpensive and may be titrated easily. Opioids to avoid are meperidine and the agonist-antagonist drugs class of narcotics. Meperidine (Demerol) is used to treat acute pain but has a toxic metabolite, normeperidine, that may cause CNS stimulation and seizures.

Tables 19.4 and 19.5 provide guidance regarding the usual starting oral or parenteral dose for moderate to severe pain. These tables also provide equianalgesic doses. After titrating the analgesic agent and determining the patient's opioid requirement, equianalgesic conversion should be used to place the patient on a long-acting agent if the pain is expected to persist for some time. Patients will be more comfortable and better able to adhere to the pain management regime if they are required to take medication every 6 or 12 hours, or every 3 days, rather than every 4 hours.

The use of mixed agonist-antagonists such as pentazocine (Talwin), nalbephine (Nubain), and butorphanol (Stadol) produce analgesia by binding to the opioid receptor site kappa. At higher doses they have less risk of respiratory depression, but also less analgesia. In the cancer population they have not been found to be useful and are not recommended. Mixed agonist-antagonists can precipitate withdrawal in opioid-dependent patients.

When initiating opioids it is essential to inform the patient of potential side effects to alleviate his fears and prepare him to manage his own care. For the purpose of minimizing barriers to effective pain control, it is important to define terms and distinguish between addiction, tolerance, and dependence. Patients receiving opioids for pain control rarely get addicted to their analgesics; however, tolerance and physical dependence are to be expected. These should not be equated with psychological depen-

Table 19.4 Equivalents for Opioid Analgesics in Opioid-Naive Adults and Children ≥50 kg[a]

Drug	Approximate Equianalgesic Dose		Usual Starting Dose for Moderate to Severe Pain	
	Oral	Parenteral	Oral	Parenteral
OPIOID AGONIST[b]				
Morphine[c]	30 mg q3–4h (repeat around-the-clock dosing) 60 mg q3–4h (single dose or intermittent dosing)	10 mg q3–4h	30 mg q3–4h	10 mg q3–4h
Morphine, controlled-release[c,d] (MS Contin, Oramorph)	90–120 mg q12h	N/A	90–120 mg q12h	N/A
Hydromorphone[c] (Dilaudid)	7.5 mg q3–4h	1.5 mg q3–4h	6 mg q3–4h	1.5 mg q3–4h
Levorphanol (Levo-Dromoran)	4 mg q6–8h	2 mg q6–8h	4 mg q6–8h	2 mg q6–8h
Meperidine (Demerol)	300 mg q2–3h	100 mg q3h	N/R	100 mg q3h
Methadone (Dolophine, other)	20 mg q6–8h	10 mg q6–8h	20 mg q6–8h	10 mg q6–8h
Oxymorphone[c] (Numorphan)	N/A	1 mg q3–4h	N/A	1 mg q3–4h

Combination Opioid/NSAID Preparations[e]				
Codeine[f] (with aspirin or acetaminophen)	180–200 mg q3–4h	130 mg q3–4h	60 mg q3–4h	60 mg q2h (IM/SC)
Hydrocodone (in Lorcet, Lortab, Vicodin, others)	30 mg q3–4h	N/A	10 mg q3–4h	N/A
Oxycodone (Roxicodone, also in Percocet, Percodan, Tylox, others)	30 mg q3–4h	N/A	10 mg q3–4h	N/A

[a]Caution: Recommended doses do not apply for adult patients with body weight less than 50 kg.

[b]Caution: Recommended doses do not apply to patients with renal or hepatic insufficiency or other conditions affecting drug metabolism and kinetics.

[c]Caution: For morphine, hydromorphone, and oxymorphone, rectal administration is an alternate route for patients unable to take oral medications. Equianalgesic doses may differ from oral and parenteral doses because of pharmacokinetic differences.

[d]Transdermal fentanyl (Duragesic) is an alternative option. Transdermal fentanyl dosage is not calculated as equianalgesic to a single morphine dose. See the package insert for dosing calculations. Doses above 25 μg/h should not be used in opiod-naive patients.

[e]Caution: Doses of aspirin and acetaminophen in combination opioid/NSAID preparations must also be adjusted to the patient's body weight. Aspirin is contraindicated in children in the presence of fever or other viral disease because of its association with Reye's syndrome.

[f]Caution: Codeine doses above 65 mg often are not appropriate because of diminishing incremental analgesia with increasing doses but continually increasing nausea, constipation, and other side effects.

Note: Published tables vary in the suggested doses that are equianalgesic to morphine. Clinical response is the criterion that must be applied for each patient; titration to clinical responses is necessary. Because there is not complete cross-tolerance among these drugs, it is usually necessary to use a lower than equianalgesic dose when changing drugs and to retitrate to response.

(Reprinted from Jacox A, Carr DB, Payne R, et al. *Management of Cancer Pain. Clinical Practice Guideline Number 9.* Rockville, MD: Agency for Health Care Policy and Research, US Department of Health and Human Services, Public Health Service; 1994:52. AHCPR publication no. 94-0593.)

Table 19.5 Equivalents for Opioid Analgesics in Opioid-Naive Adults and Children <50 kg[a]

	Approximate Equianalgesic Dose		Usual Starting Dose for Moderate to Severe Pain	
Drug	**Oral**	**Parenteral**	**Oral**	**Parenteral**
OPIOID AGONIST[b]				
Morphine[c]	30 mg q3–4h (repeat around-the-clock dosing) 60 mg q3–4h (single dose or intermittent dosing)	10 mg q3–4h	0.3 mg/kg q3–4h	0.1 mg/kg q3–4h
Morphine, controlled-release[c,d] (MS Contin, Oramorph)	90–120 mg q12h	N/A	N/A	N/A
Hydromorphone[c] (Dilaudid)	7.5 mg q3–4h	1.5 mg q3–4h	0.06 mg/kg q3–4h	0.015 mg/kg q3–4h
Levorphanol (Levo-Dromoran)	4 mg q6–8h	2 mg q6–8h	0.04 mg/kg q6–8h	0.02 mg/kg q6–8h
Meperidine (Demerol)	300 mg q2–3h	100 mg q3h	N/R	0.75 mg/kg q2–3h
Methadone (Dolophine, others)	20 mg q6–8h	10 mg q6–8h	0.2 mg/kg q6–8h	0.1 mg/kg q6–8h

COMBINATION OPIOID/NSAID PREPARATIONS[e]

Codeine[f] (with aspirin or acetaminophen)	180–200 mg q3–4h	130 mg q3–4h	0.5–1 mg/kg q3–4h	N/R
Hydrocodone (in Lorcet, Lortab, Vicodin, others)	30 mg q3–4h	N/A	0.2 mg/kg q3–4h	N/A
Oxycodone (Roxicodone, also in Percocet, Percodan, Tylox, others)	30 mg q3–4h	N/A	0.2 mg/kg q3–4h	N/A

[a]Caution: Doses listed for patients with body weight less than 50 kg cannot be used as initial starting doses in babies less than 6 months of age.

[b]Caution: Recommended doses do not apply to patients with renal or hepatic insufficiency or other conditions affecting drug metabolism and kinetics.

[c]Caution: For morphine, hydromorphone, and oxymorphone, rectal administration is an alternate route for patients unable to take oral medications. Equianalgesic doses may differ from oral and parenteral doses because of pharmacokinetic differences.

[d]Transdermal fentanyl (Duragesic) is an alternative option. Transdermal fentanyl dosage is not calculated as equianalgesic to a single morphine dosage. See the package insert for dosing calculations. Doses above 25 μg/h should not be used in opioid-negative patients.

[e]Caution: Doses of aspirin and acetaminophen in combination opioid/NSAID preparations must also be adjusted to the patient's body weight. Aspirin is contraindicated in children in the presence of fever or other viral disease because of its association with Reye's syndrome.

[f]Caution: Some clinicians recommend not exceeding 1.5 mg/kg of codeine because of an increased incidence of side effects with higher doses.

Note: Published tables vary in the suggested doses that are equianalegsic to morphine. Clinical response is the criterion that must be applied for each patient; titration to clinical responses is necessary. Because there is not complete cross-tolerance among these drugs, it is usually necessary to use a lower than equianalgesic dose when changing drugs and to retitrate to response.

(Reprinted from Jacox A, Carr DB, Payne R, et al. *Management of Cancer Pain. Clinical Practice Guideline Number 9.* Rockville, MD: Agency for Health Care Policy and Research, US Department of Health and Human Services, Public Health Service; 1994:54. AHCPR publication no. 94-0593.)

dence, known as *addiction*, which is manifested as substance abuse behavior.

Management of Common Opioid Side Effects

Side effects associated with opioid administration should be anticipated, monitored constantly, and "prophylaxed" or treated. The most common side effects of opioids include sedation, constipation, nausea and vomiting, and itching. Constipation in the HIV patient is less of a problem than in the cancer patient population. Initially nausea and vomiting should be treated aggressively with an antiemetic given on a scheduled. When nausea or vomiting persist, switch to another opioid. Management of opiod-induced nausea and vomiting based on inferred mechanisms is displayed in Table 19.6. Drowsiness usually resolves in 48 to 72 hours. Consider reducing the opioid in each dose and increasing dose frequency. If drowsiness persists, switch to another opioid or consider adding stimulants such as methylphenidate (Ritalin) 5 to 10 mg or dextroamphetamine (Dexidirine) 2.5 to 7.5 mg on rising in the morning and before 1 pm. Less common side effects include dry mouth, nightmares, confusion, sweats, difficulty urinating, and, rarely, respiratory depression.

Adjunctive Analgesics

Adjunctive analgesics include a number of classes of drugs that work to decrease side effects or have unique analgesic properties or enhance opioids. Many adjunct agents, such as anticonvulsants or antidepressants, are drugs not usually thought of in the context of pain management. Table 19.7 provides information regarding types of HIV-associated pain and suggested adjunct medications for their treatment.

Nonpharmacological Pain Management Techniques: Physical and Psychosocial Interventions

Physical Modalities

Cutaneous stimulation (the use of heat or cold and massage or vibration) has been shown to offer improved comfort in some patients. If no contraindications exist, a trial may be worthwhile. For example, heat may relieve aching joints and muscles, whereas a cold wash cloth placed on the forehead may provide some relief from headache.

Table 19.6 Management of Opioid-Induced Nausea and Vomiting Based on Inferred Mechanism

Inferred Mechanism	Clinical Features	Antiemetic Drugs of Choice
Simulation of the medullary chemoreceptor trigger zone	Nausea or vomiting or both shortly after opioid administration	Metoclopramide, prochlorperazine, chlorpromazine, haloperidol, corticosteroids, or lorazepam
Enhanced vestibular sensitivity	Prominent movement-induced nausea and vomiting or vertigo	Scopolamine, meclizine, or lorazepam
Increased gastric antral tone	Early satiety, postprandial bloating, or vomiting	Metoclopramide or cisapride
Constipation	Passage of small, hard infrequent stool, with difficulty	Proactive bowel regimen

(Reprinted with permission from McGuire DB, Yarbro CH, Ferrell BR. *Cancer Pain Management.* 2nd ed. Boston: Jones & Bartlett; 1995:114.)

Table 19.7 Adjunct Medications[a]

Type of Pain or Related Symptom	Suggested Adjunct Medication
Bone pain	NSAIDs, steroids
Increased intracranial pressure	Steroids
Postherpetic neuralgia	Tricyclic antidepressants, clonidine, carbamazepine
Nerve compression pressure pain	Steroids, anticonvulsants
Intermittent stabbing pain (demyelination)	Sodium valproate, carbamazepine, phenytoin (anticonvulsants)
Muscle spasm pain	Baclofen, benzodiazepines
Superficial dysaesthetic	Tricyclic antidepressants, steroids, anticonvulsants
Nerve destruction pain (deafferentation)	Antidepressants and anticonvulsants
Pain and depression	Tricyclic antidepressants, pemoline
Pain and anxiety	Benzodiazepines, methotrimeprazide, phenothiazines
Intestinal colic	Loperamide, scopolamine
Agitation	Chlorpromazine, benzodiazepines
Potentiate analgesic	Tricyclic antidepressants, caffeine, steroids/methotrimeprazine, dextroamphetamines, haloperidol/pemoline, antihistamines
Skin ulceration (malignant, decubitus, or infected)	NSAIDs, antibiotics, nitrous oxide inhalation; lidocaine aerosol spray for dressing changes
Stomatitis	Lidocaine viscous or jelly, artificial saliva
Sedation	Dexedrine, dextroamphetamines
Terminal agitation	Methotrimeprazine (may be useful in opioid-tolerant patient), benzodiazepines
Trigeminal neuralgia	Baclofen
Second-line approach in patients with refractory neuropathic pain	Clonidine
Headache	Caffeine

[a]This list is not all inclusive. Dosages for pain management sometimes vary from those used in treatment of primary indication.

NSAID = nonsteroidal anti-inflammatory drug.

(From Coyne, Lush L, MacMurren M, Long S, Barsanti J. Pain management: A resource manual: Virginia Commonwealth University/Medical College of Virginia Hospital. Duarte CA: Mayday Foundation. 1996.)

Counterstimulation

Transcutaneous electrical nerve stimulation (TENS), like acupuncture, provides counterstimulation. TENS therapy is an intervention typically applied by the physical therapist in an attempt to modulate pain transmission. TENS is believed to cause the peripheral nerves to activate the endogenous pain pathways. A low-voltage electrical stimulus is placed via electrodes at locations determined by nerve innervation and pain location. TENS for HIV pain requires further research to determine proper utilization, especially with peripheral neuropathy.

Cognitive-Behavioral Interventions

Psychosocial or cognitive strategies involve mental activity to alter the evaluation of sensations as painful while also perceiving greater control or self-efficacy. These interventions need to be introduced early in the disease process while the patient has sufficient strength, concentration, and energy to master the techniques, which include:

- Mental imagery
- Relaxation techniques
- Hypnosis
- Distraction: rhythmic breathing, rocking back and forth, singing or humming, conversation, music
- Cognitive reframing
- Biofeedback

Support groups or prayer and pastoral counseling may also provide supportive care that improves HIV pain management.

Patient education that provides information prior to procedures or treatments that cause discomfort, although not a replacement for adequate analgesia, will help decrease anxiety and thus increase comfort.[28] Education regarding the entire pain management program that emphasizes the roles of patients and their significant other can empower and improve symptom outcomes.

Pain Management of the HIV-Infected Individual with a History of Substance Abuse

Management of pain in the individual with an active or past history of substance abuse is challenging for any provider, but it becomes highly complex when the disease is HIV. Twenty-three to 28% of AIDS patients are reported to have been transmitted through IV drug abuse.[29] This type of patient demands that health care providers seek out and recognize their own biases and limitations, and requires answering the question: Am I treating this person ethically and morally? Most health care professionals do not relish the concept, never mind the reality, of giving narcotics to a drug abuser. However, these individuals are entitled to safe, reasonable, and good-quality HIV care. This should include appropriate and adequate pain management whenever discomfort is present. The patient's complaint of pain should be believed. Initiating drug rehabilitation when the patient is in pain is not appropriate. Pain management should never become a bargaining chip.[30]

Individuals with a history of substance abuse require special intervention that should include a detailed history of drugs used, route, frequency, side effects, and withdrawal occurrences. This should be incorporated as an integral part of the history. As part of the physical exam, an evaluation for injection marks or tracks should be conducted and recorded, both positive and negative findings. Areas that may be injected include arms, legs, feet, neck, breast, groin, and even the penis. All active abusers and those for whom there are abuse questions should have a drug screen performed for all potential drugs of abuse, including opioids, cocaine, barbiturates, and amphetamines.

The drugs that the patient is using are an integral component to understanding and predicting potential hazards that they may encounter. A heroin addict may begin to demonstrate signs of withdrawal 12 hours or earlier from the last dose. Cocaine, on the other hand, does not have a clear withdrawal syndrome and it may be difficult to detect or define, occurring hours to days after the last use. Unlike heroin and cocaine, drugs affecting the CNS (such as alcohol and benzodiazepines) are life threatening and require detoxification protocols.

Methadone therapy is frequently utilized in the opioid (heroin)-abusing patient in an attempt to decrease drug craving. Although methadone is a powerful opioid, those receiving maintenance will typically require more opioids during painful episodes. These individuals can have substantial opioid tolerance, therefore one should anticipate a greater opioid requirement than for a nonopioid abuser.

A technique that may be utilized to obtain analgesia for the individual on methadone maintenance is to continue the current daily dose of methadone but divide the dose into 6- to 8-hour intervals. This will decrease the risk of sedation because doses can be held if needed, then titrate short-acting opioids to comfort the patient. Patient-controlled analgesic devices can be utilized. When a steady state of analgesia is obtained, the opioid then can be converted easily to methadone. Methadone should be dosed every 6 to 8 hours when it is being utilized for pain control.

Individuals with a history of substance abuse have a high incidence of major psychiatric disorders, with some estimates higher than 50%.[31] These are primarily depression and affective disorders, but also include antisocial behaviors and borderline personalities. The overall treatment of the patient with HIV and a history of substance abuse requires a caring, consistent, patient, nonjudgmental approach. Treatment techniques vary, but all require assessment and evaluation of drug use, potential drug interactions, and withdrawal while initiating analgesic therapy. A contract should define activities that will not be tolerated, such as drug hoarding or diversion, and prescription forgery or theft. Limits need to be incorporated into any treatment plan, as does ensuring that the patient has a clear understanding of potential repercussions. These individuals will frequently require the help of social workers to assist in providing counseling, chaplains, support groups, and public assistance.

References

1. O'Neil WM, Sherrard JS. Pain in human immunodeficiency virus disease: a review. *Pain.* 1993;54:3–14.
2. Breitbart W. Pain management and psychosocial issue in HIV and AIDS. *Am J of Hospice-Paliative Care,* 1996;13(1):20–29.
3. Breitbart W, McDonald MV, Rosenfeld B, et al. Pain in ambulatory AIDS patients. I: pain characteristics and medical correlates. *Pain.* 1996;68:315–321.
4. Lebovits AH, Lefkowitz M, McCarthy D, Simon R, Wilpon H, Jung R, Fried E. The prevalence and management of pain in patients with AIDS: a review of 134 cases. *Clin J. Pain.* 1989;5(3):245–248.
5. Lefkowitz M, Breitbart W. Chronic pain and AIDS. *Innovations in Pain Medicine.* 1989;36:2–3.
6. Schofferman I. Pain: Diagnosis and management in the palliative care of AIDS. *J Palliat Care.* 1988;4:46–49.
7. Singer E, Zorilla C, Fahy-Chandon B, Chi S, Syndulko K, Tourtellotte W. Painful symptoms reported by ambulatory HIV-infected men in a longitudinal study. *Pain.* 1993;54:15–19.
8. Hewitt DJ, McDonald M, Portenoy RK, Rosenfeld B, Passik S, Breitbart W. Pain syndromes and etiologies in ambulatory AIDS patients. *Pain.* 1997;70:117–123.

9. Rosenfeld B, Breitbart W, McDonald MV, Passik SD, Thaler H, Portenoy RK. Pain in ambulatory AIDS patients. II: Impact of pain on psychological functioning and quality of life. *Pain.* 1996; 68:323–328.
10. McCormack JP, Li R, Zarowny D, Singer J. Inadequate treatment of pain in ambulatory HIV patients. *Clin J Pain.* 1993;9:279–283.
11. Brietbart W, Rosenfeld BD, Passik SD, McDonald MV, Thaler H, Portenoy RK. The undertreatment of pain in ambulatory AIDS patients. *Pain.* 1996;65: 243–249.
12. National Institute of Nursing Research: Priority Expert Panel on Symptom Management. 6. Symptom management: Acute Pain. : Bethesda MD, National Institutes of Health, U.S. Public Health Service, U.S. Department of Health & Human Services, NIH Pub. No. 94-2421;1994.
13. International Association for the Study of Pain Subcommittee on Taxonomy. Pain terms: a list with definitions and usage. *Pain.* 1997;6:249–252.
14. American Pain Society. *Principles of Analgesic Use in the Treatment of Acute Pain and Cancer Pain.* 3rd ed. Skokie, IL: American Pain Society; 1992.
15. McCaffery M. Nursing practice theories related to cognition, bodily pain and man-environment interactions. Los Angeles: University of California at Los Angeles Student Store; 1998.
16. Larue L, Brasseur L, Musseault P, Demeulemeester R, Bonifassi L, Berg G. Pain and symptoms in HIV disease: a national survey of France. *J Palliat Care.* 1994;10:95. Abstract.
17. Jacox A, Carr DB, Payne R, et al. *Management of Cancer Pain. Clinical Practice Guideline Number 9.* Rockville, MD: Agency for Health Care Policy and Research, US Department of Health and Human Services, Public Health Service; 1994. AHCPR publication no. 94-5-0592.
18. World Health Organization (WHO) Expert Committee. Cancer pain relief and palliative care: Report of a WHO expert committee. Technical Report Series No. 804. Geneva, Switzerland: WHO:1990.
19. Carr D, Addison R, eds. *Pain in HIV/AIDS: La douleur du SIDA/HIV.* Washington, DC: France-USA Pain Association; 1994.
20. Melzack R, Wall P. Pain mechanisms: A new theory. *Science.* 1965;150:971–979.
21. McGuire DB, Yarbro CH, Ferrell R. *Cancer Pain Management.* 2nd ed. Boston: Jones & Bartlett; 1995.
22. Melzack R, Wall P. *The Challenge of Pain.* London: Penguin Books; 1988.
23. Payne R. Anatomy, physiology and neuropharmacy of cancer pain. *Medical Clinics of North America* 1987;71(2):253–267.
24. Breitbart, Lebovits, Smith, Maignau, Lefkowitz. 1994.
25. Koppel B. Neurologic syndromes due to HIV infection. *Hosp Physician.* 1992; 12–24.
26. Coyle N, Adelhart J, Foley K, Portenoy, R. Character of terminal illness in the

advanced cancer patient: Pain and other symptoms during the last four weeks of life. Journal of Pain and Symptom Management 1995; 5(2):83–93.
27. Breitbart W. Pain in AIDS: bridging the gap between pain experts and *aids* specialists. *APS Bull.* 1995;5(4):1–4.
28. Johnson JE, Fieler VK, Jones LS, Wiasowica GS, Mitchell ML. *Self-Regulation Theory: Applying Theory to Your Practice.* Pittsburgh: Oncology Nursing Press; 1997.
29. Centers for Disease Control. *HIV Surveillance.* Atlanta: US Department of Health and Human Services; July 1993.
30. Hoyt M. Management of pain in persons with AIDS. *HIV Digest.* 1995;4(3):1–3.
31. Ross H, Glaser F, Germanson T. The prevalence of psychiatric disorders in patients with alcohol and other drug problems. *Arch Gen Psych.* 1988;45: 1023–1031.

CHAPTER 20

Night Sweats, Fever, Chills, and Shivering

Barbara Holtzclaw Ph.D. RN, FAAN

Chapter Preview

- Definition
- Biologic and Behavioral Basis
- Etiologies Related to HIV and Its Medical Treatment
- Presentation and Assessment
- Related Medical Management
- Interventions
- Information for the Patient

Definition

Fever is one of the most common of the broad and complex responses associated with HIV infection, AIDS, and the myriad of OIs that accompany these conditions. While some symptoms of fever are antigen specific, many are nonspecific host mechanisms that trigger a cascade of predictable sequelae. In persons with healthy immune systems, fever includes beneficial host responses that help combat infection. Rising body temperature and malaise are temporary and tolerable conditions that make the body less habitable to invading organisms. However, derangement of T-cell and host immune functions in HIV infection allow most distressful symptoms to persist, while failing to provide some of fever's most important benefits. Fever and inflammatory responses are activated through alternative complement pathways, but the full aggregate of defense mechanisms is no longer intact. Medical management of fever in patients with AIDS is aimed at the infectious agent, with pharmacological therapy chosen for its specificity. Nursing care, however, is directed toward predictable symptoms of fever, regardless of infectious agent. Chills, rigors, and febrile shivering characterize the onset of fever. In the case of nursing action, it is the *host response specificity* that guides the appropriate action. Understanding the underlying dynamics of fever helps caregivers understand the basis for well-justified nursing actions, even though the origin of the fever may never be known.

Even though fever is a common phenomenon to most nurses, there tends to be confusion in terms. *Fever* is defined as abnormally high body temperature that occurs as a host response to *pyrogens*. A synonym for fever is *pyrexia*, and *hyperpyrexia* refers to high fever.[1] Of importance to nursing care in fever is the understanding that pyrogens cause the hypothalamus to readjust to a higher range, but *thermoregulatory function remains intact*. Efforts to cool the body lead to distressful chilling and are counterproductive to reducing body heat. This characteristic of fever differentiates it from *hyperthermia*, a condition when high temperatures result from dysfunctional thermoregulatory functions. The inability to lose heat effectively allows the temperature to rise to lethal levels. Unlike fever, hyperthermia requires active cooling interventions to prevent irreversible brain damage.

Biologic and Behavioral Basis

The febrile response depends on several integrated physiological processes, with biochemical, neurological, and metabolic activities playing major roles. The capacity to "mount" a fever depends on (1) the ability of phagocytic cells to migrate and become activated to release fever mediators, (2) the function of the hypothalamic thermoregulatory center to activate warming responses, and (3) the ability of the vasomotor and musculoskeletal system to conserve heat by vasoconstriction and generate heat by shivering.

Fever Mediators

Fever-producing pyrogens include infectious organisms and noninfectious substances such as toxic drugs, chemical compounds, blood products, neoplastic cells, and foreign bodies. *Exogenous pyrogens* do not act directly, but trigger the release of fever mediators or *endogenous pyrogen* (EP) from cells within the body. Thus, a chain of events begins when a pyrogen enters a person's system and sends off numerous endogenous blood-borne biochemical messengers. Among these messengers are a class of closely related molecules called *cytokines*, produced by cells of the immune system. The cytokines IL-1, TNF-α, IFN-α2, IL-6, transforming growth factor, and macrophage inflammatory protein 1 are known to function as EP.[1–3] EP is released from host monocytes and macrophages, and mediates fever by increasing synthesis of hypothalamic prostaglandins of the E group (PGE). Although they recruit a variety of host defenses that are still not fully understood, their EP activity is clearly evident. EP acts on the thermostatic centers of the hypothalamus to readjust the acceptable range of body temperature to a higher level. In HIV infection, interactions between IL-1, IL-6, and TNF-α heighten febrile responses, yet immunostimulatory effects are blocked.[4] The fact that numerous exogenously introduced and endogenously produced substances are capable of inducing fever helps to explain why the origin of fever is often difficult to determine. The *fever of unknown origin* (FUO) or fever of undetermined cause usually refers to a febrile illness, of at least a 3-week duration, during which the body temperature has risen to 38.2°C or higher. In immunosuppressed populations it is sometimes necessary to treat such fevers empirically, rather than waiting for absolute confirmation of the etiology.

Hypothalamic Thermoregulatory Effects

The prevailing model for fever and thermoregulation is that of a negative feedback loop, where hypothalamic sensors and activators keep central temperatures fairly constant within a narrow range called the *set point* (approximately 36.2 to 37.8°C). Integrated feedback impulses from internal and external sensory thermoreceptors activate heat loss or heat conservation mechanisms. Preoptic regions of the hypothalamus act as a thermostat, integrating sensory information from the viscera, muscle, and skin receptors with that from the brain. Cooling of skin receptors can override stimuli from other sites, a factor particularly amenable to nursing intervention.

Vasomotor and Musculoskeletal Thermoregulatory Responses

Fever's dynamic course follows three distinct phases (Figure 20.1) directly linked to EP levels: *chill*, with its rapid production of heat; *plateau*, with a steady core temperature maintained at a higher than usual level; and *defervescence*, which is also called *crisis*, *flush*, or the *break* in fever. In

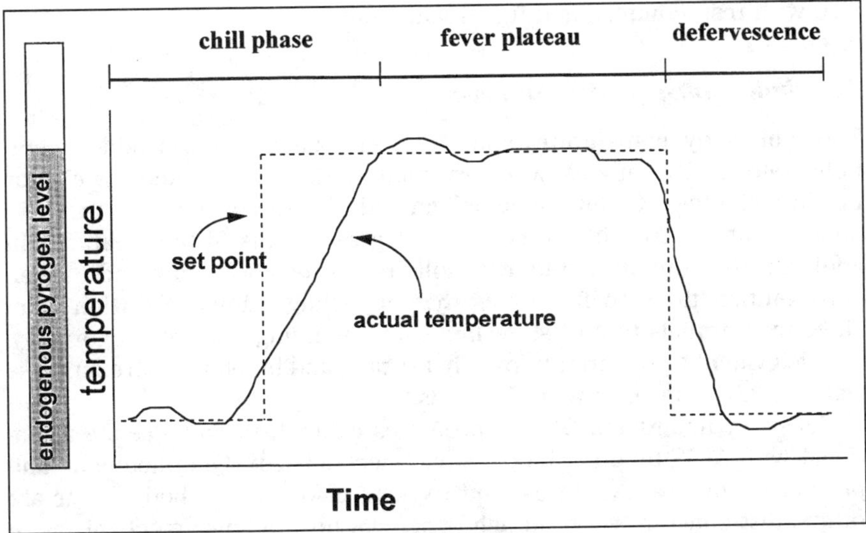

Figure 20.1 Phases of the Febrile Episode During Which Set Point Changes Are Influenced by Levels of Circulating Endogenous Pyrogen

phase 1 the pyrogen drives up the set point to a higher range, which causes the person's existing body temperature to be sensed as below the acceptable range. This triggers the chill phase of fever. Shivering and vasoconstriction are activated to generate and conserve heat to raise internal temperatures to the new set point. Shaking chills, or *rigors*, may occur while temperatures rise to febrile levels. Environmental temperatures, which are comfortable during normal conditions, feel bitterly cold during fever. In phase 2, when the body has warmed to the new set point range, chills stop and a leveling off of body temperature occurs. Subjective feelings of chill decline. In the third phase, body temperature may rise above the set point, or levels of EP decline, causing the fever to break. Subjective feelings of extreme warmth are accompanied by physiological cooling mechanisms of sweating and vasodilation. The shivering *threshold* is lower during fever, so that even beyond the chill phase, drafts or exposure to cooling stimuli is more likely to cause shivering.[5,6] Vasoconstriction, shaking chills, vasodilation, and diaphoresis are reminders that thermoregulatory mechanisms are fully functional, but operating at a higher than normal range. Subjectively, cytokines tend to promote myalgia, general malaise, irritability, and loss of appetite. These symptoms are distressful and interfere with rest, comfort, and functional ability.

Metabolic Consequences of Fever

The rising body temperature expends calories and imposes an added metabolic burden on patients who are anemic, dehydrated, and have poor nutritional intake. Cellular metabolism and oxygen consumption increase approximately 10% with every added degree Celsius of temperature.[1] In addition, shivering during febrile chills raises metabolic rate and oxygen consumption three to five times that of resting values.[7] Exertion from shivering parallels that of shoveling snow or riding a bicycle vigorously. This is evident as respiratory rate, heart rate, and blood pressure increase significantly to meet oxygen demands.[8]

Sepsis or underlying OI also promotes catabolism and wasting in patients with AIDS by other biochemical mechanisms. Hypermetabolic and proteolytic processes that expend oxygen, calories, and body water are of greatest concern. Even though beneficial host defense mechanisms of fever-producing cytokines are missing in patients with AIDS, these same biochemicals hasten disease progression in AIDS by inducing anorexia, wasting, and dehydration.[4,9] Fever has previously been underestimated as a major contributor to wasting and weight loss in AIDS. Recent studies of persons with HIV infection showed that current methods for calculating energy expenditure fail to estimate metabolic need fully.[10] Fever and sepsis are identified stress factors that can make calculations of metabolic expenditure more accurate.

Etiologies Related to HIV Infection and Its Medical Treatment

Fever as General Clinical Manifestation of Primary HIV Infection

Fever occurs as a clinical feature and consistent sign of primary HIV-1 infection in approximately 97% of adult cases.[11] Febrile "flulike" symptoms typically occur from 2 to 4 weeks after exposure, with variations ranging from 6 days to 6 weeks.[12] These findings have become known as HIV-infected persons are identified earlier in their course of disease. The actual incidence of fever in early HIV infection may be even higher, as those who have remained unaware of their seropositive status for years may have difficulty recalling an acute clinical illness near time of infection. Fever, with or without night sweats, accompanies and may contribute to several clinical features of primary HIV infection, including myalgia, anorexia, dehydration, and fatigue. Fever accompanies HIV-1 infection, OIs, and several common, noninfectious processes such as dehydration from diaphoresis or diarrhea.[13]

Immunologic Derangements Contributing to Febrile Symptoms in AIDS

The susceptibility of the HIV-infected person to OI makes the interpretation of fever difficult. Not only are a wide gamut of infections more possible, derangement in immunologic responses often causes a heightened febrile response in those with HIV infection. Fever in a severely immunosuppressed patient with AIDS reflects a derangement of part, but not all, of the immune system. Antigens that would normally stimulate host responses (ILs and TNF) are now thought to have a role in the immunopathogenesis of HIV infection.[4,14] The incidence of OIs in AIDS differs from that found in the immunosuppressed cancer patient. Infections often involve latent and previously controlled organisms, such as herpes virus, varicella zoster virus, or wild and aberrant forms of normally low-virulence pathogens that overwhelm the host.[14–17] For example, folliculitis and seborrheic dermatitis, which are mildly symptomatic in those with healthy immune systems, can cause severe chills, fever, and night sweats in HIV-infected persons.

Interactions among hormones and cytokines are particularly important to the febrile response. Contrary to earlier findings, IL-1 production is higher in persons with AIDS than in control subjects.[4,15] However, it may lack its immunostimulatory properties because of a specific inhibiting substance common to HIV infection. Low assay levels of IL-1 are thought to result from inhibitor-masked IL-1 activity, which may also block IL-1-dependent maturation of T lymphocytes. Fever and catabolism occur because the inhibitor does not alter the TNF-stimulating and catabolic effects of IL-1. IL-1 further contributes to the malnutrition of fever-induced catabolism in AIDS by decreasing albumin transcription, releasing amino acids from muscle, promoting anorexia, and stimulating adrenocorticotropic hormone (ACTH) release.[14]

Noninfectious Causes of Fever in HIV/AIDS

It is important to recognize, when considering fever, that febrile episodes may be noninfectious in origin. Any substance recognized as "foreign" by the body can elicit host-defense responses from the immune system. Several drugs specific to AIDS treatment have been associated with fever. These include trimethoprim-sulfamethoxazole (Septra), atovaquone, amphotericin B, ddI, amoxicillin-clavulanic acid, dapsone, ceftazidime, and ganciclovir. Some drugs, such as amphotericin B are inherently pyrogenic. Others may cause diarrhea and may cause fever indirectly by dehydration. Platelets and other blood products may also stimulate a febrile response, which most often represents an antigenic rather than an infectious process.

Water Loss as a Factor in Fever

While sweating provides a source for evaporative heat loss during fever, it contributes to total-body water loss. Water loss directly affects the hypothalamic set point range and indirectly reduces the ability to redistribute blood to skin to dissipate body heat. Fever is estimated to increase insensible airway and nonsweating water loss 10% for each 0.5°C temperature increase.[18] *Dehydration* (hypertonic dehydration) is known to induce fever and is common when water is lost through diarrhea. *Desiccation* (isotonic dehydration) occurs when both water and sodium are lost in profuse sweating. Cytokine-induced cellular destruction and related fluid loss contribute to only part of the energy and water expenditure in fever. Febrile shivering exerts aerobic muscle contractions, respiratory effort increases to provide oxygen and exchange heat, and sweating provides a source for evaporative heat loss. Oxygen expenditure alone is sufficient reason to control febrile chills, but loss of airway and insensible moisture make water restoration a priority.

Presentation and Assessment

Instruments for Monitoring Body Temperature

Mercury-and-glass thermometers are rapidly being replaced for general use because they are difficult to read, break easily, and the mercury is toxic. Studies show they are no more reliable than calibrated electronic thermometers. In addition, they vary in shelf life and accuracy, and they take longer in general to register.[19] Electronic thermometers have become popular alternatives and are used in hospitals, clinics, and homes to measure temperature. They vary by brand, type, and accuracy. Many clinical units can be calibrated, with accuracy guaranteed and maintained by the manufacturer. Rapid digital readout makes readings less ambiguous and frequent measurement easier. Plastic probes also resist breakage when dropped or during reflex contraction of jaws. Small hand-held, battery-powered digital thermometers are desirable for home use, as they are easier for patients and family members to read and interpret. They are about the same size and cost, as a reliable mercury-in-glass thermometer.

Tympanic membrane (TM) infrared reflectance thermometers are relatively new instruments for measuring temperature. They vary widely in accuracy and reliability, and are practically impossible for someone to use to measure their own temperature. For clinical use, however, there are accurate, easily operated units that can provide nonintrusive, rapid reading of TM temperature from the auditory canal opening in less than 10 seconds.[19] Nurses should be aware of some confusing aspects to TM measurements. Several brands give "offsets" to estimate oral, rectal, or core temperatures, and these vary from brand to brand. It is important to clarify which estimate of body temperature is being charted or reported to avoid unnecessary or inappropriate interventions arising from erroneous information. Use of TM thermometry also requires "otoscopic" training of staff to ensure accurate measurement, otherwise readings can vary with the angle in which probe is pointed. Units are expensive, and the most accurate costs more. Unfortunately, cheaper home units are most likely to appeal to patients and are often unreliable.

Diagnostic Tests in Fever

Blood cultures are sometimes collected at onset or peak of temperature spikes, which coincides with prevalence of organisms. Absolute neutrophil counts may have less diagnostic value in HIV-related fever than in other immunosuppressed states because neutropenia is common in advanced HIV disease, with or without myelosuppressive drug exposure, infections, or neoplasms. A less serious risk of bacterial infection is associated with low neutrophil counts in HIV-infected patients, than in cancer patients with therapy-induced neutropenia. Clusters of other supporting laboratory and radiological tests (e.g., fluoroscopy, ultrasound, radiography, sedimentation rates, and tumor antigens) help rule out noninfectious fevers (e.g., lymphomas, tumors, and dehydration). As in most laboratory and diagnostic tests used for evaluation and staging of HIV disease, the clinical presentation of the patient remains the most powerful tool. While CD4+ cell count, viral load, hematocrit, albumin, and pathological signs make interpretation of fever more accurate, the combined picture of fever, night sweats, and general health can better stage the progress of HIV disease.

Patient Assessment in Febrile Illness

Fever, while common in advanced HIV infection, is rarely the result of the HIV infection alone. Nose, throat, respiratory, and urinary tract infections; abscesses; gingivitis; gastroenteritis; drug reactions; and lymphoma are among the most prevalent causes. Fever, as a host response, is sometimes the only indicator of systemic infection in the severely immunocompromised person. However, deficiency of the patient's underlying immune system may interfere with beneficial cell-mediated effects of the febrile response.

Patterns of Fever

Febrile temperature variations provide few cues for diagnosis in persons with AIDS. In cases of noninfectious pyrogens, such as drugs or blood products, the onset of fever may help to isolate the causative agent. However, with infectious organisms fever patterns more often reflect the levels of specific cytokines rather than the type of infection.[14] The tendency for fevers to spike and fall at different times of the day represents the rise and decline in circulating EP. In *intermittent* fever patterns, spikes of fever are interspersed with normal levels. In *remittent* fever patterns, spikes and falls in temperatures occur, but levels do not fall to euthermic levels. Remittent fever is common in viral infections. Typically the fever spike progresses rapidly, with temperatures changing as quickly as 1°C/hour. The more rapid the rise, the more profound the feelings of chill, the vasoconstriction, and the shivering activity that preceded it. Collection of specimens for blood culture are timed to coincide with the onset or peak of temperature spikes, a time often coinciding with a prevalence of organisms. In septicemia or bacteremia, a cascade of fever-producing cellular and humoral mediators are activated by septic inflammatory response.[15] The intensity of the febrile reaction reflects both the potency of the antigen and the sensitivity of the host response. Fevers in persons with HIV infection tend to be "hectic" in nature, rising and falling abruptly and not conforming to fever patterns seen in HIV-seronegative persons. In hospital units where temperatures are only measured once per shift, febrile spikes in temperature may be missed.[20] Therefore, there is a need to monitor rate and pattern of temperature at least every 4 hours. If temperature is elevated 1°C above the last reading, wait 15 minutes and take it again to determine if it is "on the rise." Hectic fevers often rise more than 1°C within an hour.

Significance of Night Sweats

Patient complaints of disrupted sleep from awakening drenched in sweat several times per night should be evaluated for fever. The symptom of fever or night sweats alone should not be used as an indication or prognostic sign of HIV infection or AIDS. The term *night sweats* is rather imprecise in meaning because it generally refers to heavy sweating during sleep. It has little prognostic or diagnostic meaning *as a single sign* because healthy persons, those with cardiovascular, psychogenic, or hormonal alterations, and those with fever may all manifest sweating during sleep. However, fever and drenching night sweats often complicate late-stage AIDS and neoplastic diseases such as lymphoma, and present as a *cluster* of nonspecific indicators called *B symptoms* (weight loss, fever, and night sweats). B symptoms may indicate a general decline rather than a specific diagnostic predictor.

Related Medical Management

Medical management of fever in the patient with AIDS is concerned with control of the underlying infection, pathology, or fluid imbalance responsible. Hyperpyrexia is nearly always related to OI or a condition other than HIV. Drugs are aimed primarily at combating OIs with organism-specific antibiotic or antifungal therapy. When no clear etiology of fever can be found, noninfectious causes, drug toxicity, or adrenal insufficiency are considered. Supportive medical and pharmacological management include fluid replacement and antipyretics. Acetaminophen is often the antipyretic drug of choice because aspirin and potent prostaglandin inhibitors adversely affect clotting factors, platelets, and gastric mucosal integrity. These side effects are particularly problematic for patients who are anemic or who have mucosal irritation. Acetaminophen was initially implicated as increasing zidovudine (AZT) toxicity, but has been shown to be safe at current levels of AZT administration.[21] Acetaminophen has mild analgesic effects to relieve the discomfort of fever and was not found effective in reducing febrile shivering in immunosuppressed persons with cancer.

Physicians are beginning to recognize that efforts to cool the patient aggressively are seldom justified unless thermoregulatory mechanisms are impaired. Fevers are usually self-limiting, unless there is severe neurological damage impairing sweating and vasodilation. Use of conductive cooling blankets is usually reserved for treating high temperatures above 40°C that are unresponsive to antipyretic drugs, to prevent irreversible brain damage. Steep gradients between circulating fluid and body surface temperature rapidly overwhelm the patient's heat defenses and lower body temperature. Temperatures fall quickly to hypothermic levels unless heat loss is carefully controlled.

Compensatory shivering and vasoconstriction are usually severe enough to require meperidine as a suppressant. The tendency toward hypothermia adds another hazard, as the patient can become poikilothermic and subject to uncontrolled "drift."[22]

Interventions

Nursing fever management is aimed at symptomatology, regardless of etiology. The goals are to (1) maintain body temperature within a safe range, (2) maintain and restore fluid balance, (3) conserve energy and avoid fatigue, and (4) promote thermal comfort during fever. Each patient care unit needs clear standards of care for febrile symptom management because the ubiquitous nature of fever tends to make nurses and caregivers complacent toward treating its symptoms. Most nurses believe they know what to do, yet most care is based on tradition or "common sense." While fever progress is monitored closely and pharmaceutical prescriptions are followed strictly, nursing activities have been directed toward cooling the patient. This approach has seldom been well justified. Nursing textbooks frequently gloss over specific interventions for fever, stating simply to use "cooling measures." Unfortunately, the use of cooling methods such as sponge baths or fans fails to consider the thermoregulatory dynamics involved and elicits responses that are contrary to the therapeutic goal. Effects of environmental temperature, patient hydration, and physical activity on febrile responses are seldom considered.

Scientifically Based Intervention

Effective fever management is scientifically based on principles of thermoregulation. Knowledge about altered hypothalamic thermoregulatory set points in fever allows the nurse to make predictions about the patient's thermal responses to internal and external stimuli. Knowledge about the patient's physiological status, and ability to compensate and tolerate sequelae enables the nurse to plan actions that enhance, replace, suppress, or avoid thermal responses. Ability to assess nursing care outcomes critically provides the nurse a test of the efficacy of the interventions. Basic to intervention is the knowledge that fever is a *host response* and not an illness in itself. Therefore, reducing the body temperature will not relieve the underlying cause of fever. Mildly elevated temperature is less harmful than the underlying infections or disorder. Body temperatures around 39°C have been found to optimize host defenses and promote conditions less favorable to invading organisms. Two fever-related factors—fluid loss and febrile shivering—are associated with harmful effects. Both of these factors are amenable to nursing care. As long as the EP is elevated, thermoregulatory mechanisms will act to maintain temperature at higher levels. For this reason, *efforts to cool the febrile patient should be avoided,* as they tend to stimulate further warming responses and to drive up body temperatures.

Therapeutic Goals

Clarifying the therapeutic goal is essential before appropriate nursing actions can be selected. In patients for whom infection is confirmed or obvious, the febrile curve is sometimes needed to follow effectiveness of antimicrobial therapy. In this case, interventions are aimed at treating discomfort of fever, but not to bring down the temperature artificially. In late-stage AIDS, palliation and quality of life are as important a therapeutic goal as detecting the infectious or neoplastic disease. Around-the-clock antipyretics and analgesics are appropriate. Although therapeutic goals for medical management of fever may seem straightforward concerning use of antipyretics and antibiotics, supportive nursing actions are often complex. Among these, requiring knowledge beyond rote drug administration, are (1) choice and timing of drug administration, (2) adjustment of environment and protective covering to avoid chills and shivering while enabling heat loss, and (3) efforts to rehydrate and restore calories to the febrile patient. In cases when the patient's medical treatment may be the cause of fever, such as in cases of "drug fever" or blood administration, nursing care is aimed at reducing febrile shivering, maintaining fluid and energy sources, and restoring comfort during the inevitable fever.[8]

Fever tends to be self-limiting, with some biochemicals acting to limit and others acting to elicit host responses.[1] When thermoregulatory mechanisms are intact, cooling measures should be avoided during fever. However, in cases when body systems are declining, dehydration and debilitation increase risk of hyperthermia. Then the therapeutic goal may shift to preventing irreversible denaturation of cell protein and brain damage, which can occur when temperatures exceed 40°C. *Such cases are uncommon,* but when a person becomes hyperthermic and temperatures continue to climb above 40°C, cooling measures are warranted to prevent irreparable neurological damage.

Shivering Prevention

The threshold for shivering is strongly influenced by skin temperature and skin-to-core gradients. During fever, less heat loss is required to elicit shivering and vasoconstriction.[5,6] Sudden inadvertent exposure to drafts or cool bed linen may trigger an episode of chills. Failure to replace sweat-drenched bed clothing after a diaphoretic episode promotes rapid evaporative heat loss that can initiate a chill. Likewise, undressing the damp patient in a neutral or cool room causes chilling. Vigorous shivering, in turn, raises temperature higher. Protecting the patient from chills is an important measure in maintaining a safe body temperature, preventing the fatigue of shivering, and promoting thermal comfort. The febrile patient, in any stage, will be highly sensitive to any cooling activity, including drafts, bathing, or drinking cool liquid. Those in the chill phase will experience shaking chills, or rigors, and may have a subjective feeling of cold, even though they have high body temperatures. A protocol for shivering prevention during the chill phase appears in the next paragraph. Those in the plateau or defervescence phase will have subjective feelings of being overly warm, but are extremely sensitive to chilling if exposed or chilled by bathing and cooling. Nursing strategies for preventing chills and shivering during the plateau and defervescence phases of fever are listed below.

- Recognize that the shivering threshold is lower during fever, so mild heat loss promotes shivering.
- Avoid the chilling of evaporative heat loss by keeping the skin dry and covered.
- Change clothing when sweat soaked, but do so without fanning bed clothes or exposing skin.
- Avoid giving chilled or cold liquids to drink. Instead, prepare warm or room temperature liquids.
- Avoid bathing the skin *at all* during the chill phase. During the plateau or defervescence phases, use only very warm water, and use a towel to cover the area being washed to avoid convective drafts.

(continued)

- Have the patient change clothes under the covers if possible. Ambulatory patients should be shown how to remove underclothes under a robe or wrap to avoid being chilled.
- Keep bathrooms warm. Fixtures such as toilet seats are cold and can be protected by rolled towels.
- Provide slippers when ambulating on cold tile floors.

The following treatment for shivering prevention during febrile chills involves the use of warmth, insulation, and protection from sensed heat loss throughout the febrile period, while allowing heat excesses to be lost from areas, such as the chest, that do not trigger warming responses. Insulative wraps described here are easily adapted to clinical settings.[23] In home care, insulative clothing, extra socks, arm wraps, and shawls can be used to accomplish these goals. If conductive cooling blankets are warranted to reduce harmfully high temperatures, these extremity wraps diminish distress and shivering. They are applied *before* applying the cooling blanket:

1. Apply a blood pressure cuff and any monitoring equipment involving the extremities prior to beginning wrapping procedures.
2. Place three bath towels lengthwise under each arm. Bring up the lateral edges of the towels to form a seam. Secure with plastic clips (plastic nose clips like those used by respiratory therapy work well; even clothespins can be used) or wide tape along the seam, allowing IV lines, monitor leads, and blood pressure tubing to exit along the seam. Roll up excess toweling at the fingertips to form a "mitten." Secure with tape.
3. Place three bath towels lengthwise under each leg. Bring up the lateral edges of towels to form a seam. Secure with plastic clips or tape along the seam, allowing monitor leads to exit along the seam. Roll up excess toweling at toes to form a "boot." Secure with tape.
4. Do not allow towels to remain damp. If sweating is excessive or towels become damp, replace quickly with warmed towels causing as little exposure or air movement as possible.

Protecting Exposed Thermosensitive Areas

Sensitive heat-loss receptors are not uniformly distributed over the skin. Specific regions of skin—on the arms, hands, feet, and face—are more dominant in afferent influence, whereas the trunk is less sensitive.[6] Warmed blankets, cloth toweling, and protective clothing during ambulation can help prevent chills and shivering during the chill phase of fever. Warm rooms, used with febrile patients, have helped to control chills and shivering without causing increases in body temperature.[24] If conductive cooling blankets are warranted to reduce harmfully high temperatures, insulation of hands and feet prevent distress and shivering.[23,25] If aggressive cooling measures are required, such as conductive cooling blankets, extremity wraps are applied *before* applying the cooling blanket. Close monitoring of the patient is required during artificial cooling to avoid rapid descent of temperature to hypothermic levels.

Aggressive Oral Fluid Replacement

Replacement of fluid deficit helps to resensitize the hypothalamic set point while increasing the circulating blood volume. This improves perfusion of superficial tissues and enables heat to be lost more easily. Aggressive fluid replacement from oral routes must be balanced with other factors affecting the patient's appetite, oral mucosa, and sensitivity to chilling.

Sweating may have depleted sodium as well as water. Balanced electrolytes in some oral replacements, along with dietary salt, may appeal to the patient's taste. If the patient is nauseated or vomiting, forcing oral fluids may be counterproductive. Vomiting ingested fluids nearly always results in more being lost than was originally swallowed. Acidic foods or liquids may be painful or irritating to patients with mouth lesions. Jello and bland fruit juices at room temperature may be palatable to these patients. While iced foods may be more palatable when there are mouth ulcers, ingestion of cold liquids may trigger chills. Sucking or licking frozen liquids allows a more gradual intake without chilling the patient. With pharyngitis or difficulty swallowing, jelled or semisolid products may be easier to swallow than liquids.

Information for the Patient

For the patient with AIDS fever is a familiar yet baffling symptom. Fever is something experienced by nearly everyone at some time in their life, yet with HIV it can occur without warning or explanation. Explain to your patients that HIV makes fever more likely when they develop an infection.

A checklist of what to do and who to call is often helpful to send home with the patient and caregivers. An example of a checklist follows.

It is a good idea to ask your doctor or clinic nurse what they recommend if you begin to run a fever at home. Usually they will tell you to take aspirin 650 mg *or* acetaminophen (Tylenol) 650 mg every 4 hours. If there are any reasons why you should take Tylenol *instead* of aspirin, they will also tell you. Drink plenty of fluids (at least 2 or 3 quarts per day). Take your temperature if you develop any symptoms of feeling sick. If your temperature is more than 99°F, take it again in 3 to 4 hours. New onset of a fever with temperatures above 101°F should be reported to your doctor within 24 hours.

1. Call your doctor or clinic if you develop a *new* fever of more than 101°F.
2. When you call about your fever, give the following information to the receptionist or nurse:
   - If your records are not at that clinic, provide your last T-helper cell count.
   - Do you have any symptoms affecting your breathing such as shortness of breath, cough, stuffy nose, or congestion?
   - Do you have any symptoms or pain affecting your swallowing, sinuses, or throat?
   - Are there any places that have broken out? Or rashes, swelling, streaking, drainage, blisters, or hot areas on your skin?
   - Do you have any abdominal pain, pain under your breast bone, nausea, vomiting, or painful bowel movements?
   - Are you having any "cobwebs" or "curtains" blocking your vision, pain in your eyes, double vision, or pain and redness of the eyes?
   - Are you having increased headaches, problems with staying alert, numbness, or unusual sensations in feeling?

Simple explanations are best to help the patient look for associated signs and symptoms. In many clinics, algorithms for emergent, urgent, and nonurgent referral of patient symptoms are prioritized, with levels of immunocompetence playing an important factor.[26] Patients with CD4 counts of >500 cells/mm^3 may be triaged for pulmonary symptoms and fever in much the same way as patients without HIV infection. When CD4 counts are between 200 and 500 cells/mm^3 there is immunosuppression, but OIs may be infrequent. In these patients, delay in specific medical treatment may not be life threatening, but requires consideration of other risk factors. Patients with fever who have CD4 counts of <50 cells/mm^3 often have more serious implications and need immediate or same-day referral. There are also large numbers of patients living at home with indwelling venous access devices and varying degrees of neutropenia for whom new-onset fever may signal serious infection.

Patients with AIDS may look at fever as an indicator of HIV progression and may fear that higher fevers show later stages of HIV disease. Emphasize that the height of the fever is not an indicator of severity of HIV infection. Inform patients that fever is a symptom rather than an illness, and it can reflect a large number of infections or conditions. Engage patients in participating in their own care by teaching self-monitoring of temperature. This includes how to use and read the thermometer correctly. Have the patient write down normal temperature (for self) as well as febrile readings for later reference. Encourage the use of a "fever diary" for a home record of temperatures during health and illness.

References

1. Kluger MJ. Fever: role of pyrogens and cryogens. *Physiol Rev.* 1991;71:93–127.
2. Dascombe MJ. The pharmacology of fever. *Prog Neurobiol.* 1985;25:327–373.
3. Dinarello CA. Interleukin-1. *Rev Infect Dis.* 1984;6:51–95.
4. Catania A, Airaghi L, Manfredi MG, et al. Propiomelanocortin-derived peptides and cytokines: relations in patients with acquired immunodeficiency syndrome. *Clin Immunol Immunopathol.* 1993;66:73–79.
5. Strom G. Central nervous regulation of body temperature. In: Field J, Magoun HW, Hall VE, eds. *Neurophysiology.* Washington, DC: American Physiological Society; 1960:1173–1193.
6. Hellon RF. Neurophysiology of temperature regulation: problems and perspectives. *Fed Proc.* 1981;40:2804–2807.
7. Hemingway A. Shivering. *Physiol Rev.* 1963;43:397–422.
8. Holtzclaw BJ. Control of febrile shivering during amphotericin B therapy. *Oncol Nurs Forum.* 1990;17:521–524.
9. Hori T, Nakashima T, Take S, Kaizuka Y, Mori T, Katafuchi T. Immune cytokines and regulation of body temperature, food intake and cellular immunity. *Brain Res Bull.* 1991;27:309–311.
10. Anderson R, Grady C, Ropka M. A comparison of calculated energy require-

ments to measure resting energy expenditure in HIV-1-infected subjects. *J Assoc Nurs AIDS Care.* 1994;5:30–34.
11. Clark SJ, Saag M, Decker WD, et al. High titers of cytopathic virus in plasma of patients with symptomatic primary HIV-1 infection. *N Engl J Med.* 1991;324: 954–960.
12. Tindall B, Carr A, Cooper CA. Primary HIV infection: clinical, immunologic and serologic aspects. In: Sande MA, Volberding PA, eds. *The Medical Management of AIDS.* 4th ed. Philadelphia: WB Saunders; 1995:50–129.
13. Casey KC. Pathophysiology of HIV-1, clinical course and treatment. In: Flaskerud JH, Ungvarski PJ, eds. *HIV/AIDS: A Guide to Nursing Care.* 3rd ed. Philadelphia: WB Saunders; 1992:64–80.
14. Calderon E, Ramirez MA, Arrieta MI, Fernandez-Caldas E, Russell DW, Lockey RF. Nutritional disorders in HIV disease. *Prog Food Nutr Sci.* 1990;14:371–402.
15. Stroud M, Swindell B, Bernard GR. Cellular and humoral mediators of sepsis syndrome. *Crit Care Nurs Clin North Am.* 1990;2:151–160.
16. Halliburton P. Immunosuppression. In: Carrieri-Kohlman V, Lindsay AM, West CM, eds. *Pathophysiological Phenomena in Nursing.* Philadelphia: WB Saunders; 1993:420–442.
17. Krumholz H, Sande M, Lo B. Community-acquired bacteremia in patients with acquired immunodeficiency syndrome: clinical presentation, bacteriology, and outcome. *Am J Med.* 1989;86:776–779.
18. Goldberger E. *A Primer of Water, Electrolyte, and Acid Base Syndromes.* 7th ed. Philadelphia: Lea & Febiger; 1986:34.
19. Holtzclaw BJ. Monitoring body temperature. *AACN Clin Issues Crit Care Nurs.* 1993;4:44–55.
20. Taliaferro DH. Monitoring fever patterns and hydration in hospitalized PLWA. In: *Proceedings: 10th Annual Research Conference.* Miami Beach, FL: Southern Nursing Research Society; 1996:34.
21. Steffe EM, King JH, Inciardi JF, et al. The effect of acetaminophen on zidovudine metabolism in HIV-infected patients. *J Acquir Immune Defic Syndr.* 1990;3: 691–694.
22. Holtzclaw BJ. Thermal balance. In: Kinney MR, Packa D, Dunbar S, eds. *AACN's Clinical Reference for Critical Care Nursing.* 3rd ed. St. Louis: Mosby Year Book; 1993:365–378.
23. Holtzclaw BJ. Fevers, shivers get wrappings. *Reflections.* 1996;22(3):13.
24. Palmes ED, Park CR. The regulation of body temperature during fever. *Arch Environ Health.* 1965;11:749–759.
25. Holtzclaw BJ. Effects of extremity wraps to control drug induced shivering: a pilot study. *Nurs Res.* 1990;39(5):280–283.
26. Windle SL, Moore JS, Fitch NL. Giving telephone advice to people with HIV infection. *Nurse Week.* 1995;8(1):10–11.

UNIT THREE

HIV Special Treatment Considerations

CHAPTER **21**

Compliance: Challenges and Strategies

Edward V. Morse, PhD • Patricia M. Simon, MSW, PhD
JoLynn M. Pratt, MPH

Chapter Preview

- Medication Management Issues
- Mental Health Issues
- Sociocultural Issues
- Health Care Delivery System Issues

Supported in part by the following NIAID contracts: NO1-A1-45233, 1UO1A1388440, and 5UO1A132913-05.

HIV-infected individuals live with a chronic, ultimately fatal, contagious disease process that requires continual monitoring by health care providers (HCPs), sometimes extending over a decade. The HIV-infected patient thus presents a long-term management challenge to the health care team. For a patient's HIV treatment to be efficacious over time, it is essential that the nurse and other HCPs be knowledgeable of and sensitive to the multifaceted, ever-changing compliance challenges presented by patients infected with the virus. Among all the members of the health care team, it is the nurse who is most likely to have regular, repeated contact with the patient for the duration of the illness and thus it is the nurse who is in the best position to monitor patient compliance. The term *compliance* is used as an umbrella term, referring to the extent to which a patient follows prescribed prevention, treatment, or diagnostic regimens. This is sometimes also referred to as *adherence*. Although many compliance issues are generic and express themselves as patient management concerns across a wide diversity of health conditions, the stigma, chronicity, and fatality associated with HIV/AIDS brings with it special, and at times unique, compliance concerns.[1] To assist HCPs in preventing, identifying, and managing noncompliance, a brief overview of compliance dynamics is presented first. The remainder of the chapter is organized as a compliance management rapid reference guide that can be used by the clinician to identify compliance issues easily and provides strategies to address these issues.

The guiding premise of this chapter is that potential compliance management issues are best addressed proactively. All too often, issues initially ignored or set aside until the patient has settled into the HIV treatment regimen worsen rapidly and stimulate or exacerbate other latent concerns, such as social isolation, substance abuse, and lack of economic support. To best meet a patient's compliance-related needs, it is important that problems are anticipated and minimized prior to the patient starting HIV treatment. Essential background information needed to identify potential compliance issues can be gathered routinely as part of the initial assessment and, if available, the social workers' intake evaluation. Utilizing a standardized paper-and-pencil compliance screening instrument can be very helpful (Figure 21.1). Issues triggering potential noncompliance can be categorized as either (1) medication management, (2) mental health, (3) sociocultural issues, and (4) those issues associated with the health care delivery system. Frequently, issues are interrelated across categories.

COMPLIANCE RATING INSTRUMENT

SITE ______________ CRI SCORE ______

PATIENT ID# _ _ _ _ _ _ _ _ _ DATE __ __/__ __/__ __ INTERVIEWER ______ PATIENT AGE __ __

MARITAL STATUS: NM M SEP D ______ CDC STAGE ______

LEVEL OF EDUCATION ______ Date of Birth ______ SEX: M F

SCORE

☐ 1. With whom do you live? ___
*(1) Live alone (2) Roommate (3) Husband (4) Friend
(5) Lover/partner (6) Parents(s) (7) Other family *(8) Homeless
(9) Other (Specify) ______________

If the patient does not live alone, ask parts (a) and (b). If he/she __lives alone or is homeless__, skip to question #2 and score 1 point for each part in (a) and (b).

☐ (a) How long have you lived with this (these) person (people)? ___
*(1) Less than 3 months (2) 3 months to 1 year (3) 1 year +

(b) How much do you depend on this (these) person (people) for:

☐ Emotional support --------------------- *(1) Not at all (2) Somewhat (3) Very much ___

☐ Economic support ---------------------- *(1) Not at all (2) Somewhat (3) Very much ___

☐ Social support ------------------------ *(1) Not at all (2) Somewhat (3) Very much ___

☐ Help in handling day-to-day problems --- *(1) Not at all (2) Somewhat (3) Very much ___

☐ 2. How long have you lived at your current address: ___
*(1) Less than 3 months (2) 3 months to 1 year (3) 1 year +

☐ 3. Are you currently employed? *(1) No (2) Yes ___
(Specify occupation) ______________

☐ (a) If no, when were you last employed? ___
*(1) Have never been employed (2) Last employed over 1 year ago
(3) Last employed between 6 months & 1 year ago (4) Last employed less than 6 months ago

☐ (b) If yes, how long have you been on your current job? ___
(1) More than 5 years (2) Less than 5 years, but more than 1 year *(3) Less than 1 year

☐ 4. How many children do you have? ___

☐ (a) How many live with you? ___

☐ (b) Do you have any children who are HIV infected? (1) No (2) Yes ___

☐ (c) If infected, are they being treated for HIV? (1) No* (2) Yes ___

☐ 5. Beside yourself, do you know anyone who is HIV infected? *(1) No (2) Yes ___

☐ 6. How long have you known you were HIV positive? ___
*(1) < one week *(2) > one week, but < one month
*(3) > one month, but < 6 months (4) Six months, but < 1 year (5) > 1 year

☐ (a) Are you currently experiencing symptoms associated with HIV? *(1) No (2) Yes ___

☐ 7. Do you know how you became HIV infected? *(1) No (2) Yes ___

☐ (a) If yes, how: (1) ___ Needles (2) ___ Sexual Contact (3) ___ Transfusion

☐ 8. Have you been hospitalized in the last 2 years? *(1) No (2) Yes ___

☐ 9. Have you ever been put on medication for 6 months or longer? *(1) No (2) Yes ___
(Specify condition) ______________

Figure 21.1 Compliance Rating Instrument

☐ 10. In the past five years, have you been treated for a mental health problem? (1) No *(2) Yes ___ _

☐ (a) Have you been hospitalized for a mental health condition? (1) No *(2) Yes ___ _

COMPLIANCE RATING INSTRUMENT

Page 2

SCORE

☐ 11. Have you ever attempted suicide? (1) No *(2) Yes ___ _

☐ 12. Have you ever used IV drugs? (1) No *(2) Yes ___ _

☐ (a) If yes, do you use IV drugs now? (1) No *(2) Yes ___ _

☐ (b) If not currently using, when was the last time you used IV drugs?
* ____ days ago ____ months ago
* ____ weeks ago ____ years ago

☐ 13. Do you drink alcohol? (1) No *(2) Yes ___ _

☐ (a) If yes, on the average, how many days a week do you drink? ___ (*1 point if 4 or more days) _

☐ (b) If yes, on a day when you are drinking, how many drinks (cocktails or beer) do you have? ___ (*1 point if more than 4) _ _

☐ © Have you ever had a drinking problem? (1) No *(2) Yes ___ _

☐ 14. Have you ever been hospitalized or detoxed for alcohol or drug use? (1) No *(2) Yes ___ _

☐ (a) **If 13(c) or 14 is yes, ask:** Do you go to a self-help group such as AA or NA? *(1) No (2) Yes ___ _

☐ 15. Have you ever been arrested for a felony? (1) No *(2) Yes ___ _

☐ 16. Have you ever been put in jail? (1) No *(2) Yes ___ _

☐ 17. Do you have short or long term memory problems? (1) No *(2) Yes ___ _

☐ 18. Do you feel that your clinic visit must be completely confidential? (1) No *(2) Yes ___ _

☐ 19. How comfortable are you about being seen by other people in a clinic waiting room? ___
*(1) Very Uncomfortable (2) Somewhat Uncomfortable (3) Neutral
(4) Somewhat Comfortable (5) Very Comfortable (6) Not Applicable _

SCORING:

Score one point for each question answered with an asterisked response. Add up total number of points to obtain CRI Score. Scores may range from 0-33.

INTERPRETING CRI SCORE:

0-5	Low potential for compliance problem
6-9	Medium potential for compliance problem (participant worth watching)
10+	High probability for compliance problem (participant will require additional investment of time, attention and resources to remain compliant)

Use of CRI:

The Compliance Rating Instrument is "in the Public Domain," thus you are free to use the CRI in any way you chose, without obtaining our permission.

Figure 21.1 *Continued*

Medication Management Issues

The course of HIV infection presents a whole other dimension to the issues of patient management, particularly as it applies to medication management. HIV-infected individuals are normally asymptomatic for an extended period of time. They look healthy and do not feel sick even after having been diagnosed, therefore they have little or no reason to enter the sick role. It is often difficult to educate them effectively to the notion that taking prophylactic medication and changing their lifestyle are essential to maintaining their long-term health status. Later in the disease progression, treatment regimens that necessitate multiple medications, frequent transportation to the clinic, alterations in diet, and changes in living arrangements make compliance difficult if not impossible for many patients. The HCP can help to minimize and contain such problems by drawing on a variety of resources that are often overlooked, such as HIV/AIDS community support services, religious organizations, and "buddy programs."

Mental Health Issues

Issues the HCP might identify within the category of mental health include social isolation (living alone), homelessness (having no permanent or even temporary residence), drug or alcohol addiction, chronic mental illness, criminal record, and illiteracy. For example, this means that the HCP who learns, at the time of initial contact with HIV-infected patients, that the patients are homeless or living in isolation must keep in mind that patients lacking social companionship may suffer negatively from the isolation. In addition, the lack of social contact may stem from a latent drug/alcohol addiction or mental health problem. Each sociobehavioral marker commonly interacts and often additively contributes to poor compliance.[2] To complicate matters, the extent that any one factor might contribute to noncompliance is most likely to vary over the course of the patient's long and arduous course of treatment.

Within the category of mental health, other major issues that affect patient compliance are substance abuse and alternative lifestyles. Substance users are notorious for poor compliance due to drug-related behavior that is contrary to a rigid treatment regimen. While it is common knowledge that injecting drug users are at a higher risk for HIV infection, often substance abusers who are also HIV-infected are overlooked when treating the behavioral problems associated with their drug use. In addition, many individuals infected with HIV lead an alternative lifestyle that may include drug use and/or sexual orientation variations. Not only can an alternative lifestyle and risk-associated behavior put an individual at a higher risk of contracting HIV through multiple exposure, but it also further complicates issues of compliance.[3] For example, homosexual men frequently live in greater social isolation from the larger community and are disassociated from their families, and thus may have fewer familial resources on which to draw. Lovers, often infected themselves, may be too fragile socially and emotionally to play a realistic role in any treatment plan over the long term. HCPs need to be aware of issues and risks that the patient's lifestyle includes and attempt to integrate treatment (and safe sexual practices) to complement the individual's living patterns. This can be done by incorporating the patient's definition of family into the treatment process in a nonjudgmental fashion.

Sociocultural Issues

A wide range of corrective steps can be taken to mitigate potential problems with compliance. Working with the patient's family and encouraging buddy networks is an effective way to improve the patient's integration into social ties that might have deteriorated due to the consequences of previous lifestyle behaviors, such as drug use, serving time in prison, and alternative sexual preference.[2,3] This may involve interventions such as getting a family member, partner, or a close friend involved in the patient's treatment plan to assist the patient with taking medication according to the proper dose schedule, getting the patient to appointments on time, and offering social support through a difficult period in the patient's life.

If HCPs have access to other professional resources, referral to these resources can help to decrease potential patient compliance concerns. Integrating social workers or case managers into the patient's treatment plan helps to minimize compliance problems by providing social support and avenues of referral for special services or entitlements that can augment the treatment program. For people with drug and alcohol addictions, referrals to Alcoholics Anonymous (AA) or Narcotics Anonymous (NA) as part of the treatment plan saves time and money, and minimizes frustrations that providers often feel when patients fail to comply. Identification of mental health problems and referral to appropriate mental health providers for assessment and treatment maximizes compliance potential. For the patient with a criminal record, it is important to work *within* their nonpredictive world, rather than against it. Health care providers do not have to accept or approve of a patient's means of social and economic support, but they do need to recognize it and identify how it might hinder compliance inadvertently. Utilizing a multifaceted or systems approach to developing treatment plans will better address patients' individual needs, promote good patient compliance, and thus make HIV treatment a greater success.

Patient compliance can be influenced by what one might otherwise think of as insignificant or unrelated patient characteristics. For instance, very simple circumstances can make access to health care difficult. The distance between a patient's home and clinic, available transportation, the rural or urban nature of where they live, work schedule, and reading level can all play a major role in determining a patient's health care compliance patterns.[4,5] In addition, concerns of confidentiality and fear of disclosure are the invisible building material from which walls of isolation are constructed, walls that will affect treatment compliance eventually. Thus, disclosure issues are frequently associated with poor compliance in the areas of taking medication, keeping appointments, and following health care recommendations. In general, the stigma associated with HIV and AIDS makes patients socially isolated, because infected individuals are frequently outcast from their immediate communities.[6] Such isolation is devastating to patients, particularly those who lived previously surrounded by friends, family, and coworkers, and who were dependent on these people for social and emotional support.

Health Care Delivery System Issues

The nature of the health care delivery system can itself contribute to problems with patient compliance. For many HIV-infected women with children, finding child care frequently inhibits the woman from attending health care appointments. Health care facilities rarely offer child care services for patients who need them. The continuous rotation of medical staff, long wait time for appointments, and inflexibility of appointment times that exists in most clinic settings can be disturbing to an individual who may already lack stability in her life. Although the continuous rotation of health care staff is common to many health care delivery settings, frequent turnover in clinical staff makes it difficult for the patient to bond with the treatment team. Payment for health care services can also impair compliance because some services are not reimbursed by third-party payers. These individuals can benefit greatly from a relatively stable health care environment and health care providers who have time to spend with them for help with both physical health care as well as psychosocial concerns related to this very demanding disease.

Preventing poor compliance is the best way to ensure good patient compliance. However, prevention is not always enough. Even with the best of efforts to prevent compliance problems, the prolonged nature of treatment for HIV will present a variety of complications. Since patient compliance is a dynamic process, it is an important process to assess throughout HIV treatment because compliance tends to decrease over time.[4] Patient compliance can be monitored in a variety of different ways. For example, medication over- and under-compliance can be measured through laboratory tests; electronic technology, such as Medication Event Monitor System (MEMS) caps and individual reports from the patient, health care staff, family, significant others, and close friends. In addition, compliance can be estimated indirectly by monitoring patient appointments for no-shows, and canceled and rescheduled appointments.

The remainder of this chapter is devoted to a compliance management rapid reference guide, which can be used to identify and to address compliance problems of HIV-infected patients. To use the chart (Table 21.1), the clinician need only (1) locate the specific compliance issue under one of the four general headings of medication management, mental health, sociocultural issues, and health care delivery system issues, and then (2) examine proposed problem-solving strategies that can emanate from a variety of different sources, including health care staff, the patient, the patient's family, significant others, and outside referral resources.

Nurses are a key point of patient contact, especially when it comes to patients who need extra care such as those with HIV/AIDS. A nurse can have a tremendous impact on the level of compliance with a patient treatment regimen. Compliance is vital to the efficacy of medical treatment and health care in general. By being aware of compliance issues and ways to solve or minimize these problems, health care providers can influence positively the level of individual patient compliance.

Table 21.1 Compliance Management Reference Guide

Potential Compliance Problems	Compliance Enhancement Resources
A. MEDICATION MANAGEMENT	
1. Dosing, complicated schedules	
HIV patients tend to take many medications with complicated dosing schedules. This can lead to forgetting to take medication altogether, taking medication at the wrong time, or taking medication multiple times. Overdosing can also be life threatening to the patient. The role of the nurse and other health care providers (HCPs) is very important to ensuring that a patient takes the proper medication dose on the correct dosing schedule.	**Health care providers:** Most patients need to be taught the "tricks of the trade" of taking medication if they are to remain compliant when taking a large number of pills over time. The nurse can teach the patient to incorporate the dosing schedule into everyday activities, such as meals, work or school schedules, or on waking and going to sleep. Additional health care staff can assist in teaching pill-taking techniques and developing reminders for pill taking that will greatly increase compliance. Technology has provided some assistance in the form of reminder schemes that can be applied as needed by individual patients. *MEMS caps* are microelectronic monitoring devices that mark the date and time that a pill bottle is opened. *Pill boxes* allow patients to separate doses by day and sometimes even by time. This ensures that medications are taken on schedule and without duplication of dose. *Calendars and daily planners* can be useful reminders and medication can be *color coded* (on the bottle and calendar) to make it easier to remember which medication to take at what time. **Patient:** By providing the HCP with a daily schedule and a list of typical activities, the patient can work with the HCP to develop a pill-taking schedule. The patient should be taught the various tricks for medication reminders that are listed in the Health Care Staff guidelines and should provide the health care provider with feedback on the most helpful methods.

(continued)

Table 21.1 *Continued*

Potential Compliance Problems	Compliance Enhancement Resources
	Social support network: Social support will also help to increase compliance for a person taking a large number of pills. Building a network of support is vital to compliance, and these individuals can serve as gentle reminders for treatment, when feasible and with patient permission. Getting people who are in the daily surroundings of the patient to be aware of and involved in the pill-taking process will assist in patient medication compliance. It is also helpful to encourage the individual members of the patient's support system to reframe the close supervision of pill taking into an act of caring. These people are important to the patient's care, and the health care provider may need to encourage social support and suggest that daily routines be restructured to accommodate the medication regimen.
	Outside referral: Referral to support groups for HIV-infected individuals helps reinforce the importance of medication. The group support gives the patient a sense that she is not alone in having to manage complicated dosing schedules. Support group members can also share medication-taking hints with each other. Peer learning can be a powerful compliance reinforcer.
2. Side effects	
Unpleasant side effects (vomiting, diarrhea and headaches) frequently accompany medication taken by HIV-infected persons. Not taking the medications appears to the patient to have no adverse effects and is therefore seen as a better option.	**Health care providers:** An increase in perceived benefit of medication leads to an improvement in compliance.[7,8] Begin with health education. Work with the patient and ensure that the advantages to taking the medication are understood, as well as the disadvantages of not taking the medication. This should also include instruction on

Table 21.1 *Continued*

Potential Compliance Problems	Compliance Enhancement Resources
	managing side effects (e.g., taking medication with or without food, taking medication early or late in the day).
	Patient: Encourage the patient to be open and honest about symptoms and side effects, and to inform the health care team when medication schedules are not kept.
	Social support network: Solicit information from family members, significant others, and close friends (with patient permission), and provide them with education. Enlisting support through the eyes and ears of the patients' support network will enhance compliance and help the patient understand the importance of medication compliance, even under adverse circumstances.
	Outside referral: Refer patients to a health educator as necessary for further instruction on medication advantages and managing the side effects involved.
B. Mental Health	
1. Dementia	
Dementia is frequently associated with more advanced stages of HIV. Compliance is hindered as mental faculties diminish (see Chapter 9).	**Health care providers:** Dementia and other mental health problems should be assessed and managed immediately because good compliance requires full use of mental faculties. Treatment should be kept simple. Directly observed therapy by health care staff is sometimes recommended, especially in extreme cases.
	Patient: Encourage the patient to keep a treatment diary.
	Social support network: Family members and close friends may take responsibility for administering medication and getting the

Table 21.1 *Continued*

Potential Compliance Problems	Compliance Enhancement Resources
	patient to health care appointments as needed. **Outside referral:** Refer the patient to a mental health professional for assessment and consultation for treatment of dementia.
2. Emotional response, caregivers	
Caregivers experience denial, fear, and anger as reactions to a loved one with HIV. They may also have trouble dealing with the alternative lifestyle of the infected person. The alternative lifestyle may or may not have been common knowledge prior to infection disclosure and can lead to rejection or isolation.	**Health care providers:** Encourage social support and refer to mental health or family counseling as needed. Provide education to the family as needed. **Patient:** Encourage the patient to be open with family and friends. **Social support network:** Encourage family members and significant others to utilize available counseling services and support groups to deal better with emotional response. **Outside referral:** Refer to counseling or to family support groups.
3. Emotional response, patients	
Denial, fear, and anger often characterize the emotional reactions of the HIV-infected patient. Denial and anger can interfere with compliance. These coping mechanisms often result in the patient not recognizing that she is sick and thus sees little need to be compliant.	**Health care providers:** Encourage social support, listen, and try not to be defensive. Refer to mental health counseling as needed. Do not take anger personally. Denial, fear, and anger are coping mechanisms. **Patient:** Encourage participation in support groups and open communication about feelings. **Social support network:** Use family, friends, and significant others to gain important mental health information about the patient's emotional response patterns. This network can also be relied on to engage the patient in mental health care. Educate these individuals about noted responses.

Table 21.1 *Continued*

Potential Compliance Problems	Compliance Enhancement Resources
	Outside referral: Refer to mental health professionals as necessary.
4. Homelessness Homelessness and instability of the home environment are major contributors to poor compliance. Social isolation and homelessness often result from the stigma of HIV/AIDS. Homelessness is frequently a consequence of substance abuse.	**Health care providers:** Make access to health care easy and encourage the use of social services. This may require educating the patients about what social and mental health services are available. A social worker can assist in making appropriate referrals as needed. Provide a place to store medication because this may be difficult for those without a stable, permanent home. **Patient:** Encourage the patient to keep in contact with the health care team on a regular basis, because finding homeless individuals is often difficult. Encourage patients to utilize available social and mental health services. **Social support network:** If family members are available, encourage them to provide storage facilities and medication access to the patient. If the significant other is also homeless, make sure referrals are appropriate for the couple. **Outside referral:** Shelters, transitional housing, and special housing for HIV-infected individuals is available.
5. Isolation, social Social isolation is common for persons infected with HIV and is usually a by-product of the stigma associated with HIV. Isolation can lead to mental health problems because people have a need for social support and human contact. Compliance tends to be difficult for	**Health care providers:** The health care staff can minimize patient social isolation. Members of the staff should be trained to listen, enabling them to show that they care about the patient. Identifying problems and knowing when to make mental health referrals is critical to compliance. It is also important to keep patient contact with

Table 21.1 *Continued*

Potential Compliance Problems	Compliance Enhancement Resources
those who are isolated socially. It is important to get them involved socially in some way.	clinical staff consistent over time. This allows patients to bond with staff and to have at least one source of potential social contact. **Patient:** Patients should be encouraged to discuss any concerns of stigma associated with the disclosure of HIV status with health care personnel. **Social support network:** Involving family, friends, and significant others in the treatment process adds another social contact, and helps minimize social isolation. It also gives the patient support and encouragement, which helps with patient compliance. These people can provide assistance in helping patients get to appointments and remind patients of medication schedules. Patients should also be encouraged to rebuild strained or broken family ties by writing letters or calling on the telephone. Maximizing social support maximizes health care compliance.[7] **Outside referral:** Social workers can also be helpful in the compliance maximization process. A social worker can link the patient with resources that can help to create a more stable living environment. The socially isolated patient can be referred to an HIV support group in hopes of increasing socialization.
6. Substance abuse	
Substance abuse can be a barrier to patient compliance. Substance abuse and compliance have a well-known inverse relationship.[9] Most often, clinicians fail to screen for	**Health care providers:** Screening for substance abuse is an important part of the patient assessment. While encouraging the patient to refrain from substance use, it is also important for the health care staff to try

Table 21.1 *Continued*

Potential Compliance Problems	Compliance Enhancement Resources
substance abuse. It is unlikely that patients discuss their substance abuse openly, especially the use of injection drugs. Many destroy their family structure and family support system because of their substance abuse.	and work with the concerns that the patient presents. Nonjudgmental attitudes will encourage patient compliance. **Patient:** Encourage the patient to seek treatment. Support attempts to reduce substance use. **Social support network:** Frequently substance abusers destroy their family unit and isolate themselves socially from the support of the family. Encourage the rebuilding of family ties whenever possible. Check to see if the significant other is a substance abuser. If so, encourage substance abuse treatment for both, or promote Al-Anon, Narcotics Anonymous, or codependency support groups. **Outside referral:** Those patients with substance abuse problems should be referred to substance abuse programs such as Alcoholics Anonymous or Narcotics Anonymous immediately. Referrals will minimize the stress put on the nurse when a patient does not comply, as well as get treatment for those who need it.
C. SOCIOCULTURAL ISSUES	
1. Alternative lifestyle, homosexual or bisexual	
The patient's alternative lifestyle may hinder the patient/provider relationship, thus aggravating patient treatment compliance.	**Health care providers:** Be aware of the alternative lifestyle cultural differences in any individual. Treat him with respect, as you would any cultural difference. Be aware of your own prejudices. **Patient:** In a nonjudgmental way, encourage patients to share their beliefs. **Social support network:** Incorporate family members into the treatment regimen

Table 21.1 *Continued*

Potential Compliance Problems	Compliance Enhancement Resources
	to show recognition and acceptance of lifestyle choices. Significant others and close friends may be the "family" of a homosexual or bisexual individual. Make attempts to incorporate them into the treatment process. **Outside referral:** Refer to support groups that welcome individuals with alternative lifestyles and can provide social support.
2. Confidentiality concerns	
Maintaining confidentiality is frequently a major concern of the patient, especially for those infected with HIV/AIDS. Although confidentiality may not be a problem at your health care facility, patients may still have concerns. Patients may also fear disclosure of HIV infection to friends and family members who are unaware of their status.	**Health care providers:** Assure patients that confidentiality is also important to you, and that your health care facility and staff take measures to maintain confidentiality. Health care staff should be made aware of confidentiality and disclosure procedures. **Patient:** The patient should be made aware of confidentiality and disclosure procedures. **Social support network:** Respect the patient's wishes for disclosure to the family and significant other. Assure these people of confidentiality as necessary. **Outside referral:** When contacting outside referral sources, try to have the patient directly involved. Let the patient seek out the referral source so that he can control the flow of confidential information.
3. Cultural beliefs	
The cultural belief system of the patient often gets in the way of modern medical treatment. For example, individuals may choose to receive treatment from a traditional healer. Such treatment may be contrary to the prescribed modern treatment in terms of medication	**Health care providers:** Health care staff members should learn to listen to cultural differences. There may be a variety of concerns that are different. Learn to speak to a person with a different cultural background so that the patient can understand you and not feel intimidated by you. This may require the health care

Table 21.1 *Continued*

Potential Compliance Problems	Compliance Enhancement Resources
and ritual. Alternately, religious and cultural beliefs may discourage the use of modern medication and related treatment. This can be very difficult for the health care staff, but the following solutions should help to minimize frustration and maximize compliance.	provider to learn a new language and/or new terminology. It helps to work within the alternative culture's definitions of disease and treatment. When possible, incorporate modern medicine into nonharmful traditional practices. **Patient:** In a nonjudgmental way, encourage the patient to share her beliefs. **Social support network:** Incorporate family members and significant others into the treatment regimen and show respect, especially for older family members. The patient may define a significant other and close friends as family, and they should be treated as such. **Outside referral:** Work with traditional and religious healers whenever possible. This will help to increase the health care provider's understanding of the patient and the patient's cultural beliefs, and help build a relationship of trust between the provider, the traditional healer, and the patient.
4. HIV health care appointments, attending	
Transportation to and from health care appointments. No child care during medical appointments. Access to dependable and affordable child care and transportation to and from health care appointments are essential components to maintaining compliance. Often patients experience serious difficulty negotiating for basic needs by themselves resulting in serious barriers to compliance.	**Health care providers:** To maximize compliance, health service centers should consider providing transportation with taxis or bus tokens and consider providing child care. Schedules for public transportation should be made available. It is important to be aware that these issues may present compliance problems and need to be resolved for maximal compliance. **Patient:** Encourage patients to utilize available social services and public transportation.

Table 21.1 *Continued*

Potential Compliance Problems	Compliance Enhancement Resources
	Social support network: Encourage the family and significant other to provide needed transportation and/or child care. **Outside referral:** Social services may also be able to provide or locate some of these resources.
5. Illiteracy	
Illiteracy is another obstacle to compliance. Not being able to read medication labels, appointment cards, health care literature, and street maps greatly hinder an individual's ability to comply with any health care regimen. Interaction with patients may lead the nurse to suspect that inadequate reading levels exist.[10]	**Health care providers:** Keep treatment as simple as possible. Color coding of pill bottles and time tables is one option that may be helpful. Education must be delivered in a manner that is easy to understand and follow. Be aware of the reading level of educational material. A health educator can assist in reading labels and instructions. **Patient:** Encourage the patient to utilize adult education services and to ask for help with reading and understanding medication requirements. **Social support network:** Family members, significant others, and close friends can assist in reading labels and educational material. **Outside referral:** Refer to community-based adult education classes.
6. Knowledge of HIV/AIDS, lack of	
Many of the individuals infected with HIV lack specific knowledge about the disease.	**Health care providers:** Patient education that is easily comprehended will ensure basic knowledge about HIV/AIDS. Taking the time to answer any questions the patient may have will also be helpful. This will aid in patient compliance, as will keeping the treatment simple and making referrals to health educators and social workers for HIV education as needed.

Table 21.1 *Continued*

Potential Compliance Problems	Compliance Enhancement Resources
	Patient: Encourage the patient to ask questions. **Social support network:** Encourage family members and significant others to ask questions to ensure a basic comprehension about HIV. **Outside referral:** Refer patients to health education programs.
7. Stigma, disclosure	
Due to the stigma associated with HIV, patients frequently fear that their serological status will be revealed, thus making them societal outcasts.	**Health care providers:** Reassure patients of confidentiality. Discuss the pros and cons of HIV disclosure with the patient. Offer to be present when the patient discloses, to assist with emotional contact, and to provide educational information. **Patient:** Encourage the patient to talk with you about fears of HIV disclosure. **Social support network:** Respect patient's wishes for HIV disclosure to family members and significant others. **Outside referral:** Refer patients to social services as necessary.
D. HEALTH CARE DELIVERY SYSTEM	
1. HIV health care appointments, long waits	
Failure of the health care staff to schedule appointments in a timely fashion and thus make patients wait may lead to poor patient compliance. This may also increase feelings of social isolation and may be interpreted as lack of caring.[11]	**Health care providers:** Keep appointments as close to on time as possible. Make it easy for an individual to comply by being attentive and on time. This will also help to minimize feelings of isolation. Reduce waiting time in the office as much as possible. **Patient:** Encourage patients to schedule appointments when they have the most available free time.

Table 21.1 *Continued*

Potential Compliance Problems	Compliance Enhancement Resources
	Social support network: Explain the clinic situation to the family and significant others. Encourage them to attend clinic visits when possible to provide companionship and support to the patient while she waits.
	Outside referral: If your facility is over-crowded and another facility is available, refer the patient to the less crowded facility.
2. Multiple health care providers	
A patient's health care provider changes frequently, which increases instability for the patient.	**Health care provider:** Attempts should be made to keep HCPs consistent throughout treatment. This allows a patient to bond to specific staff members. The added social support will assist in compliance.
	Patient: Changes in staff need to be explained to the patient, and the patient's response and reaction to change need to be addressed.
	Social support network: Family members and significant others need to be made aware of any provider change. Encourage the patient to talk about how the change effects him.
	Outside referral: If clinician consistency is not available at your facility, consider referring the patient to a facility where consistency would be available.
3. Provider time vs. patient needs	
Unfortunately, some health care providers may ignore the patient's need to talk and share with the clinical staff. Health care providers have two kinds of time with patients—physical (the actual	**Health care providers:** Take the time to listen to patients or to make referrals if the requests for time become unreasonable. Patients need time to discuss their health care needs and concerns.
	Patient: Encourage the patient to ask for a

Table 21.1 *Continued*

Potential Compliance Problems	Compliance Enhancement Resources
medical or nursing time) and psychosocial (time to explain and listen to patient concerns). Patients need both.	doctor's or nurse's time as he needs it. **Social support network:** Family members and significant others need time to ask questions of providers. Try to account for this time when scheduling appointments. **Outside referral:** Refer to another office where time may be more available.
4. Universal precautions	
Health care providers may ignore standard precautions (see Appendix B.), thus setting a poor compliance example.	**Health care providers:** By following guidelines for standard precautions, health care providers set a good compliance example. Patients see this example and are more likely to follow the treatment plan that has been established. **Patient:** It is important that the patient realize that standard precautions are not designed just to protect the clinician from infection, but are designed to protect the patient as well. **Social support network:** Family members, significant others, and close friends who care for HIV-infected individuals need to be instructed in standard precautions. (see Appendix B.) **Outside referral:** Referral to a health educator can reinforce the need for standard precautions.

MEMS = Medication Event Monitor System.
See the following worldwide web sites for additional information.
Website course, "Evolving HIV Treatment: Advances and the Challenges of Adherence". http://www.heathcg.com/hiv/treatment/icaac97/adherence/print.html.1997.
Chesney MA. "New Antiretroviral Therapies: Adherence Challenges and Strategies". http://www.healthcg.com/hiv/treatment/icaac97/adherence/chesney.html/

References

1. Besch CL. Compliance in clinical trials. *AIDS.* 1995;9(1):1–10.
2. Morse EV, Simon PM, Balson PM. Using experiential training to enhance health professional's awareness of patient compliance issues. *Acad Med.* 1993;68(9): 693–697.
3. Elliott WJ. Compliance strategies. *Curr Opin Nephrol Hypertens.* 1994;3(3): 271–278.
4. Griffith S. A review of the factors associated with patient compliance and the taking of prescribed medicines. *Br J Gen Pract.* 1990;40:114–116.
5. Orr PR, Blackhurst DW, Hawkins BS. Patient and clinic factors predictive of missed visits and inactive status in a multicenter clinical trial. *Control Clin Trials.* 1992;13:40–49.
6. Kissinger P, Cohen D, Brandon W, Rice J, Morse A, Clark R. Compliance with the public sector HIV medical care. *J Natl Med Assoc.* 1995;87(1):19–24.
7. DiMatteo RM, DiNicola DD. *Achieving Patient Compliance: The Psychology of the Medical Practitioner's Role.* New York: Pergamon Press; 1982.
8. Morisky DE, Green LW, Levine DM. Concurrent and predictive validity of a self-reported measure of medication adherence. *Med Care.* 1986;24(1):67–71.
9. Baker A, Heather N, Wodak A, Dixon J, Holt P. Evaluation of a cognitive-behavioral intervention for HIV prevention among injecting drug users. *AIDS.* 1993;7(2):247–256.
10. Hussey LC. Minimizing effects of low literacy on medication knowledge and compliance among the elderly. *Clin Nurs Res.* 1994;3(2):132–145.
11. Morse EV, Simon PM, Besch CL, Walker J. Issues of recruitment, retention, and compliance in community based clinical trials with traditional underserved populations. *Appl Nurs Res.* 1995;8(1):8–14.

CHAPTER 22

Models of Care: Continuity Across Settings

Richard Sowell, PhD, RN, FAAN
Linda Moneyham, DNS, RN

Chapter Preview

The advent of the HIV epidemic in 1981 has single handedly created a crisis in the health care system. HIV has placed a tremendous burden on the acute-care component of the health care delivery system, and it is expected that its burden and costs will continue to increase.[1,2]

As a major public health problem, HIV has served to illuminate the fragmented nature of care coordination in the United States.[3,4] Over the past decades, the health care system has emphasized a "cure" approach to care, which has focused on technology, medical treatment, and hospital-based acute care to the exclusion of health promotion, health maintenance, and quality-of-life issues frequently encountered by individuals with long-term illnesses such as HIV. The course of HIV varies greatly, characterized by an erratic, unpredictable trajectory of sudden, unpredictable crises interspersed with long periods of relative wellness during which acute care and hospitalization are not needed.[2,5] Because of such variability, those infected exhibit a full spectrum of needs that fall outside the traditional acute model of care.

As medical treatments have improved life expectancy, the perspective of HIV as an acute terminal illness has shifted toward the view of HIV as a chronic illness.[6,7] Like other illnesses of a chronic and/or terminal nature, HIV affects every aspect of the infected individual's life and the lives of those close to them. Health care providers are faced with many questions about the type of care and services needed by infected individuals and their families.

Despite varying perspectives on the appropriate response to the HIV epidemic, it is generally agreed that a "whole-person" response is needed in the care of persons with HIV infection.[4] Major interventions necessarily must focus on both preventing OIs and promoting the highest quality of life despite the presence of an ultimately devastating and terminal disease. Consideration of the out-of-hospital needs of infected clients is emerging, with a growing emphasis on prevention, health promotion, and health maintenance issues. Morrison calls this change in perspective a shift in "attention from dying from AIDS to living with HIV."[2(p 323)] Unfortunately, the services and programs being developed and used at the current time are not always the most appropriate or efficient.[2]

The emergence of an increasingly diverse population infected with HIV has further complicated the problem of care delivery.[8] Although HIV initially emerged as a problem among urban, white, gay middle- and upper-class males, more recently the greatest growth has occurred in distinctly varied and vulnerable subpopulations including minorities, women, and IV drug users.[9–16] HIV infection is also increasingly prevalent in rural areas.[17,18] Although health care needs may be similar across these new subpopulations, available research indicates that their psychological and social issues and needs vary.[16,18–24] For example, a large number of women infected with HIV are single mothers with inadequate support systems, which requires services that are sensitive to the care and well-being of the children as well as the mother (see Chapters 25 and 26). Programs of services that are rigidly designed and unresponsive to the individual needs of clients will be ineffective in promoting quality of life. The case management (CM) model is one system of care coordination that has been promoted in order to address the problem of fragmentation of care and to meet the varied needs of affected subpopulations.[8]

Case Management: An Overview

The concept of case management (CM) as a care coordination strategy is not new. Historically the roots of CM lie in the efforts of nurses and social workers to provide coordinated services at the beginning of the twentieth century.[25] The early models were not driven by cost control issues. Over the past several decades, CM has been implemented to address care coordination problems in a number of underserved or chronically ill populations, including the elderly and chronically mentally ill.[26] These later efforts to coordinate health care services and control the cost of care have produced varied results.[27–36] Although those who receive CM services generally evaluate it,[37,38] conclusions about the effectiveness of the CM model are premature due to a paucity of controlled studies that link CM interventions with relevant, measurable outcomes.

Despite these limitations, CM continues to have widespread appeal as an answer to reducing the length of stay in hospitals and controlling the overall cost of care. Concerns about the increasing cost of health care in the 1980s saw a renewed interest in the concept of CM as a means of facilitating movement of patients through the acute-care system in a more cost-effective manner. Most often nurses were designated as case managers, with the responsibility of coordinating the many diagnostic procedures, treatments, and services patients required during hospitalization. Efforts focused on coordinating the contributions of varied disciplines to impact ultimately the course of hospitalization. Some care settings developed interdisciplinary teams with the aim of improving both the quality and cost-effectiveness of the CM approach to hospital care. While some evidence supports the conclusion that these CM approaches affected inpatient care positively, the ability to facilitate care coordination after discharge remained limited. Follow-through on discharge planning between hospital and community providers continues to be poor, often resulting in fragmentation of care and the need for clients to be readmitted for expensive inpatient care.[39]

Case Management Definition

Although frequently cited as the panacea to the woes surrounding the care of clients with HIV, little consensus is evident regarding what constitutes CM. CM is difficult to define given the diversity of CM models that have emerged.[40] In a review of relevant literature, Goodwin[40] noted that the term *case management* has been used to refer to such diverse phenomena as "a patient care delivery system, a professional practice model, a group of activities that a nurse performs within an organization setting, or a separate service provided by private practitioners."[40(p 29)] Benjamin[41] identified four models of CM: (1) the *hospital model of discharge planning*, involving only a brief monitoring of the client after an inpatient stay; (2) the *traditional CM model*, in which the client is contacted as early as possible and is provided planning, coordination of services and care, and monitoring throughout the illness, and thus spans both acute-based and community-based care needs of the client; (3) the *direct care model*, where in addition to performing the coordinating functions of the traditional model, the case manager also provides services directly to the client; and (4) the *gap-filling model*, in which the case manager plays a traditional role, while also having the resources to purchase extra services needed by clients. A number of hybrids of these models also exist.

Case Management Models

Efforts have been made to identify some of the common functions performed in the various CM models. A number of authors have identified *service coordination* and *monitoring* as major functional roles.[42–46] *Service coordination* involves linking clients to various resources and services available within the community. It may include the processing of referrals, delegation to other health care workers and providers, and coordination of services or interventions.[42] *Service monitoring* involves making sure the client receives the agreed services, which may at times entail supervision of other health care providers or a multidisciplinary team. Two major functional models of CM have been identified: the *brokerage model* and the *casework model*.[42,44]

In the brokerage model, the functions performed by case managers are limited to service coordination and service monitoring.[44] This model is consistent with the social work model of CM that is seen frequently in community-based settings. In contrast, in the casework model the case manager is also a major provider of health care services to the client. The casework model is more consistent with CM models that have evolved within hospital nursing care delivery systems, in which the care of the client is managed by a nurse provider.

CM can also be defined according to the setting or population being served.[40] Perhaps the most divergent views of CM are evident in an examination of acute, hospital-based models vs. community-based models. In community-based models, the social work or brokerage model is more commonly the norm, and the role of the case manager is focused not so much on the direct provision of services, but rather on identifying needs of clients within a given population and matching them to available services in the broad network of service organizations that exist within the community. For example, in HIV care, a community-based model of CM is frequently advocated due to a lack of organized systems that meet the needs of infected individuals and their families. HIV-infected individuals and their families present with a holistic array of needs that tend to be more functional and emotional in nature than disease oriented.[47] As a result, the major portion of care required by these individuals and families falls outside of the traditional health care system.[47]

Case Management in the Acute-care Setting

CM has only recently been adopted for use in the acute-care setting. In contrast to community-based models, the CM model most evident in acute, hospital-based settings is more self-contained. In the acute-care model, the case manager is most often a registered nurse who is part of a multidisciplinary team of providers that makes decisions about the client's care. The case manager participates in providing direct care as well as in coordinating and monitoring the overall care received by the client.[31] The case manager is also accountable for monitoring both clinical and financial outcomes for each episode of care.[31] The primary emphasis is on the acute phase of illness, although discharge planning is a critical component of the financial objectives of the plan of care. A major criticism of this model is that, for individuals with long-term conditions such as HIV, it fails to address those needs that span the illness trajectory and that exist beyond acute phases of physical illness and hospitalization. As a result, this model rarely addresses primary prevention, health promotion, and health maintenance issues occurring beyond hospitalization.

Critical Pathways and Acute-care CM

A key component of the acute-care, hospital-based model of CM is the critical pathway. The *critical path* is a method for mapping, tracking, evaluating, and modifying the patient's plan of care and its outcomes.[31,48] The critical path outlines the critical or key incidents that must occur in a particular time frame to achieve what is considered to be an appropriate length of stay as outlined by specific diagnosis-related groups.[31,49] Proponents of this method emphasize the importance of both quality of care and financial goals. As with any cost management program, critics suggest that quality of care is all too often sacrificed to meet financial goals. What is touted as CM in some systems is actually a system of utilization review. It is important to remember that the critical pathway is a tool to assist the case manager and is not a protocol to be followed blindly. Williams[50] has acknowledged that the critical thinking and assessment skills of the case manager are the core of any effective management system. The application of critical pathways to HIV is difficult because of the numerous OIs experienced by persons with HIV, and the erratic and unpredictable trajectory of the disease.

Home Health and CM

More recently CM has emerged within home health care, with nurses acting as both case managers and direct providers of care. Major emphasis is placed on improving function and quality of life by maintaining the client within the family and the community, while also cutting acute-care costs. Case managers who are employed by third-party payers to monitor and expedite client progress through the home health care system are becoming increasingly common. The emergence of this additional layer of CM raises questions concerning potential conflict of interest in the determination of what is best for the client. It can also create confusion for clients and direct care providers as to who is accountable for determining and coordinating needed services, and for monitoring patient and financial outcomes.[40]

Similar to acute-care settings, critical pathways are increasingly being developed for use in home health care.[48,49] Critical pathways are viewed as a systematic method for addressing client needs and achieving outcomes. When the critical pathways used in home health care are derived and flow from the critical pathways used in acute-care settings, there is a greater potential for achieving a seamless transition from hospital to home and continuity of care.

CM in HIV Care

CM specific to persons with HIV primarily has been community based and has varied widely in its implementation. HIV CM denotes a broad variety of activities performed by people with various disciplinary backgrounds and educational preparation in a number of different types of organizations.

Widespread application of CM in HIV care delivery had its origins in the multisite HIV demonstration projects funded by the Robert Wood Johnson Foundation, the Health Resources and Services Administration, and the United States Public Health Service (USPHS) in the mid 1980s.[51–54] Within these initiatives CM became a strategy for linking persons with HIV to existing services and preventing duplication of services within organized communities.[51,55] CM was formalized as the service model in HIV care with the passage of federal legislation—the Ryan White Comprehensive AIDS Resources Emergency Act of 1990.

In its broadest sense, HIV CM has been defined as a client-focused process that augments and coordinates existing care systems.[56] An aspect of community-based CM unique to HIV has been the need to fill the gaps in existing services through the development and provision of HIV-specific services. Success in the provision of direct services for HIV within the CM framework has been a direct result of the ability to rally HIV-affected communities to both demand and assist in providing those services most needed by persons with HIV.

The effectiveness of the CM model in HIV care is not known due to the paucity of outcome-based studies. If valid, research-based evaluation of HIV CM is to be accomplished, the structures, processes, and outcomes of the CM model relevant to HIV must first be articulated.[54,57] Such standards of service need to form the framework for the delivery and evaluation of CM. Clear outcome criteria for HIV CM needs to be developed to facilitate the evaluation process. Such outcome or evaluation criteria require that standards of service outlining the process and expected outcomes of CM services be established.

A New Model to Promote Continuity of Care: Care Management

The need for a comprehensive approach to services for persons with HIV requires new and innovative models of care management. Existence of the psychological, social, and physical issues associated with care of persons with HIV mandates a more comprehensive approach to care delivery. For example, little is gained by treating a case of pneumocystis pneumonia if the client is homeless and discharged into the streets in winter. Conversely, accessing medical care and treatment is the paramount issue for community-based case managers to assist persons who develop acute symptoms associated with HIV. The benefit of collaborative relationships across the care continuum can potentially outweigh the efforts required to break down traditional system boundaries or overcome turf control issues. To denote movement of the care delivery system toward one that is more comprehensive in scope and is more client focused, the term *care management* rather than *case management* is appropriate. Here the emphasis changes to quality care that is cost-effective from an emphasis singularly on cost. The expertise and cooperation of various social service and health care providers must be integrated for effective interdisciplinary teams. In such an interdisciplinary system, nurses, physicians, social workers, therapists, and pastoral care counselors working in conjunction with the client will be essential team members. The use of a diverse care management team allows clients to benefit from a broad perspective of service delivery not restricted by professional boundaries. Such teams will be most beneficial if they span the hospital-community continuum. A system that facilitates the exchange of client-focused information is required so that clients experience a "seamless" continuum of care.

One of the greatest challenges for health service planners and care managers has been the development of ongoing relationships between hospital and community providers. Fostering such relationships was difficult because the goals and structure of inpatient systems vary markedly from those of community-based HIV service organizations. Expertise in organizational development and conflict resolution are valuable skills when undertaking the challenges of restructuring traditional CM approaches to a system that can accommodate both hospital and community HIV care objectives. Integration across care delivery systems can be initiated by either hospital or community providers because care managers in all settings are responsible for resource development.

An Integrated Model of Care Management

Development of an integrated care management model requires the realization by providers that a broad view of care of persons with HIV is necessary. Once a broad view is embraced, care managers within either acute-care or community settings can then identify their counterparts, who are also managing care and/or coordinating services for persons with HIV. Once these targeted individuals are identified, a willingness to establish a working relationship between hospital and community care managers is essential. Too often, nurse care managers or coordinators working within inpatient agencies have inadequate knowledge of the history of the social and behavioral issues faced by a newly hospitalized client, in addition to their physical or medical problems. The movement to decrease length of stay (LOS) often makes comprehensive care coordination and, ultimately, discharge planning difficult. Likewise, the community-based care manager too often loses knowledge of his client's condition and experience once he enters the hospital. Once the client is discharged, the community-based care manager is thus faced with responding on a crisis basis to the client's social service and support needs that could have been anticipated if contact with the client during hospitalization could have been maintained. Thus, integrated systems for coordination and planning between hospital and community care managers are essential for continuous and appropriate care.

Currently, hospital CM systems exhibit a more well-defined structure and process than most community-based systems. This structural development offers the opportunity for hospital case managers to assist community HIV service organizations in developing standards and methods to better organize the process of community-based care management.

An example of a system in which nurses have guided the development of the organizational components of an integrated care management system is found in Atlanta, Georgia.[58] This community-based HIV/AIDS care management system features centralized administration while providing actual services in a variety of hospital-based clinics, public health HIV/AIDS clinics, and grass roots community-based agencies. To support continuity and consistency of care, standards of service and outcome evaluation criteria tailored to specific community needs and available resources have been developed.[4]

The first step in restructuring the Atlanta care management system was the acceptance of a consistent working definition of care management. Care management was defined as a partnership between client and care manager. This partnership was defined through mutual participation of the client and the care manager in the ongoing assessment of client needs, the planning and implementation of interventions to match clients to appropriate levels of resources, and the evaluation of interventions and reassessment of client needs (Figure 22.1).

A second step in restructuring the care management system was aimed at improving continuity of service across delivery settings. While hospital-type critical pathways were beyond the scope of this community system, standards of service that clearly outlined expectations of service were developed to provide a common ground for communication between community and acute-care agencies, as well as to provide a basis for evaluation of outcomes. Additionally, standards of service provide a framework on which documentation of services can be constructed to allow for the transfer of relevant client information across service delivery settings.

Development of Standards

Development of standards is key to the implementation of a care management system that addresses quality-of-care issues. Such standards serve as the basis for determining relevant outcomes that can be used to evaluate the quality of care delivered through the care management system. Standards of service provide guidance for care managers in developing individualized plans of service. However, unlike more structured protocols, they do not limit the care manager's ability to seek innovative solutions to complex problems. An outline for the process of development of standards of service is as follows:

- Identify the problem or client concern.
- Review existing literature.
- Define the rationale for criteria-based standards.

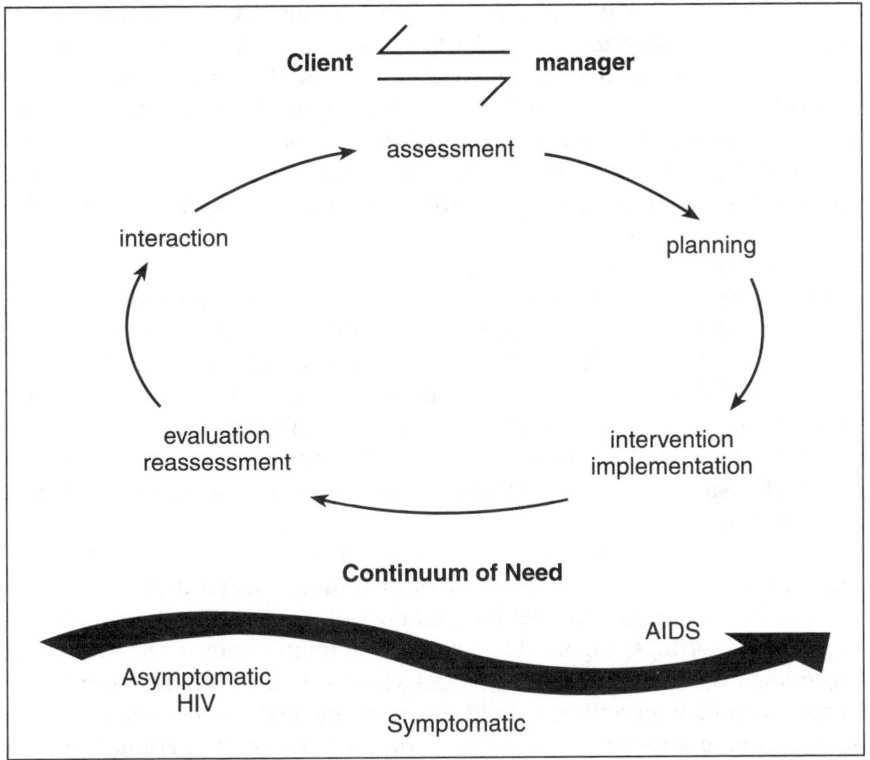

Figure 22.1 Essential Components and Interactions within Care Management

- Review HIV/AIDS CM standards existing in other agencies.
- Establish a client-centered focus for the standard.
- Define the process of care management.
- Define the characteristics of the standard.
- Identify specific client and care manager roles within the CM process.
- Identify resources.
- Develop outcome and evaluation criteria.

(From Sowell R, Meadows T. An integrated case management model: developing standards, evaluation, and outcome criteria. *Nurs Adm Q*. 1994;18(2):58. Reprinted with permission. © 1994, Aspen Publishers, Inc.):

Standards were developed for the most frequently encountered client concerns. Areas of concern included housing, financial, legal, substance use, and medical care issues. In developing each standard, the problem being addressed was identified, and care management interventions were outlined. In addition, for each standard, resources for addressing the problem were identified, and outcome and evaluation criteria were defined. An example of a standard developed within this system is presented in Figure 22.2.

Evaluation

Standards of service provide the necessary criteria by which objective evaluation can be accomplished, and support the ongoing reassessment of client needs. The unpredictable and frequently changing needs of persons with HIV makes such reassessment an essential component of HIV care management.[59] Such evaluations are not only important for ongoing adjustments or modifications of treatment and/or service, but the documentation of positive outcomes of HIV care management is necessary if funding is to be maintained.

Evaluation of care management can occur using a variety of strategies. Traditional approaches to evaluation often found in hospitals, such as chart reviews and analysis of utilization and cost of services, can be adapted to community settings. Figure 22.3 provides outcome criteria for evaluating the standard of service for homeless clients in the Atlanta model. The degree of consumer activism that has surrounded HIV mandates that client satisfaction and relevance of services offered be essential components of the evaluation of HIV service delivery. Ongoing client input into the type of services needed and the manner in which such services are delivered may represent the best source of service delivery evaluation.

Documentation

The goal of facilitating communication within and across provider agencies emphasizes the need for a well-defined documentation system. In developing a documentation system for the Atlanta care management system, the staff modified the Goal-Oriented Nursing Record prepared by King[60] to include social issues. Further, a goal-oriented problem list was established to summarize major problems and client concerns as well as short- and long-term goals. This problem list approach (Figure 22.4), based on the Weed[61] system of problem-oriented charting, is familiar to many acute-care providers, and thus served to facilitate communication between

STANDARD OF SERVICE - HOMELESS CLIENTS

Homelessness: Defined as without consistent legal access to house, apartment, room, or other domicile. Client may be homeless by choice.

Extenuating factors to be considered:
–Financial status
–Lack of support system
–Substance abuse
–Psychiatric/mental health history
–Physical disability
–History of family violence
–Literacy difficulties
–Impaired comprehension and understanding

Client's role:

1. Client must define his housing choice.
2. Client who is homeless by choice must inform the care manager and should be willing to explore the reasons.
3. Client who is homeless by circumstance will inform care manager and the process for housing should begin.
4. Client will be expected to provide documentation of income, if any.
5. Client who is marginally housed must provide documentation of need. Such documentation may be written or oral.

Care Manager's role:

1. Care Manager must complete the housing assessment (housing section of database).
2. Care Manager must assist client in exploring housing options and help client define whether the options are realistic based on health and weather conditions.
3. Care Manager will identify temporary housing for client (shelter, room, boarding house, etc.).
4. Care Manager will assist client with application process where applicable.
5. Care Manager will review financial status (disability eligibility, Emergency Assistance Fund [EAF], etc.).
6. Care Manager will review extenuating factors to determine possible contributing complications.
7. Care Manager will seek to determine how conditions of homelessness may contribute to the client's medical condition and make the appropriate referrals.
8. Care Manager will arrange EAF where applicable for temporary shelter (see EAF policy).
9. Care Manager will review EAF, housing, and financial standards to follow-up general assistance.

High-need clients. All homeless clients.

____________________ __________
Client's Signature Date

____________________ __________
Care Manager's Signature Date

Figure 22.2 Care Management Standard of Service for Homeless Clients (Used with permission: Grier J. *Standard of Service in HIV/AIDS Case Management.* Atlanta, GA: AID Atlanta, Inc.; 1995.)

HOMELESSNESS	MET	N/MET	N/A	COMMENTS
Housing assessment completed during intake process.				
Realistic housing options based on weather and health status explored with client.				
Assistance with housing application process as needed.				
Identification of client's income resources and financial status for possible housing options.				
Assessment of other extenuating factors impacting housing explored for possible contribution(s) to homelessness.				
Determination of homelessness on client's medical condition; appropriate health care referrals made.				
Arrangements for Emergency Assistance Fund (EAF) completed as necessary for temporary shelter.				
Comprehensive review completed regarding EAF, housing, and financial standards for general assistance follow-up.				
The Care Manager Generalist must complete all the usual documentation (database, assessments, referrals, applications, etc.).				
The Care Manager Generalist must exhaust the usual resources prior to referral to the Specialist.				
The Care Manager Generalist must bring complete documentation of efforts to the Specialist prior to turning over to Specialists for assistance.				
The Care Manager Specialist will staff with Generalist and resolve those cases that can be effectively managed without transfer.				
The Care Manager Specialist will assume 30-day responsibility for those complex cases requiring intense management. During the 30-day period the Specialist will seek out all alternatives for client. After the 30-day period, the client will be referred back to the Care Manager Generalist for maintenance.				
The Care Manager will keep those cases where there is no resolution and continue working to find a solution (other Specialists, referral, etc.).				
The management of complex cases will be staffed by supervisor(s) and other Specialist(s) as appropriate.				

Care Manager Generalist = care manager who provides services to a diverse caseload of persons with HIV. Expertise of this care manager is the ability to respond adequately to a wide range of problems and clients. Care Manager Specialist = care manager who has in-depth expertise in a specific area such as housing or legal issues. Caseload consists of persons with high need or high likelihood of need in a specific area. Provides consultation in area of expertise to other care managers.

Figure 22.3 Evaluation Criterion Tool for Standard of Care for Homeless Clients (Used with permission: Grier J. *Standard of Service in HIV/AIDS Case Management.* Atlanta, GA: AID Atlanta, Inc.; 1995.)

DATE: ________	PROBLEM/NEEDS/STANDARDS OF SERVICE C = Client's perception CM = Care Manager's perception	SHORT-TERM OBJECTIVES	LONG-TERM GOALS	C & CM INITIALS
INCOME	C: "Not enough money to meet my needs." CM: Need for financial counseling and management	Access to appropriate income sources; possible emergency assistance	Stable income	
INSURANCE/ MEDICAL	C: "No insurance. I receive health care at Grady Hospital." CM: Has accessed available health care	Access to medical care and medication	Medicare/Medicaid entitlement programs	
HOUSING	C: "Adequate. I live with my partner." CM: Adequate living arrangements	Home assessment	Maintain housing options	
FOOD	C: "I receive POH and food stamps." CM: Potential need for information regarding nutrition	Nutritional assessment; referral to a dietitian	Maintain food options, provide information on nutritional intake and HIV	
SOCIAL SUPPORT/ COUNSELING	C: "My family helps, but they don't want to talk about my condition." CM: Need for additional social support	Linkage to support groups	Develop stable support system	
ADDICTION/ RECOVERY	C: "I attend NA meetings daily." CM: History of substance use; presently linked to appropriate treatment source	Link to substance abuse counselor/support; monitor meeting attendance	Maintain recovery	
LEGAL	C: None noted CM:	Monitor legal status	No legal involvement	
FURNITURE/ CLOTHING	C: None noted. CM:	Monitor	Maintain current status	

Client's ID# 123456 ________ Client's Signature ________
Client's Name ________ Care Manager's Signature ________

Figure 22.4 Example of an HIV/AIDS Care Management Service Plan

hospital and community settings. A unique element of this documentation system is the formal involvement of the client in the assessment, planning, and evaluation process.

For agencies that have the resources available, computer technology allows the development of a client data base to assist care managers in documentation. Using a computer, care managers can document identified client problems, previous interventions, and ongoing assessment of the client directly in the client data base. In the emerging health care system where agencies are responsible for managing care for persons across hospital and community settings, computerized record systems that span settings have the potential for supporting communication and the continuity of service delivery.

In summary, the challenge for care management lies in the need to integrate the delivery of services across the continuum of illness and a variety of needs (physical, psychological, social, economic, and spiritual). The need for integrated services is especially important to persons with HIV. There is great need for a client-focused system that overcomes professional and organizational boundaries to assist the client in maintaining the highest possible quality of life.

References

1. Hardy A. Planning for the health care needs of patients with AIDS. *JAMA*. 1986;256:3140.
2. Morrison C. Delivery systems for the care of persons with HIV infection and AIDS. *Nurs Clin North Am*. 1993;28(2):317–333.
3. Panem S. Planning for the next health emergency. *Issues Sci Tech*. 1988;4: 59–64.
4. Sowell RL, Grier J. HIV/AIDS case management: developing an integrated community model. In: Blancett SS, Flarey DL, eds. *Case Studies in Nursing Case Management*. Gaithersburg, MD: Aspen; 1996.
5. National Center for Nursing Research. *Priority Expert Panel on HIV Infection: Delivery of Nursing Care: HIV Infection: Prevention and Care*. Bethesda, MD: National Center for Nursing Research; 1990.
6. Emini E. *HIV-1 protease inhibitors*. Presented at the Third National Conference on Retroviruses and Opportunitic Infections. Washington, DC. January 1996. Abstract no. L1.
7. Lederman M, Connick E, Landay A, et al. *Partial Immune Reconstitution after*

12 Weeks of HAART (AZT, 3TC, Ritonavir): Preliminary Results of ACTG 315. Presented at the Fourth National Conference on Retroviruses and Opportunistic Infections. Washington, DC. January 1997. Abstract no. 13.

8. Layzell S, McCarthy M. Community based health services for persons with HIV/AIDS: a view from health services perspective. *AIDS Care.* 1992;4:203–215.
9. Grmek MD. *History of AIDS: Emergence and Origin of a Modern Pandemic.* Princeton: University Press; 1990.
10. Shilts R. *And the Band Played On: Politics, People, and the AIDS Epidemic.* New York: St. Martin's Press; 1987.
11. US Department of Health and Human Services. *HIV Infection in Rural Areas: Issues in Prevention and Services.* Baltimore: Office of AIDS and Office of Rural Policy; 1990.
12. Berry DE. The emerging epidemiology of rural AIDS. *J Rural Health.* 1993;9: 293–304.
13. CDC. HIV prevalence estimates and AIDS case projections for the United States: Report based on a workshop. MMWR. 1990;39(R16): 1–31.
14. CDC. The HIV/AIDS epidemic: the first ten years. *MMWR.* 1991;40:357.
15. CDC. *AIDS Surveillance Information Report.* Atlanta, GA: CDC; May 1993.
16. CDC. *National HIV Serosurveillance Survey: Results through 1992.* Atlanta, GA: US Dept. of Health and Human Services, CDC; 1994. No. 3.
17. CDC. *HIV/AIDS Surveillance Report.* Atlanta, GA: CDC; 1995.
18. Cohn SE, Klein JD, Mohr JE. The geography of AIDS: patterns of urban and rural migration. *South Med J.* 1994;87:599–606.
19. Summer L. *Limited Access: Health Care for the Rural Poor.* Washington, DC: Center of Budget and Priorities; 1991.
20. Weinert C, Long KA. Rural families and health care: refining the knowledge base. *Marriage Fam Rev.* 1990;15:57–75.
21. Gentry JH. Women and AIDS. *Psychol AIDS Exchange.* 1992;1–2:6–7.
22. Mitchell J, Tucker J, Loftmon PO, et al. HIV and women: current controversies and clinical relevance. *J Women's Health.* 1992;1:35–39.
23. Parker M, Quinn J, Viehl M, et al. Issues in rural case management. *Fam Commun Health.* 1992;14(4):40–60.
24. Bushy A. When your client lives in a rural area. Part I: rural health care delivery issues. *Issues Ment Health Nurs.* 1994;15:253–266.
25. Fuszard B, Bowman R, Howell HT, et al. *Nursing Case Management.* Washington, DC: American Nurses Association; 1988.
26. Piette J, Fleishman JA, Mor V, et al. A comparison of hospital and community case management programs for persons with AIDS. *Med Care.* 1990;28:746–755.
27. Lamb GS, Stempel JE. Nurse case management from the client's view: growing as insider-expert. *Nurs Outlook.* 1994;42(1):7–13.
28. Cohen E. Nurse case management: does it pay? *J Nurs Adm.* 1991;20:20–25.

29. Ethridge P, Lamb G. Professional nursing case management improves quality, access, and costs. *Nurse Manager.* 1989;20:30–37.
30. Rogers M, Riordan J, Swindle D. Community-based case management pays off. *Nurse Manager.* 1991;22:30–37.
31. Zander K. Nursing case management: strategic management of cost and quality outcomes. *J Nurs Adm.* 1988;18(5):23–30.
32. Borland A, McRae J, Lycean C. Outcomes of five years of continuous intensive case management. *Hosp Commun Psychiatry.* 1989;40:369–376.
33. Kemper P. Case management agency system of administering long-term care: evidence from the channeling demonstration. *Gerontologist.* 1990;30:817–824.
34. Gillette Y, Hansen NB, Robinson JL, et al. Hospital-based case management for medically fragile infants: results of a randomized trial. *Patient Educ Couns.* 1991;17:59–70.
35. Nickel JT. *Effects of Nurse Case-Managed Home Care for HIV Patients.* Columbus, OH: College of Nursing, Ohio State University; 1993.
36. Sowell RL, Gueldner SH, Killeen M, et al. Impact of case management on hospital charges of PWA's in Georgia. *J Assoc Nurs AIDS Care.* 1992;3:24–31.
37. Fleishman J, More V, Piette J. AIDS case management: the client perspective. *Health Serv Res.* 1991;26:447–470.
38. Spitz B. A national survey of medical case management programs. *Health Aff (Millwood).* 1987;6:61–70.
39. Lowenstein AJ, Hoff PS. Discharge planning: a study of nursing staff involvement. *J Nurs Adm.* 1994;24(4):45–50.
40. Goodwin DR. Nursing case management activities: how they differ between employment settings. *J Nurs Adm.* 1994;24(2):29–34.
41. Benjamin AE, Lee PR, Solkowetz SN. Case management for persons with Acquired Immune Deficiency Syndrome in San Francisco. *Health Care Financing Review.* (annual supplement) 1988, 69–73.
42. Rheaume A, Frisch S, Smith A, Kennedy C. Case management and nursing practice. *J Nurs Adm.* 1994;24(3):30–36.
43. American Nurses' Association. *Nursing Case Management.* Kansas City: American Nurses Association; 1988. Pub. no. NS-32.
44. Stanhope M, Lancaster J. *Community Health Nursing.* 3rd ed. St Louis: Mosby Yearbook; 1992.
45. Grau L. Case management and the nurse. *Geriatric Nurs.* 1984;5(8):372–375.
46. Wahlstedt P, Blaser W. Nurse case management for the frail elderly: a curriculum to prepare nurses for that role. *Home Health Care Nurse.* 1986;4(2):30–35.
47. McGuire JF. AIDS: the community response. *AIDS.* 1989;3(suppl 1):s279–s282.
48. Hampton DC. Implementing a managed care framework through care maps. *J Nurs Adm.* 1993;23(5):21–27.

49. Goodwin DR. Critical pathways in home health care. *J Nurs Adm.* 1992;22(2): 35–48.
50. Williams DC. Is the case manager being replaced? *Nurs Case Manage.* 1996; 1(4):153.
51. Flaskerud JH, Ungvarski PJ. *HIV/AIDS: A Guide to Nursing Care.* 3rd ed. Philadelphia: WB Saunders; 1995.
52. Piette J, Fleishman JA, Mor V, et al. A comparison of hospital and community case management programs for persons with AIDS. *Med Care.* 1990;28:746–755.
53. Jellinek PS. Case-managing AIDS. *Issues Serv Tech.* 1988;4:59–63.
54. Mor V, Piette J, Fleishman J. Community-based case management for persons with AIDS. *Health Aff (Millwood).* 1989;8:139–153.
55. Sierra Health Foundation. *Coordinating HIV/AIDS care and services in the next decade.* Report of the National Symposium, Case Management and HIV/ AIDS. Sacramento CA December 16–17, 1991.
56. Agency for Health Care Policy and Research, Public Health Service, US Department of Health and Human Services. Evaluation and management of early HIV infection. *Clin Pract Guide.* 1994;7:95–100.
57. Lamb GS. Conceptual and methodological issues in nurse case management research. *Adv Nurs Sci.* 1992;15:16–24.
58. Grier J, Sowell RL. Standards and evaluation in community-based case management. *J Assoc Nurs AIDS Care.* 1993;4:32–33.
59. Sowell RL, Meadows TM. An integrated case management model: developing standards, evaluation, and outcome criteria. *Nurs Adm Q.* 1994;18(2):53–64.
60. King IM. *A Theory for Nursing: Systems, Concepts, Process.* New York: Wiley; 1981.
61. Weed LL. *Medical Records, Medical Evaluation and Patient Outcome.* Cleveland, OH: Press of Case Western University; 1969.

CHAPTER 23

Ethical Issues for the Clinician

Evan G. DeRenzo, PhD • Wende L. Levy, RN, MS

Chapter Preview

- Decisions Concerning Care
- HIV Testing of Pregnant Women
- Access to Care
- Decisions Concerning Treatment and Withdrawal of Treatment
- Decisions Related to Caregivers, Families, and Significant Others

Ethical decision making is an integral component of caring for persons with AIDS. The canons of ethical nursing practice are historically grounded in moral ideals, and today, patients depend on the integrity of the nursing professionals who care for them. Nurses and other health care professionals are in an excellent position to explore with their patients patient feelings, values, and knowledge regarding quality of life and medical interventions in the face of health and illness, especially in the case of terminal or irreversible disease. Consistent with nursing's long-standing ethical traditions of patient advocacy, educating patients, and maximizing patient autonomy and independence, AIDS patients provide nurses with rewarding opportunities and challenges to putting these traditions into action.

Decisions Concerning Care

Duty to Treat

Historically health care providers have made their own decisions about who to treat or not to treat. Although abandonment is and has been ethically and legally impermissible, the decision about beginning to care for a patient has traditionally been left up to the treating professional. Even in emergency situations and epidemics there are accounts of physicians choosing not to treat sick persons because of concerns for their own health. These ancient discretionary practices had not much changed by the time HIV appeared.

Today in the case of HIV infection and AIDS, however, such discretion has been removed. Ethically, it is generally accepted that health care workers have a duty to treat persons with HIV and AIDS.[1] Enactment of the Americans with Disabilities Act in 1990 has ensured that persons with HIV disease are treated. Although there are some occasions when health care workers can refuse, for deeply held religious or other moral reasons, not to perform a particular medical procedure (e.g., abortion), discretion does not extend to choice about caring for persons with HIV infection or AIDS.

What has been enacted into law, however, is what some have always considered ethical practice. Nurses accept, when choosing their profession, that there will be risks to them in caring for sick persons. Although caring for persons with HIV infection and AIDS can arouse concern in nurses for their own health and well-being, taking reasonable and recommended precautions can reduce the risk significantly of infection transmission from patient to nurse. This also applies to the treatment of persons who have HIV-related infectious conditions, such as TB. Even in the case of drug-resistant TB, the duty to treat is clear.

Further, not only is there a duty to treat but there is a duty to treat appropriately. This statement may seem obvious, but such is not always the case in HIV disease. For example, meeting one's obligations to treat pain in an AIDS patient with a history of substance abuse can blur one's understanding of appropriateness. Adequate pain treatment for persons with drug abuse histories may require more analgesics than for persons without previous drug use problems. Contributing to the complexity of the clinical situation is the bias some nurses feel toward those who have contracted HIV infection through drug abuse practices. Whether personal bias is recognized by nurses holding such views or not, this bias often exists and must be addressed by the nursing staff caring for these patients. That is, judgmental behaviors must be discussed openly and corrected quickly to ensure that patients receive proper medical care. Individualized systems should be put in place prospectively to address the special and difficult pain management problems these patients present to ensure that nurses can meet their duty to treat regardless of any particular nurse's beliefs about drug abuse.

Although there is consensus that professionals have a duty to treat patients, that does not translate into an obligation to take excessive risk. Health care workers must be vigilant about reducing risks to their own health and protecting the health of patients being cared for by HIV-infected health care workers. That nurses should take adequate protections against contracting the virus from patients is obvious. What requires more thoughtful attention is how such protections are instituted in a nonstigmatizing manner. That is, CDC guidelines ought not be applied in a discriminatory way. Universal precautions are just that—universal. These protective measures should be applied evenly across all patients, not simply those known or suspected to have HIV infection.

Concerning protections against HIV-infected nurse-to-patient transmission, the ethical analysis is less well articulated. Although no such case has ever been reported, public fears deserve respectful consideration. Some believe the risks (not only of transmission per se, but of loss of trust in the medical community by the public) are of sufficient concern that

HIV-infected health care providers ought not hold patient care roles, or at least ought to inform their patients of their seropositivity. In that way their patients can make informed decisions about whether or not to be cared for by an HIV-infected health care provider. Others feel such disclosure and/or voluntary withdrawal from patient care activities is unnecessary and fuels inappropriate fears about HIV transmissibility and discrimination against persons with HIV infection and AIDS. It is advisable for health care providers who find themselves to be HIV infected to learn about institutional policies on HIV-infected staff and to consult with organizations that provide confidential counseling to HIV-infected professionals.

Autonomous Choices

The autonomy principle, or the principle of respect for persons, requires that patient decision making be informed. This means that persons must have sufficient information, be able to comprehend the meaning of that information, and be free and uncoerced, if they are to make autonomous decisions. This principle also requires that appropriate protections be established in the care of persons whose autonomy is compromised, and that impaired persons' ability to be self-determining be maximized to the greatest degree possible.

In meeting this dual obligation, nurses play a critical role on the health care team. For patients who are fully capacitated decision makers (that is, they are able to understand information and there are no undue constraints on their ability to make a decision), nurses can be one of the primary sources of necessary information.

Nurses need to be careful, however, to present information in a balanced, neutral manner when it comes to information that is part of patient decision making. Making a neutral presentation can be difficult, in part because nurses are trained to be directive. This is important and necessary, for example, when nurses are educating patients on requirements of medical regimens or on how to keep various medical apparatus clean. When presenting information about treatment options, however, nurses have to shift gears and move into a nondirective stance or the risk of coercion is high. That is because the power difference between the patient and nurse places the patient in a position of dependence and vulnerability to manipulation, even when such manipulation—through presenting treatment choices in ways that clearly favor one alternative over another—is well intentioned and unconscious.

Another ethical requirement that sometimes presents difficulties for nurses is implementing the second half of the requirement of respect for persons; namely, protecting those with impaired decisional capacity. Given that HIV disease is known to cause often subtle mental status changes, it is important not to overestimate persons' decision-making capabilities. Rather, nurses need to be vigilant to changes in behaviors, mental status, and/or previously espoused values. Even in seemingly clear-headed patients, problems such as anxiety can cloud patients' thinking, limiting their ability to act in truly self-determining ways. Thus, nurses play a key role in assessment of capacity to make autonomous decisions.

Confidentiality

Patient confidentiality refers to keeping information about the patient private. Protecting patient confidentiality is an ethical requirement on the part of health care professionals. Although this obligation applies to all patients, not merely to patients with HIV infection or AIDS, the consequences of not doing so may be particularly grave in this patient population for whom the risk of stigmatization of persons with AIDS is great. Simultaneously, however, it is important to remember how difficult it is to keep medical information confidential. Many persons and entities (e.g., third-party payers) have access or can easily obtain access to patient records and charts. Nurses need to assist patients in appreciating this practicality so patients do not assume a higher degree of confidentiality than is functionally possible. Nonetheless, nurses must be careful to guard against inadvertent breaches of confidence that might occur as a result of allowing others to overhear conversations, leaving charts open, or engaging in overly expressive charting. Because the threat of discrimination is so great in this population, nurses must make an extra effort to protect the confidentiality of HIV-infected patients.

Disclosure of Status

Although nurses are required ethically to protect patient confidentiality, confidentiality is not absolute. As noted previously, constraints on confidentiality come from various directions. One of the most common limits on confidentiality relates to safety considerations for others and involves the potential appropriateness of disclosure of HIV status to sexual and/or drug-sharing partners.

Traditional medical ethics dictates that information about one person not be divulged to another. Today that strict principle has been limited to the degree that we balance protection of patient confidentiality and trust in the patient/professional relationship against professional obligations to protect identifiable others from harm posed by patients. Although far from a settled issue, there are those who believe that having a professional share a patient's HIV status with a sexual or needle-sharing partner is justifiable, if that patient is unable or unwilling to share the information herself. The justification rests on the obligation of the health care provider to do good in treating, curing, and preventing disease. Those who oppose partner notification do so on the grounds that the risk/benefit ratio, in HIV infection, tips in the wrong direction. Notification opponents point out that by the time the professional knows about a patient's HIV positivity and knows who might be at risk through sexual or needle-sharing partnership, it is likely that transmission has already occurred. This reasoning goes further to suggest that the erosion of trust in the patient/professional relationship resulting from involuntary partner notification will have a chilling effect on treatment. That is, if persons grow to fear that if they are found to be HIV infected health care providers will breach confidentiality through partner notification practices, individuals will be less inclined to be tested for HIV infection, thus exacerbating attempts to curtail disease spread.

In addition to controversies over disclosure of HIV status to identified partners, the degree to which health care workers have the right to know a patient's HIV status is also unsettled. Some think, for example, that persons within a hospital or home health care agency ought to know patient HIV status, but that this information should not be given to persons outside the organization. Some believe that knowledge of serological status is required to plan adequately for and deliver optimal health care services. Others believe that the risks to health care professionals are sufficiently great that professional caregivers should be able to obtain that information, whether through standardized testing policies in hospitals or through chart access. Some states have laws allowing disclosure of serological status to other health care providers when the patient's life is endangered. There is, however, no national or professional ethical consensus around this issue, and nurses are encouraged to learn their state laws and organizational policies on this matter.

HIV Testing of Pregnant Women

CDC guidelines call on medical professionals to provide HIV counseling and voluntary testing of all pregnant women. It remains a woman's choice whether to be tested. HIV counseling and testing during the prenatal period offer important prevention opportunities for both uninfected and infected women and their infants. Risk identification for uninfected women as well as education on risk reduction are essential. For infected women, knowledge of their HIV status provides them the opportunity to receive early treatment for themselves, allows them to make reproductive decisions with the full knowledge of the risks involved, and allows them the opportunity to be informed of the methods to reduce the risk of prenatal transmission of HIV. Clinical research clearly demonstrates that transmission of HIV from mother to child can be reduced by appropriate treatment.

It is important that health care providers ensure that all pregnant women are routinely counseled and encouraged to be tested for HIV. Consent for testing should be in accordance with the legal requirements of the jurisdiction where the testing is performed. Women who are found to be infected or who refuse testing must not be denied prenatal or other health care services.

Access to Care

Standard Care

Inequities in our national health care system present barriers to access to standard care for persons with HIV infection or AIDS. Nurses can play an important role in assisting HIV-infected persons and those with AIDS in obtaining standard care for their health needs by developing creative programs for service delivery to poor persons with HIV infection. In nurses' historic role as providers of information, nurses can assist HIV-infected persons in seeking out opportunities to obtain services. Finally, nurses can advocate for patients in their own institutions, through legislative routes in their states, and as voters.

Research Participation

The concept of access to care through research participation is relatively new and comes from three trends in modern society. The first is the reversal of how biomedical research is viewed intrinsically. That is, historically research had been considered a burden and a process in which persons must be protected from research risks. Today, in large part because of a vocal and well-organized AIDS lobby, research participation is seen by many as a benefit.

In all of medicine, there has been a major shift in how benefits and risks are understood. Over the last several decades in the United States, health care professionals have come to accept that assessment of risks and benefits is a personal matter, and only in part based on objective medical information. In research, this change has resulted in better informed consent procedures. This shift is grounded in the ethical maxim that health care professionals have an obligation to support autonomous decision making. The historical understanding of research as a burden posing risks from which subjects must be protected has given way to a view that the subject should play a central part in deciding just which risks are worth taking.

The second trend comes from increased appreciation of racial and gender imbalances in subject selection in research. While racial and gender inequities appear to exist in all sectors of our society, there has been an awakening to these inequities within the biomedical research community specifically. There is a new appreciation that as a result of women and minorities having been excluded from study populations, these populations are now receiving medical interventions based on faulty assumptions. To rectify this problem, federal guidelines on the inclusion of women and minorities[2] have been produced, and women and minority populations are being included more equitably in research.

The third trend relates to considerations of inequities in access to standard care—not research—but has implications for research participation. Because various populations within our society such as the poor, the homeless, and persons with HIV disease have problems gaining access to standard care, there has been a push to devise creative ways of providing needed care to these groups. One way that some have considered is through research participation.

Decisions Concerning Treatment and Withdrawal of Treatment

Informed Consent

Whether in research or in clinical care, informed consent is the basis of sound and ethically acceptable decision making. In the context of a terminal condition, decisions about initiating, withholding, or withdrawing medical care must be well considered. Nurses can assist patients greatly with these difficult decisions.

It is well established ethically and legally that an autonomous decision maker has the right to accept or reject any medical intervention he wishes. This moral norm is grounded in our social consensus that competent adults have the right to decide what will or will not be done with or to their bodies.

In the context of HIV infection and AIDS, nurses can assist patients in making decisions concerning initiating, withholding, or withdrawing treatment by providing adequate information in unbiased ways. Keeping in mind that informed consent is a process, a signed document is only a written manifestation of a process that takes time, patience, and sensitivity. Even when patients are fully capacitated, their ability to absorb large amounts of complex medical and/or research-related information may be compromised by fear, pain, or other distractions.

Advance Directives: Articulating Patient Preferences for Future Care

Advance directives are defined as the statement of desires, made by a competent person, directing her medical care in the event that she is unable to make decisions for herself. Formulating advance directives can assist persons with AIDS to live and die as they wish, having their decisions surrounding health and illness honored to the greatest degree possible.

There are a variety of means of documenting advance directives (as discussed in Chapter 24).

Discussions with patients, appropriately involved family members, and significant others is especially important in the population of persons who are infected with HIV. These patients are at risk for developing altered mental status and often wish to have a spokesperson other than their next of kin. The health of the appointed proxy may be an issue that needs addressing. The proxy may also be ill with HIV and his health may be failing as or more rapidly than the patient's. In this situation, further discussion with the patient is warranted to encourage the patient to designate an alternate proxy.

Do-Not-Resuscitate (DNR) and Comfort-Measures-Only (CMO) Orders

DNR and CMO orders are appropriately considered when the patient's disease has, in the words of Hippocrates, "overmastered" the patient. That is, at the point at which the disease process has progressed so that intervening in potentially reversible events is more a matter of prolonging the dying process than prolonging the living process, establishment of DNR or CMO orders is appropriate.

Optimally this is not the point at which discussion of such orders is being initiated. Health care providers should have discussions with patients sufficiently early in the course of their HIV infection that a patient's preferences can be anticipated. That way, when consideration of formally writing the order actually begins, all parties involved will be more comfortable having the discussions, and the orders will be a generally seamless extension of ongoing care.

Formalization of a DNR or a CMO order should be made in consultation with the patient. Although there may be an occasion when it is ethically permissible to write a DNR or CMO order over a patient's objection, such cases are rare and ethically controversial. Therefore, when disagreement about the timing of a DNR or CMO order arises, it is wise to call for a consultation with the facility's bioethicist or ethics committee chairperson to see if consensus can be reached.

When health care providers feel that resuscitation or other aggressive intervention is antithetical to sound and ethical medical practice, but the patient continues to request aggressive care, it may be more a matter of death anxiety in the patient than a reasoned request. In addition to calling for a bioethics consultation, if there is nursing or psychology staff specifically trained to work with dying patients, such persons should be consulted also. Practically, however, cases arise when a patient is unwilling to agree to a DNR or CMO order. Such cases can be wrenching for nurses and the rest of the health care team. But unless appropriate procedures are in place, such as an institutional ethics committee review, that permit DNR orders to be written over the objection of a patient, one can at least remember that even persons on respirators die of their disease process. No matter how aggressively we apply our technologies, eventually the disease will overmaster the patient.

Planned vs. Natural Death

Public discussion about planned vs. natural death, more commonly referred to as *suicide* and *assisted suicide*, has become more common in recent years. In the context of HIV infection and AIDS, it is not uncommon for patients to address this topic with their nurse. Regardless of one's personal views on the ethical permissibility of suicide, assisted suicide, or professional-assisted suicide, nurses are obligated ethically to protect and promote the life of their patients. Often that means providing care and compassion in an attempt to reduce pain and suffering without any attempt at retarding disease progression. Assisting in a patient's decision to withhold or withdraw medical treatment is not participating in a planned death. Such actions may simply be a matter of shifting from a curative to a palliative approach to the care of the dying. That is not, however, the same as suggesting that a nurse may assist in bringing about a patient's death. Doing so is not now permitted by any nursing code of ethics or accepted standards of ethical nursing practice.

There are occasions when methods of reducing pain and suffering can secondarily lead to a patient's death. Known as the *rule of double effect*, if a standardly used medical intervention shortens a patient's life but is administered with the intention of reducing pain and suffering, no ethical transgression has occurred. This is most commonly understood in the context of narcotic administration. Patients should be provided whatever is necessary to relieve pain. The fact that increasing doses of narcotics may depress respiration to levels incompatible with sustaining bodily functions ought not to be considered a barrier to pain relief. The goal is to keep patients comfortable through the terminal phase of their disease. If they die in the course of making that attempt then that is an ethically acceptable risk.

Decisions Related to Caregivers, Families, and Significant Others

Partner Involvement

When decisions about initiating, withholding, or withdrawing medical treatments for an HIV-infected or AIDS patient are being made, the degree to which a partner is involved should be determined by patient preferences. Meeting patient preferences in this context can influence positively the quality of patient decision making. Honoring patient preferences for the involvement of partners in decision making can increase markedly the prospects for sound decisions. The nurse's role here is to assist in clarifying the patient's preferences and then to facilitate those preferences.

The Decisionally Impaired Patient

Caring for a decisionally impaired patient can be highly complex. We use the term *decisionally impaired* interchangeably with the term *not-capacitated patient*. Neither of these terms, however, are synonymous with saying a patient is incompetent. Incompetency is a legal term that can only be applied by a court of law. Most persons who are unable to make their own decisions have never been declared incompetent. Those who have been, have a guardian (see Chapter 24). In this section we are talking about the full range of persons who, by virtue of the progression of their disease, are so decisionally impaired that they are unable to make their own health care decisions.

In the relatively straightforward case of a clearly identified surrogate with whom the patient has had detailed conversations and with whom there is no conflict with other family members, implementing patient wishes ought to present no special problems. If, however, there is conflict among family and personal caregivers, especially if such conflict is exacerbated by a lack of clearly articulated patient preferences, ascertaining what the patient might have wanted or, failing that, what is in the patient's best interest, can be difficult indeed.

Nurses can take an active, preventive role by having frank conversations with patients early in their disease process. When this is impossible, nurses can learn much about what a patient might have wanted by talking with those who have been closest to the patient. One wants to guard against the situation in which a long-standing partner, because nothing has been written down, is pushed aside by family members new on the scene. The ethical requirement is to apply a substituted judgment standard for decision making, and when that is unknown, to make a good-faith effort at approximating that standard to the greatest degree possible. For nurses this means standing firm in the face of stronger, perhaps more powerful, family members and even, perhaps, members of the health care team, attempting to make decisions for a decisionally impaired patient that seem not to be the decisions the person would have made for herself. Blood ties do not automatically identify the most ethically appropriate surrogate. The most ethically appropriate decision maker, if the patient has not identified a surrogate, will be the individual who can be expected to be best able to speak in the patient's voice. Only after vigorous attempts at meeting the substituted judgment standard should we fall back on the traditional standard of best interest.

Alternative Treatment Decisions and Sources of Information

Nurses can assist patients in coming to decisions that advance life goals by providing useful, accurate information in nonjudgmental ways. Here, like the earlier discussion of duty to treat, nurses must be self-monitoring of their own biases. Information and discussions about alternative approaches to care must be handled in a straightforward manner and with the same degree of professionalism and accuracy as discussing any orthodox treatment option. Nurses must be careful not to react judgmentally to the kinds of information that persons with HIV infection bring into the decision-making process nor dampen the empowering experience that bringing such information to the table can be for the patient. The nurse's obligation to assist patients to be self-determining agents includes tolerating and even fostering the power equalization that comes from a patient's investigations of alternative care approaches and alternative sources of information.

References

1. Cohen PT, Sande MA, Volberding PA. *The AIDS Knowledge Base.* Boston: Little, Brown; 1994.
2. Federal register. *NIH Guidelines on the Inclusion of Women and Minorities as Subjects in Clinical Research.* Washington, DC: US Government Printing Office, 1994. Part IV, March 9. Part 59 FR 11146-11151.

CHAPTER **24**

Legal Issues for the Clinician

Steven Jay Farber, PA-C, JD

Chapter Preview

- Informed Consent and the HIV Test
- Confidentiality
- Judgmental Capacity
- Advance Directives
- Guardianship Issues
- Insurance Issues

Well into the second decade of the HIV/AIDS epidemic, researchers have made great strides in identifying and developing new and often complex approaches to treating AIDS. However, there has been a continuing problem with the development of a variety of legal issues surrounding HIV/AIDS. For instance, the concept of informed consent as it applies to the HIV test itself is at times a problematic area. Confidentiality issues abound, especially concerning the privacy of one's HIV status and medical records. A medical practitioner's duty to warn those at possible risk of infection from a known positive patient continues to be a difficult issue. Competence issues surrounding an HIV/AIDS patient's decisional or judgmental capacity, especially as it relates to treatment issues, is a problematic area. Guardianship issues pertaining to the surviving children of HIV/AIDS patients, living wills, advance directives, and insurance problems are issues that are receiving more attention as of late.

A basic understanding of these difficult topics will allow nurses to approach their patients with understanding and an ability to direct and assist patients in seeking appropriate guidance and counseling.

Informed Consent and the HIV Test

In general, physicians and other medical providers must obtain a patient's consent prior to a medical procedure. However, when the procedure is the procurement of an HIV test there are more defined legal guidelines that often include statutory regulations.[1] For instance, many states require a patient's written or documented oral consent before the HIV antibody or other HIV test is performed. "Other HIV test" could include T-cell subset studies as well as viral load testing, which could presumably help make the diagnosis of HIV immunosuppression without a documented, positive HIV antibody test.

Therefore, it is clear that before a practitioner orders and a specimen is obtained for an HIV antibody or related test, except in rare exceptions, the patient must consent to such a test. There are two common scenarios for unconsented HIV testing. One case is when a patient is unable to grant or to withhold consent, no other authorized person is available to decide for the patient, and the test is needed for urgent care. In some states the test may be performed under these circumstances if informed consent is obtained as soon as practical. A second scenario for an unconsented HIV test is the case when a health care professional has had a significant exposure and the appropriate statutory criteria are met. Here too the patient must be offered, although he may refuse, informed consent. In addition, many states require not only consent but pre- and post test counseling by a trained individual.

Confidentiality

Issues concerning the confidentiality of HIV-related medical documents has been the subject of legal scholars and politicians since the early 1980s. Many states now have statutes that set forth requirements that must be met before HIV-related information can be disclosed. A general authorization for the release of medical information is not sufficient for the release of HIV-related medical records unless the release clearly indicates its request for HIV information as well as general medical information.

There are exceptions allowing HIV-related information to be released without express consent. The details vary from state to state and are set forth in the statutes. In some states, HIV-related information may be released to a health care provider or facility when it is required for appropriate care, to medical examiners, to hospital oversight review organizations, and to the patient or legal guardian as well as the ordering physician. In addition, utilizing partner notification regulations and acting within strict statutory guidelines, HIV status may be released by public health officers and physicians to partners of HIV-positive persons. A public health official may inform or warn partners that they may have been exposed to the HIV virus, without releasing the infected party's name.

Therefore, although state statutes have recognized the right of privacy of HIV-infected individuals, there are statutorily defined procedures for the release of HIV-related information to both public and private entities. Nurses should be aware of what is legal in the jurisdiction in which they practice and should not hesitate to seek legal counsel regarding specific situations before taking action.

Judgmental Capacity

The question of competence is a legal question and one that should be answered by a judge in a courtroom. People are allowed to make bad decisions and to have bad judgment. Sometimes when health care professionals disagree with a patient's decision concerning a procedure, test, or treatment, they may believe that the patient's mental status may be altered. A psychiatric consultation can comment on the patient's judgmental capacity, and this opinion, among others, will be weighed by the court making the decision.

If the patient is deemed incompetent in court, then a surrogate decision maker will be appointed. This person, depending on the state or jurisdiction, can be called several things: a *conservator*, *guardian*, or *health care agent*. The surrogate decision maker is appointed by the court, with the input of family members if there are any. The incompetent person may participate as well in the decision process, depending on the degree of dementia or incompetence. The guardian may be a member of the immediate family of the patient.

Advance Directives

The use of advance directives allows the person with HIV to choose a surrogate decision maker early in the course of the illness while her faculties are intact. In addition, through the use of a living will, she can direct the life-saving measures she would like implemented should the need arise.

Clearly if one desires to have control over one's life, to be able to make decisions even after the ability to make decisions is lost, then an advance directive in the form of a living will or durable power of attorney should be implemented. A living will may not only direct that there be no resuscitative efforts, but it may define and limit living-saving efforts and under what circumstance they may be applied. A power of attorney document or the appointment of health care agent authorizes someone else—a family member, friend, or even an attorney—to make decisions for the incompetent patient, and to manage financial, medical, or other affairs. However, both the living will and the power of attorney end with the death of the patient. At the time of death, a person's wishes can only be fulfilled through the use of a will.[2] If there is no will and someone dies intestate, then the state will impose its statutorily defined rules and distribute the deceased's estate per statute.

The documents necessary to implement a living will, health care proxy, or durable power of attorney are relatively straightforward and should be available in most hospitals' legal or social work departments. Currently, 45 states allow for both a living will and the appointment of a health care proxy.[3] Nurses who are familiar with local regulations and institutional resources can be of substantial service to patients by initiating a conversation and assisting patients in obtaining the necessary information and forms.

Guardianship Issues

It is estimated that in the United States alone more than 30,000 children have lost one or both parents to AIDS.[3] The problem is worse in other parts of the world, with more than 80,000 such orphans in Zambia alone, and estimates that by the year 2000 this number will swell to more than 625,000.[3] Figures like this and the mortality associated with AIDS make it imperative that parents with AIDS make plans for the care of their children. Further, parents with AIDS often become hospitalized and must arrange for someone to take responsibility for their children during hospitalization.

To address these troubling issues, one may utilize either permanent or temporary guardianship, or foster care. A guardian, whether permanent or temporary, acts as the child's parent, and can make decisions (including decisions for medical care) and is legally responsible for the child's well-being. Not all states have temporary guardianships. In those that do not, the parent may lose all parental rights to the child permanently by appointing a guardian, although in others the parent may retain some parental rights. In states that do have temporary guardianships, such an arrangement when documented before the fact may make a parent's hospitalization less stressful by simply knowing who will care for the children.

Foster care arrangements may be made as well, but there can be drawbacks to these arrangements. Foster homes are state controlled. Foster parents must undergo investigation by the state to meet guidelines for the safety and well-being of a child. It may be difficult for the parent to regain custody. In a so-called *kinship foster care* arrangement, the child will become the foster child of relatives. However, as foster care is state controlled, family members must be investigated as well, which can be a time-consuming process. In the interim the child will be a ward of the state.

Some relatives, although willing to care for the children, may be unwilling to undergo intense state scrutiny.

The problem with the care of a hospitalized person's children is one that allows no easy answers. The options are there, but none are as good as having the child and parent remain at home. The home care support systems that would allow this are growing, but are not yet widely available. More social programs and legislation are needed to allow for broader reimbursement for this compassionate and cost-effective program. Both the child and parent will benefit from maintaining the family structure and strengthening family bonds.

Insurance Issues

People with HIV have many concerns about insurance. The four most relevant types of insurance are health insurance, life insurance, disability insurance, and public entitlement programs. Perhaps of primary concern is getting insurance, keeping it, and benefiting from it.

Health Insurance

There are two classes of health insurance plans—those that are self-insured and those that are not self-insured. With self-insured plans, a large company insures its employees itself rather than buying insurance from an insurance company. These self-insured plans are regulated by federal law under the Employee Retirement Income Security Act.

The insurance industry has established policies and operating procedures to improve its profitability and protect itself from paying out to the insured. For instance, if one falsifies or omits a material fact on the initial insurance application form that concerns the applicant's health, the insurance company has the right to cancel the policy and return the premium. Of course if a policy is rescinded, the applicant has the right to contest the rescission. Under these circumstances, cashing a refunded premium may be construed as acceptance of the rescission.

Preexisting condition clauses are another way for insurance companies to limit their payouts. A preexisting condition is a condition that exists at the time of application for an insurance policy. Further, it may be construed to mean any condition that the applicant knew or should have known he had at the time of insurance. The preexisting condition clause lasts for a finite period of time, perhaps 6 months to 1 year. If an insured seeks to be reimbursed for a treated, preexisting condition, the insurance company will not reimburse.

Capping is a practice by which an insurance company will limit the amount of coverage for a given illness—AIDS, for instance. Capping is most prevalent in self-insured companies. In light of the Americans with Disabilities Act and several lawsuits, the practice of capping is less common than it once was.

Life Insurance

Life insurance is extremely important to many people with HIV. To limit liability, before a life insurance policy is issued an applicant will have to have an HIV test. If the applicant tests positive, in all likelihood the policy will be denied. Typically, life insurance benefits the surviving beneficiaries of the insured. That is, after the insured dies, his beneficiaries receive a cash payment. The AIDS epidemic has spawned a concept called *viatical settlements*. Here the insured can cash in the policy while alive and enjoy the proceeds. The many companies involved in viatical settlements vary as to the percentage of the policy they will cash and the number of years of life expectancy of the insured.

Disability Insurance

Disability insurance is insurance that covers an insured for a defined period of time and for a set sum should the insured be unable to work. The guidelines and protections offered to the insured as well as the insurance company are very similar to those that govern health and life insurance. Therefore, applicants should be aware of preexisting conditions and misrepresentations in the application process.

Public Insurance

In addition to private insurance there is also the availability of federal, state, or local programs. Programs like Medicare, Social Security Insurance, Medicaid, Aid For Dependent Children, and national programs like the AIDS Drug Assistance Program can help with various forms of medical and prescription drug coverage when no private insurance is available. There are strict eligibility guidelines for these programs, and the social work staff as well as the agencies involved may be very helpful. It is important that patients are aware of the availability of these options when they are in need of assistance. Further, assistance may be necessary during the often intimidating application process.

In summary, it should be clear by now that those living with HIV/AIDS, in addition to managing their illness and juggling medication schedules, medical appointments, and life's obligations in general must also face a myriad of legal issues. The following are the points of this chapter.

1. Informed consent and the HIV test is straightforward and, except for the rare exception, if there is no consent, there will be no test. In terms of the release of HIV-related medical information, generally the release must request HIV information specifically. A general medical release is not acceptable. Within statutory guidelines, specified health care professionals may legally notify the significant other of an HIV-positive patient if he believes them to be at risk.
2. A court of law determines if a person is incompetent, not a psychiatrist. A psychiatrist can comment on a patient's frame of mind and ability to make informed decisions. There are several options to have others make decisions for another person. In various jurisdictions, these options may be called *health care agent*, *power of attorney*, *conservator*, or *guardian*. If a person opts to make plans for her health care decisions while still capable of making decisions, this is called an *advance directive*. An advance directive may take several forms, including a living will, a surrogate decision maker, or health care proxy to name but a few.
3. Permanent or temporary guardianships as well as foster care arrangements can help make hospitalizations and transitions less stressful for AIDS patients with dependent children. The growing field of home care should allow more moderately ill patients to avoid hospitalization and help keep families together.
4. By avoiding misrepresentations and being aware of preexisting conditions, an HIV-positive insurance applicant can avoid unwanted surprises. Viatical settlements are allowing HIV/AIDS patients to enjoy

a degree of financial security previously unavailable. State and federal programs are available, but the application process may be tedious and the eligibility requirements strict.

Lastly, when faced with questions of a legal nature it is imperative to consult with your facility's legal department. If there is no legal department where you work, then seek an attorney familiar with medical issues. Make no medical-legal decisions on your own. The information discussed here should not be construed as legal advice. It is a general and brief overview of only a few, select legal issues.

References

1. Leonard AS, Bobinski AB, eds. *AIDS LAW and Policy: Cases and Materials.* 2nd ed. Houston: The John Marshall Publishing Company; 1995:31.
2. Terl AH. *AIDS and the Law. A Basic Guide for the Non-lawyer.* Washington, DC: Hemisphere Publishing; 1992:149–152.
3. Senak MS. *HIV, AIDS and the Law. A Guide to Our Rights and Challenges.* New York: Insight Books; 1996:221.

UNIT FOUR

HIV Special or Vulnerable Populations

CHAPTER 25

Women

Susan B. Sepples RN, CCRN, PhD

Chapter Preview

- Epidemiology
- Transmission
- Presentation and Course
- Pregnancy

Women remain especially vulnerable regarding HIV despite massive education campaigns aimed at women and health care providers who come in contact with them, a refocusing of the research agenda to include women in HIV clinical trials and treatment research, and a revision of the CDC case definition of AIDS to better incorporate women-specific manifestations of HIV infection (see Appendix A). Because women have social roles and meet social expectations that are different than those of men, and because HIV infection places different burdens on women, an understanding of the experiences of men living with HIV does not translate to an understanding of the experiences of women with HIV.

Epidemiology

In 1996, 20% of AIDS cases reported to the CDC were among women, of whom 60% were Hispanic or African-American. From 1992 thorough 1996 the proportion of women with AIDS has progressively increased (Table 25.1).[1] Through June 1995, injection drug use was reported as the primary mode of exposure in 43% of AIDS cases in white women, in 50% of cases in African-American women, and in 37% of cases in Hispanic women. In cases where heterosexual contact was the risk category (37% of cases in white women, 33% of cases in African-American women, and 44% of cases in Hispanic women), significantly more than half of white and Hispanic women, and about half of women reported sex with an injection drug user as the mode of exposure. This means that injection drug use either directly or indirectly accounts for nearly 70% of HIV infection in women. In young women, heterosexual exposure is reported in more than half of all cases as the primary risk factor. The geographic pattern of HIV among women differs little from that seen among men.[2]

In January 1993 the AIDS surveillance definition was expanded to include conditions seen frequently in HIV-infected women and injection drug users. In addition to cervical cancer and bacterial pneumonia, individuals with a positive antibody test and a CD4 lymphocyte count of <200 cells/mm^3 are included in the revised definition. As a result, 59% of AIDS cases in women in 1994 were reported based on the revised criteria.[3]

Statistics reported on women with HIV infection differ somewhat from those gathered on men. Because it is not possible to determine the actual source of transmission, all reported cases in men and women are listed

Table 25.1 Number and Percentages of Persons Reported with AIDS, by Gender–United States 1992–1996

Gender	1992	1993	1994	1995	1996
Female	6,307 (14%)	16,671 (16%)	13,830 (18%)	13,682 (19%)	13,820 (20%)
Male	40,330 (86%)	87,945 (84%)	64,730 (82%)	59,285 (81%)	54,653 (80%)

From CDC. Update: trends in AIDS incidence, deaths, and prevalence—United States, 1996. *MMWR*. 1997;46(8):316.

only once according to hierarchical exposure categories. While there is a category for men with two reported modes of exposure, sexual (men having sex with men) and blood borne (injection drug use), there is no comparable category for women who are both injection drug users and partners of injection drug users. Because women who use drugs are often engaged in relationships with men who use drugs, they may be exposed through heterosexual contact, although they are listed as injection drug users.[2]

Transmission

Women acquire HIV primarily via parenteral or sexual transmission. Regarding parenteral transmission, a number of cofactors have been shown to augment risk of parenteral transmission in women injection drug users: (1) distorted perceptions of risk related to drug use; (2) the practice of bartering sex, specifically sex without a condom, for money or drugs; and (3) a lifestyle in a culture defined by violence.[4] Women drug users may be less influenced than men by education to change unsafe behaviors. In one study of 263 men and 126 women, 19% of men continued to share needles after receiving HIV education while 42% of women receiving the same information continued to share.[5] It is not known why gender factors differ so significantly in this study. Perhaps information reaching women is not relevant (or realistic), perhaps women face different obstacles than men in changing risk practices, or perhaps they are not equally able to access harm prevention information.

The sexual partners of injection drug users are an almost invisible group of women at risk. While women injection drug users tend to be in heterosexual relationships with other injection drug users, almost 80% of male injection drug users are in relationships with women who do not use drugs.[6] The partners of injection drug users often face economic and emotional problems similar to those of women who use drugs, but are not similarly targeted for education and prevention.

HIV is transmitted sexually both from men to women and from women to women when body fluids are exchanged. Cofactors that augment sexual transmission of HIV to women include (1) adolescent physiology, (2) vaginal and cervical trauma, and (3) sexually transmitted diseases (STDs). All may affect physiologic barriers to viral infection adversely. Although HIV has been cultured in almost all body fluids, only blood, semen, and vaginal secretions have been implicated in transmission.[7] Male-to-female transmission may be more efficient because of the larger area of exposed mucosal surface in the female genital tract. The risk of heterosexual transmission to a woman is increased significantly in the presence of STDs; during anal intercourse, although vaginal intercourse is sufficient; and when her male partner has a high viral load (when HIV infection has progressed to AIDS).[8]

Trauma to the vagina increases the risk of contact between virally infected semen and blood. Trauma can occur as a result of inadequate lubrication in adolescent women or as a result of forced penetration.

STDs may both increase transmission of the virus and enhance susceptibility to transmission of HIV. STDs such as genital herpes, chancroid, HPV, and syphilis can create ulcers that disrupt the lining of the female genital tract. STDs that cause vaginal inflammation may act as local irritants and bring lymphocytes in contact with virus by initiating a systemic immune response.[9]

Prevention of Sexually Acquired HIV: Methods Women Can Use

Since 1990, to the credit of social and scientific activists, more attention has been directed toward understanding transmission to women in an effort to develop methods women can use to protect themselves from HIV infection. This research has led to advances in understanding the relationship between STDs and viral infection; uncovered the role of bacteria in transmission, indicating the need for advances in the development of microbicides as well as virucides; and demonstrated the effectiveness of barrier methods, such as the diaphragm, in protecting against gonorrhea, *Trichomonas*, and chlamydia. Unfortunately, the acceptability to women and the effectiveness of many of these methods are still open issues.[10]

Chemical Barriers

Commercially prepared, over-the-counter spermicides are probably the most accessible and effective form of protection women can use. They have been found to be active against HIV, CMV, herpes simplex type II, hepatitis B virus, *Neisseria gonorrhoea, Treponema pallidum, Trichomonas vaginalis*, and *Candida albicans*. They are most effective in preventing infection when used with a condom during intercourse. When not used with a condom and even when inserted after intercourse, they provide some effectiveness in preventing STDs.[11]

Nonoxynol-9 (N9) is perhaps the best known chemical barrier method available to women, and the active ingredient in most spermicides. N9 is a microbicide that provides protection against certain STD pathogens. N9 has been shown to reduce the spread of chlamydia and gonorrhea by as much as 50%, and has been associated with a decreased risk of cervical cancer and, inferentially, HPV.

Other microbicides are being developed that are active against a broader spectrum of pathogens than N9. Some of these, like N9, disrupt the outer membrane of pathogens. Other chemical preparations augment physiologic barriers to infection or change the acidity of vaginal secretions (Table 25.2).[12] Virucides are being investigated that would provide women wishing to conceive with protection from the virus without contraception. Dextran sulfate is a virucide that is currently being laboratory tested.[10]

Physical Barriers

Cervical caps and diaphragms, when used with a spermicide, provide both chemical and mechanical barriers to infection. While they leave a significant portion of the lower genital tract unprotected, they offer good protection against organisms that infect the cervix, such as gonococci and chlamydia, and may protect against cervical cancer and HPV.

It has been postulated that cervical ectopy, seen in adolescents and in women using oral contraceptives (OCPs), may play a role in transmission. Physical barrier methods afford protection to adolescent women and women on long-term oral contraceptives. Barrier methods may also protect a woman's sexual partners. In one study, shedding of virus was found more frequently at the cervix than in the vagina. For infected women whose partner refuses to use protection, this method provides women with a possible means to prevent transmitting the virus.[10]

The female condom offers high-level protection against STD, protecting both internal and external genitalia from exposure. It has proved imperme-

Table 25.2 Prevention: Methods Women Can Use

Method	Advantages	Disadvantages	Information for Health Care Providers
Chemical barriers	Readily available, inexpensive, safe; some effectiveness when used after intercourse; effective against a number of pathogens; provide broad-spectrum protection	May be less effective for women with multiple partners; may be irritating	Microbicides are both contraceptive and protect against infection; virucides provide protection against infection without contraception; more effective when used in conjunction with barrier methods
Physical barriers	Safe, discrete, nontoxic; diaphragm and cap provide effective protection against infections of the cervix, and protect partners from cervical viral shedding; female diaphragm can be bought over the counter; does not require fittings	Diaphragm and cervical cap are less effective protection in women who have had vaginal deliveries; female diaphragm is cumbersome and expensive	Women need teaching and practice on proper positioning; need to be "fit" and refit for internal barriers when weight is lost or gained
Natural methods	Provide alternatives to chemical and physical barriers when these are not available	Require comfort with own body and assertiveness with partner about alternative forms of intercourse; require that the woman is well educated and motivated; less effective in preventing transmission than barrier methods	Involves educating clients on the concept of relative risk; counseling on the relative risk of various sexual practices is critical

able to CMV and HIV.[11] However, it is cumbersome, visible, expensive (approximately $3.00 per condom), and difficult to find. Predictably, it has not been well received by women.

Education

Emphasizing methods women can use in preventing the transmission of HIV is important in educating and teaching women about HIV infection. Education about the use of condoms for the prevention of HIV, when comprehensive and extensive, has also proven to be an effective tool. A large multisite evaluation on the outcome of one-on-one education and counseling regarding condom use among women found that consistent condom use increased from 13% at enrollment to 36% at the 3-month follow-up. The fact that OCPs offer no protection against STDs should be emphasized. Women who are HIV infected need to be vigilant about reexposure to HIV and to other STDs.

Presentation and Course

Women are different than men in terms of HIV infection. Fat-to-muscle distribution and hormonal shifts make women respond differently to drugs. Women have different vulnerability to infection because of unique physical structures; women have different diseases, such as cervical dysplasia; and they are the ones who become pregnant.

An analysis of surveillance data through 1990 showed that even before changes in the surveillance reporting of AIDS, women and men presented with different rates of OI. Women in this study were shown to present more often with oral and esophageal candidiasis and less often with PCP than men.[13] This corroborates findings from earlier studies[14] which demonstrated that women get different infections; however, the infections limited to those in the surveillance definition before 1991 that were more prevalent in women were not particularly more hazardous. Women-specific HIV problems not discussed in other chapters of the book are considered in some detail here because they probably make up a significant portion of what is different between men and women clinically in terms of HIV infection. When relevant material is covered in another chapter of this book, the reader is referred there.

Gynecological Disease and HIV

Health care providers working in women's health clinics are on the front lines in terms of early diagnosis and treatment of HIV in women. Many women use their women's health providers as primary care providers. Recommendations for gynecologic screening and care of HIV-infected women are constantly reevaluated as more is understood about the natural history of HIV in women. An approach to the clinical care of infected women has been developed by Williams[15] and is outlined in Table 25.3.

Vaginal Candidiasis

Vaginal candidiasis is often the earliest manifestation of HIV in women, and often the harbinger of more severe OIs. Vaginal *Candida* infections are usually persistent and severe in women with HIV infection, and often they return when treatment is withdrawn. In one study,[16] 86% percent of women with recurrent, severe vaginal candidiasis developed other OIs within a 30-month period. Vaginal candidiasis is discussed in the Fungal Infections section of Chapter 4 and its treatment is discussed in the Fungal Infections section of Chapter 5.

Unfortunately, because vaginal *Candida* is not an unusual infection in healthy women and because over-the-counter treatments have become available recently, women may delay in seeking health care for these infections. Women need to be made aware that recurrent or refractory vaginal infections are an indication for follow-up care. HIV-infected women report an increase in frequency and severity of vaginal infections between 6 months and 3 years before being tested for HIV. Typically women with previous histories of vaginitis report at least a doubling of the incidence of vaginal infections after HIV infection.[17]

Human Papillomavirus

HPV is widespread in the United States, with 20% of the adult population (40 million people) harboring this virus. HPV is responsible for genital warts; vaginal, cervical, and penile lesions; precancerous conditions; and cervical and anal cancer. HPV is readily transmitted, not only sexually but through skin-to-skin contact (young women have reportedly contracted

Table 25.3 Guidelines for Gynecologic Care of the HIV-Infected Woman

Visit	History	Physical Exam	Laboratory
Initial	Sexual, menstrual, obstetric, family planning, breast, review of symptoms	Breast, abdomen, pelvic, rectal	Cervical Pap, gonorrhea screen, chlamydia screen, syphilis serology, mammography (when appropriate), microscopic examination of vaginal secretions
Interim and on every visit	Review of symptoms: vaginal discharge, pruritus, rash, genital sores, lumps, abdominal or pelvic pain, dyspareunia, dysuria, last menstrual period	As indicated by history; if any symptoms, complete pelvic exam	Microscopic examination of vaginal secretions as indicated by history and physical exam
Annual	Changes in libido or function, menstrual history, contraceptive practices, review of current symptoms (listed above under Interim and on every visit)	Breast, abdomen, pelvic, rectal	Cervical Pap smear, gonorrhea screen, chlamydia screen, syphilis serology, mammography (if indicated), microscopic examination: saline and potassium hydroxide

Williams AB. Gynecologic care of women with human immunodeficiency virus infection. *Clin Excel Nurs Pract.* 1(2):116, 1977.

HPV by sharing underwear). At the cervix, HPV causes local immune suppression, leaving women more vulnerable to other STDs. HPV causes papillations, fronds, or warts of tissue containing a capillary loop, which add to the vascular surface of the genital tract and may potentiate transmission of HIV infection. HPV is seen frequently in women with HIV infection. Risk factors for HIV and HPV infection are similar, but there is also evidence that immunosuppression may predispose women to HPV infection and cervical cancer.[18]

More than 60 molecular types of HPV have been identified. About 15 have been isolated in the genital tract; some are relatively harmless, whereas others (types 16, 18, 31, 33, 35, 45, 51, 52, and 56) have been found to be more pathogenic. The infection is not reportable and often, because it can be difficult to detect and because cell sampling techniques differ significantly, estimates from different populations may be confounding. Genital HPV is of concern because it is linked to cervical cancer—a threat that is magnified in the presence of immunosuppression. HPV is also discussed in the Viral Infections section of Chapter 4, and its treatment is discussed in the Viral Infections section of Chapter 5.

Cervical Dysplasia/Cervical Carcinoma

There is a clear association between HIV and cervical dysplasia/neoplasia that increases with advanced HIV infection (see Chapter 6).

STDs

STDs may significantly increase the woman's risk of HIV infection and the rate of transmission of HIV to sexual partners. Clinical manifestations and natural histories of STDs may be altered by HIV. STD treatment recommendations may differ in the presence of HIV infection.[1] Studies have indicated that conditions that cause genital ulcers are strongly associated with HIV-1 infection. Studies in the United States as well as abroad have determined that ulcerative disease is an independent risk factor for HIV infection. In this country the two most common ulcerative diseases believed to contribute to HIV risk among heterosexuals are genital herpes and syphilis.[19] STDs that are characterized by ulceration (including chancroid, herpes, and syphilis) may provide a direct port of entry for HIV or, because they cause an inflammatory immune response resulting in a migration of lymphocytes to the area, may facilitate viral infection of circulating lymphocytes.[20]

HSV occurs more frequently in women with HIV infection, resulting in lesions that become more persistent, widespread, and painful as the immune system deteriorates. HSV is discussed in the Viral Infections section of Chapter 4, and its treatment is discussed in the Viral Infections section of Chapter 5.

Because STDs are often seen in combination, when treating one STD it is always critical to consider the possibility of others. HIV-infected women seem to be at increased risk of pelvic inflammatory disease (PID), and infections associated with PID are more severe in this population.

Menstrual Irregularities and Infertility

Research on menstrual irregularities and HIV is difficult to assess because of confounding variables. The incidence of amenorrhea among women with HIV has been described alternately as significant and as coincidental. Amenorrhea may be related to HIV symptoms, such as profound weight loss in women with wasting syndrome, or treatment with certain drugs.[21] A large-scale study conducted to look at menstrual irregularities found that women with asymptomatic and mildly symptomatic HIV infection were more likely to have both menstrual abnormalities and clinically defined amenorrhea (longer than 3 months without menstruating).[22] Other findings from this research suggest that HIV-infected women may have more anovulatory cycles. On the other hand, menstrual irregularities were not apparent in a US study of 55 HIV-infected women when compared with a matched control group. This study controlled for confounding variables of injection drug use, methadone maintenance, and weight loss, and failed to confirm reports of the higher prevalence of menstrual symptoms in HIV-infected women. As early recognition and more effective treatment of HIV becomes available, long-term follow-up studies will be necessary to determine if menstrual irregularities are a late presenting symptom in HIV-related illness.[23]

Infertility in women with HIV is not well understood. Except for reports of an increased incidence of anovulatory cycles in HIV-infected women, there has been little in the literature about the effect of HIV on fertility. Women concerned about menstrual changes and irregularities should be encouraged to keep menstrual diaries. Obtaining a detailed menstrual history will help in ruling out treatable causes of menstrual irregularities such as anxiety, impaired nutrition, and drug-related effects.

Pregnancy

By far the greatest focus of all research on women with HIV has surrounded reproductive issues, which is in large part because a significant proportion of women have been diagnosed as HIV infected only when they became pregnant. Women traditionally seek health care in significant numbers primarily for reproductive issues. In general, young women are known to avoid prenatal care when their self-care behaviors, such as smoking, drinking, and drug use, will be questioned. For this reason, prenatal care is poorest in women with the highest risk pregnancies. This tends to hold true for HIV-infected women. Since the effectiveness of Zidovudine in preventing vertical transmission of HIV has been demonstrated, mandatory or at least routinized screening of all women for HIV has again become a focus of debate.

Changes in the immune system during normal pregnancy are in some respects similar to those seen in HIV infection. HIV-infected women have a greater and more sustained drop in CD4 lymphocytes during pregnancy and may not recover immune mechanisms as readily as seronegative women. Maternal lymphocyte production is decreased by the lack of HLA antigens in the placenta. Other nonspecific immunosuppressive effects of pregnancy include the production of pregnancy-specific beta-1 glycoprotein, human placental lactogen, human chorionic gonadotropin, estrogen, and progesterone. Pregnancy is a mildly immunosuppressive state because of a decrease in the number and functioning of CD4 lymphocytes. The ratio of helper to suppressor lymphocytes (usually 1.7:2.3) decreases to 0.9:1.92. While these factors may influence the development of infection and its response to treatment, they are also mitigated by factors such as age, nutritional status, and substance abuse.[24]

Early in the epidemic many clinicians were concerned about the effect of pregnancy on the health of HIV-infected women. However, despite the potential for progression of HIV due to immunologic changes in pregnancy, this has not been completely the case. Although women with advanced HIV infection may have a rapid progression of disease and ultimately a poor prognosis, in women with asymptomatic disease pregnancy does not aggravate the course of HIV infection.[24]

HIV-infected pregnant women will require more thorough physical examinations, and should be followed closely by both their obstetric practitioner and an infectious disease specialist. Physical exam should include careful monitoring for weight loss, as second- and third-trimester weight loss of more than 10% can be indicative of wasting syndrome. Any increase in temperature is cause for a full workup, as this is often the earliest indication of an OI. Skin and mouth exams, and lymph node assessment, which are not routinely preformed in pregnancy, are part of routine prenatal care for HIV-infected women.

CD4+ levels are monitored closely and pregnant women are treated prophylactically with trimethoprim-sulfamethoxazole or pentamidine for *Pneumocystis carinii* pneumonia when CD4+ levels drop below 200 cells/mm^3, or less than 20% of the total lymphocyte count. Zidovudine, once recommended for prophylaxis for CD4+ levels below 500 cells/mm^3, is now recommended as a means of preventing vertical transmission even in the presence of normal CD4+ counts. Zidovudine suppresses bone marrow, exacerbating pregnancy-related anemia. Headache, nausea, fever, and fatigue are other common side effects. Zidovudine in crossing the placenta, may affect fetal marrow as well.[25]

Vertical transmission is considered to occur mainly from transplacental exchange of blood. Potential mechanisms may include (1) infection of the placental macrophage, (2) infection of the syncytiotrophoblastic layer of the placenta, or (3) complete passage of maternal blood into fetal circulation. At delivery, transmission of the virus may occur as a result of microscopic injuries that allow for the mixing of maternal and fetal blood. The virus has also been detected in and apparently passed via breast milk.[26] Maternal factors associated with an increased risk of vertical transmission include (1) low CD4 counts, (2) high maternal viral titer, (3) advanced HIV infection, (4) the presence of p24 antigen in maternal serum, (5) placental membrane inflammation, (6) intrapartum complications resulting in fetal exposure to maternal blood, and (7) ruptured membranes for more than 4 hours. The rate of transmission is estimated to be between 13 and 40%.[27]

In February 1995, results were reported from the National Institutes of Health AIDS Clinical Trial Group ACTG-076 on reducing vertical transmission with Zidovudine.[28] Zidovudine was found to reduce perinatal transmission of HIV by as much as two-thirds in women with CD4+ counts higher than 500 cells/mm^3. The CDC published guidelines for HIV counseling and testing for pregnant women; the goal being to provide early intervention for both the health of the mother and to reduce the likelihood of fetal transmission. It was proposed that early recognition in pregnant women might translate to a better survival rate for women in general. However, opponents of routine testing were concerned that women, worried about being HIV infected, might put off seeking prenatal care, ultimately a greater risk to their health and the health of their baby. At present, recommendations state that all women should be offered the option of HIV testing when they seek prenatal care.[26] Prenatal counseling is far from standardized. It is critical that health care providers working in prenatal care be versed in current counseling recommendations. Counseling and testing courses are offered at the state level for health care providers.

The long-term effects of Zidovudine for both treated mothers and infants are not yet known, and health care providers must encourage women to consider the benefits and the risks in making a decision. As few as 13% of infants born to HIV-infected women are infected, thus the high proportion of infants needlessly exposed to potentially teratogenic drugs is under scrutiny. Research on viral load and transmission rates suggests there is a difference in the relationship between viral load and transmission in women with early HIV infection (less immunocompensation) and women with significant immunosuppression.[29] For some women, the risk of taking Zidovudine when so little is known about its effect is too high, whereas for others this risk is minimized when it is considered in light of the risk of having an HIV-infected child. It is a significant burden for women to make these decisions.

In the postpartum period women must be instructed carefully about the risks of infection. Worsening of fatigue, anorexia, weight loss, cough, skin lesions, or vaginitis are reportable problems. Contraceptive counseling, with information on methods of safer sex women can employ, should be provided to women before discharge. Nutritional teaching and information about gynecologic follow-up according to the guidelines of the American College of Obstetrics and Gynecology (ACOG) should be provided. Women may be overwhelmed by the care of their HIV-infected infant and may require additional follow-up and support after discharge.[26]

In summary, women with HIV have specific and unique needs. The issues affecting them are only beginning to be understood. There is little in the literature on the specific legal and social assistance needed by women with HIV. Although only anecdotally reported, the social isolation of HIV-infected women may have significant implications for their care. Women represent a population whose HIV-related needs are becoming evermore apparent.

References

1. CDC. Update: trends in AIDS incidence, deaths, and prevalence—United States, 1996. *MMWR.* 1997;46(8):166–173.
2. CDC. *HIV/AIDS surveillance report.* Atlanta, GA: CDC, Division of HIV/AIDS Prevention. 1995. no. 1.
3. CDC. Update: AIDS among women—United States, 1994. *MMWR.* 1995;44(5): 81–84.
4. Des Jarlais DC, Friedman SR, Hopkins W. Risk reduction for the acquired immunodeficiency syndrome among intravenous drug users. *Ann Intern Med.* 1985;103:755–759.
5. Saalfield C, Chris C, Lurie R, Pearl M. Intravenous drug use, women and HIV. In: *Women AIDS and Activism.* New York: The ACT UP/NY Women & AIDS Book Group; South End Press 1990:123–129.
6. Des Jarlais DC, Friedman SR, Novick DM, et al. HIV-1 infection among intravenous drug users in Manhattan, New York City, from 1977–1987. *JAMA.* 1989; 261:1008–1012.
7. Holman S. Epidemiology and transmission of HIV infection in women. *J Nurse Midwifery* 1989;34:233–241.
8. Ickovics JR, Rodin J. Women and AIDS in the United States: epidemiology, natural history, and mediating mechanisms. *Health Psychol.* 1992;11:1–16.
9. Smeltzer SC, Whipple B. Women with HIV infection: the unrecognized population. *Health Values.* 1991;15:41–48.
10. Stein Z. HIV prevention: an update on the status of methods women can use. *Am J Public Health.* 1993;83:1379–1381.
11. Rosenberg MJ, Gollub EL. Commentary: methods women can use that may prevent sexually transmitted disease, including HIV. *Am J Public Health.* 1992; 82:1473–1477.
12. Cohen J. Women: absent term in the AIDS research equation. *Science.* 1995; 269:777–780.
13. Murrain M. Differences in opportunistic infection rates in women with AIDS. *J Women's Health.* 1993;2:243–248.
14. Carpernter CJ, Mayer KH, Fisher A, et al. Natural history of acquired immunodeficiency syndrome in women in Rhode Island. *Am J Med.* 1989;86:771–775.

15. Williams AB. Gynecological care of women with immunodeficiency virus infection. *Clin Excel Nurs Pract.* 1997;1(2):115–123.
16. Rhoads JL, Wright CD, Redfield RR, Burke DS. Chronic vaginal candidiasis in women with human immunodeficiency virus infection. *JAMA.* 1987;257: 3105–3107.
17. Baker DA. Management of the female HIV infected patient. *AIDS Res Hum Retroviruses.* 1994;10:935–938.
18. Franke-Ruta G. Women & AIDS. Cervical cancer in women with HIV. *QW.* 1992; 52–53.
19. Hook EW, Cannon RO, Nahmias AJ, et al. Herpes simplex virus infection as a risk factor for human immunodeficiency virus infection in heterosexuals. *J Infect Dis.* 1992;165:251–255.
20. Leonard Z. HIV-antibody testing and legal issues for HIV positive people. In: Banzahaf M. ed. *Women, AIDS and Activism.* New York: The ACT UP/NY Women and AIDS Book Group; South End Press 1990:55–56.
21. Anderson JR. Early intervention for HIV in a gynecologic setting. *J Women's Health.* 1993;2:343–347.
22. Chirwig KD, Feldman J, Muneyyici-Delale O, Landesman S, and Minkoff H. Menstrual function in human immunodeficiency virus-infected women without acquired immunodeficiency syndrome. *J Acquir Immun Syndr Human Retrov.* 1996;12:489–494.
23. Shah PN, Smith JR, Wells C, et al. Menstrual symptoms in women infected by the human immunodeficiency virus. *Obstet Gynecol.* 1994;83:397–400.
24. Tinkle MB, Amaya MA, Tamayo OW. HIV disease and pregnancy. Part 1. Epidemiology, pathogenesis, and natural history. *JOGNN.* 1992;21:86–93.
25. Acosta YM, Goodwin C, Amaya MA, et al. HIV disease and pregnancy. Part 2. Antepartum and intrapartum care. *JOGNN.* 1992;21:97–103.
26. Bastin N, Tamayo OW, Tinkle MB. HIV disease and pregnancy. Part 3. Postpartum care of the HIV positive woman and her newborn. *JOGNN.* 1992;21:105–110.
27. CDC. *U.S. Public Health Service Recommendations for HIV Counseling and Testing for Pregnant Women.* Atlanta, GA; 1995.
28. Conner EM, Sperling RS, Gelber R, et al. Reduction of maternal-infant transmission of human immunodeficiency virus type 1 with zidovudine treatment. Pediatric AIDS Cinical Trials Group. *N Engl J Med.* 1994;331:1173–1180.
29. Thea, DM et al. Maternal viral load and perinatal transmission. *AIDS.* 1997; 11(4):435–444.

CHAPTER 26

Infants, Children, and Adolescents

Arlene Manns Butz, RN, CPNP, ScD
Alain Joffe, MD

Chapter Preview

- HIV Infection in Infants and Children
- Adolescents and HIV Infection
- Resources

HIV Infection in Infants and Children

Perinatal HIV infection continues to have a profound impact on young children in the United States. HIV infection is now the fifth leading cause of death in children less than 15 years of age and the seventh leading cause of death in children age 1 to 4 years in the United States.[1] HIV infection in children is similar to childhood cancers, cystic fibrosis, sickle cell disease, and other pediatric chronic illnesses in that it is treatable but not curable.[2] Although a variety of treatment interventions are available, early diagnosis of HIV infection in children is the key to providing the highest quality and duration of life. This chapter addresses pediatric and adolescent HIV infection.

Epidemiology of Pediatric HIV Infection

As of June 1997, 7,902 children less than 13 years of age have been diagnosed with AIDS.[3] The epidemic in children less than 13 years of age closely parallels the HIV epidemic in women (see Chapter 25 p. 614) because the predominant mode of transmission is mother to infant or perinatal transmission.[4] The racial/ethnic distribution of pediatric HIV infection is overrepresented in minority populations, specifically African-Americans (55%) (see Chapter 29) and Hispanics (20%) (see Chapter 28).

In children the primary routes of transmission of HIV infection are (1) mother to infant or perinatal transmission; (2) transfusion acquired, such as children with hemophilia; (3) sexual intercourse by consensual agreement or through sexual abuse; and (4) IV drug use. Perinatal transmission, the predominant mode of transmission, is believed to occur at three different times during a pregnancy: (1) antepartum, transplacentally in utero accounting for 30 to 50% of perinatal transmission; (2) intrapartum, during the delivery process by exposure to infected maternal blood in 50 to 70%; or (3) postpartum, by ingestion of breast milk in 10 to 15%.[5] The overall perinatal transmission rate from an HIV-infected mother to her infant is between 20 to 30%,[5–8] with the majority of infants who are born to an HIV-infected mother being uninfected.[9] Risk factors associated with an increased rate of perinatal transmission include the viral load of HIV in the mother at time of conception, low maternal CD4+ lymphocyte count, overall maternal health status, placental factors such as maternal chorioamnionitis, and fetal and newborn factors.[5,6] Because the impact of breast-feeding on the overall mother to child transmission rate is uncertain, HIV-infected women should be counseled not to breast-feed.[10]

Older children may be exposed to HIV through sexual abuse and child prostitution. Sexual abuse is often overlooked as a route of transmission in children. The high prevalence of sexual abuse in HIV-infected children also has important implications for siblings of these children.[11,12]

Diagnosis of HIV Infection in Infants and Children

Optimal outcomes for infants and children rely on early diagnosis of HIV infection, starting ideally early in the pregnancy. The importance of early diagnosis is to identify HIV-infected infants so they can receive prompt PCP prophylaxis to prevent PCP, which is sometimes fatal in young infants. Testing for HIV during pregnancy allows HIV-infected pregnant women the opportunity to benefit from medical interventions to maintain or improve their own health and decrease the risk of transmission of HIV infection to their infants. The ACTG-076 study demonstrated that use of zidovudine given orally to the mother during the second and third trimesters of pregnancy, intravenously during labor and delivery, and orally to the infant during the first 6 weeks of life reduced the HIV perinatal transmission rate by two-thirds from 25% to 8%.[13] However, long-term risks of zidovudine therapy, as administered in the ACTG-076 protocol, are unknown.

Because some HIV-infected children may not be identified at birth, health care providers (HCPs) should be familiar with clinical signs and symptoms of HIV infection in infants and children. Clinical indicators for testing infants and children born to mothers with an unknown HIV status are:

- Failure to thrive
- Generalized lymphadenopathy
- Recurrent bacterial infections
- Chronic diarrhea
- Hepatosplenomegaly
- Developmental delay
- Recurrent oral candidiasis
- Radiographic evidence of persistent, diffuse lung disease
- Maternal risk factors for HIV infection: substance abuse, multiple sexual partners, history of sexual contact with known infected partner

Specific HIV Tests for Infants and Older Children

The specific HIV tests used to detect HIV infection in infants and children are described in Table 26.1. The most commonly used tests are enzyme-linked immunoassay (EIA) plus Western blot, PCR, and HIV culture.

Laboratory Evaluation for HIV Infection in Infants and Children

Testing for the presence of HIV in infants less than 18 months of age is complicated by the presence of maternal HIV antibody from passive transfer that may not accurately reflect the infant's HIV status. Several laboratory tests to diagnose HIV infection are available for infants and children. HIV culture and PCR are the preferred laboratory tests for diagnosing HIV infection in infants. Recommendations for testing infants and children for HIV are the following:[14,15]

- HIV culture or PCR should be performed three times: once at 4 days of age, once at ≥1 month of age and once at ≥4 months of age. If the result of any test is positive, testing should be repeated to confirm the diagnosis of HIV infection.
- The diagnosis to rule out HIV infection in infants is based on two or more negative viral diagnostic tests (HIV culture or PCR), both of which are performed at ≥1 month of age and one of which is performed at ≥4 months of age.
- For clinical centers that do not have access to the viral diagnostic tests such as HIV culture and PCR, HIV infection can be ruled out based on two or more negative HIV antibody tests performed at ≥6 months of age.

For children older than 2 years of age, the standard HIV antibody tests of EIA plus Western blot are adequate for detecting HIV infection.

Ensuring voluntary and informed consent for HIV testing is the responsibility of the health professional caring for the child and family. Interpretation of the test results is very important, especially until a definite diagnosis is reached. Clarifying misconceptions of infants being "carriers" of HIV infection or misunderstanding the loss of maternal antibody is difficult for many families.[16]

Monitoring Immune Status in Infants and Children

Other laboratory tests used to monitor HIV disease progression include the CD4+ count and percentage. Monitoring the CD4+ cell counts

Table 26.1 HIV Diagnostic Tests for Infants[a]

HIV Test Name	Availability, Time to Results, and Cost
EIA	Standard antibody HIV test that is highly sensitive and specific; useful after 18 months of age; positive EIA test requires confirmation with a follow-up Western blot test **Time to result:** 1–2 days up to 1 week **Cost:** For a positive specimen, $50 ($3–$5 for EIA + $40–$50 for Western blot)
PCR	Sensitive test if performed in qualified lab for early diagnosis of HIV; more sensitive than p24 antigen; less expensive than HIV viral culture; available at most referral centers for HIV **Time to result:** 1–2 days **Cost:** $175
HIV culture	Gold standard in virology testing in infants; expensive, labor intensive, and results not available for 4–6 weeks after processing; positive result is diagnostic of HIV infection, but negative culture does not always rule out infection; sensitivity[b] of HIV culture and PCR combined: ≤50%, at 1 week of age; >90%, at 3 months of age; >99%, at 6 months of age[16,17] **Time to result:** 15–35 days **Cost:** $250[c]
p24 antigen	Helpful in establishing diagnosis of HIV but not a reliable prognostic indicator for HIV infection; less sensitive than either HIV culture or PCR, especially when anti-HIV antibody levels are high because it fails to detect immune-complexed p24 antigen **Time to result:** 1–2 days **Cost:** $25[c]
anti-HIV IgA antibodies	Useful after 4 months of age; not available in many settings, not commonly used; less sensitive than HIV culture and PCR **Time to result:** 1–2 days **Cost:** $10–$50[c]

[a]Data culled from various sources.[5,14–17]

[b]Number of subjects with the disease who have a positive HIV test.

[c]Cost was quoted from Pizzo & Wilfert, 1994 and from specific hospital laboratory at time of chapter submission.[5]

EIA = enzyme-linked immunosorbent assays; PCR = polymerase chain reaction; Ig = immunoglobulin.

and percentages every 3 months in HIV-infected infants and children is useful to (1) assess the status of the HIV infection, (2) determine when to initiate antiretroviral therapy (ART), (3) measure the response to therapy, and (4) provide a criterion for when to alter therapies. Table 26.2 includes normal age-specific CD4+ counts and percentages. Viral load testing is performed when available to monitor disease progression and to measure response to therapy. Standard norms for viral load in children have not been established.

Prognosis of HIV Infection in Infants and Children

In comparison to HIV-infected adults, perinatally infected infants develop immunodeficiency and related diseases faster.[17] The median survival age has increased to 9 years of age for the majority of perinatally HIV-infected children. Shorter survival is associated with early onset of OIs, growth retardation, recurrent oral candidiasis, and encephalopathy.[12] Based on longitudinal studies of HIV-infected children, two patterns of disease progression—early and late symptomatic onset of HIV infection—have been described in perinatally infected children[5]:

- **Early onset** (**<2 years old;** 10 to 25% of infected children)
  - Survival <6 years old
  - Severe failure to thrive
  - Developmental delay
  - Progressive encephalopathy
  - Severe candidiasis (oral esophageal infection)
  - PCP
  - Severe, life-threatening bacterial infections
- **Late onset** (**>4 years old;** 75 to 90% infected children)
  - Survival >8 years old
  - Growth failure (mild to moderate)
  - Chronic multisystem disease
  - PGL
  - Lymphoid interstitial pneumonitis
  - Malabsorption syndrome
  - Malignancies

These patterns have different survival times, as indicated. Some (less than 50%) perinatally infected children remain asymptomatic or mildly symptomatic throughout adolescence.[17]

Table 26.2 Age-Specific CD4+ Counts and Percentages by Level of Immune Suppression

	CD4+ Counts and Percentages					
	No Suppression		Moderate Suppression		Severe Suppression	
Age	CD4+ µl	CD4+%	CD4+ µl	CD4+%	CD4+ µl	CD4+%
<12 mo	≥1,500	≥25	750–1,499	15–24	<750	<15
1–5 yr	≥1,000	≥25	500–999	15–24	<500	<15
6–12 yr	≥500	≥25	<500	15–24	<200	<15

From CDC. 1994 Revised classification system for human immunodeficiency virus infection in children less than 13 years of age. *MMWR.* 1994;43:RR-12:1–10.

HIV Classification System for Children <13 Years

An HIV infection classification system for children <13 years was devised in 1987 and revised in 1994.[18] According to the CDC revised guidelines, children who are perinatally exposed or infected with HIV may be classified into one of four mutually exclusive clinical categories based on signs, symptoms, or diagnoses of the HIV infection (Table 26.3).[18] Each category (N, A, B, and C) is described here.

- Category N—Not symptomatic; includes children with no signs or symptoms considered to be the result of HIV infection or with only one of the conditions listed under category A
- Category A—Mildly symptomatic; includes children with two or more of the conditions listed below but none of the conditions listed in categories B and C
  - Lymphadenopathy (≥0.5 cm at more than two sites; bilateral = one site)
  - Hepatomegaly
  - Splenomegaly
  - Dermatitis
  - Parotitis
  - Recurrent or persistent upper respiratory infection, sinusitis, or otitis media
- Category B—Moderately symptomatic; includes children who have symptomatic conditions other than those listed for category A or C that are attributed to HIV infection
  - Anemia (≤8 g/dl), neutropenia, or thrombocytopenia ≥ 30 days
  - Bacterial meningitis, pneumonia, or sepsis
  - Candidiasis, oropharyngeal, persisting >2 months in children >6 months of age
  - Cardiomyopathy
  - CMV infection, with onset before 1 month of age
  - Diarrhea, recurrent or chronic
  - Hepatitis
  - HSV stomatitis
  - HSV bronchitis, pneumonitis, or esophagitis with onset before 1 month of age

Table 26.3 Pediatric HIV 1994 Revised Classification[a]

Immunologic Categories[b]	Clinical Categories			
	N: No Signs/ Symptoms	A: Mild Signs/ Symptoms	B: Moderate Signs/ Symptoms	C: Severe Signs/ Symptoms
No evidence of suppression	N1	A1	B1	C1
Moderate suppression	N2	A2	B2	C2
Severe suppression	N3	A3	B3	C3

[a]Children whose HIV infection status is not confirmed are classified by using this grid with a letter E (for perinatally exposed) placed before the appropriate code (e.g., EN2). For example, a 4-year-old asymptomatic child who has a CD4+ percent of 30% and count of 1,120 ul would be classified as N1. Whereas, a 2-year-old child who has been diagnosed with recurrent, serious bacterial infections and has a CD4+ percent of 20% and CD4 count of 750 would be classified as C2.

[b]See Table 26.2 for a definition of level of immunsuppression based on CD4+ cell count and percent.

From CDC. 1994 Revised classification system for human immunodeficiency virus infection on children less than 13 years of age. *MMWR.* 1994;43:RR-12:24.

    - Leiomyosarcoma
    - Lymphoid interstititial pneumonitis (LIP)
    - Nephropathy
    - Nocardiosis
    - Persistent fever (lasting >1 month)
    - Toxoplasmosis, onset before 1 month of age
    - Varicella, disseminated
- Category C—Severely symptomatic; children who have any condition listed in the 1987 surveillance case definition for AIDS with the exception of LIP
    - Serious bacterial infections, multiple or recurrent
    - Candidiasis, esophageal or pulmonary
    - Coccidioidomycosis, disseminated
    - Cryptococcosis extrapulmonary
    - Cryptosporidiosis or isosporiasis with diarrhea persisting >1 month
    - CMV disease with onset of symptoms at age >1 month (at site other than liver, spleen, or lymph nodes)
    - Encephalopathy
    - HSV infection causing mucocutaneous ulcer that persists >1 month
    - Histoplasmosis, disseminated
    - KS
    - Lymphoma, primary in brain
    - Lymphoma (Burkitt's) or large cell of unknown immunologic phenotype
    - *M. tuberculosis*, disseminated or extrapulmonary
    - *Mycobacterium*, other species, disseminated
    - *M. avium complex* or *M. kansasii*, disseminated
    - Toxoplasmosis, onset before 1 month of age
    - PCP
    - PML
    - *Salmonella* (nontyphoid) septicemia, recurrent
    - Toxoplasmosis of the brain with onset at >1 month of age
    - Wasting syndrome

Any child diagnosed with LIP, any condition in category C, or a CD4+ percentage less than 15% is defined as having an AIDS-defining condition and must be reported to state and local health departments.

Manifestations of HIV Infection in Infants and Children

The most common complications of HIV infection in infants and children are described by organ system. For each organ system, complications are listed in order of most common to least common occurrence.

Respiratory

PCP. **Epidemiology:** PCP is the most common OI in children infected with HIV. It occurs most often in infants 3 to 6 months of age and presents as an acute pneumonia and results in a poor prognosis for the infant.

Clinical features: Features are low-grade fever and increased respiratory rate. Initial chest X-ray may be normal, but progression of the pneumonia results in bilateral perihilar or interstitial infiltrates.

Treatment and prevention: Trimethoprim-sulfamethoxazole is the preferred treatment for PCP. Current guidelines for PCP prevention are presented in Table 26.4. The decision to continue PCP prophylaxis for HIV-

Table 26.4 PCP Prophylaxis for HIV-Exposed Infants and HIV-Infected Children, by Age and HIV Infection Status

Age and HIV Infection Status	PCP Prophylaxis
Birth to 4–6 weeks for *all* infants exposed to HIV (HIV indeterminate or infected)	No prophylaxis
6 weeks to 4 months for *all* infants exposed to HIV (HIV indeterminate or infected)	Prophylaxis
4–12 months	
HIV infected or indeterminate	Prophylaxis
HIV noninfected (HIV infection reasonably excluded with two or more negative HIV diagnostic tests)	No prophylaxis
1–5 years (HIV infected)	Prophylaxis if CD4+ count <500 cells/μl or CD4% < 15%
6–12 years (HIV infected)	Prophylaxis if CD4+ count <200 cells/μl or CD4% <15%

PCP = *Pneumocystis carinii* pneumonia.
From CDC. 1995 Revised guidelines for prophylaxis against *Pneumocystis carinii* pneumonia for children infected with or perinatally exposed to human immunodeficiency virus. *MMWR.* 1995;44:RR-4: I-II.

infected children older than 12 months is based on CD4+ cell counts and percentages.[19] The PCP prophylaxis medication regimen for infants and children ≥4 weeks of age is seen in Table 26.5. PCP prophylaxis should not be administered to infants <4 weeks of age due to (1) low risk of PCP in this age group; (2) adverse effects from use of sulfa drugs in this age group resulting from immature bilirubin metabolism; and (3) unknown effects of concurrent use of sulfa drugs in infants also receiving zidovudine during the first 6 weeks of life, which can potentiate anemia in some children receiving zidovudine.

Table 26.5 PCP Prophylaxis Medication Regimen for Infants and Children ≥4 Weeks of Age

Medication Name	Dosage, Route and Frequency of Use
TMP-SMX	150 mg TMP/M^2/day with 750 mg SMX/M^2/day, orally, bid three times a week *on consecutive days* (Monday, Tuesday, Wednesday) *Acceptable alternative TMP-SMX dosing schedules:* • 150 mg TMP/M^2/day with 750 mg SMX/M^2/day administered orally as a single daily dose three times per week *on consecutive days* • 150 mg TMP/M^2/day with 750 mg SMX/M^2/day orally divided bid and administered 7 days per week • 150 mg TMP/M^2/day with 750 mg SMX/M^2/day administered orally divided bid and administered three times per week *on alternate days* (Monday, Wednesday, Friday)[14]
If TMP-SMX is not tolerated, alternative medications are dapsone or aerosolized pentamidine	Dapsone 2 mg/kg (not to exceed 100 mg), orally, *once daily* *or* Aerosolized pentamidine, 300 mg via Respirgard II inhaler *monthly* (children >5 years of age)

TMP-SMX = trimethoprim-sulfamethoxazole.
From CDC. 1995 Revised guidelines for prophylaxis against *Pneumocystis carinii* pneumonia for children infected with or perinatally exposed to human immunodeficiency virus. *MMWR.* 1995;44:RR-4:8.

LYMPHOID INTERSTITIAL PNEUMONITIS (LIP) **Epidemiology:** LIP is one of the most frequent forms of pulmonary involvement of HIV infection in children and is an AIDS-defining illness in children less than 13 years of age.[5]

Clinical features: Tachypnea, cough (see Chapter 12), wheezing, and hypoxemia are the usual signs of LIP. Clubbing is a sign of advanced disease. CXR findings diagnostic of LIP usually indicate symmetric, bilateral reticulonodular interstitial infiltrates with or without hilar adenopathy that persists on CXR for 2 months or longer and that are unresponsive to antimicrobial therapy. The definitive diagnosis of LIP is made by lung biopsy.

Treatment and prevention: Treatment consists of antiretroviral agents to control underlying HIV infection, and monitoring pulmonary function. Supplemental oxygen and corticosteroids may be required to suppress pulmonary lymphocytic infiltration. Prevention of LIP is linked to prevention of HIV.

M. TUBERCULOSIS. **Epidemiology:** Mycobacterial infections *(M. tuberculosis* and *M. avium intercellulare)* are increasingly important in HIV-infected children, although the incidence of mycobacterial infections in infants and children is still low. Most of the *M. tuberculosis* infections are seen among inner-city populations of lower socioeconomic status. Children with primary TB tend to have more disseminated disease rather than the classic pulmonary TB seen in HIV-infected adults.

Clinical features: Prolonged low-grade fever, cough (see Chapter 12), weight loss (see Chapter 10), night sweats (see Chapter 20), and failure to thrive are typical features. Due to the bronchial obstruction, specific pulmonary symptoms include wheezing, decreased breath sounds, tachypnea, and respiratory distress. CXR findings indicate localized or diffuse infiltrates. In contrast to HIV-infected adults, most TB in HIV-infected children is the result of primary infection rather than reactivation of latent infection seen in HIV-infected adults.

Treatment and prevention: The recommended medications for initial treatment of TB in children include isoniazid, rifampin, pyrazinamide, streptomycin, and ethambutol. Isolation with appropriate ventilation should be instituted in areas with high prevalence of TB (see Chapter 4 and Appendix B). All HIV-infected and uninfected children who live in the household with HIV-infected individuals should have an annual TB skin test beginning at age 1 year using only the Mantoux test.[20] The Mantoux test contains five tuberculin units of purified protein derivative.[21] In the United States, multipuncture skin tests should not be used.

RESPIRATORY SYNCYTIAL VIRUS (RSV). **Epidemiology:** RSV is a common respiratory viral infection seen in infants and children. The peak seasons are fall and early spring.

Clinical features: The typical clinical course includes rhinitis for 1 to 2 days, dry cough (see Chapter 12) and mild to moderate fever (see Chapter 20). These symptoms usually resolve in 3 to 7 days. However, approximately 30 to 40% of children progress to pneumonia or bronchiolitis, which may lead to respiratory distress. Children infected with RSV pose a very challenging diagnostic dilemma because the symptoms of RSV are difficult to distinguish from PCP. Obtaining RSV cultures is one tool to assist in diagnosing RSV.

Treatment and prevention: Most children with HIV infection tolerate RSV without complications, but children with concurrent pneumonia or PCP infection may develop respiratory distress and require ART with ribavirin.[22] Shedding of the RSV has been prolonged in some HIV-infected children, as long as 56 days[5] vs. the usual 3- to 8-day shedding period in HIV-noninfected children.

GI and Nutritional (See Chapter 10)

Epidemiology: Wasting or failure to thrive may be due to reduced intake resulting from (1) infectious complications of the oral cavity and esophagus, such as candidiasis; (2) excessive weight loss due to GI malabsorption from acute and chronic diarrhea; and (3) increased metabolic demand due to chronic or recurrent GI or systemic infections.[23]

Clinical features: Features include diarrhea, anorexia, abdominal pain, malabsorption, weight loss, vomiting, dysphasia, and eventually death.

Treatment and prevention: Aggressive diagnostic methods should be used to determine the cause of the malnutrition, followed by measures to promote good nutrition. Intervention for adequate nutrition ranges from stepwise progression starting with oral dietary supplements or via nasogastric tube or gastrostomy tube feedings. This emphasizes the need for the HIV multidisciplinary team to include a child nutritionist to assist with nutritional assessment, special diets, and feeding techniques.[24]

Neurological

Epidemiology: The true incidence of CNS abnormalities in HIV-infected children is unknown, but is reported to range from 20 to 40% of children.[5] CNS involvement, ranging from mild to severe, presents with either acute meningoencephalitis, seizures, brain atrophy with subsequent microcephaly, or encephalopathy.[24] Encephalopathy is the most common clinical manifestation of CNS abnormalities in HIV-infected children. The two patterns of HIV encephalopathy are static (nonprogressive) and progressive. Static encephalopathy has been observed in approximately 25% of HIV-infected children.[5] (See Chapter 9 for a discussion of neurology and HIV.)

Clinical features: Progressive encephalopathy is the most severe manifestation of CNS disease in children, as evidenced by progressive deterioration in cognitive, motor, language, and adaptive functioning, and by the loss of previously obtained milestones. Children with the more frequent type of encephalopathy, static encephalopathy, gain little or no developmental skills over time, with a decline in IQ, but have no loss of previously acquired developmental skills. CNS abnormalities may result from primary infection of the brain, secondary complications resulting from OIs (CMV, toxoplasmosis), CNS lesions (neoplasms or vascular lesions), or other organ involvement resulting in CNS complications (thrombocytopenia).[16]

Treatment and prevention: Recent studies indicate that early intervention with ART is associated with significant improvement in CNS function in HIV-infected children. However, long-term CNS complications may be inevitable because the exact timing of HIV invasion into the CNS in infants and children is unknown.[5] The best preventive measure is repeated clinical neurological and psychological assessments to evaluate the need for change in types of medical therapies.

Cardiac

Epidemiology: With the increased survival time of HIV-infected children, more cardiac abnormalities have been detected. The most common cardiac manifestation in HIV-infected children is left ventricular dysfunction, including left ventricular dilation with systolic dysfunction and congestive heart failure.[5]

Clinical features: Generalized signs and symptoms of cardiac disease include unresponsive or unexpected respiratory symptoms that last more than 7 days (oxygen desaturation, rales, cough), persistent tachycardia, poor feeding, poor perfusion, presence of arrhythmias, and cyanosis.

Treatment and prevention: All asymptomatic HIV-infected children should receive a baseline cardiac evaluation including electrocardiography and echocardiography at time of HIV diagnosis. Follow-up includes echocardiography every 6 to 12 months and electrocardiography at 1-year intervals.[5] Treatment is dependent on the type of cardiac disease, however it is important to correct any factor that may be contributing to cardiac symptoms, including anemia, malnutrition, and electrolyte imbalance.

Hematologic

Epidemiology: The most common hematologic problems—anemia, neutropenia, and thrombocytopenia (see Chapter 7)—are related to both HIV disease and drug-associated toxicities. Anemia is the most common hematologic disorder seen in HIV-infected children.[5] The etiology of anemia in HIV-infected children is multifactorial and is related to severity of HIV disease, ART, and age. Neutropenia, which has an absolute neutrophil cout (ANC) of <1,500 cells/mm^3, can increase with HIV disease progression in children. Thrombocytopenia has been reported in 19% of HIV-infected children[25,26] and is probably a result of both shortened platelet life span and suppressed platelet production.[27] Significant bleeding may occur resulting in CNS complications and anemia.

Listed below are the clinical features, treatment and prevention of anemia, neutropenia, and thrombocytopenia seen in HIV-infected children.

Clinical features (laboratory):

- Anemia—microcytic and hypochromic
- Neutropenia—ANC of <1,500 cells/mm^3
- Thrombocytopenia—platelet count of <50,000 cells/mm^3

Treatment and prevention:

- **Anemia**
  - If iron deficient, treat with ferrous sulfate. Chronic anemia may require periodic packed cell transfusion.
  - If recurrent transfusion (>2 months required) while on zidovudine, consider dose reduction, switch to another antiretroviral agent, or treat with erythropoietin 3 days each week.
- **Neutropenia**
  - ANC of 800 to 1,500 cells/mm^3: follow closely

- ANC of <800 cells/mm^3 and on zidovudine: reduce dose, switch to other antiretroviral agent, or treat with G-CSF
- **Thrombocytopenia**
  - Platelet count >50,000 cells/mm^3: follow closely
  - Platelet count of 20,000 to 50,000 cells/mm^3: follow closely; if on zidovudine, consider switch to ddI
  - Platelet count of <20,000 cells/mm^3: treat with IV Ig for 1 to 5 days[5] (Often HIV-infected children with thrombocytopenia require corticosteroids and eventually a splenectomy.)

Infections

Children diagnosed with recurrent serious bacterial OIs (at least two culture-confirmed infections within a 2-year period) are defined as having an AIDS-defining condition.[18,28] Other major OIs include *Candida albicans*, VZV, HSV, measles, CMV, and congenital syphilis (see Chapter 4). These infections are described in Table 26.6.

Primary Care Considerations of HIV-Infected Infants and Children

HIV-infected children need continuity of care by one provider whenever possible. Specialty care can be provided through consultation and coordination with the child's primary care provider. The usual primary care needs of any child, including immunizations; monitoring of nutrition, growth and development, and behavior; standard precaution education (see Appendix B); and psychosocial needs require attention by one individual for HIV-infected children.

Immunizations

Both HIV-infected and HIV-exposed infants should receive standard pediatric immunizations such as diphtheria-pertussis-tetanus, hepatitis B vaccine, and *Haemophilus influenzae* as listed in Table 26.7.[29] Inactivated polio is administered to prevent transmission of polio to an HIV-infected household member. Varicella vaccine is not recommended for HIV-infected children.[20]

General Nutritional Assessment and Counseling

Nutritional assessment and counseling are recommended for all HIV-risk children. This assessment includes monitoring their weight, height, weight for height, and head circumference on growth charts at every visit,

Table 26.6 Major Opportunistic Infections Associated with HIV Infection in Infants and Children

Infection	Epidemiology	Clinical Manifestations	Treatment
Bacterial infections	Common pathogens: pneumococcus, *Salmonella*, *Enterococcus*, *Staphylococcus aureus*, *Pseudomonas aeruginosa*, *Haemophilus influenzae*	Fever, increased WBC count, tachypnea, gastroenteritis, localized infections (otitis media, sinusitis, meningitis, urinary tract and soft-tissue infections)	Antibiotics based on culture and sensitivity of causative organism
Candida albicans	Oral candidiasis occurs in 15–40% of HIV-infected children	Oral candidiasis (whitish plaque on oral mucosa) may progress to esophagitis	Oral: oral nystatin, clotrimazole, ketoconazole, fluconazole with nystatin failure
		Cutaneous (diaper): dermatitis	Cutaneous: nystatin or ketoconazole cream
		Disseminated	Disseminated: amphotericin B
VZV	Incubation period 10–21 days for normal and immunocompromised children; HIV-infected children can suffer from chronic and persistent VZV	Vesicular lesions on face and trunk and spread centripetally; pneumonitis and life-threatening bacterial infections may be common among HIV-infected children, but the true incidence is unknown	Acyclovir 500 mg/m^2 q8h for 7–10 days Postexposure: varicella zoster immune globulin 1.25 ml for each 10 kg of body weight within 96 hours of exposure may reduce severity of infection

(continued)

Table 26.6 *Continued*

Infection	Epidemiology	Clinical Manifestations	Treatment
HSV-1	Transmitted primarily by oral secretions; 5–10% of children with AIDS have frequent HSV-1 recurrences	Gingivostomatitis, esophagitis, disseminated disease (liver, adrenals, lungs, spleen, kidney, and brain)	Acyclovir 250 mg/m^2 orally q6h or IV q8h
Measles	Severe illness in HIV-infected children	Maculopapular rash begins at hairline and spreads downward over face and body within 3 days; interstitial pneumonitis; can be fatal in HIV-infected children	IV immuneglobulin 0.5 ml/kg (maximum 15 ml) IV or IM as soon as possible after exposure up to 6 days; prevention: measle immunization
CMV	Approximately 60% of HIV-infected children with AIDS have either systemic CMV or asymptomatic CMV shedding[28]	Chorioretinitis, hepatitis, pneumonitis, encephalitis, esophagitis, and colitis[24]	Ganciclovir 7.5–15 mg/kg/day divided into two or three doses for 10–21 days

VZV = varicella zoster virus; HSV = herpes simplex virus; CMV = cytomegalovirus.
Source: Pizzo PA, Wilfert CM. *Pediatric AIDS: The Challenge of HIV Infection on Infants, Children and Adolescents.* 2nd ed. Baltimore: Williams & Wilkins; 1994:241–250, 326–329, 346–352, 352–356, 356–360, 371–374.

Table 26.7 Immunization Schedule for Healthy and HIV-Infected Infants and Children

	Immunizations Required	
Age	**Healthy Child Schedule**	**HIV-Infected Child Schedule**
Birth (newborn)	HBV	HBV
1–2 mo	HBV	HBV
2 mo	DTP, OPV, HIB	DTP, IPV, HIB
4 mo	DTP, OPV, HIB	DTP, IPV, HIB
6 mo	DTP, OPV (optional), HIB, HBV	DTP, IPV (optional), HIB, HBV
7 mo	None	Influenza virus vaccine #1 (annually after 6 months of age)
8 mo	None	Influenza virus vaccine #2
12 mo	MMR (in high-risk areas)	MMR (in high-risk areas)
15–18 mo	MMR (if not administered at 12 mo), DTP*, OPV	MMR (if not administered at 12 months of age), DTP*, IPV
24 mo	None	Pneumococcal vaccine (after age 2 years)
4–6 yr	DTP*, OPV, MMR (second dose)	DTP, IPV, MMR (second dose)
14–16 yr	dT,	dT,

*or DTaP = A cellular pertusis vaccine

HBV = hepatitis B vaccine; DTP = diphtheria, tetanus, and pertussis; OPV = oral polio vaccine; HIB = *Haemophilus influenzae* type B conjugate; IPV = inactivated (nonreplicating) polio vaccine; MMR = measles, mumps, and rubella; dT = diphtheria, tetanus.

Source: Pizzo PA, Wilfert CM. *Pediatric AIDS: The Challenge of HIV Infection in Infants, Children and Adolescents.* 2nd ed. Baltimore: Williams and Wilkins; 1994:862–866.

as well as screening for iron deficiency anemia. Failure to thrive is one common manifestation of HIV infection, which can often be treated with nutritional supplementation if diagnosed early and treated promptly. Other nutritional counseling includes teaching the families to avoid raw eggs, milk, shellfish, and undercooked meat to avoid food poisoning.

Developmental Assessment

Because neurological abnormalities have been reported in 20 to 40% of HIV-infected children[5] and developmental delay is a hallmark of pediatric

HIV infection, developmental assessment should be conducted on a regular basis by a clinical psychologist skilled in administering standard developmental testing scales. Neurodevelopmental testing, including a comprehensive neurological exam with deep-tendon and primitive reflexes, and developmental milestone testing, are recommended to be performed every 6 months to detect any neurological complications.

Frequency of Follow-up

ASYMPTOMATIC HIV-INFECTED INFANTS. Infants younger than 18 months of age who are diagnosed with HIV infection but do not have symptoms should be followed for routine visits at 1, 2, 4, 6, 9, 12, 15, and 18 months of age and every three month thereafter. A careful physical exam and developmental and psychosocial assessment should be performed at each visit. Immunizations should be administered as detailed in Table 26.7.

SYMPTOMATIC HIV-INFECTED CHILDREN. HIV-infected children with symptoms including LIP, failure to thrive, recurrent bacterial infections, hepatosplenomegaly, and neurological abnormalities require close follow-up. The primary care provider can arrange the follow-up with any specialist that may need to be consulted regarding the child's care. Coordination between inpatient, outpatient, and home care teams is vital to ensuring comprehensive care to HIV-infected children (see Chapter 22). Dental examinations should be scheduled starting at age 2 years.[5]

LABORATORY FOLLOW-UP OF HIV-INFECTED INFANTS AND CHILDREN. Laboratory tests are obtained to monitor HIV disease progression. They should be obtained as described in Table 26.8.

Treatment of HIV Infection in Infants and Children

Antiretroviral Therapy (ART)

Any child with a confirmed diagnosis of HIV infection should be evaluated for treatment with ART. For optimal patient care, the primary care provider should decide when to start ART in collaboration with physicians and researchers knowledgeable in the management of pediatric HIV infection. The decision to start ART in children is based on CD4 lymphocyte counts and percentages viral load, and clinical criteria. ART is indicated for children who have laboratory evidence of significant immunodeficiency

Table 26.8 Laboratory Tests and Frequency of Testing for HIV-Infected Infants and Children

Laboratory Test	Frequency of Testing
CD4+ counts and percents	Every 3 months or more often if indicated (e.g., decreasing CD4 counts)
Complete blood count and platelets	Initially every 2–4 weeks for 2 months then every 2–3 months
Chemistry panel including liver function tests	Every 3–6 months
Urinalysis	Every 3–6 months (cytomegalovirus urine at birth: 2, 4, and 6 months)
Viral load	Every 2–3 months for monitoring disease progression (when available)
Quantitative immunoglobulins (IgG, IgA, and IgM)	Every 3–6 months

Source: Pizzo PA, Wilfert CM. *Pediatric AIDS: The Challenge of HIV Infection in Infants, Children and Adolescents.* 2nd ed. Baltimore: Williams and Wilkins; 1994:665–681.

Table 26.9 CD4+ Lymphocyte Percentage and Count Criteria for Initiation of Antiretroviral Therapy

Age of Child	CD4+%	CD4+ Count (cells/mm³)
<1 yr	<30%	<1,750
1–2 yr	<25%	<1,000
>2 yr	<20%	<750

Source: Pizzo A, Wilfert CM. *Pediatric AIDS: The Challenge of HIV Infection in Infants, Children and Adolescents.* 2nd ed. Baltimore: Williams and Wilkins; 1994:664.

(Table 26.9) or who have developed any AIDS-defining disease manifestations or clinical conditions indicative of immunosuppression. Due to the continual expanding knowledge of antiretroviral drugs and the availability of multiple new retroviral drugs, current recommendations for the type of ART are being revised. Listed in Table 26.10 are the most frequently used antiretrovirals in children, the dosage, major toxicities, and how to monitor the child on each type of antiretroviral medication. Zidovudine (AZT),

Table 26.10 Antiretroviral Therapies for HIV-Infected Infants and Children

Drug Name	Description	Dosage	Major Toxicities	Monitor for Toxicities
Zidovudine (AZT, Retrovir)	Benefits in infants and children: improvement in activity, growth, neurological and cognitive functioning[5]	0–2 weeks of age: 2 mg/kg orally q6h; 3–4 weeks of age: 3 mg/kg q6h; 4 weeks–13 years of age: 160 mg/m^2/q8h; ≥13 years of age: the adult dose (500 mg/day) is recommended, although specific dosing data are lacking	Anemia, neutropenia, myositis, headache, nausea, hepatic transaminitis	CBC, differential, and platelet count every 4–6 weeks; liver function tests every 8–12 weeks
Didanosine (ddI, Videx)	Used in HIV-infected children who are symptomatic when zidovudine is not tolerated, or used in combination with zidovudine when symptoms such as growth failure or CNS disease are progressing	90 mg/m^2 twice daily in combination with other ARTS	Pancreatitis, peripheral neuropathy, retinal depigmentation	Liver function tests every 8–12 weeks; retinal examinations (dilated) every 6 months or if visual change occurs

Zalcitabine (ddC)	Use in children is limited	Up to 0.03 mg/kg orally every 6 hours	Peripheral neuropathy, pancreatitis, mouth sores, rash	CBC, differential, and platelet count every 4–6 weeks; liver function tests every 8–12 weeks
Lamivudine (3TC, Epivir)	An analog of ddC; exhibits less cytotoxicity than either ddC or zidovudine	3 months–12 years: 4 mg/kg twice daily; ≥12 years: 150 mg twice daily	Pancreatitis, peripheral neuropathies	CBC, differential, and platelet count every 4–6 weeks; liver function tests every 8–12 weeks

didanosine (ddI), zalcitabine (ddC), and lamivudine (3TC) are the only approved antiretroviral agents for use in children. Two protease inhibitors are now approved for use in children—noravir and viracept. Whenever possible, children should enroll in clinical trials. Information on these trials is available by calling 1-800-TRIALS-A (AIDS Clinical Trials Groups).

Other Therapies

NEVIRAPINE. Nevirapine is a nonnucleoside reverse transcriptase inhibitor that has a high degree of antiretroviral activity with minimal toxicity.[30] This drug may have use in combination with zidovudine and/or didanosine. Several clinical trials examining combination therapy using nevirapine are underway in adults and children.

GRANULOCYLZ COLONY-STIMULATING FACTOR (G-CSF). Use of G-CSF may be highly effective in treating neutropenia by increasing the WBC count, which in turn prevents infections associated with neutropenia. G-CSF is administered subcutaneously and the dose is titrated as necessary between 1 to 20 μg/kg daily.

Psychosocial Needs of Pediatric HIV Patients

Pediatric HIV is a family disease afflicting multigenerations in one family. To treat the HIV-infected child optimally, one must attend to the numerous psychosocial and family-oriented issues surrounding the HIV infection in the family. Wherever there is an HIV-infected child, there is almost always an infected mother (see Chapter 25). When the mother dies she leaves behind not only her infected children but also uninfected children. In a study of older children and adolescents living with perinatally acquired HIV infection, 76% of these older children were orphaned as a result of maternal death.[31] Often the father of the children is also infected and may have died before or around the same time as the mother.

Specific issues relating to the mother include maternal guilt, secrecy of not telling anyone about her HIV diagnosis, neglecting her own health care, concurrent substance abuse, and inadequate social support systems.[32] Although often not verbalized, HIV-infected mothers experience tremendous guilt knowing they may have infected their infant. The uncertainty of the child's diagnosis until 4 to 9 months of age further contributes to the stress of feeling guilty about infecting her child. This uncertainty can sometimes lead either to (1) lack of bonding with the infant if the mother believes the child will die at a young age or (2) increased protection of the infant in which the mother overprotects the child and does not allow the child to experience a "normal" childhood. Either scenario requires listening and support by the health care provider.

The mother is also a patient. Encouraging the mother to seek health care for herself may be difficult. She may only have the emotional and time resources to seek health care for her child. For many HIV-infected women, support systems are lacking and the health care provider may be the only support system available to the mother. As the mother's HIV infection progresses, she may manifest AIDS dementia (see Chapter 9). Health care providers for the child may be the first staff to detect AIDS dementia in the mother based on subtle cues such as inappropriate care of the child manifested by inability to report medication administration for the child or inability to provide any details about the child's daily routine. If AIDS dementia is diagnosed in the mother, surrogate care for the child should be approached with the mother and other supportive family members. Investigating the possibility of other family members caring for the child must be addressed cautiously.

In planning for the ongoing care of the child, several considerations need to be addressed with the mother, including (1) care of the child when the mother dies, (2) care of the child if the mother becomes physically and mentally incompetent to care for the child alone, (3) disclosing the child's HIV diagnosis to the child, and (4) disclosing the HIV diagnosis of herself and the child to other family members. Addressing these issues can only be accomplished when the mother trusts the child's health care provider. It is preferable that these issues be addressed in conjunction with the mother's health care provider to ensure that all members of the health care team are informed of the mother's requests. Family sessions with the mother, health care providers for the child and the mother, and supportive family members can be arranged to establish the optimal plan for each family member's needs.

Due to the continued stigma of HIV, many families refuse to disclose the HIV diagnosis to the child (see Chapter 29). In the study of older children and adolescents living with perinatally acquired HIV infection, 43% of the children had not been told their diagnosis.[31] This raises the ethical question regarding how older children and adolescents can participate in decisions regarding their life choices and health care if they are unaware of their diagnosis.[31] The practitioner must acknowledge any of their own biases that may conflict with the family's requests. If there are reasons for the child to know his diagnosis, the health care provider should state these concerns directly to the family. If and when the family decides to disclose the diagnosis to the child or adolescent, the practitioner must be available and supportive to the child and family.

Parental drug use often accompanies children with HIV infection. Parental drug use must be addressed when caring for the child. Familiarity with substance abuse clinics, detox programs, and 12-step programs is the best approach for parents who continue to use illicit drugs. Substance abuse treatment is complex and can require enormous amounts of time by specialists in this area. The role of the child's health care provider is to be direct but supportive to the parent to seek treatment for their substance abuse.

School Issues for HIV-Infected Children

The natural history of pediatric HIV infections reveals that children are surviving longer after perinatal HIV infection, so more HIV-infected children attend school. School attendance raises several issues for biologic as well as adoptive families of these children. Caregivers are often reluctant to disclose the HIV diagnosis to the child or to school personnel due to the stigma of HIV illness. A low disclosure rate of the child's HIV diagnosis to school personnel raises many concerns for primary health care providers. Health needs of HIV-infected children at the school include assessment of the child's limitations for the physical and educational demands of school, and administration of medications during school hours. Monitoring exposure of the child to pathogens such as varicella or measles while in school can be conducted only if school personnel are aware of the child's HIV infection. It has been suggested that the school nurse, when available in schools, is a safe person within the school setting to provide emotional and psychological support for stresses related to HIV disease.[31] Encouraging the caregiver to disclose the child's diagnosis is recommended and may require the primary care provider to facilitate this interaction by arranging a meeting with the child's caregiver and school nurse.

Adolescents and HIV Infection

HIV infection in adolescents poses challenges distinct from those of adult or pediatric HIV infection and is a serious health threat to many US adolescents. In 1991 AIDS was the sixth leading cause of death among adolescents age 15 to 24 years.[33] Because adolescence is a period of biologic and psychosocial development involving sexual curiosity and experimentation, adolescents are placed at increased risk for HIV infection. Since infection may occur as long as 10 years before an AIDS diagnosis, many adults with AIDS were likely infected with HIV either as adolescents or young adults. All adolescent health care providers can play an important role in providing appropriate health care to the HIV seropositive adolescent, and offering prevention and risk reduction information to all adolescents.

Epidemiology of HIV Infection in Adolescents

Although the prevalence of HIV infection in adolescents is unknown, 2,953 cases of AIDS among adolescents 13 to 19 years of age had been reported to the CDC as of June 1997.[3] While adolescents account for only 0.4% of the total number of cases of AIDS in the United States (612,078), the incidence of AIDS has increased in this age group from 0.20 per 100,000 in 1985 to 0.72 per 100,000 diagnosed in 1992.[35] These data suggest that many adolescents may be infected with HIV but are not ill, and some are unaware of their infection.[34]

Seroprevalence Data

Adolescents are a heterogenous group with different risks for and rates of HIV infection. Overall the seroprevalence rates of HIV infection in adolescents less than 20 years of age attending adolescent medicine clinics, STD clinics, juvenile detention/correctional facilities, and homeless and runaway youth centers were low (0.2–1.1%).[36] HIV infection rates are highest in homeless and runaway youth.[35]

Demographic Characteristics

The incidence of AIDS cases in adolescents increases by year of age. The majority (74%) of AIDS cases reported in the United States were among 17- to 19-year-old adolescents, with 26% among 13- to 16-year-old adolescents.[35] Among adolescents, the ratio of males to females with AIDS is lower (2:1) than among adults (8:1). Seroprevalence rates among males and females are similar across a variety of settings, suggesting that a large proportion of adolescent HIV cases have been contracted by heterosexual transmission.

In 1992, black (see Chapter 29) and Hispanic (see Chapter 28) males accounted for 31% and 21% respectively of AIDS cases in adolescent males age 13 to 19 years in the United States.[33] During the same time period in adolescent females with AIDS, blacks and Hispanics make up a larger proportion of the female cases—57% black and 17% Hispanic.[34]

Modes of Transmission

Until recently the most frequent mode of transmission of HIV among adolescents was the treatment for coagulation disorder—hemophilia. However, since the advent of nationwide screening of blood and blood products for HIV in 1985, this mode of transmission has been virtually eliminated.[34] Currently the more common modes of adolescent transmission include males who have sex with males, injection drug use, and heterosexual contact. Transmission risks differ for male and female adolescents. Most adolescent females infected with HIV acquired their infection through heterosexual contact. National data indicate that an increasing proportion of adolescents have initiated sexual activity at an earlier age and perform unprotected sexual activity more often.[36]

Transmission rates by race/ethnicity indicate that the majority (62%) of white male adolescents infected with HIV were exposed through treatment for a coagulation disorder as compared with black male adolescents who reported males who have sex with males as the highest transmission route (56%). One other trend noted is that younger adolescents have acquired their infection from receipt of HIV-contaminated blood products, whereas older adolescents and young adults have primarily acquired their HIV through sexual transmission or injection drug use.[34] Sexual abuse is another mode of transmission often overlooked in adolescents. The absolute number of adolescents acquiring HIV infection by sexual abuse is unknown.[37]

Survival Data

Survival data for adolescents with HIV infection is sparse. In 1991 HIV infection and AIDS was the sixth leading cause of death among youth 15 to 24 years of age.[33] A more rapid onset of AIDS is associated with having hemophilia and an older age at becoming infected with HIV.[38]

Delay in diagnosis and treatment for HIV in adolescents is one suggested explanation for the shortened survival time in adolescents, rather than an inherently rapid disease progression. This may also explain the reported increased number of adolescent patients who present with serious immune dysfunction at their initial clinic visit.[39]

HIV Testing in Adolescents

The traditional tests (EIA and Western blot, HIV culture) used in adults (see Chapter 2) are the tests used to identify HIV infection in adolescents. In contrast with adults, several complex ethical and legal issues are raised when testing adolescents for HIV.

Pretest Counseling

Pretest counseling in the adolescent involves covering several issues:[40] (1) Assess the adolescent's motivation for HIV testing. (2) Describe the HIV test, what a positive or negative test means, and the benefits and associated risks to being tested. The adolescent should understand that a positive HIV test result means that she is infected with the virus that causes HIV infection, but it does not indicate whether she has AIDS. (3) HIV infection is now considered a chronic illness, which can be managed with medications and is not an end-of- life sentence. (4) Assess the adolescent's coping ability by asking: Is there anyone you can tell about getting tested? How do you think you might react to a positive result? (5) Help the adolescent develop a support system for the waiting period and thereafter if the test result is positive.[41]

Informed Consent

Adolescents 18 years of age or older and who are competent can give informed consent for HIV testing after the risks and benefits, implications, and alternatives to the test are discussed. The informed consent for HIV testing by an adolescent should include the following: (1) comprehensive, age-appropriate, and culturally relevant explanation of the risks and benefits of HIV testing; (2) what information will be disclosed in the patient record; (3) who will have access to the medical record information; and (4) identification of a significant adult for support for the adolescent.[41] For adolescents age 12 to 17 years, laws vary considerably by state as to whether the adolescent can give his or her consent if judged competent to do so. In some states minors can give consent under the minor consent statutes for treatment of STDs or substance abuse problems. For children age 12 years and younger or judged to be incompetent adolescents, the law states that a third party (parent or guardian) should authorize the HIV testing.[41] Because of the complex consent and confidentiality issues, nurses and physicians should be certain of state laws regarding informed consent and disclosure of HIV test results prior to testing any adolescent. Specific information regarding confidentiality of HIV test results for adolescents should also include (1) who receives the test results, (2) where the test results are recorded, and (3) what is written in the adolescent's chart regarding HIV testing and results.

Disclosure

Disclosure to other involved individuals including parents, siblings, and school personnel requires discussion with the adolescent prior to testing. Local law may dictate to whom the HIV test results can be disclosed after testing. Health care providers need to know who can receive HIV test results when testing adolescents.

Developmental Stage

Understanding the pattern of cognitive maturity during adolescence influences the effectiveness of HIV counseling. Cognition evolves from concrete operational thinking during early adolescence to formal operational or "abstract thinking" during late adolescence.[41] With young adolescents, it is best to use simple, concrete messages and to avoid intellectual reasoning.[42] For older adolescents, the explanation of HIV testing and consequences of the testing can be more in depth. It is essential to remember that physical maturity does not necessarily correlate with cognitive maturity.

Posttest Counseling

Posttest counseling is important. When counseling adolescents it is important to (1) review transmission, risk behaviors, and the meaning of HIV test results, and (2) assess the support systems of each adolescent.

Clinical Manifestation of HIV Infection in Adolescents

Recognizing the common clinical manifestations of HIV infection in adolescents is critical for early diagnosis. In general, the development of AIDS-defining conditions for HIV-infected adolescents is similar to that of adults. The initial clinical evidence of HIV infection is usually a mild mononucleosislike or flulike syndrome followed by seroconversion 3 to 6 months after exposure. As the disease progresses, the immune system is eventually destroyed, which results in OIs and/or malignancies and AIDS.[41] Early clinical manifestations of HIV infection in adolescents are listed below.[41,43]

- Generalized lymphadenopathy
- Unexplained weight loss, fatigue, and malaise
- Cervical dysplasia as noted on Pap smear
- Oral hairy leukoplakia
- Oral candidiasis
- Lingering viral infections
- Extensive genital warts
- Severe *molluscum contagiosum*
- Seborrheic dermatitis
- Psoriasis exacerbations
- Thrombocytopenia
- Periodontal disease (i.e., gingivitis, mouth or gum sores, and inflammation, tooth decay)

An HIV health history for the initial evaluation should include a review of systems[41] specific to HIV as follows:

- General: failure to gain weight, weight loss, fatigue, fever, poor appetite,
- Head, ears, eyes, nose,and throat (HEENT):
  eyes, visual changes, blurring vision, or double vision;
  mouth, dysphagia, mouth sores and ulcers on gums, tooth decay;
  nose and sinuses, sinusitis
- Respiratory: persistent cough and shortness of breath
- Gastrointestinal: diarrhea, abdominal pain or masses, anal pain, experience with anal-receptive intercourse
- Neurological: weakness, myalgia, aches and pains or abnormal sensations
- Neuropsychiatric: personality changes, dementia, depression, anxiety and headaches, substance abuse, alcohol consumption

The HIV-specific physical exam for an adolescent should assess nutritional status and growth, lymph nodes, skin, head, ears, eyes, nose and throat, cardiovascular, respiratory, abdominal, genital, and neurological systems.[5,44] Specific exam items for each body system are listed below.

The physical examination for adolescents is different from the adult exam for the following body systems.

General appearance: Changes in somatic growth and cognitive function should be noted because adolescence is characterized by increased growth and enhanced cognitive capabilities. Height and weight velocity should be included in the growth assessment. Note any weight loss *or* failure to gain expected weight. Record sexual maturity staging (Tanner stage) based on pubic hair distribution, testicular size, and breast development. Vital signs including blood pressure should be recorded.

Skin: Some common dermatologic problems are seen with HIV infection and may indicate disease progression. Note any lesions consistent with subacute bacterial endocarditis (SBE).

Lymph nodes: A description of the location, number, size, consistency, temperature, and persistence of lymphadenopathy should be recorded. Adolescence is a time when lymph tissue begins to regress. One sign of advanced AIDS is regression of adenopathy.[41]

HEENT: Visual acuity and funduscopic exam may reveal any retinitis or other ophthalmologic changes. Oral candidiasis may present as erythematous and denuded patches on the mucous membranes rather than the typical whitish plaques. Dental decay and gingivitis are other common manifestations of HIV infection in adolescents. Sinuses should be assessed for tenderness.

Respiratory: Note any abnormal breath sounds and respiratory rate.

Cardiovascular: Note pulse rate and any abnormal cardiac sounds.

Genitalia: Females 18 years or older, or who have had sexual intercourse, or who complain of unexplained pelvic pain require a yearly or twice yearly pelvic exam with appropriate laboratory tests and inspection for lesions such as herpes or warts. Gynecologic complaints are common in HIV-infected adolescents. With declining CD4+ counts, vaginal candidiasis and genital herpes simplex may present more frequently and severely.[46]

Adolescent males also require inspection of genitals for any lesions. Anal inspection is important to detect herpes, warts, or other lesions

(continued)

even in those adolescents who deny anal intercourse.[5] A rectal exam should be performed on any HIV-seropositive adolescent with GI symptoms.

Neurological: The neurological exam, including a mental status assessment, may detect subtle changes in neurological functioning. Test for cranial nerves, reflexes, strength, sensation, and cerebellar function. Data are sparse regarding how HIV infection affects cognitive development in adolescents.

The most common AIDS-defining clinical conditions in adolescents with AIDS are displayed in Table 26.11.[34] Their occurrence is different than in adults.

Medical Treatment of HIV Infection in Adolescents

Effective medical care for HIV-infected adolescents blends the specialization of infectious disease with the basics of adolescent health care to offer the most current treatment options in a relevant and practical manner, as well as offering prevention strategies for all adolescents.[44,46] Access to

Table 26.11 The Most Common AIDS-Defining Clinical Conditions in Adolescents

AIDS-Defining Condition	Percentage of Patients
Pneumocystis carinii	41
Candida esophagitis	22
Wasting syndrome	19
Mycobacterium avium complex	9
Extrapulmonary cryptococcosis	9
Chronic herpes simplex	8
HIV encephalopathy	6
Toxoplasmosis of brain	5

Source: From Lindegren ML, Hansen C, Miller K, Byers RH, Onorato AI. Epidemiology of human immunodeficiency virus infection in adolescents, United States. *Pediatr Infect Dis J.* 1994;13:528.

health care is the key to increasing survival time in adolescents infected with HIV.

Monitoring Disease Progression

Until recently, CD4+ lymphocyte counts and percentages, CD4+/CD8+ ratio, and p24 antigen tests were the most useful markers for HIV disease progression in adolescents. The normal CD4+ count for an adolescent is 800 to 1,050 cells/mm^3. CD4+ counts of <500 cells/mm^3 indicate immune dysfunction and need for ART.[5] Currently, use of tests measuring viral load are used in addition to the CD4+ count as a marker of disease status and progression. Lab tests include

- CBC
- CD4+ and CD8+ percent and absolute count
- Viral load
- Chemistry panel
- Urinalysis
- STD evaluation including (1) screening for gonorrhea, syphilis, chlamydia, hepatitis B, and trichomonas (anatomic sites to be cultured depend on the sexual behavior of the adolescent); (2) a Pap smear for females; (3) evaluation for other STDs (e.g., herpes) depending on the adolescent's history and clinical presentation; and (4) adolescent females with vaginal discharge should be evaluated for bacterial vaginosis and vaginal candidiasis.

Follow-up for asymptomatic adolescents should be every 3 months, with more frequent monitoring when symptoms start to develop.[44] Close monitoring may be indicated for some adolescents, particularly when compliance with prescribed treatment regimen is low. (See p.667. Promoting adherence of the adolescent to HIV Treatment Plan) Staff need to track patients actively, especially asymptomatic adolescents who do not feel ill and therefore may not believe they need ongoing medical care.

Medications

Use of Tanner staging is the method preferred over chronological age for determining appropriate dosage of antiretroviral medications for adolescents. In general, adolescent patients at Tanner stage 1 should be given pediatric doses, and adolescents at Tanner 5 should be given adult doses regardless of their chronological age. Dosages for adolescents at stages 2 through 4 remain undetermined.[5] Some clinicians calculate medication dosages for adolescents based on weight and surface area despite their Tanner stage. Use of alcohol, tobacco, and illicit drugs can alter medication efficacy and toxicity, which must be considered when prescribing antiretroviral medications.[44]

ANTIRETROVIRALS. Based on extrapolation from adult HIV therapy data, initial therapy for adolescents with CD4+ counts of <500 cells/mm^3 should be zidovudine in combination with either lamivudine (Epivir, 3TC), didanosine (ddI), or zalcitabine (ddC)[47] (Table 26.12).[49] At present, combination therapy (AZT and Epivir, AZT and DDI) and new treatment options such as protease inhibitors appear most promising for increasing the survival rate for HIV-infected adolescents (see Chapter 3).

OPPORTUNISTIC INFECTIONS. Adolescents with a previous episode of *Pneumocystis* pneumonia or a CD4+ cell count of <200 cells/mm^3 require prophylaxis.[40] For adolescents in Tanner stage 5, the initial prophylaxis for PCP includes trimethoprim-sulfamethoxazole prescribed at adult dosages (see Chapter 5). For Tanner stage 1 or 2, pediatric dosing of trimethoprim-sulfamethoxazole is recommended (see the discussion of PCP prophylaxis in this chapter and see Chapter 4).

Promoting Adherence of the Adolescent to the HIV Treatment Plan

(Adapted with permission from Anderson and Morris[49])

Promoting adherence in adolescents with HIV presents a challenge for health care providers. Familiarity with the developmental level of each adolescent will assist in a user-friendly treatment plan. To enhance adherence, consider the following tips:

- Simplify health care treatment to fit the adolescent's lifestyle.
- Provide written instructions at reading levels appropriate to the patient.
- Enlist the adolescent's cooperation in the treatment plan by eliciting ideas from the adolescent for enhancing adherence. Suggest ways to remember to take the medication, including a medication diary, calendar, and associating the medication with daily activities such as showering or mealtimes.

Table 26.12 HIV Antiretroviral Therapy in Adolescents[a]

Antiretroviral	Dosage	Indications
AZT (zidovudine, Retrovir)	200 mg tid q8h *or* 100 mg q4h (five times daily)	CD4+ of <500 cells/mm^3 *or* >30,000 to 50,000 HIV RNA copies per milliliter, or with rapidly declining CD4+ cell counts, or any HIV-related symptoms.
ddI (didanosine, Videx)	*If weight is >60 kg*, 200 mg q12h or twice daily; *if weight is <60 kg*, 125 mg q12h or twice daily	Intolerance to or worsening clinical status on Zidovudine for >6 months
ddC (dideoxycytidine, zalcitibine)	0.75 mg q8h or tid	Intolerance to or worsening clinical status on Zidovudine for >6 months
Lamivudine (Epivir, 3TC)	Combination therapy with Zidovudine: >16 years, 150 mg bid; <16 years, use pediatric dosing, 4 mg/kg bid	Intolerance to or worsening clinical status on Zidovudine for >6 months

[a]Data culled from various sources.[45,49]
RNA = ribonucleic acid.

- Make the adolescent responsible for their treatment as much as possible. Assist the adolescent in finding techniques to enhance self-management such as a diary, pill box, or watch with an alarm. Encouraging the adolescent to improve self-management may also increase their self-esteem.
- Share that you understand the difficulties in adhering to the prescribed daily regimen and encourage the adolescent to share with you any difficulties he may be having in doing so. If it is necessary to enlist the cooperation of other adults to assist with the adolescent's care, obtain the adolescent's permission and participation. Encourage the adult and adolescent to work as a team and have the same goals.
- Incorporate the adolescent's stage of cognitive development into the treatment plan. Early adolescents require use of concrete reasoning using simplified discussions and avoiding didactic lecture. Older adolescents may request a more in-depth explanation of the rationale for each component of the treatment plan. Self-esteem issues and feeling "similar to other adolescents" affect adherence in adolescents. When medications or other HIV treatments make the adolescent feel different from his or her peers, adherence to the treatment plan will become difficult.

Prevention of HIV Infection in Adolescents

Until a vaccine is developed to prevent HIV, prevention education is the main tool available to reduce the risk of HIV infection in adolescents. HIV prevention education for adolescents begins with recognizing high-risk behaviors. Several adolescent behaviors place these youth at increased risk for HIV infection, as described next.

Sexual Intercourse (Vaginal, Anal, and Orogenital)

Adolescent pregnancy and STDs, indicating unprotected sexual intercourse, are markers of risky sexual behavior. The presence of STDs (including syphilis, genital ulcer disease, and herpes infection), multiple sex partners, and substance and/or alcohol abuse increases the risk of acquiring HIV infection.[50,51] Adolescents are having sexual intercourse earlier and often in serial monogamous relationships resulting in an increase in STDs. Although anal intercourse is most often observed in male-to-male sex, many women also experience this form of sexual intercourse,[5] using it sometimes as a form of birth control.

Sexual Abuse

Sexual abuse is a risk factor for HIV infection. The absolute number of adolescents who have acquired HIV through sexual abuse is unknown due to the multiple barriers to diagnosing sexual abuse.[37] However, adolescents being evaluated for sexual abuse are probably at greater risk for HIV infection than nonabused adolescents.[37]

Injection Drug Use

Accurate estimates of adolescent injection drug use are difficult to obtain; however, studies indicate that the rates are low. For adolescent males the rate of injection drug use is 2.3 to 3.7% and for adolescent females the rate is 0.7 to 1.8%.[52] More commonly, adolescents engage in other forms of drug use such as snorting or smoking illegal drugs. The link between noninjection types of drug use and transmission of HIV is unclear. It is suggested that crack cocaine is linked to an increase in the rate of STDs in adolescents[46] caused by impaired judgment and inappropriate decisions concerning sex and other risky behavior.[53]

Recommendations for Successful HIV Prevention Education

Health professionals need to provide a consistent message of simple facts regarding preventing HIV infection to all adolescents. *Simple information messages* include the following:

- If you are sexually active now or in the future, you can become HIV infected.
- Sexual abstinence and avoiding injection drug use reduce the risk of HIV transmission.
- If you are sexually active, limit your number of partners, avoid high-risk sexual practices including anal intercourse, and use barrier protection such as a condom.

Several factors shown to reduce adolescents' risk for HIV infection include (1) helping youth perceive HIV as a problem, (2) motivating youth to act safely, (3) providing coping skills to assist in implementing safe behavior, (4) providing access to condoms, and (5) providing access to health care.[54]

Effective HIV prevention programs for adolescents should include the following strategies.[55]

- Programs need to go beyond education. The adolescent must be able to process complex information. Adolescents need skills to think into the future, discuss and negotiate condom use with their partner, and resist peer pressure.
- Use groups for education and support. Many adolescents are more comfortable in group meetings than one-on-one presentations. Group rules should be established and followed.[47]
- Programs should be based on a theoretical framework and guided by theory, including the Health Belief Model, Social Learning Theory, Self-Efficacy Theory, or other established principles of behavior change.
- HIV prevention programs should be multimethod (didactic, skills building) and multimedium (video, role playing, computer assisted).
- Effective programs are based on up-to-date health care and epidemiological information regarding HIV.
- Programs need to account for cultural, religious, and sexual differences among adolescents. Focus groups can be used to determine within-group differences.
- Programs need to be accessible to adolescents. Many high-risk adolescents do not attend school. Recommended sites include community-based settings and family planning, STD, and adolescent clinics.
- Use community outreach strategies, including building relationships with community service agencies, providing consultation and expertise to schools, and advocating public policy for safe sex and drug use prevention.[47]
- Use of peer educators and counselors, school-based clinics with a defined HIV educational component, and educational programs that combine communication skills with decision making and HIV information have demonstrated a positive impact in modifying adolescent behavior.[42]

Resources

Information about HIV Infection in Children

National AIDS/HIV Hotline
English: 1-800-342-2437 (24 hours)
Spanish: 1-800-344-7432

National AIDS Information Clearinghouse
1-800-458-5231

National Pediatric HIV Resource Center
1-800-362-0071

National Association of People with AIDS
1-202-898-0414

To obtain *written materials* about HIV/AIDS, contact
The Centers for Disease Control (CDC)
National AIDS Clearinghouse
PO Box 6003
Rockville, MD 20849-6003
1-800-458-5231

Resources for Adolescents

AIDS Hotline
US Public Health Service
English: 1-800-342-AIDS
Spanish: 1-800-344-SIDA

American Academy of Child and Adolescent Psychiatry
"Children, Adolescents and HIV/AIDS"
http://www.cmhcsys.com

National AIDS Network
2033 M Street, NW, Suite 800
Washington, DC 20036
202-293-2437

Teens Teaching AIDS Prevention Program
1-800-234-8336

Camps

The Hole in the Wall Gang Camp
565 Ashford Center Road
Ashford, CT 06278
860-429-3444

Camp Heartland
4564 N. Green Bay Avenue
Milwaukee, WI 53209
1-800-724-HOPE

Camp Chrysalis
PO Box 990
Belfast, ME 04915
207-338-5089

Herbert G. Birch Residential Children's Center
594 E. 53rd Street
Brooklyn, NY 11203
718-763-3198

Camp Good Days and Special Times, Incorporated
1332 Pittsford Mendon Road
Mendon, NY 14506
716-624-5555

References

1. National Center for Health Statistics. *Annual Summary of Births, Marriages, Divorces and Deaths: United States, 1992. Monthly Vital Statistics Report.* Vol. 42, no. 2 suppl. Hyattsville, MD: Department of Health and Human Services, 1993.
2. Pizzo PA, Wilfert CM. Antiretroviral therapy and medical management of the human immunodeficiency virus-infected child. *Pediatr Infect Dis J.* 1993;12: 513–522.
3. CDC, USDHHS. *HIV/AIDS Surveillance Report.* Vol. 9, No. 1, June 1997. Atlanta: Centers for Disease Control.
4. CDC. *HIV/AIDS Surveillance Report.* 1995;7:1. Atlanta: Centers for Disease Control.
5. Pizzo PA, Wilfert CM. *Pediatric AIDS: The Challenge of HIV Infection in Infants, Children and Adolescents.* 2nd ed. Baltimore: Williams & Wilkins; 1994.
6. Oxtoby MJ. Perinatally acquired human immunodeficiency virus infection. *Pediatr Infect Dis J.* 1990;9:609–619.
7. European Collaborative Study. risk factors for mother-to-child transmission of HIV-1. *Lancet.* 1992;339:1007–1012.
8. Tovo PA, de Martino M, Gabiano C, et al. Prognostic factors and survival in children with perinatal HIV-1 infection. *Lancet.* 1992;339:1249–1253.
9. Mofenson L. Epidemiology and determinants of vertical HIV transmission. *Semin Pediatr Infect Dis.* 1994;5:252–265.

10. Ruff AJ, Halsey NA, Coberly J, et al. Breast-feeding and maternal-infant transmission of HIV type 1. *J Pediatr.* 1992;121:325–329.
11. Gutman LT, St Claire KK, Weedy C, et al. Human immunodeficiency virus transmission by child sexual abuse. *Am J Dis Child.* 1991;145:137–141.
12. Oleske JM. The many needs of the HIV-infected child. *Hosp Pract.* 1994;29: 81–87.
13. CDC. Zidovudine for the prevention of HIV transmission from mother to infant. *MMWR.* 1994;43:285–287.
14. McIntosh K, Pitt J, Brambilla D. Blood culture in the first 6 months of life for the diagnosis of vertically transmitted human immunodeficiency virus infection. *J Infect Dis.* 1994;170:996–1000.
15. Borkowsky W, Krasinski P, Pollack H, et al. Early diagnosis of human immunodeficiency virus infection in children <6 months of age: comparison of polymerase chain reaction, culture and plasma antigen capture techniques. *J Infect Dis.* 1992;166:616–619.
16. O'Hara MJ. Care of children with HIV infection. In: Kelly P, Holman S, Rothenberg R, Holzemer SP, eds. *Primary Care of Women and Children with HIV Infection.* Boston: Jones and Bartlett; 1995:103–131.
17. Wilfert CM, Wilson C, Luzuriaga K, et al. Pathogenesis of pediatric human immunodeficiency virus type-1 infection. *J Infect Dis.* 1994;170:286–292.
18. CDC. 1994 Revised classification system for human immunodeficiency virus infection in children less than 13 years of age. *MMWR.* 1994;43:RR-12:1–10.
19. CDC. 1995 Revised guidelines for prophylaxis against *Pneumocystis carinii* pneumonia for children infected with or perinatally exposed to human immunodeficiency virus. *MMWR.* 1995;44:RR-4:1–11.
20. American Academy of Pediatrics. Evaluation and medical treatment of the HIV-exposed infant. *Pediatrics.* 1997;99:909–917.
21. CDC. Purified protein derivative (PPD)-tuberculin anergy and HIV infection: guidelines for anergy testing and management of anergic persons at risk for tuberculosis. *MMWR.* 1991;40:27–32.
22. Stephenson KS. Pediatric HIV infection. In: Muma RD, Lyons BA, Borucki MJ, Pollard RB, eds. *HIV, Manual for Health Care Professionals.* Norwalk, CT: Appleton & Lange; 1994:177–202.
23. Grubman S, Oleske J. The maturation of an epidemic: update on pediatric HIV infection. *AIDS.* (suppl 1) 1993;7:S225–S234.
24. Frenkel LD, Gaur S. Perinatal HIV infection and AIDS. *Clin Perinatol.* 1994; 21:95–107.
25. Ellaurie M, Burns ER, Bernstein LJ. Thrombocytopenia and human immunodeficiency virus in children. *Pediatrics.* 1988;82:905–908.
26. Perkocha LA, Rodgers GM. Hematologic aspects of human immunodeficiency

virus infection: laboratory and clinical considerations. *Am J Hematol.* 1988; 29:94–105.
27. Ballem PJ, Belzberg A, Devine D. Pathophysiology of thrombocytopenia associated with HIV infection in homosexual men. *Blutcalkohol.* 1989;59:111–114.
28. Scott GB, Buck BE, Letterman JG. Acquired immunodeficiency syndrome in infants. *N Engl J Med.* 1984;310:76–81.
29. American Academy of Pediatrics. In: Peter G, ed. *1997 Red book: Report of the Committee on Infectious Diseases.* 24th ed. Elk Grove Village: American Academy of Pediatrics; 1997.
30. Pizzo PA, Wilfert CM. AIDS commentary. Antiretroviral therapy for infection due to human immunodeficiency virus in children. *Clin Infect Dis.* 1994;19: 177–196.
31. Grubman S, Gross E, Lerner-Weiss N, et al. Older children and adolescents living with perinatally acquired human immunodeficiency virus infection. *Pediatrics.* 1995;95:657–663.
32. Butz AM, Hutton N, Joyner M. HIV-infected women and infants. Social and health factors impeding utilization of health care. *J Nurse Midwifery.* 1993; 38:103–109.
33. National Center for Health Statistics. *Advance Report for Final Mortality Statistics, 1991. Monthly Vital Statistics Report.* Vol. 42, no. 2 suppl. Hyattsville, MD: Public Health Service; 1993.
34. Lindegren ML, Hanson C, Miller K, Byers RH, Onorato AI. Epidemiology of human immunodeficiency virus infection in adolescents, United States. *Pediatr Infect Dis J.* 1994;13:525–535.
35. Sweeney P, Lindegren ML, Buehler JW, Onorato IM, Janssen RS. Teenagers at risk of human immunodeficiency virus type 1 infection. *Arch Pediatr Adolesc Med.* 1995;149:521–528.
36. CDC. Premarital sexual experience among adolescent women: United States 1970–1988. *MMWR.* 1991;39:929–932.
37. Gutman LP, St Claire KK, Weedy C. Human immunodeficiency virus transmission by child sexual abuse. *Am J Dis Child.* 1991;145:137–141.
38. Goedert JJ, Kessle CM, Aledort LM. A prospective study of human immunodeficiency virus type 1 infection and the development of AIDS in subjects with hemophilia. *N Engl J Med.* 1989;321:1141–1148.
39. Remafedi G, Lauer T. Survival trends in adolescents with human immunodeficiency virus infection. *Arch Pediatr Adolesc Med.* 1995;149:1093–1096.
40. Futterman D, Hein H, Kunins H. Teens and AIDS. Identifying and testing those at risk. *Contemp Pediatr.* 1993;9:68–93.
41. Neinstein LS. *Adolescent Health Care. A Practical Guide.* 2nd ed. Baltimore: Urban & Schwarzenberg, Inc; 1991.

42. Jay MS, Durant RH. Compliance. In: McAnarney ER, Kreipe RE, Orr DP, Comerci GD, eds. *Textbook of Adolescent Medicine.* Philadelphia: WB Saunders; 1992: Chapter 26, pages 206–209.
43. Futterman D, Hein K, Kunins H. Teens and AIDS. Treating the HIV-positive adolescent. *Contemp Pediatr.* 1993;9:55–71.
44. Futterman D, Hein K. Module three: HIV/AIDS medical management. *J Adolesc Health.* 1993;14:36S–52S.
45. Fullilove RE, Fullilove MT, Bowser BP, Gross SA. Risk of sexually transmitted disease among black adolescent crack users in Oakland and San Francisco. *JAMA.* 1990;263:851–855.
46. Hein K, Futterman D. Medical management in HIV-infected adolescents. *J Pediatr.* 1991;119:518–520.
47. Futterman D, Hein H, Kunins H. Teens and AIDS. Reducing AIDS risk in adolescents. *Contemp Pediatr.* 1993;9:67–80.
48. Carpenter CJ, Fischl MA, Hammer SM, et al. Antiretroviral therapy for HIV infection in 1996. Recommendations of an international panel. *JAMA.* 1996; 276:146–154.
49. Anderson MM, Morris RE. HIV and adolescents. *Pediatr Ann.* 1993;22:436–446.
50. Hook EW, Canon RO, Nahmias AJ. Herpes simplex virus infection as a risk factor for human immunodeficiency virus infection in heterosexuals. *J Infect Dis.* 1992;165:251–255.
51. Lyon ME, Richmond D, D'Angelo LJ. Is sexual abuse in childhood or adolescence a predisposing factor for HIV infection during adolescence? *Pediatr AIDS HIV Infect.* 1995;6:271–275.
52. Holtzman D, Anderson JF, Kann L. HIV instruction, HIV knowledge and drug injection among high school students in the United States. *Am J Public Health.* 1991;81:1596–1601.
53. Zabin LS, Hardy JB, Smith EA, Hirsch MB. Substance use and its relation to sexual activity among inner-city adolescents. *J Adolesc Health Care.* 1986;7: 320–331.
54. Rotheram-Borus MJ, Mahler KA, Rosario M. AIDS prevention with adolescents. *AIDS Educ Prev.* 1995;7:320–336.
55. Boyer CB. Psychosocial, behavioral and educational factors in preventing sexually transmitted disease. *Adolesc Med: State of the Art Reviews.* 1990;1:597–613.

CHAPTER 27

Substance Abusers

Mary Jo Hoyt, RN, MSN, FNP

Chapter Preview

- Effect of Substance Abuse on HIV Disease
- Medical Complications of Injection Drug Use
- Major Drugs of Abuse
- Nursing History, Physical Exam, and Management
- Treatment Programs for Substance Abusers

Nurses caring for patients with HIV infection must increasingly be aware of substance abuse disorders, their treatment, and sequelae. Substance abuse is a risk factor for HIV infection through the use of infected injection equipment among injection drug users and through high-risk sexual practices associated with abuse of other drugs and alcohol. Sexual partners of substance users and their children are also at high risk for HIV infection through sexual and perinatal transmission.

HIV can be transmitted through injection drug use when the blood of an HIV-infected drug user is transferred to a drug user who is not yet HIV infected. Needles and syringes are the primary drug injection equipment involved in transferring HIV-infected blood between drug injectors. This transfer of HIV-infected blood occurs almost exclusively through the multiperson use, or sharing, of drug injection equipment.

HIV transmission also is occurring among people who trade sex for noninjected drugs. Recent reports suggest that "crack" cocaine smokers may be at very high risk of acquiring HIV infection heterosexually. Data from one study[1] revealed a 15.7% HIV seroprevalence rate among 1,137 young, inner-city men and women who smoked crack regularly but never injected drugs. The association between crack smoking and high-risk sexual practices and HIV infection was stronger among women than men in the study, with the prevalence of HIV infection as high as 29.6% among crack-smoking women in New York City.[1]

The use of noninjected drugs or alcohol also places a person at risk for HIV transmission because these substances lessen inhibitions and reduce reluctance to engage in unsafe sex. These drugs can reduce inhibition, cloud judgment, result in memory lapses or "blackouts," and may lead to false feelings of safety and lack of concern about HIV.

Drug addict: A person who is physically dependent on one or more psychoactive substances, whose long-term use has produced tolerance, who has lost control over his intake, and who would manifest withdrawal phenomena if discontinuance were to occur

Addiction: A chronic disorder characterized by the compulsive use of a substance resulting in physical, psychological, or social harm to the user and continued despite the harm

Alcoholic: A person who has experienced physical, psychological, social, or occupational impairment as a consequence of habitual, excessive consumption of alcohol

Chemical dependency: Generic term relating to psychological or physical dependency, or both, on an exogenous substance

Drug abuse: Any use of drugs that causes physical, psychological, economic, legal, or social harm to the individual user or to others affected by the drug user's behavior

Substance abuse: The use of a psychoactive substance in a manner detrimental to the individual or society but not meeting criteria for substance or drug dependence

Tolerance: Physiological adaptation to the effect of drugs, so as to diminish effects with constant dosages or to maintain the intensity and duration of effects through increased dosage

Detoxification: A process of withdrawing a person from an addictive substance in a safe and effective manner

Withdrawal: Cessation of drug or alcohol use by an individual in whom dependence is established

Withdrawal syndrome: The onset of a predictable constellation of signs and symptoms involving altered activity of the CNS after the abrupt discontinuation of or rapid decrease in dosage of drug

Enabling behavior: Any action by another person or an institution that intentionally or unintentionally has the effect of facilitating the continuation of abuse or dependence

Recovery: A process of overcoming both physiological and psychological dependence on a drug or alcohol

Relapse: Recurrence of alcohol- or drug-dependent behavior in an individual who has previously achieved and maintained abstinence for a significant time beyond the period of detoxification

Rinaldi RC, Steindler EM, Wilford BB, et al. Clarification and standardization of substance abuse terminology. *JAMA*. 1988;259:555–557.

Effect of Substance Abuse on HIV Disease

The question of whether substance abuse alters the rate of progression of HIV disease and length of survival is complex and has not been clearly answered. What is known is the following:

- Substance abuse increases the risk of acquiring HIV infection
- Some drugs of abuse, particularly opiates and alcohol, have immunosup-

pressive effects that increase the risk of acquiring infectious disease with or without HIV infection
- Injection drug use increases the risk of exposure to blood-borne diseases in addition to HIV
- Other behaviors associated with drug use increase the risk of exposure to infectious diseases (such as STDs and TB)
- Lifestyle factors associated with drug use effect health adversely by interfering with the ability to comply with treatment, eat a healthy diet, and perform basic self-care activities

Medical Complications of Injection Drug Use

The following lists HIV-related and other diseases commonly seen in injection drug users.[2] The asterisks indicate conditions seen in injection drug users that are also common HIV-related opportunistic diseases.

- Bacterial infections
  - Pneumonia*
  - Endocarditis/sepsis (with metastatic abscesses)
  - Skin and soft-tissue infections
  - Osteomyelitis and other skeletal infections
- TB; latent and active (pulmonary and extrapulmonary)*
- STDs
  - Syphilis, gonorrhea, chlamydia
  - Chancroid, herpes simplex,* HPV
- Hepatitis
  - Hepatitis A, B, C, and alcoholic hepatitis
  - HIV-related OIs*
- Nervous system diseases
  - CNS (e.g., drug-related CNS effects, stroke, pyogenic infections, OIS*)
  - Peripheral nervous system (e.g., toxic, nutritional, traumatic, and HIV-related peripheral neuropathies*)
- Other retroviruses; human T-lymphocytic retroviruses types I and II (degenerative neurological diseases, T-cell leukemia/lymphoma, HIV disease progression)

- Malignancies
  - Lymphomas*
  - Solid tumors (e.g., lung, cervix, oropharynx, larynx)
- Miscellaneous
  - Renal disease
  - Constitutional symptoms*
  - Lymphadenopathy*

(Selwyn PA, O'Connor PG. Diagnosis and treatment of substance users with HIV infection. *Prim Care.* 1992;19:120.)

There is significant overlap between the spectrum of opportunistic disease associated with HIV infection and the spectrum of infectious disease associated with injection drug use. Any of the potential complications of injection drug use can occur in conjunction with HIV infection, and HIV may have a negative impact on outcomes associated with these complications.

Bacterial pneumonia and *sepsis* tend to occur in the earlier stages of HIV-related immunosuppression and may be predictors of subsequent HIV-related illness in previously asymptomatic patients. These infections occur more frequently in the HIV-infected injection drug user, even when drug use has been discontinued. *Endocarditis* and *soft-tissue infections* are strongly associated with injection drug use and may be more severe and complicated in the setting of HIV infection. *TB* is more common among drug users, and since both injection drug use and HIV infection are known to produce anergy, tuberculin skin testing for evidence of infection may not be reliable. TB should be considered strongly in the differential diagnosis whenever pulmonary symptoms are present, and providers should have a high index of suspicion for TB in its more uncommon, occult, or disseminated forms with other undiagnosed febrile syndromes.[2]

Manifestations and complications of substance use may overlap closely with those of HIV infection in the area of nervous system dysfunction and disease. *Altered mental status* and some *neuropsychiatric syndromes* can result from the acute or chronic effects of substance use. *Peripheral neuropathies* are associated with substance abuse. In addition to HIV infection, they can be related directly to alcoholism, nutritional deficiencies, or trauma.

Human T-lymphotropic retrovirus (HTLV) types I and II have routes of transmission believed to be similar to those of HIV, and HTLV-I has been found to be concentrated among IV drug users, especially among blacks.[3] HTLV-I is associated with adult T-cell leukemia/lymphoma, with the chronic degenerative neurological disease tropical spastic paraparesis, and with HTLV-I-associated myelopathy. HTLV-I coinfection with HIV has been reported to be associated with a pattern of rapid HIV disease progression.[4]

Major Drugs of Abuse

Heroin

Heroin is an opioid and is the most common opioid to be used intravenously. Heroin may also be smoked, "snorted" (intranasal), or "skin popped" (intradermal injection). Since heroin is generally sold in single-dose "bags," addicts generally report the number of "bags" per day they use. The duration of action of heroin is 3 to 4 hours, so that addicts must inject four to six times per day to avoid withdrawal symptoms.

The following is some drug-related street terminology.

Mainlining: Injecting drugs directly into a vein
Skin popping: Injecting drugs intradermally
Snort: Short inhalation of heroin through the nose
Sniff: Short inhalation of cocaine through the nose
Booting: Process of drawing blood back into the syringe and mixing it with the drug before injecting
Spike: Needle
Works: Syringe, needle, and cooker
Cooker: Spoon or metal soda can top that is used to prepare heroin for injection; the heroin is mixed with water, heated over a flame to dissolve it, cooled, and then drawn into the syringe through a piece of cotton
Shooting gallery: A place, frequently an abandoned building, where drugs are sold and bought, along with the equipment needed for injecting; sex for drugs and money is also frequently available
Tracks: Needle marks on the skin
Speedball: Heroin and cocaine taken together

Freebase: Kit used to remove impurities from cocaine so that the fumes can be inhaled
Freeze: Cold feeling in the throat after sniffing cocaine
Line: Cocaine powder or flakes in a line on a smooth, hard surface so that it may be sniffed

(From Narcotic and Drug Research, Inc. AIDS: Medical Management of the HIV-Infected/Chemically Dependent Client. New York: Narcotic and Drug Research, Inc.; 1989:XV.)

The primary effect sought by users is an immediate euphoria. Euphoria is followed by sedation ("nodding") and then withdrawal ("kicking"). Chronic heroin use leads to a loss of the euphoric effects, and use becomes more a matter of avoiding withdrawal. To counteract the sedative effect of heroin, some addicts mix it with cocaine to make a "speedball."

Heroin withdrawal begins within 4 to 6 hours, peaks between 2 and 3 days, and the acute syndrome lasts 7 to 12 days. In severe withdrawal, agitation, muscle cramps, and diarrhea predominate. Table 27.1 lists the signs and symptoms of opioid withdrawal.

Management of Heroin Overdose

Symptoms of heroin (as well as other opiates) overdose are primarily respiratory and CNS depression. Initial management involves an assess-

Table 27.1 Signs and Symptoms of Opioid Withdrawal

Affected System	Sign/Symptom
General	Anxiety, opioid craving
Vital signs	Hypertension, tachycardia, fever
Nervous system	Restlessness, irritability, tremor, chills, insomnia, muscle cramps, yawning
Skin	Perspiration, "goose flesh"
Ear, nose, throat (ENT)	Pupillary dilation, lacrimation, rhinorrhea
Gastrointestinal	Anorexia, nausea, vomiting, hyperactive bowel sounds, diarrhea

Selwyn PA, O'Connor PG. Diagnosis and treatment of substance users with HIV infection. *Prim Care.* 1992;19:133.

ment of the neurological and pulmonary dysfunction, with intubation and assisted ventilation provided if indicated. The mainstay of pharmacological management is naloxone, a short-acting opioid antagonist that is given in doses of up to 0.4 mg IV and repeated as indicated.[2] Urine toxicology should be performed. It should be determined whether the overdose was unintentional or suicidal, and follow-up drug treatment and/or psychiatric treatment should be arranged.

Management of Heroin Withdrawal

The acute opioid withdrawal syndrome can be very uncomfortable and is a strong stimulus for continued drug use. In deciding the type and extent of management necessary to manage withdrawal, both physical signs and a patient's subjective symptoms should be evaluated. Mild withdrawal may not require any pharmacological intervention, whereas more severe opioid withdrawal may require more aggressive inpatient management. Three approaches can be employed as needed.

1. Methadone is a synthetic opioid. Because of its properties of cross-tolerance with heroin, its oral availability, and its relatively long half-life (24–36 hours), methadone can block withdrawal symptoms and provide a comfortable detoxification. Starting daily doses range from 10 to 30 mg, and then the dose is tapered over 5 to 14 days. Methadone detoxification can only be used in the inpatient setting or in the setting of a methadone maintenance program.[2]
2. Clonidine can suppress signs and symptoms of opioid withdrawal. Doses are generally 0.2 mg of clonidine orally every 4 hours for a total daily dose of up to 1.4 mg. (Higher doses of clonidine are needed for detoxification than for hypertension.) Peak doses are usually used on day 2 or 3, with a taper over subsequent days and discontinuation by 7 to 14 days. Clonidine can be useful in the ambulatory care setting, when methadone detoxification is not possible, or in the inpatient setting. In an outpatient setting, it must be supervised carefully by daily dispensing and careful monitoring for hypotension.[2]
3. Clonidine in combination with naltrexone can provide rapid detoxification. Naltrexone is a potent, long-acting narcotic antagonist. Patients are "preloaded" with clonidine on day 1 and are then given a small dose of naltrexone (12.5 or 25.0 mg) to induce opioid withdrawal. This induced withdrawal is generally more severe than pa-

tients would experience otherwise, but it is relatively brief and patients are detoxified in 2 to 4 days rather than in the 7 to 14 days required for clonidine alone.[2]

Cocaine

Cocaine is both a stimulant and an anesthetic. It can be "sniffed," smoked as "crack," or injected intravenously. Crack cocaine gained widespread use in many urban neighborhoods in the mid 1980s. Although injection drug use is practiced predominantly by men, the use of crack cocaine is widespread among both men and women.

Users describe intense pleasure, feeling of well-being, heightened energy and sexuality, and lowered anxiety. Tolerance does not develop to cocaine as it does with opioids. IV cocaine and crack users often take the drug in binges lasting for hours or days. The effects of cocaine administered intravenously last 20 to 40 minutes; the duration of effect for crack cocaine is shorter.

Abrupt discontinuance of the use of cocaine does not lead to a physiologically disruptive state as seen with opioids. There is, however, a recognized and prolonged withdrawal syndrome with three distinct phases. "Crash" is a period of extreme exhaustion, sleep, and lethargy lasting for several days postbinge. The "withdrawal" period, characterized by depression with anhedonia can then follow, lasting for several weeks. "Extinction" occurs with prolonged abstinence, when patients experience cocaine craving with conditioned cues (people, places, and circumstances associated with cocaine use).[5]

Management of Cocaine Emergencies

Acute cocaine intoxication is generally associated with binge cocaine use. Symptoms are primarily behavioral, including disinhibition, psychomotor activation, impulsiveness, anxiety, irritability, paranoia, and delusions. Acutely psychotic patients should be hospitalized. Many of these symptoms can be treated with targeted medical interventions, such as benzodiazepines for anxiety and antipsychotic agents for delusions and paranoia. In general, these symptoms resolve within several days after cocaine use is discontinued. Often, symptoms can be managed without specific medical therapy in a supportive environment.

Treatment of cocaine overdose can be a medical emergency. Cocaine toxicity produces hypertension, tachycardia, tonic-clonic seizures, dyspnea, and ventricular arrhythmias. IV diazepam in doses up to 0.5 mg/kg administered over an 8-hour period has been shown to be effective in controlling seizures. The systemic concomitants of a hypermetabolic state produced by cocaine toxicity with concurrent ventricular arrhythmias have been managed successfully by administration of 0.5 to 1.0 mg of propranolol IV.[6]

Management of Cocaine Withdrawal

A physiological withdrawal syndrome is less of an issue with cocaine than with opiate withdrawal, and outpatient detoxification is often employed. In comparison to opioids, standard medical therapies for managing cocaine withdrawal and relapse prevention are relatively undeveloped. Agents with cocaine-blocking and cross-tolerance properties are not currently available for treatment of cocaine addiction. With high levels of binge use, however, inpatient detoxification may be necessary to interrupt cocaine use. Medical therapy has been employed experimentally to promote detoxification and relapse prevention. The tricyclic antidepressants have been studied most extensively for this purpose. Early uncontrolled studies and subsequent randomized trials have suggested that desipramine may result in decreased cocaine craving, milder withdrawal, and decreased cocaine use.[7]

Nursing History, Physical Exam, and Management

The most effective way of getting people to minimize the harmful effects of their drug use is to provide user-friendly services that attract them and empower them to change their behavior toward a suitable, healthier, intermediate objective. For example, one appropriate intermediate objective is to keep the client engaged in care. Providing nonjudgmental services is one way to achieve that goal. It is often helpful for nurses to think of substance use as a chronic disease, with features common to other chronic diseases with which we are more familiar, such as diabetes or chronic lung disease. Like these conditions, substance use is characterized by exacerbation and remissions. Being able to anticipate and accept relapses, and becoming familiar with the treatment options that are available helps to alleviate frustration for health care providers, and helps them to provide better care.[2]

Drug users often feel inadequate to hold their own with professionals, and are accustomed to experiencing contempt from human service and health care workers. It is helpful for nurses to try to set up an egalitarian relationship rather than a hierarchical one, and to try to convey to the client that you do not have an agenda of your own regarding the client's drug use.

To engage drug-using clients, it is important to provide services that give a direct, immediate benefit. For example, if a drug user is admitted to the hospital and her first complaint is that she is cold and hungry, provide a blanket and a meal whenever possible before proceeding with your work. In the outpatient setting, ask the client what she really wants. Validate what it is and then tell her what is available and what you can do to help her. Although it is very appropriate to let the client know the rules, do not begin your relationship with threats and warnings.

Problematic Behavior

In their day-to-day lives, chemically dependent clients have difficulty setting limits on their behaviors. The pain and anxiety that accompany acute or chronic illness can further decrease their ability to exercise control over their behaviors. For nurses dealing with inappropriate behaviors, it is helpful first to identify which behavior changes are of the highest priority and then to be very specific about what is expected from the client, as well as what is expected from the staff. Set limits without judgment and anger.

The health care team should devote the time and effort required to develop a simple, realistic plan of care and to follow through with the plan consistently. Inconsistency on the part of staff may fuel attempts at manipulation and result in staff frustration and anger. To avoid inconsistency it may be helpful for the staff to discuss how easy it is to become involved inadvertently in either "rescuing" or angry behaviors. Anticipate specific problems that may occur with a particular client and identify what should be done, in contrast to what may be a tempting, yet detrimental, response.[8]

Sometimes the client's unacceptable behavior is the only way the client knows how to respond. Foul language and verbal rudeness may be common in the client's daily life, and there may be a lack of exposure to more appropriate means of communication. The events that precipitated the behavior should be explored, and the desired behavior stated clearly. For example, the nurse can state that foul language in not acceptable, and then ask the client if something specific has caused the client to be angry. The nurse can also assist the client to learn the new behavior. The nurse can acknowledge the client's anger, and then suggest an alternative response such as, "Rather than use words that upset the nurses, you might try telling the nurse that you are experiencing uncomfortable symptoms, and would appreciate it if your methadone dose could be brought to you as soon as possible."[8]

Written agreements that include mutually agreed-on goals and behaviors expected of both the patient and the nurse may also be useful. Contracts should be kept very simple, dealing only with the degree of behavioral change that is absolutely required, and should be carefully reviewed verbally with the client. The contract also needs to include what the client can expect from caregivers. For example, the client can agree to refrain from abusive language, and the nurses can agree to deliver the methadone dose within 10 minutes of its scheduled administration time. The most difficult consideration in such contracts is deciding what can be done if the client violates the contract. A client's failure does not mean that the staff fails in their professional responsibilities.

Nursing History

Nurses can develop a consistent method of taking a substance abuse history on all patients that is thorough yet brief, and asking questions in a nonjudgmental fashion to nurture trust and to encourage honesty. The history should include information on five major aspects of substance use: types of drugs used, route of administration, pattern of use, treatment, and complications. In identifying types of substances, it is important to ask about each specific drug used. Specific information should be requested regarding route of administration and pattern of use for each drug used. To determine recent use, ask: When did you last use . . . ?[2]

The following is a sample drug history guide.

- Substances used
  - Opioids: heroin; methadone; prescription analgesics: codeine, fentanyl, hydromorphone (Dilaudid), meperidine (Demerol), oxycodone (Percocet, Percodan), propoxyphene (Darvon)
  - Stimulants: cocaine; prescription stimulants: dextroamphetamine (Dexedrine), methamphetamine (Desoxyn), methylphenidate (Ritalin)
  - Alcohol: beer; "spirits"; wine
  - Anxiolytics: benzodiazepines: alprazolam (Xanax), chlordiazepoxide (Librium), clonazepam (Klonipin), diazepam (Valium), flurazepam (Dalmane), lorazepam (Ativan)
  - Other sedatives/hypnotics: barbiturates: phenobarbital, secobarbital; chloral hydrate
  - Marijuana and hashish hallucinogens, LSD; phencyclidine (PCP)
  - Others: inhaled solvents (glues), nonprescription drugs: sleeping pills, weight-loss products
- Administration
  - Intravenous ("shooting")
  - Subcutaneous ("skin popping")
  - Intranasal ("snorting," "sniffing")
  - Inhaled ("smoking")
  - Oral ("popping")
- Patterns of use
  - Duration
  - Frequency
  - Most recent use
  - Amount (usual and highest)
  - Polysubstance use
- Treatment history
  - Detoxification and relapse prevention
  - Outpatient: self-help groups (Alcoholic Anonymous, Narcotics Anonymous), counseling (individual, group, family), medically supported (e.g., clonidine, methadone, naltrexone, disulfiram [Antabuse]), employee assistance program

(continued)

  - Inpatient: hospital based, residential therapeutic communities
- Complications
  - Medical: needle-induced complications (e.g., endocarditis, hepatitis, soft-tissue infections), drug-induced complications (e.g., overdose, withdrawal, chronic toxicity)
  - Social: marital and family disruption, legal problems, employment problems

(Selwyn PA, O'Connor PG. Diagnosis and treatment of substance users with HIV infection. *Prim Care.* 1992;19:135.)

The CAGE Questionnaire is used to screen for alcohol abuse. A positive response to one of the four questions has a sensitivity of 85% and a specificity of 89% in detecting alcohol abuse.

1. Have you ever felt you ought to CUT DOWN on your drinking?
2. Have people ANNOYED you by criticizing your drinking?
3. Have you ever felt GUILTY about your drinking?
4. Have you ever had a drink first thing in the morning to steady your nerves (EYE OPENER)?

(Ewing, JA Detecting alcoholism, the CAGE Questionaire, *JAMA* 1984;252:1905)

Nursing Physical Examination

A physical examination can be helpful in assessing patients with HIV infection for the effects of acute or chronic substance use. Routine assessment of patients should include special attention for the presence of following signs: injection marks or "tracks," usually found in the antecubital fossae, on the forearms, hands, neck, legs, or feet, and less commonly involving such sites as the breasts or the dorsal vein of the penis. These may be fresh (appearing as fresh punctate marks, often with mild surrounding erythema) or old (linear, hyperpigmented scars). Also, be alert for redness and lymphedema of the hands ("puffy-hand" sign), cigarette burns; fresh or old abscesses and soft-tissue infections; hyperemia or erosion of the nasal septum; hepatosplenomegaly; and the stigmata of chronic alcohol abuse and cirrhosis.[2]

Nursing Management of Clients on Methadone Maintenance

When methadone-maintained patients are admitted to the hospital, their methadone dose should be confirmed with the program as soon as possible. Unless medically contraindicated, the same dose, given at the same time, should be continued in the inpatient setting without interruption. Some drugs may interfere with methadone metabolism, and the dose of methadone must be altered accordingly (as described later). A maintenance dose of methadone should not be considered a substitute for adequate pain management in acute medical or surgical conditions. Methadone-maintained patients may require analgesics in higher than usual doses because of their high opioid tolerance.

Rifampin increases the elimination of methadone and reduces methadone plasma levels, probably because of the induction of hepatic microsomal enzymes. This effect results in the rapid onset of classic opioid withdrawal symptoms, usually within the first several days of rifampin initiation. This can be prevented by increasing patients' daily methadone doses, usually by 10 mg every 1 to 2 days, beginning on the day that rifampin is started and finally reaching a new steady state at a dosage level that is often at least 50% greater than the original daily dose. These rapid dosage increases should be monitored closely, titrated to oversedation. It may be useful to divide the daily methadone dose, giving two thirds in the morning and one third in the evening, to prevent the occurrence of withdrawal symptoms at the end of the 24-hour dosing interval.[2]

Phenytoin and *phenobarbital* may also result in opioid withdrawal symptoms when used in methadone-maintained patients. The effects are usually less dramatic than those of rifampin, and generally occur over days to weeks rather than over the first few days of therapy. Accordingly, methadone dosage increases usually do not need to be as great nor as rapid as with rifampin.[2]

Nursing Management of Pain

A number of studies[9,10] have documented both a high prevalence and intensity of pain in persons with HIV disease, and managing such pain is an important component of nursing care for persons with AIDS. The care of chemically dependent patients with pain is not only often challenging, but also potentially frustrating. Planning care for these patients is best accomplished with a team approach that includes the expertise of several specialties, particularly pain and addiction. However, sufficient information from research now exists to support suggestions for guidelines that can help nurses manage pain successfully in this special population. Pain management guidelines for persons with a history of substance abuse are as follows.

- Accept and respect the report of pain in spite of the possibility of being duped. Pain is subjective, and it will never be possible to know if the patient is telling the truth about pain.
- Remember that 50 to 90% of persons with AIDS experience pain, regardless of HIV transmission factor or history of addiction.
- Rehabilitation from addiction is not appropriate when it is not the patient's goal and/or when an acute medical problem exists.
- Prevent or minimize withdrawal symptoms in acutely ill patients.
- Pain ratings given by the patient are regarded as the single most reliable indicator of pain. Use a consistent pain rating scale so that assessments can be compared. Behaviors and vital signs cannot be used to discount what the patient reports about pain.
- Relieve pain. Utilize the World Health Organization's analgesic ladder for all patients. Withholding opioid analgesics from chemically dependent patients with pain has never been shown to increase the likelihood of recovery from addiction.
- For all patients with severe pain, increase the dose of opioid until the patient reports satisfactory pain relief or until unmanageable side effects occur.
- The preferred route of administration in all patients is oral. This helps to avoid the peaks and valleys associated with parenteral administration, and slows the development of tolerance to opioids.
- Keep all patients informed about what drugs are being used, the doses, and the intervals between. Let them know if and when changes will be made, especially if the anticipated change is from parenteral to oral dosing. Keeping this information a secret only serves to promote feelings of distrust and anxiety in the patient.
- When pain is present most of the day, analgesics should be administered at specific times around the clock.
- If the patient is chemically dependent on opioids, it is very likely that the doses of opioid required to relieve pain will be higher than those

usually required for patients who have not been taking opioids for weeks or longer.
- Never use placebos. It is deceitful and yields no useful information.
- Never use pain relief as a bargaining chip.
- Remember that methadone maintenance treatment is used to stem heroin craving and not to provide analgesia.

(McCaffery M, Vourakis C. Assessment and relief of pain in chemically dependent patients. *Orthop Nurs.* 1992;11:232.)

Pain management in patients with AIDS with a history of substance abuse is complicated by concerns about potential drug-seeking behavior, or contribution to or renewal of inappropriate drug use. While important, such concerns sometimes interfere with good clinical judgment concerning appropriate management of pain and the use of narcotic analgesics. Frequency and intensity of pain have been found to be similar in patients with AIDS with or without a history of chemical dependency.[9,10] All patients who complain of pain must be assessed carefully to identify potential disease processes that may benefit from specific therapy along with analgesia.

As in all patients with pain, the primary goal in management is to maximize comfort while minimizing side effects. If adequate relief can be obtained with non-narcotic drugs such as nonsteroidal anti-inflammatory agents, then these drugs are preferred. If narcotics are required, then they should be used, even in narcotic-dependent patients. Pain relief is a legal, medical reason for taking opioids, and it is important to realize that taking opioid analgesics for pain relief is not addiction. As with other patients, addicts are often undertreated for acute pain. Because of tolerance, opiate addicts generally require higher total doses of narcotics at more frequent dosing intervals for effective analgesia.[8] This requirement is especially true for patients maintained on methadone.

When addicts are started on narcotics for acute pain syndromes, the reasons for their use and the treatment plan must be clear to both provider and patient. It is critical that patients feel that their pain is taken seriously, but also that such narcotic use not be extended beyond the period required for analgesia. Adjustment in dosage of analgesia should be discussed with patients beforehand and, when appropriate, tapering should proceed in a consistent and explicit manner. Abrupt or undisclosed drug discontinuation easily promotes patient distrust.

Nursing Management Using the Harm Reduction Model of Care

The Harm Reduction Model of care was developed as a response to HIV/AIDS and the growing harmful consequences caused by the use of prohibited drugs. A fundamental principle of the model is that abstinence from drugs should not be the only objective of services to drug users because it excludes a large proportion of the people who deny that substance abuse is a problem, who are not motivated to discontinue drug use, or who are unable to maintain abstinence. The Harm Reduction Model also assumes that HIV and other disease prevention should take priority over absolute prevention of drug use because it presents a greater threat to the drug user, to the public health, and to the national economy.[11] The techniques of this model can be helpful in nursing care and management of drug users in acute or ambulatory care settings who refuse or fail drug treatment, and who need to be taught safer drug use techniques.

Cleaning Needles

While nurses should stress the strategy of not sharing clean injection equipment, they must also be realists and teach injectors how to clean equipment with bleach in case works are shared, and in cases when the origin of the equipment is not clear. Nursing instructions should also include skin-cleaning techniques, and avoiding arterial sticks or injury. Directions on cleaning equipment are simple.

Step 1: Use fresh bleach. Fill and empty the syringe and needle with bleach twice. Dip the spoon in bleach.

Step 2: Use fresh water. Fill and empty the syringe and needle with water twice. Dip the spoon in water.

Needle Exchange Programs

The alternative to cleaning needles with bleach is to refer the patient to a needle exchange program. These programs distribute clean needles, dispose of used ones safely for injection drug users, and offer referrals to drug treatment and HIV counseling and testing. Call the AIDS service organizations in your area to determine if such a program is available for your patients.

Alternate Ways of Taking Drugs

Another strategy is to try to convince injectors to try other routes of drug administration. Intranasal use may be less desirable for users because the drug effect comes on more slowly with snorting, and there is a loss of some of the drug, whereas with injecting in a vein, the drug is felt almost immediately and none is wasted. Nonetheless, intranasal use is safer than injection use. Cocaine and heroin can also be smoked with pipes, which involves a very quick effect and little drug waste.

Treatment Programs for Substance Abusers

When a substance use problem is identified, acceptance of the diagnosis and motivation for treatment on the part of the client are required before treatment can be initiated or be successful. Nurses should be sensitive (1) to the issues that promote denial, such as guilt, shame, and fear of social stigma; and (2) to those that interfere with motivation, such as a sense of hopelessness, lack of faith in the treatment system, depression, fear of failure, and lack of social support. Job loss; loss of other income; having children removed from the home; and loss of support from medical providers, family, and friends are realistic fears that can be addressed and discussed with the nurse or drug counselor.[2]

Nurses can also assist patients and substance abuse professionals by helping to match patients to the most appropriate treatment program. Elements to consider are addiction severity, medical status, psychiatric status, treatment history, social support, financial status/insurance coverage, and living situation.

Detoxification Programs

Patients who need to be detoxified from a single drug might be detoxified as outpatients, whereas those addicted to multiple drugs may be detoxified more safely in an inpatient setting. Patients who are unstable medically will also require an initial inpatient approach, as will those with moderate to severe psychiatric morbidity. Detoxification programs may be affiliated with a hospital or may be independent. The length of stay varies from 3 days to more than 30 days, depending on the substances involved and the program.

Therapeutic Communities (TCs)

TCs provide a highly structured living environment and a lengthy time commitment (up to 2 years). TCs are based on the theory that the problem is not just one of addiction, but of a personality deficit that leads to addiction. The individual is viewed as an infant who needs to learn adult ways of coping to replace the coping mechanism of chronic drug use. The TC environment consists of a steady stream of confrontational group therapy, community sharing of household chores, and increasing responsibilities that, successfully completed, lead to increased freedom. Through this process, personality restructuring is thought to occur. Not all TCs accept symptomatic HIV-infected individuals.

Self-Help Groups

These groups are generally based on the model of AA. Chapters of AA, NA, and Cocaine Anonymous have been organized worldwide. Members must admit they are addicts, recognize that they will always be addicts, and understand that "recovery" is a lifelong process. Recovery is a commitment to a drug- and alcohol-free lifestyle, and adherence to the values and concepts set forth in the 12-step program first developed in AA. Meetings are open and can be attended as frequently as needed by the individual. In meetings, individuals share their experiences with drugs or alcohol, and through this process and with the help of a sponsor (a fellow member), obtain mutual support to remain drug or alcohol free.

Methadone Maintenance

Methadone is a long-acting opiate that possesses almost all the physiologic properties of heroin. Chronic use of methadone blocks the withdrawal symptoms of opioid discontinuation without creating euphoria or sedation. Drug maintenance is not aimed at "curing" opiate addiction, but at providing a substitute drug that is legally accessible, safer, can be taken orally, and has a long half-life so that it can be taken once a day. Methadone can help the addict who cannot succeed in drug-free programs to improve functioning within the family and job, to decrease legal problems, and to improve health. Methadone is administered once a day at the program center, with weekend portions taken by the patient at home.

References

1. Edlin R, Irwin KL, Faruque S, et al. Intersecting epidemics—crack cocaine use and HIV infection among inner-city young adults. *N Engl J Med.* 1994;331: 1422–1453.
2. Selwyn PA, O'Connor PG. Diagnosis and treatment of substance users with HIV infection. *Prim Care.* 1992;19:119–156.
3. Robert-Guroff M, Weiss SH, Giron JA, et al. Prevalence of antibodies to HTLV-I-II and III in intravenous drug abusers from an AIDS-endemic region. *JAMA.* 1986;255:3133–3137.
4. Weiss SH, French J, Holland B, et al. HTLV-I/II coinfection is significantly associated with risk for progression to AIDS among HIV(+) intravenous drug abusers. Presented at the Fifth International Conference on AIDS. Montreal, Canada, June 1989, Abstract no. Th.A.O.23.
5. Lowenstein DH, Massa SM, Rowbotham MC, et al. Acute neurologic and psychiatric complications associated with cocaine abuse. *Am J Med.* 1987;83:841–845.
6. Mendelson JH, Mello NK. Cocaine and other commonly abused drugs. In: Isselbacher KJ, Braunwald E, Wilson JD, et al, eds. *Harrison's Principles of Internal Medicine.* 13th ed. Vol. 2. New York: McGraw-Hill; 1994:2429–2431.
7. Gawin FH, Ellinwod EH. Cocaine and other stimulants. Actions, abuse, and treatment. *N Engl J Med.* 1988;318:1173–1179.
8. McCaffery M, Vourakis C. Assessment and relief of pain in chemically dependent patients. *Orthop Nurs.* 1992;11:13–27.
9. Newshan G, Wainapel S. Pain characteristics and their management in persons with AIDS. *J Assoc Nurses AIDS Care.* 1993;4:53–59.
10. Hoyt MJ, Nokes K, Newshan G. The effect of chemical dependency on pain perception in persons with AIDS. *J Assoc Nurses AIDS Care.* 1994;5:33–38.
11. Springer E. Effective AIDS prevention with active drug use: the harm reduction model. In: Shernoff M, ed. *Counseling Chemically Dependent People with HIV Illness.* Haworth Press: Binghamton, NY; 1991:141–157.

CHAPTER 28

Culturally Diverse Populations: Hispanic

Barbara Aranda-Naranjo, PhD, RN

Chapter Preview

- Demographics
- HIV Infection among Hispanics
- Hispanics as a Vulnerable Population
- Health Care Needs for Hispanic Families Living with HIV Infection
- Case Management Approach for Hispanic Families Living with HIV Infection
- Recommendations
- Resources
- Hispanic Resources

Demographics

The Hispanic population is made up of four main subgroups: Mexican-American, Puerto Rican, Cuban, and Central and South American. The Mexican-American group accounts for the largest and fastest growing subgroup. Of the 23 million Hispanics living in the United States, 63% are Mexican-American, 12% are Puerto Rican, 13% are Central and South American, 5% are Cuban, and 8% are "other Hispanic."[1] The two subgroups with the highest poverty level are Puerto Ricans and Mexican-Americans.[1] The median age of Hispanics residing in the United States is 26.2 years, making this population one of the youngest US ethnic/racial groups. Based on current demographics, it is predicted that Hispanics will be the largest national ethnic/racial population in the United States by the year 2000, accounting for 42% of this country's new population growth.[1]

Social History

Hispanics originate from a number of areas in Latin America and most speak Spanish. The term *Hispanic* is more of a generic term and does not identify specifically the essence of the subgroups that comprise this aggregate. Besides the term *Hispanic, Latin Americans* have also been called *Latino, Chicano* (only Mexican-American descendants), *Spanish-American, Spanish-surnamed, Spanish origin,* and *Spanish speaking.*[2] Most Hispanics live in poverty in urban areas, and reside in overcrowded and substandard housing. These conditions add to the vulnerability of this population to health-related problems. The adequacy of health care among low socioeconomic status (SES) Hispanics is limited by several factors, such as (1) problems of access related to poverty, including financial and knowledge barriers; (2) cultural and language differences that may affect the quality of patient-provider interaction and may have an inhibiting effect on health care utilization; and (3) the use of folk medicine as an alternative coping strategy when problems with access occur.

Hispanic Subgroups

The migration of Mexicans, Puerto Ricans, Cubans, Central and South Americans, and other Hispanic groups to the United States resulted in varied experiences for the people that make up these subgroups. Understanding these different migration experiences will assist the health care provider in further "contextualizing" health care behaviors and attitudes exhibited by Hispanic individuals with HIV infection. *Contextualizing* refers to the identification of variables such as cultural values and beliefs, socioeconomic conditions, sociopolitical issues, and environmental factors that need to be considered when assessing a Hispanic patient and family.

Mexican-American Experience

In 1848 Mexico lost the northern half of its territory, including California, Arizona, Utah, and Nevada, to the United States. Mexicans living in this territory were given the choice of becoming citizens of the United States or returning to Mexico. Many twentieth century Mexican-Americans are descendants of the approximately 80% who chose to remain in the United States. Since then, availability of work has been the driving force behind Mexican immigration to the United States.

From the time of the earliest contact between Mexican and Anglo populations, tension has existed between them. Anglo-Americans were driven by their belief that it was their "manifest destiny" to conquer and occupy land in America. This belief was one of the forces that led ultimately to disrespect of the Mexicans who had once inhabited the northern part of Mexico, which is now part of the United States. At the end of the Mexican War, the Treaty of Guadalupe Hidalgo was signed. The treaty was supposed to guarantee that Mexicans had a right to keep their property, language, religion, culture, and customs, but this treaty was violated continually.[3] The displacement that occurred secondary to violation of the treaty has led to distrust of Anglos by present-day Mexican-Americans.

Mexicans continued to migrate to the United States in the following years for a variety of factors, primarily socioeconomic, including the instability created by the Mexican Revolution of 1910 and the emerging demand for cheap labor in this country.[4] Today the most pressing problem is the migration of "illegal aliens," Mexicans migrating illegally to the United States. A national debate about illegal migration is currently occurring. The majority of Mexican-Americans during the first half of the twentieth century remained heavily concentrated in low-skill, low-pay rural and urban employment.[5] These socioeconomic conditions and their historical context have influenced the perceptions and attitudes of Mexican-Americans in every aspect of their lives today.

Puerto Rican Experience

At the end of the Spanish-American War in 1898, the United States acquired Puerto Rico from the Spaniards as "compensation." Since then, the US dominance of the island's economic and political existence is a classic model of colonialism.[6] Like many other Hispanics, Puerto Ricans migrated to the United States for socioeconomic factors and for a better life. As a result of US trade and economic policies in the 1940s ("Operation Bootstrap"), the island's economy became increasingly geared to industrialization and away from agriculture. This created an unemployed labor pool that could not be absorbed, so people were "pushed" from their Puerto Rican homeland to the United States.[2] Like the Mexican-Americans, Puerto Ricans suffer racial prejudice in their interactions with Anglo-Americans, even though they are US citizens.[6]

Cuban Experience

In the 1900s the first wave of Cuban immigrants from all economic and social classes entered the United States. They settled primarily in Florida. The second wave of immigrants came when Fidel Castro took power in 1959. Of the 273,000 immigrated by 1973, the majority were from business and professional classes. Cubans were the only Hispanic subgroup to receive assistance from the US federal government in the form of housing, health care, and food. Cubans, unlike any other Latino group in the United States to date, gained significant political power due to dual efforts between the anti-Castro Cuban exiles and the US Central Intelligence Agency to overthrow Castro's government in the Bay of Pigs invasion.

Central and South American Experience

The most recent Hispanic arrivals have been from Central American countries, particularly El Salvador and Nicaragua. Like the Mexicans, Puerto Ricans, and Cubans, many of these immigrants are fleeing from political violence, war, and poverty in their homelands.[2] Presently these new Hispanic immigrants are denied recognized refugee status and therefore do not have access to needed health and human services. These new immigrants pose the greatest challenge to health and human service providers because they do not have consistent health care and usually wait until they are very sick before accessing a physician. Their struggles to maintain their basic needs almost always take precedence over their health care.

HIV Infection among Hispanics

AIDS is the seventh leading cause of death among Hispanics.[7] Through June 1993 the CDC had received reports of 315,390 cases of AIDS among persons in the United States, including 52,531 among Hispanics.[8] The prevalence rate among Hispanics accounts for 17% of AIDS cases in the United States, although they represent approximately 10% of the total US population.[7] The mortality attributable to AIDS was 22 deaths per 100,000 among Hispanics compared with nine deaths per 100,000 among non-Hispanic whites.[9] The major modes of transmission for Hispanics are injectable drug use and heterosexual transmission (see also the discussion in Chapter 2 on epidemiology and ethnicity).

Hispanics as a Vulnerable Population

Hispanics in the United States often do not have adequate access to primary, secondary, or tertiary health care. Lack of economic resources accompanied by cultural and institutional barriers are the primary reasons for poor access to health care.[10] The absence of health insurance is one of the most serious barriers to Hispanics to obtaining access to health care, especially preventive services.[11–13] Hispanic-Americans are more likely than blacks or Anglo-Americans to be without health insurance coverage (32% of Hispanics, 20% of blacks, and 13% of Anglos). This is accounted for by the large number of Hispanic-Americans, frequently referred to as *the working poor*, who are the first generation in the United States and thus are forced to seek low-wage employment without health insurance benefits.[14]

Institutional barriers are another major factor contributing to the underutilization of health care by Hispanics, including lack of (1) health care personnel who can speak and write Spanish, (2) cultural sensitivity to Hispanic clients' values and beliefs, and (3) Hispanic community input into the structuring of the health care system. These barriers are inherent in the US health care system and in the ways health care resources are distributed.[15] Many Hispanics seek services at public institutions, such as county hospitals, public health clinics, and health and human service agencies, which have long waiting periods and are not user friendly. This health care setup is not conducive to people experiencing an array of problems associated with poverty, illiteracy, housing, and unemployment. Health care systems in the past have not collaborated with Hispanic communities to develop user-friendly services. Health care coverage coupled with socioeconomic variables such as employment, housing, and education place the Hispanic community at risk for both acute and chronic medical diseases.

Current health policies regarding the care of HIV-infected Hispanic women were developed based on what health care providers perceived to be the needs of this population. Because this population consists of individuals from various ethnic subgroups, sociocultural differences exist that were not taken into consideration when health care policies were developed.[16] Health policy addressing the needs of non-Anglo population groups was handled under the rubric of "minority health."[17] Health care providers who interact with patients and their families on a one-on-one basis may see various aspects of this picture more clearly and can act as patient advocates to plan and provide care that is effective, humane, and respects the dignity of the patient.

Health Care Needs for Hispanic Families Living with HIV Infection

The major needs of Hispanic families living with HIV infection are similar to those without HIV living in poverty and are "basic needs," such as food, housing, transportation, and a source of income. Many of the subgroups making up the Hispanic population lack the basic resources to meet their survival needs.[18] In addition, many do not have health insurance and have thus experienced poor access to health care. With lower socioeconomic status, many families do not consider health care a priority and usually seek care only in emergency situations. "Minorities, the poor, and those with less education tend to experience more health problems in general over the course of their lives, than do their socioeconomically advantaged counterparts."[16(p 50)]

Poor access ranges from absence of a consistent health care provider to utilization of emergency rooms as a source of primary health care. The Hispanic experience as it relates to health care access is very serious for those individuals who have been infected with HIV and do not have a consistent health care provider. Early HIV diagnosis becomes difficult, as does accurate determination of HIV-related morbidity and mortality.

Other variables contributing to poor access are the array of social problems that Hispanic families must face such as poor housing, lack of transportation and finances for medication and other treatments, and no child care. Unless these needs are addressed in the initial assessment, many families will not return to HIV care. Kalichman et al[19] recommend that HIV prevention and care must integrate the array of needs that minority populations are experiencing to have a greater efficacy in reducing HIV infection. Because many Hispanic patients may present late for care due to poor access and lack of adequate knowledge about HIV, their basic needs, and needs arising from HIV infection must be addressed simultaneously. This scenario can be overwhelming for the health care providers as well as the patients and their families.

The continued secrecy and discrimination about HIV found in Hispanic communities can be best addressed by informing and recruiting Hispanic members of the community to participate in the HIV arena at the local HIV consortium level as well as in state HIV planning councils. Both infected and affected members representative of the Hispanic community must be involved at these two levels. Health care providers can assist the Hispanic community by ensuring representation of these individuals and the affected community at large.

Case Management Approach for Hispanic Families Living with HIV Infection

Advocacy and Coordination

Case management is a process by which health care providers can provide a continuum of services for individuals or families with a coordinated, culturally competent approach. Because of the array of needs among Hispanic subgroups, case management is a useful tool to assess systematically the needs of the entire family while keeping the Hispanic community and culture in perspective (see also Chapter 22). Coordinating the efforts of multiple agencies in a culturally appropriate manner ensures maximum utilization of appropriate resources in a community. For this coordination to be effective among Hispanics, the networks need to include community planning, community organization, community empowerment, and consumer participation.[20]

Intergenerational Infection

The phenomenon of *intergenerational infection* among Hispanic families creates a challenge for every health care provider and the system. Families will be coming to health care later in the stages of HIV, and more than one family member will be infected. Multiple-member infection creates diverse experiences and needs among family members. Many of these experiences can be categorized as (1) interfamilial affects, such as intergenerational dying; (2) intergenerational crisis of infected family members; and (3) interfamilial crisis with siblings and extended family members. *Intergenerational dying* is defined as two or more members of different generations in the same family dying of HIV infection. *Intergenerational crisis* is defined as two or more members of different generations of the same family experiencing a crisis at the same time. This can be seen when a child is in the hospital with an OI and the mother may be in jail for drug trafficking. *Interfamilial crisis* is defined as crisis experienced by siblings and/or the extended family at the same time. Health care providers must be prepared to establish a care plan that addresses the needs of multiple Hispanic family members. Working with the family and primary caregiver, they need to develop a coordinated, culturally sensitive, and culturally competent care plan. This should include anticipatory guidance related to HIV-related health problems and social issues. The anticipatory guidance interventions should be carried out in such a way that they respect the Hispanic cultural beliefs of a person and family. Among Hispanics, the cultural values of *simpatia*, *familialism*, and *personalismo* need to be incorporated in all interventions if they are to be perceived as relevant.[21] These values are defined as follows. *Simpatia* is to act in a polite, nonconfrontational manner. *Familialism* is the importance of the family to the individual. *Personalismo* is preference to be with other persons of the same ethnic group.[22]

Recommendations

For health care providers to be effective, HIV intervention and prevention efforts for Hispanic patients should incorporate the following recommendations:

- Health care providers who care for HIV-infected patients and families from differing ethnic and cultural backgrounds need to recognize that culture affects how people define their quality of life, their health, and how they will accept the treatments and interventions offered to them. Assessment instruments need to include factors such as the level of acculturation, the languages spoken, and the cultural meaning of health.
- Case management needs to be provided to each family to coordinate and establish trust and rapport. It is not necessary that the case manager share the same ethnic background as the patient, but that person should be aware and respectful of the patient's Hispanic culture and willing to learn more about it. In areas where Spanish is the primary language spoken at home, it is preferable that the health care provider speak Spanish.
- Home visits should be conducted at least once a year on all families. The case manager should set aside 2 hours for each visit. The first part of the visit should be devoted to some "social" time and the remainder to encouraging the family to review and identify their needs.
- The case manager should create a culturally appropriate teaching plan aimed at educating all family members about HIV infection signs and symptoms. Interactive teaching strategies and repeated verbalizations are useful to communicate facts about treatment and medications. Be aware that a person may not have disclosed their status to family members, so ask before implementing the teaching plan.
- The health care provider should be prepared to discuss and assess patient and family spiritual orientation and include this facet in the treatment plan.

Current social issues such as mandatory testing for pregnant women, welfare reform, and changing health care infrastructures are affecting health policy. Health care providers need to be involved in developing and/or revising health policies. Specific recommendations related to health policy include the following:

- Advocate for developing community coalitions and infrastructures to assist in meeting the complex health and human service needs of Hispanic women and families living with life-threatening diseases and chronic conditions such as HIV infection.
- Develop, in the cities that border Mexico, public health programs in communicable disease control, health services provision, environmental sanitation, systems development, and improved communication and standards between the health departments of the United States and Mexico.
- Provide programs to educate Hispanic men and women in participating in community advisory boards, such as the Ryan White Consortia, that prioritize and distribute money for AIDS care in every community.

Resources

National and International Organizations

American Red Cross National Headquarters, Customer and Program Support, Hispanic HIV/AIDS Program
8111 Gatehouse Road
Falls Church, VA 22042
(703)-206-7408
(703)-206-7602 (Fax)

ASPIRA Association, National Office
1444 Eye Street, NW, 8th Floor
Washington, DC 20006
(202)-835-3600
(202)-835-3613 (Fax)

National Coalition of Advocates for Students, Viviremos HIV Education Project
100 Boylston Street, Suite 737
Boston, MA 02116
(617)-357-8507
(617)-357-9549 (Fax)

National Council of La Raza (NCLR)
1111 19th Street, NW, Suite 1000
Washington, DC 20036

(202)-785-1670
(202)-785-0851 (Fax)

National Latino/a Lesbian and Gay Organization (LLEGO), Incorporated
1612 K Street, NW, Suite 500
Washington, DC 20006
(202)-466-8240
(202)-466-8530

National Puerto Rican Coalition (NPRC), Office of Policy Development
1700 K Street, NW, Suite 500
Washington, DC 20006
(202)-223-3915
(202)-429-2223

Internet Resources

AIDS & the Latino Community
http://clnet.ucr.edu/research/aids/aidscomm.html
This site provides AIDS-related resources for the Latino community, including bibliographies, fact sheets, a glossary, news items, and statistics.

CONASIDA
http://cenids.ssa.gob.mx/conasida/index.html
This Web site provides information from Consejo Nacional de Prevencion y Control del SIDA. Text is in Spanish.

Health Emergency: The Spread of Drug-Related AIDS Among African Americans and Latinos
http://www.soros.org/lindesmith/emergenc/eindex.html
This is a special report written by Dawn Day, PhD, and sponsored by Common Sense for Drug Policy, Criminal Justice Policy Foundation, Dogwood Center, Drug Policy Foundation, Harm Reduction Coalition, and the Lindesmith Center. Among other topics, it covers health risks, the connection between drug abuse and AIDS, and ways to stem the epidemic, including needle exchange.

Minority Health Project
http://www-bios.sph.unc.edu/WWW/minority/ or *www.minority.unc.edu*
This site provides statistics related to minority health issues and other information on the Minority Health Project.

Hispanic Resources

Books and Booklets

***AIDS: A Guide for Hispanic Leadership* (COSSMHO) 1989. English/Spanish. National Coalition of Hispanic Health and Human Services Organizations**
This booklet offers effective guidelines on how one can become an effective leader and advocate for the Hispanic community in its fight against AIDS. Information includes basic facts about transmission of HIV, how the crisis is affecting the Hispanic community, and how one can assess community needs. Graphics illustrate AIDS patients in the Hispanic community. The booklet is one of many resources available through COSSMHO. The cost of the booklet is $2.00. To order, or for more information on other resource materials, contact COSSMHO, 1030 15th Street, NW, Washington, DC 20005; (202)-371-2100.

***Getting Started. Becoming Part of the AIDS Solution.* National Council of La Raza. 1989. Spanish.**
This 35-page booklet is a guide for Hispanic community-based organizations that are working with Hispanics and AIDS. The booklet outlines a 16-step process, with beginning steps including learning the basics about AIDS, educating your organization, and identifying local players; middle steps including deciding your agency's role, developing a plan of action, and developing networks; and final steps including becoming a Hispanic voice, finding the money you need, and making a difference. The booklet includes several worksheets and a list of additional resources. Single copies are free. Multiple copies are $3.00 each. To request this resource, contact the National Council of La Raza, 810 First Street, NE, Suite 300, Washington, DC 20002; (202)-289-1380.

***La Mujer Marcada: La Tragedia De Una Mujer Moderna.* Hispanic AIDS Committee for Education and Resources. 1989. Spanish/English.**
This book looks at the tragedy of Gloria, a woman who contracts AIDS

by making a mistake. Booklets are $4.25 per copy and are available through HACER (Hispanic AIDS Committee for Education and Resources), 132 W. Grayson, San Antonio, TX, 78212; (210)-227-2204.

***Mi Hermano/My Brother.* The American Red Cross. March 1990. Spanish/English.**
This fotonovela tells the story of a Hispanic family confronted with the death of a son from AIDS. The story tells how AIDS is spread and there is a quiz on AIDS knowledge included. Copies of the fotonovela are available through local chapters of the American Red Cross.

***Prevencion del HIV/SIDA Para La Familia.* Sabogal F, Otero-Sabogal, R. For the American Red Cross. 1990. Spanish.**
This four-color booklet is illustrated with photos of Latinos. Each page poses a question and the answers are given as bullets. Copies of this booklet are available through local chapters of the American Red Cross.

Catalogs

***Nationwide Directory of Bilingual AIDS Educational Materials.* Hispanic Health Alliance. June 1989. English.**
This catalog breaks down materials available by target audiences, including adolescents, AIDS patients, Latino communities, children and their parents, mothers-to-be, and women. For more information contact the Hispanic Health Alliance, 1608 North Milwaukee Avenue, Suite 912, Chicago, IL 60647; (312)-252-6888.

***Novela Health Education.* Novela Health Education. English.**
This booklet catalogs the educational resource materials available through the Novela Health Foundation. Resources include training videos, fotonovelas, charts, and comic books. To get a copy of the catalog, contact Novela Health Education, 2524 16th Avenue South, Seattle, WA 98144; (206)-325-9897.

Information Packets

***Adelantel.* Hispanic AIDS Program. 1990. English.**
This newsletter provides information about the AIDS Prevention Program for Hispanic youths and families. The March 1990 issue covers a broad

overview of the Hispanic AIDS Prevention Program components, as well as available training and informational materials published by the American Red Cross. *Adelante* is free and available through the Hispanic HIV/AIDS Program, National Headquarters, American Red Cross, 1550 Sutter Street, San Francisco, CA 94109; (415)-776-1500.

***Guia Para La Prevencion del SIDA/AIDS Prevention Guide.* CDC. Control. Spanish/English.**
This information is directed at adults who will be sharing AIDS information with youths. The folder contains more than a half-dozen flyers and brochures, each informing about various AIDS issues—how a person can be infected with AIDS, deciding what to say to younger children, deciding what to say to teenagers, common questions and accurate answers, and how to join the community response. The information packet is free and is part of the *America Responde al SIDA* series. Contact the National AIDS Information Clearinghouse, PO Box 6003, Rockville, MD 20850; (800)-458-5231.

Journals

***Hispanic Journal of Behavioral Sciences.* Sage Periodicals Press. English.**
This professional journal is published four times a year and features articles relating to the US Hispanic population, with most studies identifying Hispanic subgroups. Materials include the fields of anthropology, economics, education, linguistics, political science, psychology, psychiatry, public health, and sociology. Past issues have included "Hispanic Families Learning and Teaching About AIDS: A Participatory Approach to the Community Level" and "Differences Between Hispanics and Non-Hispanics in Willingness to Provide AIDS Prevention Advice" (May 1990). Subscription rates are $30.00 for individuals and $60.00 for institutions. Contact Sage Publications, Inc., 2111 West Hillcrest Drive, Newbury Park, CA 91320; (415)-781-7430.

Manuals

***AIDS Education and the Latino Community.* Chicano Studies Research Center, UCLA; 1990. English.**
The table of contents for this publication includes bibliographic materials

on Latino AIDS, statistical materials on Latino AIDS, health education efforts on Latino AIDS, Latino AIDS policy development, and a directory of Latino AIDS services for the Greater Los Angeles area. For information, contact AIDS Education and the Latino Community, Chicano Studies Research, UCLA, 180 Haines Hall, 405 Hilgard Avenue, Los Angeles, CA 90024-1544; (213)-825-4484.

***Hablando del SIDA. Una Guia Para Trabajar En La Comunidad.* Gordon G, Klouda T. For the Federacion Internacional de Planificacion de la Familia. May 1990. Spanish.**
This guide was developed for all who are working in the field of sex education and the prevention of AIDS. The material can be adapted easily to suit individual needs. The book is illustrated with cartoons that underscore the written text. For more information, contact the Federacion Internacional de Planificacion de la Familia, Region del Hemisferio Occidental, Inc., 902 Broadway, 10th Floor, New York, NY 10010; (212)-995-8800.

***Hispanics & HIV/AIDS: A Guide to Selected Resources.* CDC National AIDS Clearinghouse; June 1996.**
This guide gives specific information regarding organizations, newsletters, Internet resources, and funding resources.

Newsletters

***NMAC Healer.* National Minority AIDS Council. Issued bimonthly.**
The *NMAC Healer* provides organizations and individuals with information concerning the effects of and responses to HIV/AIDS in ethnic and racial minority communities. Special emphasis is given to Project HEAL, a program of the National Minority AIDS Council. A "conference calendar" is a special feature of the newsletter. For more information on the *NMAC Healer*, contact the National Minority AIDS Council, 300 I Street, NE, Washington, DC 20002; (202)-544-1076.

***Pagina de Salud.* Amigos Volunteers In Education and Services, Inc. Issued monthly. Spanish.**
This newsletter is produced to educate Spanish-speaking, HIV-positive individuals on how to maintain their health. Issues address nutrition, stress,

and exercise. The information is also available in audio cassette for those who cannot read. For more information, contact the Amigos Volunteers in Education and Services, Inc., 210 Broad Street, Suite 200, Houston, TX 77087; (713)-640-2837.

***The COSSMHO AIDS Update.* COSSMHO. Issued quarterly. English.**
Produced especially for health care professionals, each issue provides important updated information on the AIDS crisis in the Hispanic community. Features include a data update. Subscription price is $40.00. COSSMHO member subscription is $30.00. For more information, contact COSSMHO Publications, 1030 15th Street, NW, Suite 1053, Washington, DC 20005; (202)-371-2100.

Videos

***Alicia's Story.* VHS. Spanish.**
This is the story of Alicia, a woman who has AIDS and whose baby is also infected through the IV drug use of her husband. The presentation is informative and also effective in communicating basic information on the transmission, symptoms, and prevention of AIDS. The tape includes a written discussion guide to encourage the use of the tape as a learning tool. The tape is available for $12.00 per copy through the National AIDS Information Clearinghouse, PO Box 6003, Rockville, MD 20850; (800)-458-5231.

***Face to Face With AIDS.* Novela Health Foundation. 1988. English.**
This is the story of how a teenager, Ana Sanchez, her family, and her friends face AIDS for the first time. Ana's father contracts AIDS and his death dramatically personalizes AIDS for them. Through Ana's experience, viewers explore common misconceptions about AIDS and its transmission. Arturo, a peer counselor at the local clinic, answers many of the questions Ana and her friends have about their own behaviors and risk. The tape is $250.00 ($10.00 for shipping). For more information, contact Select Media, Inc., 74 Varick Street, #305, New York, NY 10013; (212)-431-8923.

***La Historia de Olga/Olga's Story.* Latino Consortium/KCET. 1990. VHS. Spanish/English.**
This is the story of Olga, who has AIDS, and how her plight affects her family. A study guide to encourage discussion on HIV after viewing the

video is included. Tapes are $12.00 each and are available through the National AIDS Information Clearinghouse, PO Box 6003, Rockville, MD 20850; (800)-458-5231.

***Musicians for Life*. National AIDS Network. VHS and ¾″. Spanish/English. Audio versions also available.**
There are ten spots in this series, featuring recording artists Madonna, Los Lobos, Julie Brown, Ice T, M.C. Lyte, Gwen Guthrie, Whoopi Goldberg, Al B. Sure!, and Apollonia. Audio cassettes are $10.00. VHS is $35.00. ¾″ (tape size) is $50.00. Member rates are also available. Contact the National AIDS Network, 2033 M Street, NW, Suite 800, Washington, DC 20036; (202)-797-3503.

References

1. *The Hispanic Population in the United States: March 1991. Current Population Reports.* Washington, DC: US Bureau of the Census; 1991. Series P-20, no. 455.
2. Aguirre-Molina M, Molina CW. Latino populations: who are they? In: Aguirre-Molina CW, Molina CW, eds. *Latino Health in the United States: A Growing Challenge.* Washington, DC: American Public Health Association; 1995:1–21.
3. Catalano J. *The Mexican-Americans.* New York: Chelsea House Publishing; 1988.
4. Dieppa I, Montiel M. *An Exploration in Hispanic Families: Critical Issues for Policy and Programs in Human Services.* Washington, DC: Doubleday; 1978.
5. Meier MS, Ribera F. *Mexican-Americans, American-Mexicans: From Conquistadors to Chicanos.* Washington, DC: Hill & Wang; 1993.
6. Feagin JR, Feagin CB. *Racial and Ethnic Relations.* Englewood Cliffs, NJ: Simon & Schuster; 1993.
7. CDC. *HIV/AIDS Surveillance: U.S. AIDS Cases Reported through December, 1994.* Atlanta, GA: CDC; 1995.
8. CDC. *HIV/AIDS Surveillance Report.* Atlanta, GA: CDC; 1993.
9. CDC. Update: acquired immunodeficiency syndrome in the United States, 1989. *MMWR.* 1990;39:81–86.
10. Giachello AL. Hispanics and health care. In: Cafferty PM, Creaty W, eds. *Hispanics in the U.S.: The New Social Agenda.* Piscataway, NJ: Transaction Publishers; 1994:159–194.
11. Anerson R, Lewis S, Giachello A, Aday LA, Chiu G. Access to medical care among the Hispanic population of the southwestern United States. *J Health Soc Behav.* 1981;22:78–89.

12. Roberts R, Lee E. Health practices among Mexican-Americans: further evidence from the human population laboratory studies. *Prev Med.* 1980;9:675–688.
13. Trevino F, Moss A. *Health Insurance Coverage and Physician Visits among Hispanic and Non-Hispanic People.* Washington, DC: US Government Printing Office; 1983.
14. General Accounting Office. *Significant Gaps in Hispanic Access to Health Care* (GAO/PEMD-92-6). Washington, DC: US Government Printing Office; 1992.
15. Rodriguez-Trais H, Ramirez de Arellano AB. The health of children and youth. In: Molina CW, Aguirre-Molina M, eds. *Latino Health in the U.S.: A Growing Challenge.* Washington, DC: American Public Health Association; 1994:115–133.
16. Aday LA. *At Risk in America: The Health and Health Care Needs of Vulnerable Populations in the United States.* San Francisco: Jossey-Bass; 1993.
17. Hayes-Baulista DE, Gonzalez-Blode MA. AIDS: the silent threat to the binational security. *Salud Publica Mex.* 1991;33(4):360–370.
18. Arocena M, Vargas-Adams E, Davis PF. The under utilization of social and health services by Hispanic families. In: Center for Health Policy Development, ed. *Hispanics Health Status Symposium.* San Antonio: CHPD Inc.; 1988: 190–204.
19. Kalichman SC, Hunter TL, Kelly JA. Perceptions of AIDS susceptibility among minority and non-minority women at risk for HIV infection. *J Consult Clin Psychol.* 1992;60(5):725–732.
20. Randolph LA, Sherman BR. Project connect: an interagency partnership to confront new challenges facing at risk women and children in New York City. *J Commun Health.* 1993;18(2):73–81.
21. Marin BV, Gomez CA. Latinos, HIV disease and culture: strategies for AIDS prevention. In: Cohen PT, Sande MA, Volberding PA, eds. *The AIDS Knowledge Base.* Boston: Little, Brown; 1994:11.1.6.1–11.1.6.7.
22. Marin B, Marin G. Special issue: AIDS and Hispanics. *Hisp J Behav Sci.* 1990; 12(2):110–112.

CHAPTER 29

Culturally Diverse Populations: African-Americans

Sonia Baker, PhD, RN • Emma J. Brown, PhD, RNC

Chapter Preview

- AIDS and HIV Differences among African-Americans
- Disclosure Issues within the African-American Community
- Obstacles to Accessing Health Care
- Community-Based Health Care Programs

Although the category Black non-Hispanic is used by the CDC to capture all blacks irrespective of national origin, the focus of this chapter is on those born in the United States and not blacks from the West Indies, Haiti, or Africa. The cultural diversity of all blacks living in the United States is too vast to address in this chapter.

AIDS and HIV Differences among African-Americans

The term *black* will be used in this section to discuss statistics regarding HIV and AIDS because the CDC uses this term. Blacks are disproportionally affected by AIDS, as reported by the CDC in 1996 (see Chapter 2). They represent 41% of 1996 reported adult/adolescent AIDS cases, exceeding the proportion that is white for the first time.[1] The AIDS incidence rates per 100,000 population were 89.7 among blacks, 41.3 among Hispanics, and 13.5 among whites[1] (see Chapter 28). According to the CDC, the 1996 rate per 100,000 of AIDS among all males age 13 years and older was 51.9, whereas the rate for black males was 177.6. In contrast, the 1996 rate of AIDS per 100,000 for all females was 12.3, whereas it was 61.7 for black females (see Chapter 25). Temporal trends continue to show a rise in the incidence of AIDS among black females and a leveling off or decrease among other females and all males. Sexual transmission to females is usually acquired from partners who are injecting drug users or bisexual.[1] Similar patterns in the incidence of HIV infection are evident among blacks.

HIV Knowledge and Attitudes among African-Americans

The African-American community is not homogeneous in its knowledge or attitudes about HIV. Research has shown that HIV knowledge level varies within and among specific African-American groups formed by age, gender, geographic locale, and risk group (sexual and drug use behavior).[2–5] The following discussion of these issues focuses on the broader African-American community with the knowledge that all of the information does not apply to all African-Americans.

Knowledge Level About HIV among African-Americans

It is difficult to compare the HIV knowledge level of specific groups within the African-American community due to the variability in instruments used to collect the data. Of the studies conducted regarding African-Americans, some researchers[3,6,7] used as few as six or eight items, whereas others[2,8] used 55 items to assess HIV knowledge. Most HIV knowledge assessments were reported for adolescents, creating a lack of information about HIV knowledge among African-American adults. HIV knowledge has been collected from various samples of African-Americans: inner-city adolescents,[2,8,9] low-income adolescents,[4] incarcerated adolescents and young adults,[6,10] college students,[5] adult females,[7,11] individuals who use drugs,[12] and bisexual and homosexual males.[3,13]

Generally, the results from most studies revealed that African-Americans are knowledgeable about HIV mode of transmission—unprotected sexual activity and contaminated drug paraphernalia—and selected prevention measures, use of condoms, and use of new or clean drug works.[2–13] The most common misconceptions were those related to the transmission of HIV by mosquito bites and the donation of blood.[6,7,11] When HIV knowledge was compared by ethnicity among adolescents, African-Americans scored below whites but above Hispanics.[14,15] Although African-Americans possess moderate to high knowledge about HIV modes of transmission and prevention measures, knowledge alone has proven inadequate to change health behavior.

HIV Attitudes: Stigmatization within the African-American Community

The focus of HIV-related stigma[16–22] within the African-American community tends to be based on beliefs about the mode of contact.[11,21,22] Much of the written information on the stigma of HIV was secured from newspaper articles and abstracts from international conferences on AIDS because it was not found in mainstream journals. Even though not all African-Americans harbor negative attitudes about persons with HIV, the phenomenon must be addressed because it can impede the efficacy of HIV prevention efforts.

Stigmatization of Gay Males among African-Americans

The belief that individuals who acquire HIV are associated with alternate sexual lifestyles still exists. Homosexuality remains stigmatized within the African-American community. It is postulated that black gay males who continue to live within African-American communities alter their public behavior to avoid stigmatization.[17] The stigmatization is so powerful that HIV-infected individuals, practitioners, and researchers may be hesitant to become involved with HIV prevention and treatment efforts or research for fear of being labeled HIV-infected themselves or condoners of the gay lifestyle.[8] Other adverse consequences of homophobia related to HIV stigmatization among African-Americans are the:

- Tendency of African-American males who engage in same-sex or bisexual behavior to avoid discussing their sexual behavior with professionals, their wives, or their girlfriends[17]
- Avoidance and reluctance of getting tested for HIV[17]
- Tendency to avoid asking the community for help once HIV infected[17]
- Lag in the black gay and bisexual community to educate themselves and the public about HIV[17]

A partial explanation for the historic homophobia within the African-American community is the view that homosexual behavior is a sin. However, Dunlap (personal communication, October 12, 1995) refutes the assertion that homophobia is pervasive in the African-American community. She posits that homophobia is problematic in the religious community rather than the broader African-American community.

Nevertheless, the black Christian church (from now on called *the church*) has historically condemned homosexuality and drug use as immoral acts.[20–22] As the black church is diverse in its religious character and function, it is also diverse on its views of social and moral issues such as HIV.[23] Not all African-American church members view homosexuality and drug use as immoral. The stigma associated with homosexuality and HIV may affect black gays more than white gays. This may explain why the white gay and lesbian communities galvanize around HIV and sexuality issues, unlike the black gay and lesbian communities.

Stigmatization of Female Crack Users among African-Americans

Females who use crack are another group stigmatized because of their behavior. Those who use crack cocaine are especially stigmatized by the African-American community, even by individuals who themselves are drug users.[24] Women with children who abuse drugs are perceived as unfit mothers.[25] Women of color who are diagnosed with HIV are stigmatized as sufferers of a disease associated with promiscuity, illicit drug use, and death. However, little literature exists regarding the impact of stigmatization on the perceptions of women who use crack and how their perceptions influence their behavior. Women who are HIV-infected may be reluctant to ask for assistance, such as drug treatment or HIV-related services.

An integral part of maintaining and eventually eradicating HIV within the African-American population will require mobilizing organizations within the church and community to support HIV prevention efforts and HIV support services for those who are stigmatized. Recommendations for HIV prevention within African-American churches and the community made by researchers, practitioners, and community leaders are detailed in the next section.

Tailored HIV Prevention Strategies

Prevention programs for African-American adolescents and adults must be designed in a historical, cultural, religious, social, and political context specific to an African-American community because not all African-American communities are homogeneous.[16,18] HIV prevention strategies targeted toward African-Americans are not necessarily different from strategies geared toward other ethnic groups, but the context in which these strategies are formulated and presented should differ. The most effective prevention efforts among African-Americans share the following commonalities. They are (1) presented in African-American communities; (2) managed by members of the African-American communities who serve as advocates for African-American concerns; (3) Afrocentric in context and content, both language and message; (4) focused on process more than outcome, and on family and community more than the individual; and (5) comprehensive.

This is not to say that prevention programs for African-Americans that do not incorporate all these aspects are ineffective or that HIV prevention programs for African-Americans should never be led by non-African-Americans. When directed by non-African-Americans, the directors should acknowledge their lack of cultural unity. They should work earnestly to ensure that the essential historical, social, cultural, political, and spiritual Afrocentric aspects are designed into the HIV prevention program for the specific African-American community by working or consulting with members from that targeted community.

Spirituality

Attitudes of the church such as "AIDS is a punishment from God" and "persons with AIDS have not lived right" must change before the development and achievement of effective prevention and treatment efforts.[27] Such attitudes will change successfully when health educators and practitioners work with community members to encourage the church to view HIV as a health problem rather than a moral problem.[25] The Afrocentric perspective encourages the incorporation of spirituality into prevention and treatment programs. Spirituality is defined in the broad sense and includes Christianity, Muslim, and other beliefs, although the literature focuses on Christianity. Some, but not all, Christian churches have a history of remaining uninvolved and uncommitted to the eradication of HIV within the African-American community. This stance results from the attempt to deny that HIV is a problem in the African-American community.[28,29] When acknowledged, it is deemed a problem for those exhibiting immoral behavior (homosexuality and drug use) and therefore not worthy of true commitment.[17,20,29] Well-established churches are more inclined to offer HIV support because they are not as vulnerable to decreased donations because of taking a controversial stance.[17] In addition, churches where clergy have college degrees are more involved in HIV prevention. One study indicated that African-American Baptist ministers who received HIV prevention and educational training felt more comfortable counseling persons with AIDS, and were more likely to support and/or sponsor HIV workshops and training for their members.[29]

Family-Focused HIV Prevention

Intergenerational family involvement in HIV prevention efforts is postulated to be paramount for the most efficacious outcome.[16] Considering the demographic changes of persons with HIV among African-Americans, one realizes that women, adolescents, children, and also self-identified heterosexual men are increasingly affected. Thus, the development of prevention programs that target risk reduction for the entire family, however defined, is needed. Specific messages that encourage changes in HIV risk behavior to ensure the survival of the family are recommended. Prevention approaches that focus on African-American community and family issues are more likely to assist participants in passing HIV information on to family and friends.[9] African-American families and communities are the foundation for subjective norms, and thus affect motivation to comply with HIV prevention strategies.[17,28]

Disclosure Issues within the African-American Community

It is crucial to understand how patterns of support in the African-American community affect disclosure. Likewise it is important to know that beliefs about HIV may differ within the culture of African-Americans. African-American families traditionally extend help and support to other family members in times of need.[30–32] In order for help to be offered or provided, there must be knowledge that there is a need for assistance or support. Among some African-Americans, fear of revealing their diagnosis may exceed fear of the consequences of being infected. Because of this fear and perception of stigmatization, they may choose not to tell anyone about their need for support. Fear of being ostracized and judged about a previous lifestyle and at-risk behavior are factors that may increase reluctance to reveal their HIV status, as well as the thought of becoming a burden to others. Also, reluctance to disclose to partners has been reported among some HIV-infected women who have experienced domestic violence in their relationships.[33–35] Lastly, despite educational efforts related to how the HIV virus is spread from one person to another, there is still fear among some African-Americans of contracting the virus via casual contact. This is relevant because the infected person will not disclose his HIV diagnosis to those people who are fearful of casually contracting the virus.

Obstacles to Accessing Health Care

Factors that need to be addressed as potential obstacles to accessing health care among African-Americans are (1) education, (2) socioeconomic status, (3) attitude of the health care provider, (4) communication, (5) client-provider relationship, and (6) difficulties in negotiating the health care system. Factors such as lower socioeconomic status and education have been linked with poor health outcomes and higher mortality rates.[36,37] This continues to be a major concern in the United States because they are factors that interfere with accessing health care.

Education Issues

Being uneducated is not synonymous with being African-American. However, among the less educated, their ability to access health care is influenced in many ways, such as (1) misperception of risk for HIV infection, (2) lack of knowledge about HIV transmission, (3) lack of information regarding the need for follow-up or referrals, (4) lack of information regarding available health care services, and (5) reluctance to ask questions or request clarification of instructions.

Socioeconomic Status

Socioeconomic status influences the ability to access health care. The label of being poor should not be equated with being an African-American[16] because levels of income within the African-American community vary. However, HIV researchers report the demographics of African-Americans who participate in their studies as poor and less educated.[11,38,39] The patients in those studies were reached through clinics, public health services, and community service organizations. Less is known about middle and upper income-level HIV-infected African-Americans.

Attitude of the Health Care Provider

Attitudes of the providers can greatly influence how well they relate to their clients and the type of therapeutic relationship established. African-American patients who are already sensitive to how they are treated are particularly sensitive because of their HIV diagnosis. Due to the stigma in the African-American community about HIV, and particularly how one became infected, patients may also interpret the provider's attitude as judgmental, particularly those patients who are drug abusers, homosexuals, and prostitutes.

Communication

The manner in which the health care provider communicates with the patient is another important matter. Communication concerns discussed in this section are applicable to clients in the African-American community and other ethnic/racial groups. The providers' ability to explain medical jargon using language that the patient understands is key to successful prevention and treatment. In addition, the provider must also understand the client, the manner in which he speaks, and be sensitive to their nonverbal behavior.

Patient-Health Care Provider Relationship

A crucial component of health care for the African-American is the quality of the relationship between the health care provider and the patient. Efforts on behalf of the provider to develop a therapeutic relationship may be overwhelmed by the patient's feeling of mistrust of non-African-American health care providers, previous negative experiences in the health care system, the stigma of HIV, and sociocultural differences between the provider and the patient. The belief in some segments of the African-American community about the suspicious origin of HIV and whether they are being prescribed treatment that is more harmful than effective contribute to these problems. Some African-Americans believe that HIV was man made and targeted to minority groups in a national plan of genocide, and that the treatment being offered to them is more harmful to their health than effective.[40] To the non-African-American health care provider, these beliefs may be dismissed as hysterical or an uneducated way of thinking. To the African-American, these beliefs about the origin of HIV and questionable treatment are rooted in the historical Tuskegee Syphilis Study conducted from 1932 to 1972.[28,41–44]

Difficulties in Negotiating the Health Care System

Some HIV-infected patients may be asymptomatic, essentially healthy, and able to fulfill their own caregiving needs independently for a long time. On entering the health care system for HIV treatment they are faced with myriad of health care appointments; referrals to specialists such as dermatologists, neurologists, and psychiatrists; frequent laboratory and diagnostic tests; and appointments with social or case workers. For many African-Americans diagnosed with HIV, it may be the first health care experience in which they are expected to comply with regular appointments, follow-up referrals, and return for frequent diagnostic tests. Sometimes patients have to complete forms to receive continued services or entitlements. The forms may be complicated and may require the assistance of a social or case worker.

Services may be contained in a localized area or dispersed within an institution that may seem overwhelming or intimidating to the new African-American patient. The fact that health care providers rely on the results of laboratory and diagnostic tests on which to base treatment may not be understood fully by the African-American patient. The patient may not have followed up on obtaining prescribed tests or may be reluctant to ask for clarification. Many African-American HIV patients who are having difficulty dealing with the stigma within their own community have additional concerns about their diagnosis being revealed in the clinical setting. Although they have taken great lengths to keep their diagnosis a secret from others, as the circle of referrals increases there is a potential threat to keeping the diagnosis a secret. This is especially true when they run into others from their own community in the waiting room, or their name may be inadvertently overheard concerning HIV-related information at the clinic.

The experience of waiting for long periods before being called to be seen by the provider is common in the clinic setting. This can be a source of irritation and frustration, and may influence whether the patient returns for follow-up and treatment. The problem of waiting is magnified especially if the patient is not feeling well.

Today, the mandate that researchers include women and minority groups in clinical trial studies may pose a major problem for researchers and patients from the African-American community. Despite creative recruitment strategies and the use of monetary incentives to join HIV studies, many African-Americans may be reluctant to join research projects for reasons related to Tuskegee Syphilis Study. Their reluctance potentially places them at a disadvantage for receiving the latest treatment for HIV.

Community-Based Health Care Programs

Community-based social and health care programs are an invaluable way to bring needed services to the African-American community. In fact, the general trend regarding the provision of needed HIV services has moved from the acute care setting to the community.[45,46] As community health care planners, nurses and other health care providers must be ready to accept and answer many questions and concerns from the community about risks, benefits, and the ethics of new community programs. Questions concerning the efficacy of present community-based programs may be raised by African-American community members due to the failure of well-meaning plans to increase African-American access to health care. This may in part explain the reluctance of some individuals to accept and participate in new community HIV programs.

The African-American community must be involved from the inception of new HIV community programs and continue throughout the planning, implementation, and evaluation phases of these programs. Clinicians who are involved in HIV health planning must consider the values, beliefs, and dynamics of the African-American community. The identification of formal and informal leaders such as clergy, politicians, school board members, community activists, and planning board members is important. Understanding the relationship between the African-American community and its recognized leaders is very critical. Some leaders in the community may not truly represent the community. Therefore, the politics of leadership, organizations, and people in the African-American community must be understood. Focus groups and informal discussions with community members is a way of gaining additional insight into the dynamics of the community. Recruiting participants for these discussions can be achieved by accessing religious organizations, hair salons, barbershops, and community and recreation centers.

In summary, today's health care providers are challenged by the impact of HIV in many segments of our society. Understanding the commonalities and distinctiveness of African-American groups affected by HIV helps provide information that the provider çan incorporate in the plan of care. For the African-American patient who is infected with the HIV virus, there are additional challenges rooted in problems that are unique to this group. This chapter has introduced a brief look at these unique problems, along with recommendations for meeting the needs of this population.

References

1. CDC. *HIV/AIDS Surveillance Report, Year-end Edition.* Atlanta, GA: U.S. Department of Health and Human Services, Public Health Service, CDC; 1996.
2. Jemmott LS, Jemmott JB III. Increasing condom-use intentions among sexually active black adolescents. *Nurs Res.* 1992;41(5):273–279.

3. Peterson JL, Coates TJ, Catania JA, et al. High-risk sexual behavior and condom use among gay and bisexual African American men. *Am J Public Health.* 1992; 82(11):1490–1494.
4. St. Lawrence JS, Brasfield TL, Jefferson KW, et al. Social support as a factor in African-American adolescent's sexual risk behavior. *J Adolesc Res.* 1994; 9(3):292–310.
5. Thomas SB, Gilliam AG, Iwrey CG. Knowledge about AIDS and reported risk behaviors among black college students. *J Am Coll Health.* 1989;38:61–66.
6. Belgrave FZ, Randolph SM, Carter C, et al. The impact of knowledge, norms, and self-efficacy on intentions to engage in AIDS-preventive behaviors among young incarcerated African American males. *J Black Psychol.* 1993;19(2): 155–168.
7. Ehrhardt AA, Yingling S, Zawadzki R, et al. Prevention of heterosexual transmission of HIV: barriers for women. *J Psychol Human Sex.* 1992;5(1–2):37–67.
8. Jemmott JB III, Jemmott LS, Spears H, et al. Self-efficacy, hedonistic expectancies, and condom-use intentions among inner-city black adolescent women: a social cognitive approach to AIDS risk behavior. *Soc Adolesc Med.* 1992;(6): 512–519.
9. Damond ME, Breuer NL, Pharr AE. The evaluation of setting and a culturally specific HIV/AIDS curriculum: HIV/AIDS knowledge and behavioral intent of African American adolescents. *J Black Psychol.* 1993;19(2):169–189.
10. DiClemente RJ, Lanier MM, Horan PF, et al. Comparison of AIDS knowledge, attitudes, and behavior among incarcerated adolescents and public school sample in San Francisco. *Am J Public Health.* 1991;81(5):628–630.
11. Nyamathi A, Bennett C, Leake B, et al. AIDS-related knowledge, perceptions, and behavior among impoverished minority women. *Am J Public Health.* 1993; 83(1):65–71.
12. Lewis KL, Watters JK. Sexual risk behavior among heterosexual intravenous drug users: ethnic and gender variations. *AIDS.* 1991;5(1):77–83.
13. Rotheram-Borus MJ, Koopman C. Sexual risk behavior, AIDS knowledge, and beliefs about AIDS among predominantly minority gay and bisexual male adolescents. *AIDS Educ Res* 1991;3(4):305–312.
14. Bell D, Feraios A, Bryan T. Adolescent males' knowledge and attitudes about AIDS in the context of their social world. *J Appl Soc Psychol.* 1990;20(5): 424–448.
15. DiClemente R, Boyer C, Morales E. Minorities and AIDS: knowledge, attitudes, and misconceptions among black and Latino adolescents. *Am J Public Health.* 1988;78:55–57.
16. Chatters LM. HIV/AIDS within African American communities: diversity and interdependence. A commentary on "AIDS and the African American women: the triple burden of race, class, and gender." *Health Educ Q.* 1993;20(3): 321–326.

17. Wright JW. African-American male sexual behavior and the risk for HIV infection. *Hum Organ.* 1993;52(4):421–431.
18. Randolph SM, Banks HD. Making a way out of no way: the promise of Afrocentric approaches to HIV prevention. *J Black Psychol.* 1993;19(2):204–214.
19. Mays VM, Cochran SD. Issues in the perception of AIDS risk and risk reduction activities by black and Hispanic/Latino women. *Am Psychol.* 1988;43:949–957.
20. Quimby E, Friedman SR. Dynamics of black mobilization against AIDS in New York City. *Soc Prob.* 1989;36:403–415.
21. Moragna T. African American churches—evaluation and KAB collection. Presented at the 8th International Conference on AIDS. July 19–24, 1992.
22. Satcher D. Crime, sin, or disease: drug abuse and AIDS in the African-American community. *J Health Care Poor Underserved.* 1990;1(2):212–218.
23. Taylor RJ, Thornton MC, Chatters LM. Black Americans' perceptions on the socio-historical role of the church. *J Black Studies* 1987;18:123–138.
24. Fullilove MT, Lown EA, Fullilove RE. Crack 'hos and skeezers: traumatic experiences of women crack users. *J Sex Res.* 1992;29(2):275–287.
25. Quinn SC. Perspective on AIDS and the African American woman: the triple burden of race, class and gender. *Health Educ. Q.* 1993;20(3):305–320.
26. Land H. AIDS and women of color. *Families in Society: The Journal of Contemporary Human Services.* vol 75. 1994;June:355–361.
27. Bell AP, Weinberg M. *Homosexualities: A Study of Diversity Among Men and Women.* New York: Simon and Schuster; 1978.
28. Guinan M. Black communities' belief in "AIDS as genocide": a barrier to overcome for HIV prevention. *Ann Epidemiol.* 1993;3:193–195.
29. Crawford I, Illison KW, Robinson WL, et al. Attitudes of African American Baptist minister toward AIDS. *J Commun Psychol.* 1992;20(4):403–408.
30. Martin E, Martin J. *The Black Extended Family.* Chicago: University of Chicago Press; 1978.
31. Burton L. Black grandparents rearing of children of drug-addicted parents: stressors, outcomes, and social service needs. *Gerontologist.* 1992;6:744–751.
32. Taylor R. Receipt of support from family among black Americans: demographic and familial differences. *J Marriage Fam.* 1986;48:67–77.
33. Geilen A, O'Campo P, Faden R, et al. Women with HIV: disclosure concerns and experiences. In: *HIV Infection in Women Conference.* 1995:S25. Abstract.
34. Maroney T, Brown W. HIV, women and violence. In: *HIV Infection in Women Conference.* 1995:S35. Abstract.
35. Shannon M, Benson M, Dahroughe M, et al. Domestic violence in HIV-infected pregnant women. In: *HIV Infection in Women Conference.* 1995;S36. Abstract.
36. Pappas G, Queen S, Hadden W, et al. The increasing disparity in mortality

between socioeconomic groups in the United States, 1960 and 1986. *N Engl J Med.* 1993;2:103–109.
37. Rice D. Ethics and equity in U.S. health care: the data. *Int J Health Serv.* 1991; 4:637–651.
38. Hobfoll S, Jackson A, Lavin J, et al. Safer sex knowledge, behavior, and attitudes of inner-city women. *Health Psychol.* 1993;6:481–488.
39. Lawrence J. African American adolescents' knowledge, health-related attitudes, sexual behavior, and contraceptive decisions: implications for the prevention of adolescent HIV infection. *J Consult Psychol.* 1993;1:104–112.
40. Bates K. AIDS: Is it genocide. *Essence.* 1990;21:77–116.
41. Jones J. *Bad Blood: The Tuskegee Syphilis Experiment—A Tragedy of Race and Medicine.* New York: The Free Press; 1981.
42. Thomas S, Quinn S. Public health then and now: the Tuskegee Syphilis Study, 1932 to 1972: implications for HIV education and AIDS risk educational programs in the black community. *Am J Public Health.* 1991;11:1498–1505.
43. Jones J. The Tuskegee legacy: AIDS and the black community. *The Hastings Center Report.* 1992;December:38–40.
44. Spigner C. Sociology of AIDS within black communities: theoretical considerations. *Intern Q Commun Health Educ.* 1989–90;4:285–296.
45. Hellinger F. Forecasting the personal medical care cost of AIDS for 1988 through 1991. *Public Health Rep.* 1988;103:309–323.
46. Morrison C. Delivery systems for the care of persons with HIV infection and AIDS. *Nurs Clin North Am.* 1993;28:317–331.

APPENDIX A

1993 Revised Classification System for HIV Infection and Expanded Surveillance Case Definition for AIDS Among Adolescents and Adults

The following CDC staff members prepared this report:

National Center for Infectious Diseases
Division of HIV/AIDS
Kenneth G. Castro, M.D. • John W. Ward, M.D. •
Laurence Slutsker, M.D., M.PH. • James W. Buehler, M.D. •
Harold W. Jaffe, M.D. • Ruth L. Berkelman, M.D.

Office of the Director
Associate Director for HIV/AIDS
James W. Curran, M.D., M.P.H.

From CDC. 1993 Revised classification system for HIV Infection and expanded surveillance case Definition for AIDS Among Adolescents and Adults. MMWR 1992;41(No. RR-17):1–16.

Chapter Preview

CDC has revised the classification system for HIV infection to emphasize the clinical importance of the CD4+ T-lymphocyte count in the categorization of HIV-related clinical conditions. This classification system replaces the system published by CDC in 1986[1] and is primarily intended for use in public health practice. Consistent with the 1993 revised classification system, CDC has also expanded the AIDS surveillance case definition to include all HIV-infected persons who have <200 CD4+ T-lymphocytes/μL, or a CD4+ T-lymphocyte percentage of total lymphocytes of <14. This expansion includes the addition of three clinical conditions—pulmonary tuberculosis, recurrent pneumonia, and invasive cervical cancer—and retains the 23 clinical conditions in the AIDS surveillance case definition published in 1987[2]; it is to be used by all states for AIDS case reporting effective January 1, 1993.

Revised HIV Classification System for Adolescents and Adults

The etiologic agent of acquired immunodeficiency syndrome (AIDS) is a retrovirus designated human immunodeficiency virus (HIV). The CD4+ T-lymphocyte is the primary target for HIV infection because of the affinity of the virus for the CD4 surface marker.[3] The CD4+ T-lymphocyte coordinates a number of important immunologic functions, and a loss of these functions results in progressive impairment of the immune response. Studies of the natural history of HIV infection have documented a wide spectrum of disease manifestations, ranging from asymptomatic infection to life-threatening conditions characterized by severe immunodeficiency, serious opportunistic infections, and cancers.[4–13] Other studies have shown a strong association between the development of life-threatening opportunistic illnesses and the absolute number (per microliter of blood) or percentage of CD4+ T-lymphocytes.[14–21] As the number of CD4+ T-lymphocytes decreases, the risk and severity of opportunistic illnesses increase.

Measures of CD4+ T-lymphocytes are used to guide clinical and therapeutic management of HIV-infected persons.[22] Antimicrobial prophylaxis and antiretroviral therapies have been shown to be most effective within certain levels of immune dysfunction.[23–28] As a result, antiretroviral therapy should be considered for all persons with CD4+ T-lymphocyte counts of

<500/μL, and prophylaxis against *Pneumocystis carinii* pneumonia (PCP), the most common serious opportunistic infection diagnosed in men and women with AIDS, is recommended for all persons with CD4+ T-lymphocyte counts of <200/μL and for persons who have had prior episodes of PCP. Because of these recommendations, CD4+ T-lymphocyte determinations are an integral part of medical management of HIV-infected persons in the United States.

The classification system for HIV infection among adolescents and adults has been revised to include the CD4+ T-lymphocyte count as a marker for HIV-related immunosuppression. This revision establishes mutually exclusive subgroups for which the spectrum of clinical conditions is integrated with the CD4+ T-lymphocyte count. The objectives of these changes are to simplify the classification of HIV infection, to reflect current standards of medical care for HIV-infected persons, and to categorize more accurately HIV-related morbidity.

The revised CDC classification system for HIV-infected adolescents and adults* categorizes persons on the basis of clinical conditions associated with HIV infection and CD4+ T-lymphocyte counts. The system is based on three ranges of CD4+ T-lymphocyte counts and three clinical categories and is represented by a matrix of nine mutually exclusive categories (Table 1). This system replaces the classification system published in 1986, which included only clinical disease criteria and which was developed before the widespread use of CD4+ T-cell testing.[1]

CD4+ T-Lymphocyte Categories

The three CD4+ T-lymphocyte categories are defined as follows:

- **Category 1**: ≥500 cells/μL
- **Category 2:** 200–499 cells/μL
- **Category 3:** <200 cells/μL

*Criteria for HIV infection for persons ages ≥13 years: a) repeatedly reactive screening tests for HIV antibody (e.g., enzyme immunoassay) with specific antibody identified by the use of supplemental tests (e.g., Western blot, immunofluorescence assay); b) direct identification of virus in host tissues by virus isolation; c) HIV antigen detection; or d) a positive result on any other highly specific licensed test for HIV.

Table 1. 1993 Revised Classification System for HIV Infection and Expanded AIDS Surveillance Case Definition for Adolescents and Adults*

	Clinical Categories		
CD4+ T-cell Categories	(A) Asymptomatic, Acute (primary) HIV or PGL†	(B) Symptomatic, Not (A) or (C) Conditions‡	(C) AIDS-indicator Conditions§
(1) ≥500/μL	A1	B1	C1
(2) 200–499/μL	A2	B2	C2
(3) <200/μL AIDS-indicator T-cell count	A3	B3	C3

*The categories listed below illustrate the expanded AIDS surveillance case definition. Persons with AIDS-indicator conditions (Category C) as well as those with CD4+ T-lymphocyte counts <200/μL (Categories A3 or B3) will be reportable as AIDS cases in the United States and Territories, effective January 1, 1993.

†PGL = persistent generalized lymphadenopathy. Clinical Category A includes acute (primary) HIV infection.[29, 30]

‡See text for discussion.

§See Subappendix B.

These categories correspond to CD4+ T-lymphocyte counts per microliter of blood and guide clinical and therapeutic actions in the management of HIV-infected adolescents and adults.[22–28] The revised HIV classification system also allows for the use of the percentage of CD4+ T-cells (Subappendix A).

HIV-infected persons should be classified based on existing guidelines for the medical management of HIV-infected persons.[22] Thus, the lowest accurate, but not necessarily the most recent, CD4+ T-lymphocyte count should be used for classification purposes.

Clinical Categories

The clinical categories of HIV infection are defined as follows:

Category A

Category A consists of one or more of the conditions listed below in an adolescent or adult (≥13 years) with documented HIV infection. Conditions listed in Categories B and C must not have occurred.

- Asymptomatic HIV infection
- Persistent generalized lymphadenopathy
- Acute (primary) HIV infection with accompanying illness or history of acute HIV infection[29,30]

Category B

Category B consists of symptomatic conditions in an HIV-infected adolescent or adult that are not included among conditions listed in clinical Category C and that meet at least one of the following criteria: a) the conditions are attributed to HIV infection or are indicative of a defect in cell-mediated immunity; or b) the conditions are considered by physicians to have a clinical course or to require management that is complicated by HIV infection. **Examples** of conditions in clinical Category B include, **but are not limited to:**

- Bacillary angiomatosis
- Candidiasis, oropharyngeal (thrush)
- Candidiasis, vulvovaginal; persistent, frequent, or poorly responsive to therapy
- Cervical dysplasia (moderate or severe)/cervical carcinoma in situ
- Constitutional symptoms, such as fever (38.5°C) or diarrhea lasting >1 month
- Hairy leukoplakia, oral
- Herpes zoster (shingles), involving at least two distinct episodes or more than one dermatome
- Idiopathic thrombocytopenic purpura
- Listeriosis
- Pelvic inflammatory disease, particularly if complicated by tubo-ovarian abscess
- Peripheral neuropathy

For classification purposes, Category B conditions take precedence over those in Category A. For example, someone previously treated for oral or persistent vaginal candidiasis (and who has not developed a Category C disease) but who is now asymptomatic should be classified in clinical Category B.

Category C

Category C includes the clinical conditions listed in the AIDS surveillance case definition (Subappendix B). For classification purposes, once a Category C condition has occurred, the person will remain in Category C.

Expansion of the CDC Surveillance Case Definition for AIDS

In 1991, CDC, in collaboration with the Council of State and Territorial Epidemiologists (CSTE), proposed an expansion of the AIDS surveillance case definition. This proposal was made available for public comment in November 1991 and was discussed at an open meeting on September 2, 1992. Based on information presented and reviewed during the public comment period and at the open meeting, CDC, in collaboration with CSTE, has expanded the AIDS surveillance case definition to include all HIV-infected persons with CD4+ T-lymphocyte counts of <200 cells/μL or a CD4+ percentage of <14. In addition to retaining the 23 clinical conditions in the previous AIDS surveillance definition, the expanded definition includes pulmonary tuberculosis (TB), recurrent pneumonia, and invasive cervical cancer.* This expanded definition requires laboratory confirmation of HIV infection in persons with a CD4+ T-lymphocyte count of <200 cells/μL or with one of the added clinical conditions. This expanded definition for reporting cases to CDC becomes effective January 1, 1993.

In the revised HIV classification system, persons in subcategories A3, B3, and C3 meet the immunologic criteria of the surveillance case definition, and those persons with conditions in subcategories C1, C2, and C3 meet the clinical criteria for surveillance purposes (see Table 1).

Commentary

Revised Classification System

The revised classification system for HIV infection is based on the recommended clinical standard of monitoring CD4+ T-lymphocyte counts, since

*Diagnostic criteria for AIDS-defining conditions included in the expanded surveillance case definition are presented in Subappendix C.

this parameter consistently correlates with HIV-related immune dysfunction and disease progression and provides information needed to guide medical management of persons infected with HIV.[14–18,22–28] The classification system also allows for use of the percentage of CD4+ T-cells instead of absolute CD4+ T-lymphocyte counts (Subappendix A). Other markers of immune status—such as serum neopterin, beta-2 microglobulin, HIV p24 antigen, soluble interleukin-2 receptors, immunoglobulin A, and delayed-type hypersensitivity (DTH) skin-test reactions—may be useful in the evaluation of individual patients but are not as strongly predictive of disease progression or as specific for HIV-related immunosuppression as measures of CD4+ T-lymphocytes.[14–21,31] DTH skin-test reactions are often used in conjunction with the Mantoux tuberculin skin test to evaluate HIV-infected patients for TB infection and anergy.[31–33]

Other systems have been proposed for classification and staging of HIV infection.[1,31,34–39] In 1990, the World Health Organization (WHO) published an interim proposal for a staging system for HIV infection and diseases that was based primarily on clinical criteria and included the use of CD4+ T-lymphocyte determinations.[34] The WHO system incorporates a performance scale and total lymphocyte counts to be used in lieu of CD4+ T-lymphocyte determinations in countries where CD4+ T-lymphocyte testing is not available.

The accuracy of CD4+ T-lymphocyte counts is important for medical care of individual patients. To assure reliability, laboratories conducting CD4+ T-lymphocyte measurements should be experienced with test procedures, have established quality assurance methods, and participate in proficiency testing programs conducted by CDC or other organizations.[22,40] CDC has published guidelines for the performance of CD4+ T-cell determinations for HIV-infected persons.[41] To assure that test results are indicative of a patient's medical condition, the health-care provider should evaluate the results with those of earlier tests and with the patient's clinical condition. In clinical practice, repeat CD4+ testing may be judged necessary in guiding therapeutic decisions for individual patients. For surveillance purposes, however, a requirement for repeat CD4+ determinations is impractical for population-based monitoring.

The revised classification system of the clinical and immunologic manifestations of HIV infection provides a framework for categorizing HIV-related morbidity and immunosuppression and will assist efforts to evaluate the overall impact of the HIV epidemic. Knowledge of the spectrum of clinical conditions and the extent of immunosuppression that may occur during the course of HIV infection is important for prompt evaluation and for provision of appropriate health services. Clinicians should be aware of the clinical conditions suggestive of HIV infection and the need for prophylactic and therapeutic interventions.

This revised HIV classification system should be used by state and territorial health departments that conduct HIV infection surveillance. Because AIDS surveillance data will continue to represent only a portion of the total morbidity caused by HIV, surveillance for HIV infection may be particularly useful in depicting the total impact of HIV on health-care and social services.[42] More accurate reporting and analysis of CD4+ T-lymphocyte counts, together with HIV-related clinical conditions, should facilitate efforts to evaluate health-care and referral needs for persons with HIV infection and to project future needs for these services.

Expanded AIDS Surveillance Case Definition

The population of HIV-infected persons with CD4+ T-lymphocyte counts of <200/μL is substantially larger than the population of persons with AIDS-defining clinical conditions.[43] The inclusion in the AIDS surveillance definition of persons with a CD4+ T-lymphocyte count of <200 cells/μL or a CD4+ percentage <14 will enable AIDS surveillance to reflect more accurately the number of persons with severe HIV-related immunosuppression and those at highest risk for severe HIV-related morbidity. Since the AIDS surveillance case definition was last revised in 1987, the increasing use of prophylaxis against PCP and antiretroviral therapy for persons infected with HIV has slowed the rate at which HIV-infected persons develop AIDS-defining clinical conditions.[2,22–25] For example, among homosexual/bisexual men with AIDS reported to CDC, the proportion with PCP decreased from 62% in 1988 to 46% in 1990.[44] This trend is expected to continue.

The ability of clinicians to report HIV-infected persons on the basis of CD4+ T-lymphocyte counts may also simplify the case-reporting process. A simplified AIDS surveillance case definition will be particularly important for outpatient clinics in which the availability of staff to conduct surveillance is limited and from which an increasing proportion of AIDS cases are being reported. For example, from pre-1985 to 1988, the proportion of AIDS cases reported from outpatient sites in the state of Washington increased from 6% (9/155) to 25% (55/219).[45] A similar increase occurred in Oregon (25% [44/171] before 1987 to 38% [40/105] in the first half of 1989).[46]

Pulmonary Tuberculosis

Throughout the world, pulmonary TB is the most common type of TB in persons with HIV infection.[47] The addition of pulmonary TB to the list of AIDS-indicator diseases is based on the strong epidemiologic link between HIV infection and the development of TB.[48–50] Persons co-infected with HIV and TB have a substantially increased risk of developing active TB compared with persons without HIV infection.[48,49] In a prospective evaluation of injecting-drug users (IDUs) with positive tuberculin skin tests, the estimated annual incidence of active TB among 49 HIV-infected IDUs was 7.9 cases/100 person-years; however, no cases of active TB occurred among 62 tuberculin-positive but HIV-seronegative IDUs followed for as long as 30 months.[48]

There is also a substantial immunologic association between HIV-infected persons and pulmonary TB when compared with HIV-infected persons with extrapulmonary TB (a condition included in the 1987 surveillance definition). In a recent review, median CD4+ T-lymphocyte counts in HIV-infected patients with pulmonary TB ranged from 250 to 500 cells/μL.[51] In comparison, the median CD4+ lymphocyte count was 242 cells/μL in one study of persons with localized extrapulmonary TB and ranged from 70 to 79 cells/μL in two studies of patients with disseminated or miliary TB.[51–53] In CDC's Adult and Adolescent Spectrum of HIV Disease (ASD) Project, 69% of HIV-infected persons with pulmonary TB had CD4+ T-lymphocyte counts of <200/μL, compared with 77% of persons with extrapulmonary TB (CDC, unpublished observations).

The addition of pulmonary TB to AIDS surveillance criteria will require continued collaboration between state and local TB and HIV/AIDS programs. Knowledge of a patient's HIV status is important for the proper medical management of TB because longer courses of therapy and prophylaxis are recommended for HIV-infected patients with TB.[54] Furthermore, HIV-infected TB patients should be a priority for epidemiologic investigation because these persons are more likely to have HIV-infected contacts than are seronegative TB patients. TB contact follow-up among HIV-infected persons will help to ensure delivery of a full course of preventive therapy to these contacts, who are at greatly increased risk of developing active TB themselves.

Recurrent Pneumonia

With the exception of conditions included in the 1987 AIDS surveillance case definition, pneumonia, with or without a bacteriologic diagnosis, is the leading cause of HIV-related morbidity and death.[55,56] In addition, several studies have shown that persons with HIV-related immunosuppression are at an increased risk of bacterial pneumonia.[57–59] For example, one study found that the yearly incidence rate of bacterial pneumonia among HIV-infected IDUs without AIDS was five times that found in non-HIV-infected IDUs.[58] Recurrent episodes of pneumonia (two or more episodes within a 1-year period) are required for AIDS case reporting because pneumonia is a relatively common diagnosis and multiple episodes of pneumonia are more strongly associated with immunosuppression than are single episodes. For example, data from the ASD Project indicate that the risk of an HIV-infected person having had one episode of pneumonia in a 12-month period is approximately five times higher among infected persons with CD4+ T-lymphocyte counts of $<200/\mu L$ (320/2,411) than among those with higher CD4+ T-lymphocyte counts (90/2,792). In contrast, data from the same study indicate that the risk for multiple episodes of pneumonia in a 12-month period is approximately 20 times higher among HIV-infected persons with CD4+ T-lymphocyte counts of $<200/\mu L$ (67/2,411) than among those with higher CD4+ T-cell counts (4/2,792) (CDC, unpublished observations).

Invasive Cervical Cancer

Several studies have found an increased prevalence of cervical dysplasia, a precursor lesion for cervical cancer, among HIV-infected women.[60,61] In a study of 310 HIV-infected women attending methadone maintenance and sexually transmitted disease clinics in New York City and Newark, New Jersey, cervical dysplasia was confirmed by biopsy and/or colposcopy in approximately 22%, a prevalence rate 10 times greater than that found among women attending family planning clinics in the United States (Wright TC, personal communication).[62] Several studies have documented that a higher prevalence of cervical dysplasia among HIV-infected women is associated with greater immunosuppression (Wright TC, personal communication).[61,63] In addition, HIV infection may adversely affect the clinical course and treatment of cervical dysplasia and cancer.[64–69]

Invasive cervical cancer is a more appropriate AIDS-indicator disease than is either cervical dysplasia or carcinoma in situ because these latter cervical lesions are common and frequently do not progress to invasive disease.[70] Also, cervical dysplasia or carcinoma in situ among women with severe cervicovaginal infections, which are common in HIV-infected women, can be difficult to diagnose. In contrast, the diagnosis of invasive cervical cancer is generally unequivocal.

Invasive cervical cancer is preventable by the proper recognition and treatment of cervical dysplasia. Thus, the occurrence of invasive cervical cancer among all women—including those who are HIV-Infected—represents missed opportunities for disease prevention. The addition of invasive cervical cancer to the list of AIDS-indicator diseases emphasizes the importance of integrating gynecologic care into medical services for HIV-infected women.

Impact on AIDS Case Reporting

The expanded AIDS surveillance case definition is expected to have a substantial impact on the number of reported cases. The immediate increase in case reporting will be largely attributable to the addition of severe immunosuppression to the definition; a smaller impact is expected from the addition of pulmonary TB, recurrent pneumonia, and invasive cervical cancer, since many persons with these diseases will also have CD4+ T-lymphocyte counts of <200 cells/μL. If all of the approximately 1,000,000 persons in the United States with HIV infection were diagnosed and their immune status were known, it is estimated that 120,000–190,000 persons who do not have AIDS-indicator diseases would be found to have CD4+ T-lymphocyte counts of <200 cells/μL.[71] However, not all of these persons are aware of their HIV infection and of those who know their HIV infection status, not all have had an immunologic evaluation; thus, the immediate impact on the number of AIDS cases will be considerably less than 120,000–190,000. If AIDS surveillance criteria were unchanged, approximately 50,000–60,000 reported AIDS cases would be expected in 1993. Based on current levels of HIV and CD4+ testing, CDC estimates that the expanded definition could increase cases reported in 1993 by approximately 75%. Early effects of expanded surveillance will be greater than long-term effects because prevalent as well as incident cases of immunosuppression will be reported following implementation of the expanded surveillance case definition. In subsequent years, the effect on the number of reported cases is expected to be much smaller.

Uses of the HIV Classification System or AIDS Surveillance Case Definition

The revised HIV classification system and the AIDS surveillance case definition are intended for use in conducting public health surveillance. The CDC's AIDS surveillance case definition was not developed to determine whether statutory or other legal requirements for entitlement to Federal disability or other benefits are met. Consequently, this revised surveillance case definition does not alter the criteria used by the Social Security Administration in evaluating claims based on HIV infection under the Social Security disability insurance and Supplemental Security Income programs. Other organizations and agencies providing medical and social services should develop eligibility criteria appropriate to the services provided and local needs.

Confidentiality

The confidentiality of AIDS case reports—including laboratory reports of HIV test results, CD4+ T-lymphocyte test results, and medical records under review by health department staff—is of critical importance to maintaining effective HIV/AIDS surveillance. CDC and state health departments have implemented procedures and policies to maintain confidentiality and security of HIV/AIDS surveillance data.[72] CDC's efforts include a federal assurance of confidentiality, the removal of names before encrypted records are transmitted to CDC, strict guidelines for the release of aggregate data, and the inclusion of confidentiality and security safeguards as evaluation criteria for federal funding of state HIV/AIDS surveillance activities.[73] These strict criteria will continue to apply to cases reported under the expanded definition. CDC funding of surveillance cooperative agreements is dependent on the recipient's ability to ensure the physical security of case reports and on state policies or laws to protect the confidentiality of persons reported with AIDS. Failure to ensure the security and confidentiality of personal identifying information collected as part of AIDS or HIV surveillance activities will jeopardize federal surveillance funding.

CD4+ T-lymphocyte test results reported by laboratories will be an important adjunct to medical record review and provider-initiated reporting in order to increase completeness, timeliness, and efficiency of AIDS surveillance. Information from a laboratory-initiated report of a CD4+ T-lymphocyte count is insufficient for reporting a case of AIDS. Confirmation of HIV infection status and receipt of other surveillance information from the health-care provider or from medical or public health records will remain necessary.

Every effort should be made by health-care providers, laboratories, and public health agencies to protect the confidentiality of CD4+ T-lymphocyte test results, including the review of record-keeping practices in laboratories and health-care settings. Some states have considered additional means to assure the confidentiality of CD4+ T-lymphocyte test results. For example, a proposal in Oregon would allow health-care providers to send specimens to laboratories for CD4+ T-lymphocyte testing with a unique code for each person being tested. If the test result indicates a CD4+ T-lymphocyte count of <200 cells/μL, the health department would notify the health care provider that an AIDS case report is required if the person is HIV-infected, the CD4+ T-lymphocyte count is valid, and the case has not been previously reported. Informed consent for CD4+ T-lymphocyte testing should be obtained in accordance with local laws or regulations. CD4+ T-lymphocyte test results alone should not be used as a surrogate marker for HIV or AIDS. A low CD4+ T-lymphocyte count without a positive HIV test result will not be reportable since other conditions may result in a low CD4+ T-lymphocyte count. Health-care providers must ensure that persons who have a CD4+ T-lymphocyte count of <200/μL are HIV-infected before initiating treatment for HIV disease or reporting those persons as cases of AIDS.

Conclusion

The revised HIV classification system provides uniform and simple criteria for categorizing conditions among adolescents and adults with HIV infection and should facilitate efforts to evaluate current and future health-care and referral needs for persons with HIV infection. The addition of a measure of severe immunosuppression, as defined by a CD4+T-lymphocyte count of <200 cells/μL or a CD4+ percentage of <14, reflects the standard of immunologic monitoring for HIV-infected persons and will enable AIDS surveillance data to more accurately represent those who are recognized as being immunosuppressed, who are in greatest need of close medical follow-up, and who are at greatest risk for the full spectrum of severe HIV-related morbidity. The addition of three clinical conditions—pulmonary TB, recurrent pneumonia, and invasive cervical cancer—to AIDS surveillance criteria reflects the documented or potential importance of these diseases in the HIV epidemic. Two of these conditions (pulmonary TB and cervical cancer) are preventable if appropriate screening tests are linked with proper follow-up. The third, recurrent pneumonia, reflects the importance of pulmonary infections not included in the 1987 definition as leading causes of HIV-related morbidity and mortality. Successful implementation of expanded surveillance criteria will require the extension of existing safeguards to protect the security and confidentiality of AIDS surveillance information.

Subappendix A. Equivalences for CD4+ T-lymphocyte Count and Percentage of Total Lymphocytes

Compared with the absolute CD4+ T-lymphocyte count, the percentage of CD4+ T cells of total lymphocytes (or CD4+ percentage) is less subject to variation on repeated measurements.[18,74] However, data correlating natural history of HIV infection with the CD4+ percentage have not been as consistently available as data on absolute CD4+ T-lymphocyte counts.[14–16,18,19,21,31] Therefore, the revised classification system emphasizes the use of CD4+ T-lymphocyte counts but allows for the use of CD4+ percentages.

Equivalences (Table A1) were derived from analyses of more than 15,500 lymphocyte subset determinations from seven different sources: one multistate study of diseases in HIV-infected adolescents and adults[59] and six laboratories (two commercial, one research, and three university-based). The six laboratories are involved in proficiency testing programs for lymphocyte subset determinations. In the analyses, concordance was defined as the proportion of patients classified as having CD4+ T-lympho-

Table A1. Equivalences for Absolute Numbers of CD4+ T-lymphocytes and CD4+ Percentage*

CD4+ T-cell Category	CD4+ T-cells/μL	CD4+ Percentage (%)
(1)	≥500	≥29
(2)	200–499	14–28
(3)	<200	<14

*The percentage of lymphocytes that are CD4+ T-cells.

cyte counts in a particular range among patients with a given CD4+ percentage. A threshold value of the CD4+ percentage was calculated to obtain optimal concordance with each stratifying value of the CD4+ T-lymphocyte counts (i.e., <200/μL and ≥500/μL). The thresholds for the CD4+ percentages that best correlated with a CD4+ T-lymphocyte count of <200/μL varied minimally among the seven data sources (range, 13%–14%; median, 13%; mean, 13.4%). The average concordance for a CD4+ percentage of <14 and a CD4+ T-lymphocyte count of <200/μL was 90.2%. The threshold for the CD4+ percentages most concordant with CD4+ T-lymphocyte counts of ≥500/μL varied more widely among the seven data sources (range, 22.5%–35%; median, 29%; mean, 29.1%). This wide range of percentages optimally concordant with ≥500/μL CD4+ T-lymphocytes makes the concordance at this stratifying value less certain. The average concordance for a CD4+ percentage of ≥29 and a CD4+ T-lymphocyte count of ≥500/μL was 85% (CDC, unpublished data). Clinicians and other practitioners must recognize that these suggested equivalences may not always correspond with values observed in individual patients.

Subappendix B. Conditions Included in the 1993 AIDS Surveillance Case Definition

- Candidiasis of bronchi, trachea, or lungs
- Candidiasis, esophageal
- Cervical cancer, invasive*
- Coccidioidomycosis, disseminated or extrapulmonary
- Cryptococcosis, extrapulmonary
- Cryptosporidiosis, chronic intestinal (>1 month's duration)
- Cytomegalovirus disease (other than liver, spleen, or nodes)
- Cytomegalovirus retinitis (with loss of vision)
- Encephalopathy, HIV-related
- Herpes simplex: chronic ulcer(s) (>1 month's duration); or bronchitis, pneumonitis, or esophagitis
- Histoplasmosis, disseminated or extrapulmonary
- Isosporiasis, chronic intestinal (>1 month's duration)
- Kaposi's sarcoma
- Lymphoma, Burkitt's (or equivalent term)
- Lymphoma, immunoblastic (or equivalent term)
- Lymphoma, primary, of brain
- *Mycobacterium avium* complex or *M. kansasii*, disseminated or extrapulmonary
- *Mycobacterium tuberculosis*, any site (pulmonary* or extrapulmonary)
- *Mycobacterium*, other species or unidentified species, disseminated or extrapulmonary
- *Pneumocystis carinii* pneumonia
- Pneumonia, recurrent*
- Progressive multifocal leukoencephalopathy
- *Salmonella* septicemia, recurrent
- Toxoplasmosis of brain
- Wasting syndrome due to HIV

*Added in the 1993 expansion of the AIDS surveillance case definition.

Subappendix C. Definitive Diagnostic Methods for Diseases Indicative of AIDS

Diseases	Diagnostic Methods
Cryptosporidiosis Isosporiasis Kaposi's sarcoma Lymphoma *Pneumocystis carinii* pneumonia Progressive multifocal leukoencephalopathy Toxoplasmosis Cervical cancer	Microscopy (histology or cytology)
Candidiasis	Gross inspection by endoscopy or autopsy or by microscopy (histology or cytology) on a specimen obtained directly from the tissues affected (including scrapings from the mucosal surface), not from a culture
Coccidioidomycosis Cryptococcosis Cytomegalovirus Herpes simplex virus Histoplasmosis	Microscopy (histology or cytology), culture, or detection of antigen in a specimen obtained directly from the tissues affected or a fluid from those tissues
Tuberculosis Other mycobacteriosis Salmonellosis	Culture
HIV encephalopathy (dementia)	Clinical findings of disabling cognitive or motor dysfunction interfering with occupation or activities of daily living, progressing over weeks to months, in the absence of a concurrent illness or condition other than HIV infection that could explain the findings. Methods to rule out such concurrent illness and conditions must include cerebrospinal fluid examination and either brain imaging (computed tomography or magnetic resonance) or autopsy.

References

1. CDC. Classification system for human T-lymphotropic virus type III/lymphadenopathy-associated virus infections. *MMWR.* 1986;35:334–339.
2. CDC. Revision of the CDC surveillance case definition for acquired immunodeficiency syndrome. MMWR. 1987;36:1–15S.
3. McDougal JS, Kennedy MS, Sligh JM, et al. Binding of the HTLV-III/LAV to T4+ T cells by a complex of the 110K molecule and the T4 molecule. *Science.* 1985; 231:382–385.
4. Moss AR, Bacchetti P. Natural history of HIV infection. AIDS 1989;3:55–61.
5. Rutherford GW, Lifson AR, Hessol NA, et al. Course of HIV-1 in a cohort of homosexual and bisexual men: an 11 year follow-up study. *Br Med J.* 1990; 301:1183–1138.
6. Muñoz A, Wang MC, Bass S, et al. Acquired immunodeficiency syndrome (AIDS)—free time after human immunodeficiency virus type 1 (HIV-1) seroconversion in homosexual men. *Am J Epidemiol.* 1989;130:530–539.
7. Rezza G, Lazzarin A, Angarano G, et al. The natural history of HIV infection in intravenous drug users: risk of disease progression in a cohort of seroconverters. *AIDS.* 1989;3:87–90.
8. Selwyn PA, Hartel D, Schoenbaum EE, et al. Rates and predictors of progression to HIV disease and AIDS in a cohort of intravenous drug users (IVDUs), 1985–1990 (abstract F.C.111). VI International Conference on AIDS, San Francisco, CA, June 22, 1990;2:117.
9. Medley GF, Anderson RM, Cox DR, Billard L. Incubation period of AIDS in patients infected via blood transfusion. *Nature.* 1987;328:719–721
10. Ward JW, Bush TJ, Perkins HA, et al. The natural history of transfusion-associated infection with human immunodeficiency virus. *N Engl J Med.* 1989;321: 947–952.
11. Goedert JJ, Kessler CM, Aledort LM, et al. A prospective study of human immunodeficiency virus type 1 infection and the development of AIDS in subjects with hemophilia. *N Engl J Med.* 1989;321:1141–1148.
12. Auger I, Thomas P, De Gruttola V, et al. Incubation periods for paediatric AIDS patients. *Nature.* 1988;336:575–577.
13. Krasinski K, Borkowsky W, Holzman RS. Prognosis of human immunodeficiency virus in children and adolescents. *Pediatr Infect Dis J.* 1989;8: 216–220.
14. Goedert JJ, Biggar RJ, Melbye M, et al. Effect of T4 count and cofactors on the incidence of AIDS in homosexual men infected with human immunodeficiency virus. *JAMA.* 1987;257:331–334.
15. Nicholson JKA, Spira TJ, Aloisio CH, et al. Serial determinations of HIV-1 titers in HIV-infected homosexual men: association of rising titers with CD4 T cell depletion and progression to AIDS. AIDS Res Hum Retroviruses 1989;5:205–215.

16. Lang W, Perkins H, Anderson RE, Royce R, Jewell N, Winkelstein W. Patterns of T lymphocyte changes with human immunodeficiency virus infection: from seroconversion to the development of AIDS. *J Acquir Immune Defic Syndr* 1989;2:63–69.
17. Lange MA, de Wolf F, Goudsmit J. Markers for progression of HIV infection. *AIDS.* 1989;3(suppl.1):S153–160.
18. Taylor JM, Fahey JL, Detels R, Giorgi J. CD4 percentage, CD4 numbers, and CD4:CD8 ratio in HIV infection: which to choose and how to use. *J Acquir Immune Defic Syndr.* 1989;2:114–124.
19. Masur H, Ognibene FP, Yarchoan R, et al. CD4 counts as predictors of opportunistic pneumonias in human immunodeficiency virus (HIV) infection. *Ann Intern Med.* 1989;111:223–231.
20. Fahey JL, Taylor JMG, Detels R, et al. The prognostic value of cellular and serologic markers in infection with human immunodeficiency virus type 1. *N Engl J Med.* 1990;322:166–172.
21. Fernandez-Cruz E, Desco M, Garcia Montes M, Longo N, Gonzalez B, Zabay JM. Immunological and serological markers predictive of progression to AIDS in a cohort of HIV-infected drug users. *AIDS.* 1990;4:987–994.
22. National Institutes of Health. State-of-the-art conference on azidothymidine therapy for early HIV infection. *Am J Med.* 1990;89:335–344.
23. CDC. Guidelines for prophylaxis against *Pneumocystis carinii* pneumonia for persons infected with human immunodeficiency virus. *MMWR.* 1992;41(No. RR-4):1–11.
24. Fischl MA, Richman DD, Hansen N, et al. The safety and efficacy of zidovudine (AZT) in the treatment of subjects with mildly symptomatic human immunodeficiency virus type 1 (HIV) infection: a double blind, placebo controlled trial. *Ann Intern Med.* 1990;112:727–737.
25. Volberding PA, Lagakos SW, Koch MA, et al. Zidovudine in asymptomatic human immunodeficiency virus infection: a controlled trial in persons with fewer than 500 CD4-positive cells per cubic millimeter. *N Engl J Med.* 1990;322:941.
26. Lagakos S, Fischl MA, Stein DS, Lim L, Volberding PA. Effects of zidovudine therapy in minority and other subpopulations with early HIV infection. *JAMA.* 1991;266:2709–2712.
27. Easterbrook PJ, Keruly JC, Creagh-Kirk T, et al. Racial and ethnic differences in outcome in zidovudine-treated patients with advanced HIV disease. *JAMA.* 1991;266:2713–2718.
28. Hamilton JD, Hartigan PM, Simberkoff MS, et al. A controlled trial of early versus late treatment with zidovudine in symptomatic human immunodeficiency virus infection. *N Engl J Med.* 1992;326:437–443.
29. Ho DD, Sarngadharan MG, Resnick L, et al. Primary human T-lymphotropic virus type III infection. *Ann Intern Med.* 1985;103:880–883.

30. Tindall B, Cooper DA, Primary HIV infection: host responses and intervention strategies. *AIDS.* 1991;5:1–14.
31. Redfield RR, Wright DC, Tramont EC. The Walter Reed Staging Classification for HTLV-III/LAV Infection. *N Engl J Med.* 1986;314:131–132.
32. CDC. Guidelines for preventing the transmission of tuberculosis in health-care settings, with special focus on HIV-related issues. *MMWR.* 1990;39(No. RR-17): 1–29.
33. CDC. Purified protein derivative (PPD)-tuberculin anergy and HIV infection. *MMWR.* 1991;40(No. RR-15):37–43.
34. WHO. Interim proposal for a WHO staging system for HIV infection and diseases. Weekly Epidemiol Record 1990;65:221–224.
35. Chaisson RE, Volberding PA. Clinical manifestations of HIV infection. In: Mandell GL, Douglas RG, Bennett JE, eds. Principles and practice of infectious diseases. New York, NY: Churchill Livingstone, 1990:1061.
36. Haverkos HW, Gottlieb MS, Killen JY, Edelman R. Classification of HTLV-III/LAV-related diseases. *J Infect Dis.* 1985;152:1905.
37. Zolla-Pazner S, DesJarlais DC, Friedman SR, et al. Nonrandom development of immunologic abnormalities after infection with human immunodeficiency virus: implications for immunologic classification of the disease. Proc Natl Acad Sci USA 1987;84:5404–5408.
38. Royce RA, Luckmann RS, Fusaro RE, Winkelstein W Jr. The natural history of HIV-1 infection: staging classifications of disease. *AIDS.* 1991;5:355–364.
39. Justice AC, Feinstein AR, Wells CK. A new prognostic staging system for the acquired immunodeficiency syndrome. *N Engl J Med.* 1989;320:1388–1393.
40. Valdiserri RO, Cross GO, Gerber AR, Schwartz RE, Hearn TL. Capacity of US labs to provide TLI in support of early HIV-1 intervention. *Am J Public Health.* 1991;81:491–494
41. CDC. Guidelines for the performance of CD4+ T-cell determinations in persons with human immunodeficiency virus infections. *MMWR.* 1992;41(No. RR-8):1–12.
42. CDC. Surveillance for HIV infection—United States. *MMWR.* 1990;39:853, 859–861.
43. Brookmeyer R. Reconstruction and future trends of the AIDS epidemic in the United States. *Science.* 1991;253:37–42.
44. Ciesielski CA, Fleming PL, Berkelman RL. Changing trends in AIDS-indicator diseases in the U.S.—role of therapy and prophylaxis? (abstract 254). 31st Interscience Conference on Antimicrobial Agents and Chemotherapy, Chicago, IL, 1991:141.
45. Hopkins S, Lafferty W, Honey J, Hurlich M. Trends in the outpatient diagnosis of AIDS: implications for epidemiologic analysis and surveillance (abstract T.A.P.72). V International Conference on AIDS, Montreal, Canada, 1989:111.

46. Modesitt S, Espenlaub C, Klockner R, Fleming D. AIDS cases diagnosed as outpatients (abstract Th.C.736). VI International Conference on AIDS, San Francisco, CA, 1990;1:309.
47. Raviglione MC, Narain JP, Kochi A. HIV-associated tuberculosis in developing countries: clinical features, diagnosis, and treatment. Bull WHO 1992;70: 515–526.
48. Selwyn PA, Hartel D, Lewis VA, et al. A prospective study of the risk of tuberculosis among intravenous drug users with human immunodeficiency virus infection. *N Engl J Med.* 1989;320:545–550.
49. Selwyn PA, Sckell BM, Alcabes P, Friedland GH, Klein RS, Schoenbaum EE. High risk of active tuberculosis in HIV infected drug users with cutaneous anergy. *JAMA.* 1992;268:504–509.
50. Braun MM, Badi N, Ryder R, et al. A retrospective cohort study of the risk of tuberculosis among women of childbearing age with HIV-infection in Zaire. Am Rev Resp Dis 1991;143:501–504.
51. De Cock KM, Soro B, Coulibaly IM, Lucas SB. Tuberculosis and HIV infection in sub-Saharan Africa. *JAMA.* 1992;268:1581–1587.
52. Shafer RW, Chirgwin KD, Glatt AE, Dahdouh MA, Landesman SH, Suster B. HIV prevalence, immunosuppression, and drug resistance in patients with tuberculosis in an area endemic for AIDS. *AIDS.* 1991;5:399–405.
53. Barber TW, Craven DE, McCabe WR. Bacteremia due to *Mycobacterium tuberculosis* in patients with human immunodeficiency virus infection: a report of 9 cases and review of the literature. *Medicine.* 1990;69:375–383.
54. CDC. Tuberculosis and human immunodeficiency virus infection: recommendations of the Advisory Committee for the Elimination of Tuberculosis (ACET). *MMWR.* 1989;38:236–8, 243–250.
55. Buehler JW, Devine OJ, Berkelman RL, Chevarley FM. Impact of the human immunodeficiency virus epidemic on mortality trends in young men, United States. *Am J Public Health.* 1990;80:1080–1086.
56. Chu SY, Buehler JW, Berkelman RL. Impact of the human immunodeficiency virus epidemic on mortality in women of reproductive age, United States. *JAMA.* 1990;264:225–229.
57. Polsky B, Gold JW, Whimbey E, et al. Bacterial pneumonia in patients with the acquired immunodeficiency syndrome. *Ann Intern Med.* 1986;104:38–41.
58. Selwyn PA, Feingold AR, Hartel D, et al. Increased risk of bacterial pneumonia in HIV-infected intravenous drug users without AIDS. *AIDS.* 1988;2:267–272.
59. Farizo KM, Buehler JW, Chamberland ME, et al. Spectrum of disease in persons with human immunodeficiency virus infection in the United States. *JAMA.* 1992;267:1798–1805.

60. Laga M, Icenogle JP, Marsella R, et al. Genital papillomavirus infection and cervical dysplasia—opportunistic complications of HIV infection. *Int J Cancer.* 1992;50:45–48.
61. Schafer A, Friedmann W, Mielke M, Schwartlander B, Koch MA. The increased frequency of cervical dysplasia-neoplasia in women infected with the human immunodeficiency virus is related to the degree of immunosuppression. *Am J Obstet Gynecol.* 1991;164:593–599.
62. Sadeghi SB, Sadeghi A, Robboy SJ. Prevalence of dysplasia and cancer of the cervix in a nationwide Planned Parenthood population. *Cancer.* 1988;61: 2359–2361.
63. Feingold AR, Vermund SH, Burk RD, et al. Cervical cytologic abnormalities and papillomavirus in women infected with human immunodeficiency virus. *J Acquir Immune Defic Syndr.* 1990;3:896–903.
64. Maiman M, Fruchter RG, Serur E, Remy JC, Feuer G, Boyce J. Human immunodeficiency virus infection and cervical neoplasia. *Gynecol Oncol.* 1990;38:377–382.
65. Klein RS, Adachi A, Fleming I, Ho GYF, Burk R. A prospective study of genital neoplasia and human papillomavirus (HPV) in HIV-infected women (abstract). Vol. 1. Presented at the VIII International Conference on AIDS/III STD World Congress, Amsterdam, The Netherlands, July 19–24, 1992.
66. Fruchter R, Maiman M, Serur E, Cuthill S. Cervical intraepithelial neoplasia in HIV infected women (abstract). Vol. 1. Presented at the VIII International Conference on AIDS/III STD World Congress, Amsterdam, The Netherlands, July 19–24, 1992.
67. Richart RM, Wright TC. Controversies and the management of low-grade cervical intraepithelial neoplasia. Cancer (in press).
68. Rellihan MA, Dooley DP, Burke TW, Berkland ME, Longfield RN. Rapidly progressing cervical cancer in a patient with human immunodeficiency virus infection. *Gynecol Oncol.* 1990;36:435–438.
69. Schwartz LB, Carcangiu ML, Bradham L, Schwartz PE. Rapidly progressive squamous carcinoma of the cervix coexisting with human immunodeficiency virus infection: clinical opinion. *Gynecol Oncol.* 1991;41:255–258.
70. Richart RM. Cervical intraepithelial neoplasia: a review. In: Sommers SC, ed. Pathology annual, 1973. New York: Appleton-Century-Crofts, 1973:301–328.
71. CDC. Projections of the number of persons diagnosed with AIDS and the number of immunosuppressed HIV-infected persons—United States, 1992–1994. *MMWR.* 1992;41(No. RR-18) (in press).
72. US Congress, Office of Technology Assessment. The CDC's case definition of AIDS: implications of the proposed revisions. Background Paper, OTA-BP-H-89. Washington, DC: US Government Printing Office, August 1992.

73. Torres CG, Turner ME, Harkess JR, Istre GR. Security measures for AIDS and HIV. *Am J Public Health.* 1991;81:208–209.
74. Kessler HA, Landay A, Pottage JC, Benson CA. Absolute number versus percentage of T-helper lymphocytes in human immunodeficiency virus infection. *J Infect Dis.* 1990;161:356–357.

APPENDIX B

Guidelines for Isolation Precautions Related to HIV Infection

The "CDC Guideline for Isolation Precautions in Hospitals" was originally established by the Centers for Disease Control and Prevention (CDC) and the Hospital Infection Control Practices Advisory Committee in 1991 to help hospitals maintain up-to-date isolation practices. These guidelines were revised in 1996 and contain two parts: Part I, Evolution of Isolation Practices and Part II, Recommendations for Isolation Precautions in Hospitals. Highlights of Part II recommendations are summarized here.

The revised recommendations were developed primarily to be used in patient care in acute-care hospitals, although some recommendations may be relevant for some patients who obtain their care in subacute-care or extended-care facilities. They are not for program use in daycare, well care, or domiciliary care.

The "Guideline for Isolation Precautions in Hospitals" was revised to

From Garner JS. Hospital Infection Control Practices Advisory Committee. Guideline for isolation precautions in hospitals. *Infect Control Hosp Epidemiol.* 1996;17:53–80.

meet the following objectives: (1) to be epidemiologically sound; (2) to recognize the importance of all body fluids, secretions, and excretions in the transmission of nosocomial pathogens; (3) to contain adequate precautions for infections transmitted by the airborne, droplet, and contact routes of transmission; (4) to be as simple and user friendly as possible; and (5) to use new terms to avoid confusion with existing infection control and isolation systems. (pp 54–55)

Two levels of precautions are contained in the revised guideline. The first level contains precautions designed for the care of all hospital patients despite diagnosis or infection status. The first-level precautions are now called *standard precautions.* Their use is the primary approach for effective nosocomial infection control. The second level of precautions, *transmission-based precautions,* are for those patients with proved or suspected infection or colonization with pathogens that are important in epidemiology and can be transmitted by airborne or droplet transmission, or by contact with dry skin or contaminated surfaces.

Standard precautions combine *universal* (blood and body fluid) *precautions* (which were intended to reduce the risk of transmission of bloodborne pathogens) and *body substance isolation* (which was intended to reduce the risk of transmission of pathogens from moist body substances). Standard precautions pertain to (1) blood; (2) all body fluids, secretions, and excretions *except sweat,* whether they contain visible blood or not; (3) nonintact skin; and (4) mucous membranes.

Transmission-based precautions are of three types: (1) airborne precautions, (2) droplet precautions, and (3) contact precautions. These can be combined for conditions with multiple sources of transmission. They can be used in addition to standard precautions.

Isolation precautions in hospitals are instituted to block transmission of infection. Transmission requires three factors: (1) a source of the infecting microorganisms, human or otherwise; (2) a susceptible host; and (3) a means of transmitting the microorganism. The five main routes of transmission are (1) contact transmission—direct and indirect; (2) droplet transmission during coughing, sneezing, and talking, and during performance of certain procedures such as suctioning and bronchoscopy that do not remain suspended in air; (3) airborne transmission of either airborne droplet nuclei of evaporated droplets containing microorganisms that remain suspended in air for long periods or dust particles containing the infectious agent; (4) common vehicle transmission; and (5) vectorborne transmission. Common vehicle and vectorborne methods of transmission do not play a major role in nosocomial infections that are typical in hospitals.

A number of infection control measures are adopted to decrease the risk of transmission of microorganisms. Those fundamental to isolation precautions include (1) handwashing and gloving; (2) patient placement; (3) movement and transportation of infected patients; (4) masks, respiratory protection, eye protection, and face shields; (5) gowns and protective apparel; (6) patient care equipment and articles; (7) linen and laundry; (8) dishes, glasses, cups, and eating utensils; and (9) routine and terminal cleaning. Some information is particularly relevant to HIV care. Table B1

Table B1. Standard Precautions: Use for the Care of All Patients(pp. 68–69)

Isolation Precaution Category	Recommendations
Handwashing	Wash hands after touching blood, body fluids, secretions, excretions, and contaminated items, whether or not gloves are worn.
	Wash hands immediately after gloves are removed, between patient contacts, and when otherwise indicated to avoid transfer or microorganisms to other patients of environments.
	It may be necessary to wash hands between tasks and procedures on the same patient to prevent cross-contamination of different body sites.
	Use plain nonantimicrobial soap for routine handwashing.
	Use an antimicrobial agent or a waterless antiseptic agent for specific circumstances, as defined by the infection control program.
Gloves	Wear gloves when touching blood, body fluids, secretions, excretions, and contaminated items. Clean, nonsterile gloves are adequate.
	Put on clean gloves just before touching mucous membranes and nonintact skin.

Table B1. *Continued*

Isolation Precaution Category	Recommendations
	Change gloves between tasks and procedures on the same patient after contact with material that may contain a high concentration of microorganisms.
	Remove gloves right after use, before touching noncontaminated items and environmental surfaces, and before going to another patient, and wash hands immediately to avoid transfer of microorganisms to other patients or environments.
Mask, eye protection, face shield	Wear a mask and eye protection or a face shield to protect mucous membranes of the eyes, nose, and mouth during procedures and patient care activities that are likely to generate splashes or sprays of blood, body fluids, secretions, and excretions.
Gown	Wear a gown to protect skin and to prevent soiling of clothing during procedures and patient care activities that are likely to generate splashes or sprays of blood, body fluids, secretions, or excretions. A clean nonsterile gown is adequate. Select a gown that is appropriate for the activity and amount of fluid likely to be encountered.
	Remove a soiled gown as promptly as possible, and wash hands to avoid transfer of microorganisms to other patients or environments.
Patient care equipment	Handle used patient care equipment soiled with blood, body fluids, secretions, and excretions in a manner that prevents skin and mucous membrane exposures, contamination of clothing, and transfer of microorganisms to other patients and environments.
	Ensure that reusable equipment is not used for the care of another patient until it has been cleaned and reprocessed appropriately.
	Ensure that single-use items are discarded properly.

Table B1. *Continued*

Isolation Precaution Category	Recommendations
Environmental control	Ensure that the hospital has adequate procedures for the routine care, cleaning, and disinfection of environmental surfaces, beds, bedrails, bedside equipment, and other frequently touched surfaces, and ensure that these procedures are being followed.
Linen	Handle, transport, and process used linen soiled with blood, body fluids, secretions, and excretions in a manner that prevents skin and mucous membrane exposures and contamination of clothing, and in a manner that avoids transfer of microorganisms to other patients and environments.
Occupational health and blood-borne pathogens	Take care to prevent injuries when using sharp instruments or devices.
	Never recap used needles or any other action that directs the needle toward any part of the body.
	Place sharp objects in appropriate puncture-resistant containers.
	Use mouthpieces, resuscitation bags, or other ventilation devices as an alternative to mouth-to-mouth resuscitation.
Patient placement	Place a patient who contaminates the environment or who does not or cannot be expected to assist in maintaining appropriate hygiene or environmental control in a private room.

summarizes details regarding standard precautions as designated in the "Guideline for Isolation Precautions in Hospitals."

The following lists the types of precautions and patients requiring those precautions as recommended in the "Guideline for Isolation Precautions in Hospitals." Table B2 lists clinical syndromes or conditions that call for additional empiric precautions to prevent transmission of epidemiologically important pathogens when confirmation of diagnosis is pending.

Table B2. Clinical Syndromes or Conditions Warranting Additional Empiric Precautions to Prevent Transmission of Epidemiologically Important Pathogens Pending Confirmation of Diagnosis*(p. 67)

Clinical Syndrome or Condition†	Potential Pathogens‡	Empiric Precautions
Diarrhea		
Acute diarrhea with a likely infectious cause in an incontinent or diapered patient	Enteric pathogens§	Contact
Diarrhea in an adult with a history of recent antibiotic use	*Clostridium difficile*	Contact
Meningitis	*Neissera meningitidis*	Droplet
Rash or exanthems, generalized, etiology unknown		
Petechial/ecchymotic with fever	*Neissera meningitidis*	Droplet
Vesicular	Varicella	Airborne and contact
Maculopapular with coryza and fever	Rubeola (measles)	Airborne
Respiratory infections		
Cough/fever/upper lobe pulmonary infiltrate in an HIV-negative patient or a patient at a low risk for HIV infection	*Mycobacterium tuberculosis*	Airborne
Cough/fever/pulmonary infiltrate in any lung location in an HIV-infected patient or a patient at high risk for HIV infection	*Mycobacterium tuberculosis*	Airborne
Paroxysmal or severe persistent cough during periods of pertussis activity	*Bordetella pertussis*	Droplet

Table B2. *Continued*

Clinical Syndrome or Condition†	Potential Pathogens‡	Empiric Precautions
Respiratory infections, particularly bronchiolitis and croup, in infants and young children	Respiratory syncytial or parainfluenza virus	Contact
Risk of multidrug-resistant microorganisms		
History of infection or colonization with multidrug-resistant organisms¶	Resistant bacteria	Contact
Skin, wound, or urinary tract infection in a patient with a recent hospital or nursing home stay in a facility where multidrug-resistant organisms are prevalent	Resistant bacteria	Contact
Skin or wound infection		
Abscess or draining wound that cannot be covered	*Staphylococcus aureus*, Group A Streptococcus	Contact

*Infection control professionals are encouraged to modify or adapt this table according to local conditions. To ensure that appropriate empiric precautions are implemented always, hospitals must have systems in place to evaluate patients routinely according to these criteria as part of their preadmission and admission care.

†Patients with the syndromes or conditions listed here may present with atypical signs or symptoms (e.g., pertussis in neonates and adults may not have paroxysmal or severe cough). The clinician's index of suspicion should be guided by the prevalence of specific conditions in the community, as well as clinical judgment.

‡The organisms listed in this column are not intended to represent the complete, or even most likely diagnoses, but rather possible etiologic agents that require additional precautions beyond standard precautions until they can be ruled out.

§These pathogens include enterohemorrhagic *Escherichia coli* O157:H7, *Shigella*, hepatitis A, and rotavirus.

¶Resistant bacteria judged by the infection control program, based on current state, regional, or national recommendations, to be of special clinical or epidemiological significance.

Standard Precautions*

Use standard precautions for the care of all patients

Airborne Precautions

In addition to standard precautions use airborne precautions for patients known or suspected to have serious illnesses transmitted by airborne droplet nuclei. Examples of such illnesses include

- Measles
- Varicella (including disseminated zoster)†
- Tuberculosis

Droplet Precautions

In addition to standard precautions, use droplet precautions for patients known or suspected to have serious illnesses transmitted by large particle droplets. Examples of such illnesses include

- Invasive *Haemophilus influenzae* type b disease, including meningitis, pneumonia, epiglottitis, and sepsis
- Invasive *Neissera meningitidis* disease, including meningitis, pneumonia, and sepsis
- Other serious bacterial respiratory infections spread by droplet transmission, including
  - Diphtheria (pharyngeal)
  - Mycoplasma pneumonia
  - Pertussis
  - Pneumonic plague
  - Streptococcal pharyngitis, pneumonia, or scarlet fever in infants and young chilren
- Serious viral infections spread by droplet transmission, including
  - Adenovirus†
  - Influenza
  - Mumps
  - Parvovirus B19
  - Rubella

Contact Precautions

In addition to standard precautions, use contact precautions for patients known or suspected to have serious illnesses easily transmitted by direct patient contact or by contact with items in the patient's environment. Examples of such illnesses include

- Gastrointestinal, respiratory, skin or wound infections or colonization with multi-drug-resistant bacteria judged by the infection control program, based on current state, regional, or national recommendations, to be of special clinical and epidemiologic significance

Enteric infections with a low infectious dose or prolonged environmental survival, including
- *Clostridium difficile*
- For diapered or incontinent patients: enterohemorrhagic *Escherichia coli* O157:H7, *Shigella*, hepatitis A, or rotavirus

Respiratory syncytial virus, parainfluenza virus, or enteroviral infections in infants and young children

Skin infections that are highly contagious or that may occur on dry skin, including
- Diphtheria (cutaneous)
- Herpes simplex virus (neonatal or mucocutaneous)
- Impetigo
- Major (noncontained) abscesses, cellulitis, or decubiti
- Pediculosis
- Scabies
- Staphylococcal furunculosis in infants and young children
- Zoster (disseminated or in the immunocompromised host)†

Viral/hemorrhagic conjunctivitis

Viral hemorrhagic infections* (Ebola, Lassa, or Marburg*

*See Appendix A "Guideline for Isolation Precautions in Hospitals" (p. 73–80) for complete list of infections requiring precautions, including appropriate footnote.

†Certain infections require more than one type of precaution.

From Garner JS. Hospital Infection Control Practices Advisory Committee. Synopsis of types of precautions and patients requiring these precautions. *Infect Control Hosp Epidemiol.* 1996;17:53–80.

Index